GE[...]
ALTERNATIVES TO BRAND-NAME DRUGS

Diane Nitzki-George,
RPh, MBA, BCNSP

Basic Health
PUBLICATIONS, INC.

The information contained in this book is based upon the research and personal and professional experiences of the author. It is not intended as a substitute for consulting with your physician or other healthcare provider. Any attempt to diagnose and treat an illness should be done under the direction of a healthcare professional.

The publisher does not advocate the use of any particular healthcare protocol but believes the information in this book should be available to the public. The publisher and author are not responsible for any adverse effects or consequences resulting from the use of the suggestions, preparations, or procedures discussed in this book. Should the reader have any questions concerning the appropriateness of any procedures or preparations mentioned, the author and the publisher strongly suggest consulting a professional healthcare advisor.

Editor: Carol Rosenberg • Typesetting/Book Design: Gary A. Rosenberg
Cover Design: Mike Stromberg

Basic Health Publications, Inc.
28812 Top of the World Drive
Laguna Beach, CA 92651
949-715-7327 • www.basichealthpub.com

This book was originally published as *Generic Alternatives to Prescription Drugs* (© 2004 Basic Health Publications, Inc.)

Library of Congress Cataloging-in-Publication Data

Nitzki-George, Diane.
    Generic alternatives to brand-name drugs / Diane Nitzki-George.
      p. cm.
    Includes index.
    ISBN 978-1-59120-098-7
  1. Generic drugs. 2. Drugs—Generic substitution. I. Title.
    RS55.2.N547   2009
    615'.19—dc22

                              2009027669

Copyright © 2009 Basic Health Publications, Inc.

All rights reserved. No part of this publication may be reproduced, stored in a retrieval system, or transmitted, in any form or by any means, electronic, mechanical, photocopying, recording, or otherwise, without the prior written consent of the copyright owner.

Printed in the United States of America

10 9 8 7 6 5 4 3 2 1

Contents

A Note
from the Author

This book is for people who take prescription drugs. In addition to generic drug and pricing information, it includes helpful drug information that teaches people how to take their prescription drugs safely and effectively. But medicine is not an exact science. Although the science of medicine is predictable in most cases, do not be surprised if something unexpected happens. It is possible for people to have an unusual or unidentified response to their drug. Healthcare professionals, especially doctors, are trained to anticipate and respond to the unexpected. This is the reason that changing the dose of your prescription or giving someone else your prescription drug is unsafe. This book does not include all the information needed by healthcare professionals to safely prescribe and monitor patients who take prescription drugs. The information in this book is not intended to diagnose, treat, or cure a disease. Instead, *Generic Alternatives to Brand-Name Drugs* is a reference to guide people toward making well informed and cost effective decisions about their prescription drugs.

Introduction

In 1967, a new definition for the word "generic" was recognized in the English language. The new definition was a product that did not have a brand name or trademark. Generic products became familiar to people through grocery stores. Stores carried their house brand in addition to other name brands of the same product type. These generic products may have been a little different from the original brand-name products although they were basically the same type of product. Sometimes the taste or texture was different. But despite their differences, generic products were well accepted and became associated with a less expensive alternative.

The same concept applies to drugs. A generic drug product has the same active ingredient as the original brand-name drug. The taste or texture may be a little different. But the generic product is almost always a less expensive alternative. The U.S. Congressional Budget Offices has estimated that generic drugs save consumers $8 to $10 billion a year at retail pharmacies.

During the 1960s, several drug manufacturers began selling generic drug products to pharmacies. Many of these drugs were sold without the proper government paperwork that made sure the drug was safe and effective. Healthcare professionals challenged the reliability of generic drug products and were hesitant to dispense them. In the 1970s, the government began regulating generic drug products more closely to ensure that they were as effective as the original brand-name product.

It was not until 1985 that changes in government regulations were made to ensure that generic drug products met the same purity, quality, and potency standards required by the original brand-name drugs. All generic manufacturers must now submit a file to the U.S. Food and Drug Administration (FDA) that demonstrates the acceptability of their generic product.

As a consumer, finding out about generic drug products is not always easy. There are more than 600 prescription drugs sold through retail pharmacies in the United States. Many drugs come in different forms such as a tablet, liquid, or cream. Also, there can be more than one manufacturer for many of the drugs. The result is thousands of different drug products available by prescription. The pharmacy cannot stock every possible product, so the pharmacist decides which generic and brand-name products to carry.

What steps can you take to ensure you get the product you want? *Generic Alternatives to Brand-Name Drugs* will help guide you. It will provide insight into the availability of generic products and let you know if your prescription drug is available without a prescription at a lower strength. It also offers ideas on how you can speak with your doctor and pharmacist to be more involved in your prescription decisions. But most important, this book includes a brief summary of nearly 500 prescription drugs. It will give you an overview of substitutes that you can discuss with your doctor as possible alternatives to your prescription, and will allow you to assess whether the drug you are taking is doing what you expect or is causing side effects.

Having the knowledge to manage your prescription drug is very powerful. Aside from helping to optimize disease treatment, your involvement may result in fewer complications and greater savings.

Getting the Terminology Straight

In the United States, a drug can be sold only after it is reviewed by the Food and Drug Administration (FDA). The FDA is the regulating authority that establishes laws, standards, and guidelines to help keep the public safe. Aside from prescription drugs, the FDA also regulates cosmetics, food, food additives, herbs, supplements, over-the-counter (OTC) drugs, medical devices, blood products, radiation-emitting appliances, and veterinary drugs. Their involvement provides a broad range of scrutiny over everything we consume.

The FDA has established minimum criteria that all foods and drugs must meet. These criteria vary according to the type of product to be sold. In general, foods, herbs, and supplements can be sold without notifying the FDA in advance. However, all drugs must meet rigid safety and efficacy criteria before they can be sold. Understanding how the products are grouped based on FDA criteria helps provide a common terminology and an appreciation for the similarities and differences between products. The term "generic" means much more than the dictionary describes.

BRAND NAME VERSUS GENERIC NAME

Just like with grocery-store products, drugs can be called by more than one name. For example, Kleenex can also be called Puffs, or facial tissues, and Tylenol can also be called APAP, or acetaminophen. One name defines the active drug ingredient, while the other is a brand or trade name. Trade names are specific to the company that makes the product, while all companies use the active drug ingredient name. In the pharmacy, the name of the active drug ingredient is also referred to as the generic name. For example, the generic name for Benadryl is diphenhydramine. Both of these names can be used to describe the same product, but the generic name may also apply to other products that contain the same active drug ingredient. The generic drug name is the reference name used by healthcare professionals for all interactions and clinical information, which makes it important for people to learn the generic names of their prescription drugs.

Generic drug names are not simple. Sometimes a drug has a one-word name, but many times a generic drug is called by a two-word name. For example, the generic drug called enalapril is actually enalapril maleate. The second word in the name is specific to the chemical structure of the drug (also known as the salt form) that allows the drug to be made into different product types, such as a liquid or a tablet. In casual conversation, the second word is often dropped from the generic name, but the full drug name may be an extremely important aspect of dosing. The dose of oral tablets and oral solutions is not always the same.

GENERIC NAME VERSUS GENERIC PRODUCT

The word "generic" has turned into a type of pharmacy slang. In a broad sense, a generic name refers to the active drug ingredient in a product. However, the stricter definition of a generic drug is a product developed to copy an original brand-name drug. A generic product has the same active ingredient and is considered equivalent to the original brand-name product. So, knowing the generic name of your prescription drug is not enough to meet the criteria of being a generic product. A pharmacy can only fill your prescription with a generic product that is considered equivalent to the original drug.

For all generic products sold in the United States, an Abbreviated New Drug Application (ANDA) must be filed with the Office of Generics at the FDA. An ANDA must include evidence that the chemistry, manufacturing, and stability of the product is the same as the reference brand-name product. But the manufacturer is not required to repeat the costly clinical trials that were used to demonstrate safety and efficacy when the original drug was first developed. A generic-drug file must show that the product has:

- The same active ingredients as the original drug (inactive ingredients may vary).

- Identical strength, dosage form, and route of administration as the original drug product.

- The same indications for use as the original drug product.

- The same absorption characteristics as the original drug product.

- The same identity, strength, purity, and quality as the original drug product.

- Been manufactured under the FDA's strict standards for good manufacturing.

In general, a generic product will have the same name as the active drug ingredient or generic name. For example, the generic product of ampicillin is called ampicillin. However, the manufacturer may choose to trademark a generic product. For example, a generic form of ampicillin is called Totacillin, but the original drug brand name for ampicillin is Omnipen. If a generic manufacturer has branded the product, an additional name is added to the confusion that already exists with finding a generic product. To further complicate the naming process, an original drug product may choose to use the generic drug name.

Another point of confusion with generic drugs is the repackaging of branded drugs. The FDA allows a drug manufacturer to contract with another company for repackaging of their product. This process involves moving a drug from a larger container to smaller container. The repackaged products may not officially be generic products but are often considered the same as generic products if they carry the generic drug name.

Finally, a drug may be sold from one company to another. This happens during corporate acquisitions and mergers. In many cases, the drug has been available for an extended period of time and competition has eroded the price. When a company sells the drug, the official FDA files become the responsibility of the new company. The new company can submit an amendment to the FDA file requesting a change in the branded name if desired. These products are also not officially generic products but are routinely considered the same as generic products, especially if the new companies label the product by the generic name.

While the definition of a generic drug product is clear from an FDA standpoint, the common use of the term is less clear. Insurance companies have different co-pays for brand-name drugs and generic drugs, but the criteria they use may differ from the criteria used by the FDA. The perception that generic drug products are a less expensive alternative is not part of the official regulatory definition. In many cases, more than one generic product is available for a single drug. Generic products are priced competitively, which can range from very low to the same as the original drug product.

Generic products have not been developed for all drugs, even those available for more than twenty years. In these cases, the amount of money a company can earn by selling the drug is not enough to offset the development cost. This is true for drugs that are used to treat a small number of patients and for drugs that are expensive to manufacture.

OVER-THE-COUNTER DRUGS
VERSUS PRESCRIPTION DRUGS

The majority of drugs are sold only by prescription. However, there is one group of drugs that can be sold without a prescription called over-the-counter (OTC) drugs or nonprescription drugs. A drug can be sold over the counter when there is enough data to allow a consumer to safely and effectively use the drug without help from a healthcare professional.

OTC drugs are approved through the FDA by one of two processes. In the first process, the drugs go through the same FDA process of approval as all other drugs. Evidence of safety and efficacy is reviewed before approval. These drugs are almost always sold by prescription only before changing to OTC.

As an alternative, the FDA has developed a set of OTC drug monographs. The monographs include safety and efficacy information about the active drug ingredient but are not specific regarding the dose, formulation, labeling, and so on. Each OTC monograph stipulates manufacturing and marketing requirements that must be met for the OTC product eliminating the need for pre-approval by the FDA. Strict labeling standards apply to all OTC drugs to ensure that the consumer easily understands the label.

SUPPLEMENTS AND HERBS

Not every pill you buy in the pharmacy is a drug. Many are considered dietary supplements, which are regulated by the FDA more like food products than like drugs. The Dietary Supplement Health and Education Act (DSHEA) of 1994 defined a dietary supplement as a product taken by mouth, intended to supplement the diet, that is made from "dietary ingredients." The "dietary ingredients" include vitamins, minerals, herbs, botanicals, amino acids, and substances such as enzymes, organ tissues, glandulars, and metabolites.

Sales of dietary supplements exceed $10 billion per year. Consumers use dietary supplements to improve their health and prevent disease. Some dietary supplements are used to treat mild cases of disease, such as St. John's wort for depression. While this practice is assumed to be safe, dietary supplements should be viewed by the consumer like OTC drugs. There may be drug interactions, side effects, and toxicity associated with these products. Make sure your doctor knows all the dietary supplements and OTC drugs that you take regularly.

Since the FDA does not regulate dietary supplements in the same manner as drugs, the responsibility for safety and efficacy falls to the manufacturer. The manufacturer promoting the product is put into the position of self-regulation. This includes the physical aspects of the product, such as purity and potency, good manufacturing practices, and any claims about product health benefits. Many cases have been cited in which a product does not contain what the label says. Nobody but the manufacturer knows if shortcuts were taken during production or if promotional material overstates the value of taking the product.

There is some consistency to the labeling of dietary supplements because of standards issued by the FDA. Labels should state that a product is indeed a dietary supplement, include a list of all ingredients, provide information about the manufacturer, and state the "Supplemental Facts." These facts should clearly identify both the actual ingredient added as well as any indirect reason it is added. For example, if rose hips are added to a product, the Supplemental Facts must also state that rose hips are a source of vitamin C. Dietary supplements cannot claim to prevent, diagnose, treat, or cure a disease.

Dietary supplements are sold without the need for FDA approval. Instead, the active ingredient used in a dietary supplement must be "Generally Recognized as Safe" (GRAS). A list of GRAS ingredients was started by the FDA in 1958 to control additives put into food. Ingredients including sugar, spices, and vitamins were the foundation of the GRAS list, based on extensive, long-term use. New ingredients are added to the GRAS list each year based on published scientific evidence. In 1997, the FDA formalized the process of expanding the list by allowing manufacturers to submit new ingredients. After the FDA reviews the scientific evidence, the ingredient is either added to the list or temporarily rejected pending additional information. The list currently contains more than 1,000 ingredients with several new additions each year. If new evidence suggests that an ingredient is no longer safe, it may be removed from the GRAS list and products containing that ingredient can no longer be sold.

The dietary-supplements industry is managed primarily through self-regulation by the manufacturers. This means that products are only as good as the manufacturer. The product label does not include any special words or symbols to help identify a good manufacturer from a poor manufacturer. In 2003, it was proposed that the FDA should regulate manufacturing and labeling of dietary supplements. The intention is to provide the consumer with the confidence that a dietary supplement is manufactured correctly, contains the right ingredients, does not contain contaminants, and is labeled accurately. The outcome of the FDA proposal will not be final until the end of 2003.

The regulation of dietary supplements parallels the early days of generic drugs. Consistency of products and reliability of effects are not predictable. While some products might not be acceptable, several are manufactured with high-quality standards. Health benefits continue to be researched and information continues to evolve.

Your Prescription Cost

Do you know the actual price of your prescription? If you are like many Americans, you are not paying the full amount. Over the past ten years, there has been a shift in the payment of prescription drugs. Many insurance programs now offer drug coverage, charging you only a small portion of the overall price. There is even a government Medigap program that allows Medicare recipients to buy into health plans that help pay for prescription drugs. But even with insurance, the co-pay is higher for a brand-name drug than for a generic. And the co-pay for these programs is rising.

The price of your prescription, no matter who pays, comes from two different base costs. First is the pharmacy charge for processing your prescription, and second is the actual cost of the drug. Neither of these costs is standardized from pharmacy to pharmacy nor between drugs at the same pharmacy. Understanding more about prescription pricing may provide clues to saving money.

INSURANCE CO-PAY

Insurance companies generally have a two-tiered co-pay for prescription drugs. One price applies to brand-name drugs and a lower price applies to generic drugs. Insurance companies compile a list of drugs, called a formulary, that identifies both generic and brand-name drugs by manufacturer and gives their associated co-pay. If a drug is not included on the list, it will not be paid for by insurance. Be aware that insurance programs may not offer coverage for all prescription drugs on the market. In some cases, the insurance drug list may limit the doctor's ability to prescribe the drug of choice. If there are multiple drugs in a single category that are used to treat the same condition, the insurance company may only pay for one of the drugs. The identification of only one drug in a category is called therapeutic substitution.

A therapeutic substitute is a different drug with similar effects and side effects, but usually costs less. If the insurance program has limited the formulary to therapeutic substitutes, the doctor must write the prescription accordingly. The pharmacist is not allowed to fill a prescription with a therapeutic substitute. Don't confuse a generic substitute with a therapeutic substitute. A generic substitute is the same drug made by a different manufacturer.

Insurance companies usually have a printed formulary that they can provide to people enrolled in their plan and to the participating pharmacies. Bringing a copy of your insurance drug formulary to your doctor's appointment may save time at the pharmacy. When presenting your prescription to the pharmacy, ask if the drug is covered by insurance before the prescription is filled.

Aside from formulary limitations, insurance companies also limit the quantity of a drug that can be filled on a prescription. For example, a two-month supply may be the limit you can get with a single co-pay. In some cases, the co-pay may be higher than the actual prescription price. Comparing the price of a prescription with and without insurance may be a method of saving money. This is especially true for older drugs, drugs that are taken for a short period of time, or prescriptions that are written for a small quantity.

PHARMACY FEES

Every pharmacy has established a processing fee to ensure that they make money on each prescription. The fee is necessary to pay for the supplies, the staff, and the overall business. The fee structure is specific to an individual business model and is not consistent between pharmacies. For example, the pharmacy may charge a fee of 10 percent on the cost of the drug. So, if the drug costs $20, the pharmacy fee would be $2, resulting in a prescription price of $22. Some pharmacies will set up a variable fee structure depending on the cost of the drug—for example, a fee of 10 percent on all drugs less than $20 with only a 5 percent fee on drugs more than $20. This type of fee structure will still earn the pharmacy money, but not add excess cost to the prescription. More frequently, pharmacies charge a single fee for all prescriptions—for example, a fee of $5 no matter what the prescription cost. Pharmacy fees are not billed separately from the cost of the drug and are hidden from the consumer.

The importance of the pharmacy fee system is related to the number of visits you make to the pharmacy. Each time you get refills on your prescription, you are charged another fee. You may be able to reduce the fees paid by making sure that the "ideal quantity" of a drug is dispensed with each prescription.

Most prescriptions, with the exception of controlled drugs, are good for one year from the date written. Some prescription drugs are used as needed when symptoms develop, while others are used on a regular schedule to manage a disease or condition. Regulating the quantity of doses filled in a prescription is one method of cost savings.

If you are taking a drug on a regular schedule over an extended period of time, the "ideal quantity" is usually limited by the drug's effectiveness, side effects, cost, insurance, and your next appointment with the doctor. A three-month supply is the most common "ideal quantity," although six months may be associated with greater savings.

When first starting on a drug, make sure the drug works before stocking up on a supply. The last thing you want is to have leftover prescription drugs sitting in your medicine cabinet. Is the drug effective? Are you having side effects? Usually a one-month trial is prescribed to get answers to those questions. Many doctors get drug samples that may be given to patients during the trial period.

When taking a drug to manage occasional symptoms, such as a migraine headache, the "ideal quantity" is related to the frequency of your symptoms and the number of doses needed to alleviate those symptoms. For example, if you have six headaches a year and take four doses of a drug to get rid of your headache, the ideal prescription quantity is twenty-four doses for the year. Compare the prescription price for twenty-four doses to the co-pay fee. In some cases, you will spend less money if you do not use insurance, especially if the drug has been available for a long time and generic products are available.

Some drugs are associated with severe side effects and require frequent monitoring. In those cases, your prescription quantity is likely to be limited by the monitoring period. For example, if you need to have a blood test every month, the doctor may only prescribe a one-month supply of the drug at a time. By complying with the monitoring program, you may provide the doctor with the evidence needed to prescribe a greater quantity.

Over the past five years, there has been an increase in the shortage of prescription drugs. Among the many causes of shortages are increased demand for the drug, insufficient supply, lack of raw materials, or poor inventory control. The government has set up a special task force within the FDA to work with manufacturers during shortage periods to ensure that the drug is distributed where it is needed the most. Manufacturers may put an allocation program in place, which causes pharmacies to ration the number of doses in your prescription. If this happens, talk to your pharmacist and/or insurance company about the fee or co-pay.

The price of a prescription depends greatly on the amount a pharmacy pays for the drug. Volume discounts, special incentives, and backorders all affect the cost to a pharmacy. This cost fluctuation is generally not passed along to the consumer. Instead, the pharmacy will establish a single price for each drug. For that reason, the price of a prescription drug will vary from one pharmacy to another. There is no guarantee that one pharmacy will always have the lowest price for all drugs. It pays to shop around if price is the highest priority. But some people are willing to spend a little more to shop at the same pharmacy because of the service and support provided by their pharmacist.

THE COST OF DRUGS

The cost of a drug used to fill your prescription comes from four primary sources: the raw-material supplier, the drug manufacturer, the sales and marketing business, and the company that sells the drugs to a pharmacy (called the wholesaler, distributor, or dealer). Each drug has a price established, called the Average Wholesale Price or AWP, as a means of price communication and comparison. AWP is similar to the Average Retail Price used in the garment industry. AWP makes sure there are profits to raw-material suppliers, manufacturers, sales and marketing businesses, and wholesalers.

A pharmaceutical company spends anywhere from $5 million to $80 million and more than five years developing a new drug. This cost accounts for research, development, clinical trials, and filing with the FDA. Marketing costs may account for another $5 million to $10 million depending on the drug. Marketing pays for the television commercials, the websites, the magazine ads, plus all of the educational material provided to healthcare professionals. In addition to the high cost spent to develop and market a drug, the cost of a drug must also pay for the business overhead and other sunk costs. A pharmaceutical company can spend millions of dollars on research, development, and clinical trials only to find out that a drug is not safe and effective and cannot be sold. Those costs are buried within the AWP of other drugs as a part of normal business expenditure.

The investment and risk taken by pharmaceutical companies to develop new drugs is high. In contrast, a generic drug company has little risk. These companies are able to identify a drug for which sales are already established. With less than $1 million and a one- to two-year investment, a generic drug can be sold. The process includes submission of basic manufacturing information to the FDA and referencing the safety data already on file for the brand-name drug. In some cases, a bioequivalency study is required to demonstrate that the generic drug works the same as the brand-name drug. The investment is smaller, so the price is also lower.

The financial returns for the generic drug company are usually very good initially when the drug product can be priced just below the brand-name product, but there are dozens of generic-drug companies. These companies compete with one another by manufacturing the same generic drugs. So there are multiple product choices even when generics are used. Over time, competition among the generic drug companies results in rock-bottom prices and may even force some generic companies out of the market.

In order to protect the high risk, high investment made by pharmaceutical companies, the FDA has established a rule called "exclusivity." The concept prevents generic drugs from using the clinical studies that support the brand-name drug for five years from the date of FDA approval. This allows the pharmaceutical company enough time to earn back their investment with a profit. Exclusivity is necessary to ensure the continued development of new drugs.

Another method that pharmaceutical companies use to protect their investment is patents. Patents are good for seventeen years and may be written in a way that prevents another company from selling a generic drug. Pharmaceutical companies have become very savvy with their patents and tend to file multiple patents while the drug is being developed. The goal is to have seventeen years of patent protection starting from the time the drug is first available for sale.

In October of 2002, President Bush announced that a new FDA guideline would limit the number of legal delays that could apply to patent-infringement lawsuits on generic drugs. The intention was to make a generic drug available sooner and help consumers save money. While this action is commendable, pharmaceutical companies continue to find ways to protect their investment. Small changes in a product formula, such as developing an extended-release product, may be enough to qualify for a new patent. Although these small changes may be expensive and require a submission to the FDA, they often result in fluctuations in prescribing patterns that make the market less attractive to the generic-drug manufacturer.

The Steps to Managing Your Health

Wellness is a major focus in today's living. We have modified our diets, stopped smoking, gotten flu shots, and listened to health reports on the nightly news. We are more conscious of healthy living and preventing disease than we are educated on how to live with disease.

What steps do you take when you get sick? Do you ignore the symptoms and hope they will go away? Do you go to the drugstore and look for something to take for the symptoms? If the symptoms get worse, do you talk to a friend or family member? Are you the type of person who will read up on the symptoms instead of going to the doctor? Why is the first instinct to figure things out for ourselves?

There are many possible reasons why we avoid the doctor when we first get sick. Maybe we:

- Do not have insurance.
- Had a bad experience in the past.
- Cannot afford the fee.
- Do not think it is serious.
- Are afraid to acknowledge that we are sick.
- Do not want to spend the money.
- Do not want to spend the time.
- Think we know how to treat ourselves.
- Do not want to seem like a hypochondriac.

Some people will run to the doctor for everything while others will wait until their disease or symptoms have progressed to a critical stage. Some people will take any drug available while others do not want to take anything. Managing your health warrants a collaborative approach to the health care system.

To optimize your role in managing illness, it is helpful to follow the same course of action taken by healthcare professionals. First, know what disease you are treating. Second, know the stage of the disease and how it progresses. And finally, know the recommended treatment and expected results. While these steps are greatly simplified, they outline three basic steps to get you involved in managing your wellness.

SEEKING PROFESSIONAL HELP

The pharmacies are stocked with supplements and herbs that are associated with use in disease. Frequently, patients will assess their symptoms and decide which supplement or herb should be used for treatment. While this might be okay in some cases, it may also be the wrong treatment. In 1950, Dr. Seuss wrote a children's story called *Gertrude McFuzz* about a bird who decides to self-medicate and ends up with more trouble than she bargained for. Eventually, a doctor is needed to correct her troubles. (Dr. Suess, *Gertrude McFuzz*, In *Yertle the Turtle and Other Stories*. Random House, 1958.) One of the key roles you play in managing your health is to know your diagnosis. You could be treating an enlarged prostate when your actual diagnosis is prostate cancer. Getting a diagnosis from your doctor will help you avoid spending money and wasting time on the wrong treatments.

Consulting a doctor for a diagnosis is very important. Doctors are taught to evaluate an illness in a way that can differentiate between several diseases. For example, if you tell your doctor that you have been getting headaches, it could indicate a number of things, including a sinus infection, high blood pressure, migraines, or even, in rare cases, a brain tumor. Only by asking questions and running tests can the right diagnosis be reached. We expect doctors to take care of us when we have trouble but tend to avoid their advice before then. Doctors are trained to know which questions to ask and which test to run to get the right diagnosis.

Some people delay going to the doctor until their symptoms get very bad. This approach to saving money may actually cost you more in the long run. When a disease is left untreated, it will often progress to a more serious condition and may cause complications. The treatment is often more complex and the cost higher. Aside from cost, there may be permanent harm done to your body as a result of the disease.

Having an annual physical exam can help detect some diseases before they cause symptoms. Other diseases do not have symptoms until they start causing complications. These can also be diagnosed during an annual physical exam. Early diagnosis of a disease can avoid unnecessary complications and advancement of the disease. Health screening has become a popular alternative to seeing the doctor every year. With a simple blood test and your personal history, a health screen can identify many of the major health risks. If anything out of the ordinary is identified in the screening, the report will recommend that you see a doctor. These programs are often mobile and may be offered periodically at your pharmacy or grocery store. Check with your local pharmacy, hospital, or your insurance company to find out if this type of program is available to you.

There are some common illnesses that people often treat successfully without going to the doctor. These include colds, flu, rash, and allergies, to name a few. Although it is not necessary to run to your doctor at the first symptom of a common illness, you do not want to wait too long. If your symptoms last longer than you expect or if you do not see any improvement in your condition with nonprescription treatment, go to the doctor. If your instinct tells you that something is wrong, have it checked. Seeking professional care may avoid wasting your time, your health, and your money.

UNDERSTANDING YOUR DIAGNOSIS

Once you have the right diagnosis, you may immediately want to jump to the treatment options. But a diagnosis is not as simple as putting a disease or condition name to your symptoms. Many times, a disease name has extra words added to it, such as stage I breast cancer. The extra words help to identify the severity of the disease, or what caused the disease, or where the disease is located, and so on.

A disease is larger than a diagnosis. A diagnosis is very specific to your body and your signs and symptoms. Your diagnosis may be just a small portion of the disease, suggesting that the disease has not advanced. Or your diagnosis may include a large portion of the disease signs and symptoms, indicating the severity of your diagnosis.

Understanding the diagnosis helps you to identify what may happen to your body if the disease gets worse. It will also help to clarify what you need to do when you feel sick again. Are your symptoms a side effect of the treatment or is the treatment not working?

The best source of disease and diagnosis information is your doctor. Doctors are the experts in diseases and they know your medical history. When you are diagnosed, do not be afraid to ask questions like:

- How severe is the disease?

- Can this disease be cured?

- How long will the symptoms last?

- Should I call you if the symptoms do not go away?

- How long will I have to take the treatment?

- What complications are there?
- What happens when the disease gets worse?

In addition to your doctor, there are other ways to find out more about your diagnosis. Check your local library or bookstore for disease-related books. The Internet is full of disease information, but do not trust everything you read on the Internet unless you are sure it comes from a reliable source. Reliable information is found through professional organizations, such as the National Kidney Foundation or the American Diabetes Association. Even drug manufacturers can be a source of reliable disease information because the FDA closely regulates their information. Another good source of disease information is a support group. These groups will allow you to share what you have learned about the disease as well as learn from others. Check with your doctor or pharmacist for names of professional organizations, drug manufacturers, and support groups.

Understanding your diagnosis is also important to help identify the lifestyle changes that need to be made to prevent advancement of the disease. Most drugs cannot cure a disease, but can only treat the symptoms and/or slow the advancement of the disease. Many people need to supplement their drug treatment with dietary changes, exercise programs, a change in habits, or a change in surroundings. These lifestyle changes, no matter how small, should be discussed with your doctor to make sure your care is managed properly. If your doctor recommends a nondrug treatment plan that just happens to be free, such as exercise, it is to your benefit to follow the recommendation. Without a change in lifestyle, the drug-treatment plan may be less effective.

WHAT TO EXPECT FROM DRUGS

Once you understand your diagnosis, the next step is to consider treatment. In some cases, the treatment is not a drug but a procedure. In other cases, a nurse administers the drug in a clinic. Although these treatments are managed by a healthcare professional, it is very important for you to help them with information. Let the doctor know all the herbs, supplements, and over-the-counter drugs that you take. This is particularly important when you see a specialist, go to the dentist, or have surgery. Some nonprescription products may cause drug interactions or interfere with treatment, allowing your disease to get worse.

The most common treatment option is self-medication with a prescription drug. When the doctor gives you a prescription, you have a choice. Will you fill the prescription or will you look for another way to treat your disease? While a change in lifestyle and diet is often a recommendation that accompanies a diagnosis, these changes alone may not be enough to prevent the advancement of your disease. Many people are hesitant to take prescription drugs. We think we can "tough it out" or do not want to put chemicals in our bodies. Many times, the drugs are costly or have side effects that we do not know about or cannot tolerate. Let your doctor know if you do not plan to follow his or her recommendation or if you would like to try a nondrug approach first. Proposing alternative treatment options is happening more frequently. Your doctor will advise you if there are risks or concerns.

There is a new concept in healthcare called Evidence Based Medicine. This concept basically says that if enough people say that something is happening to their disease as a result of a treatment (drug or nondrug) then it should be believed. This concept evolved primarily from the availability of dietary supplements since 1994. The evidence is not gathered in a controlled, scientific manner, but there is enough evidence to give it power. Evidence Based Medicine has taught doctors to view treatment options differently and has made them more receptive to alternative therapy. It also allows doctors to prescribe drugs for reasons that differ from their originally intended use.

There are more than 1,000 drugs on the United States market. In many cases, there is more than one drug that can be used to treat a given disease. If a prescription drug is required to treat your disease, do you agree to take it? Do you know the alternatives? Is your drug the most cost effective one available? Do you know how it can have the maximum impact on your disease? Do you know the side effects? Understanding some drug information basics and getting a perspective on choices can be the key to successfully treating your disease. Remember that most drugs cannot cure a disease but can only treat the symptoms and/or slow the advancement of the disease.

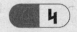

After You Swallow

Have you ever been curious to know what happens to your prescription drug after you swallow it? How does something that you put in your stomach help your headache? What can you do to make the drug more effective? How can side effects continue two weeks after a drug is stopped?

A science called pharmacokinetics, or more commonly referred to as kinetics, explains the answers to these questions and many more. Kinetics describes how the drug is handled as it passes through the body. Kinetic information is gathered through clinical studies, which evaluate four different phases:

1. Entrance to the Body
2. Movement
3. Chemical Changes
4. Removal

Kinetic information is not the same for every drug, which is why there are different actions, warnings, and precautions associated with different drugs. Kinetics is also not a precise science, since there may be a small degree of variability between patients and even within the same patient. But kinetics can set up guidelines that doctors and pharmacists use to project the expected effects, side effects, and interactions of a drug.

ENTRANCE TO THE BODY

A drug enters the body through the process of absorption. A skin cream must be absorbed into the layers of the skin to have an effect. An oral drug must pass through the mouth, down the esophagus, and into the stomach and intestines where absorption can take place along the path. The path is called the gastrointestinal (GI) tract. When taken orally, a drug is usually moved from the GI tract into the bloodstream where it continues throughout the body.

Drugs are absorbed at different places along the GI tract. Some drugs are absorbed in the mouth, some in the stomach, and others are absorbed lower in the intestines. Many drugs are absorbed all along the path. The drug characteristics, the product, GI acidity, and absorptive surface are key to where a drug is absorbed.

The reason absorption is important is because food in the stomach causes a change in the acidity of the GI tract. If you take a drug with food when it should be taken on an empty stomach, the drug may be degraded, causing the amount of drug absorbed to be lower than expected. In this case, the drug may not be effective in treating your illness. Food may also interfere with the GI absorptive surfaces and block a drug from being fully absorbed. The drug summaries in Chapter 6 provide guidance on when to take your prescription drug relative to food and if necessary which foods to avoid.

Interference with absorption is not limited to food. Other drugs, herbs, and supplements may also interfere with drug absorption, resulting in a lower that expected effect. In some cases, drugs and nutrients can increase the absorption of a drug, putting patients at risk for toxicity. Interference with absorption is only one of several types of interactions possible between drugs and nutrients.

Before a drug can be absorbed, it must be released from the product. A tablet or capsule must dissolve before the drug is available for absorption. One major concern in pharmacy is that a drug made by more than one manufacturer will have the same effect or bioequivalence. If a product made by company A dissolves slower than a generic product made by company B, the absorption may be different, resulting in a higher or lower drug effect. Most drug manufacturers test to ensure that their products are acceptable, but there may still be a slight product-to-product difference.

Drug manufacturers have used the absorption of drugs to further enhance products. Delayed- and extended-release products are made to release the drug slowly as it passes through the entire GI path. Crushing, opening, or breaking a slow-release product can result in toxicity since the entire dose may be absorbed right away. Some slow-release products are formulated in a capsule with coated pellets inside that can be sprinkled on food. In this case, the pellets contain the slow-release feature and should not be crushed or chewed.

One unique method of drug manufacturing includes creating a very fine, microsize powder of the drug that, even when made into a tablet or capsule, is absorbed quickly and more completely. Some products contain the same active drug ingredient, but are made with different powder forms (either regular or microsize). These products *are not considered generic products* since the dosing will differ.

Most topical drugs, eyedrops, and ear drops work directly at the site they touch. These products are used to get high doses of drug to a specific spot on the body. But some drugs can be absorbed through the skin, eye, or ear into the bloodstream. Be alert to the possibility of developing side effects even when using drugs not taken by mouth. Absorption of drugs through the skin is the reason that some drugs are available as topical patches. Be sure to follow the instructions for use, since moisture in the skin as well as the site of placement can influence the absorption of drugs from topical patches.

The chemical characteristics of a drug may prevent it from being absorbed into the body from the GI tract. Some of these drugs work directly at the site of contact in the GI tract; others must be given another way. Since the goal of most drugs is to be absorbed into the bloodstream, many drugs are only available as an injection in which the entire dose is injected directly into the bloodstream. Another way drugs are absorbed into the body is through the nose and lungs. A few drugs are available both as oral and inhalation products. Be aware that doses of these drugs may be different since a higher dose must be given orally to compensate for the poor absorption. An oral drug that is not absorbed passes through the GI tract and is eliminated in the feces.

MOVEMENT

Following absorption, a drug must move through the blood to the site of action, or where it works. But before it can start to follow the movement of the blood, it must reach the main circulatory path. If you think of the bloodstream as a group of continuous loops throughout the body that start at the heart, you can imagine one loop reaching the arms, another circulating to the legs, another to the lungs, and so on. Since the site of drug absorption is the GI tract rather than the heart, blood must first move back to the heart to reach other parts of the body.

Before reaching the heart, blood from the GI tract is circulated through the liver. The liver is the primary organ for causing chemical changes to a drug, as you will read in the following section. Some drugs lose a high percentage of their strength the first time they pass through the liver. In those cases, a relatively high dose of the drug must be taken to achieve the desired effects. If you have liver disease, the anticipated chemical changes and loss of drug strength may not occur. People with liver disease often require lower drug doses.

Some drugs attach themselves to proteins found in the blood, in what is called "plasma protein binding." This action may help move the drug throughout the body, but it may also be the cause of drug interactions or side effects. Often, the doctor must draw blood levels of a drug to indicate if therapy is safe or may be reaching toxic levels. These blood levels usually measure the amount of free drug in the blood, but not the amount that is plasma protein bound. So plasma protein binding may provide an unpredictable measure of safety. Typically, plasma proteins carry other blood substrates and drugs throughout the body. Since there are a limited number of binding sites on a protein, the drug may bump the blood substrate or other drug off the protein. This results in blood levels of the substrate or drug that are higher than expected, leading to possible side effects or drug interactions.

Drugs also have an inclination to move to certain areas in the body based on the characteristics of the drug. For example, some drugs have a preference for fatty areas, others move toward certain chemicals, and others flow to wherever the blood moves. This is why some drugs work in one area of the body and not in others. This is also one of the ways that drugs are released if attached to proteins. The drug may have a greater need to move into a specific tissue than to bind with the plasma protein.

Some drugs move to several different areas of the body at the same time. So you may be taking a drug for a headache that can also reduce the swelling in your sprained wrist and treat your sore back at the same time. The drug is not limited to movement in one area of the body just because it is used to treat a specific disease or condition. This is why drugs can have side effects that involve so many different areas of the body. For example, a heart medication may have an inclination to move into the eyes in addition to the heart. Vision changes and other eye problems may need to be checked regularly and may be a reason for you to stop taking the drug.

CHEMICAL CHANGES

As a drug is absorbed into the bloodstream, it begins to adjust to the chemical properties of the blood. Some drugs are called "prodrugs," which means that they are designed to improve absorption, but as soon as a drug reaches the bloodstream, it is converted to another active drug. A couple of examples of this are valganciclovir, which is converted to ganciclovir, and ba-campicillin, which is converted to ampicillin. Substrates in the blood are able to break a simple bond that connects the main drug from the carrier. Prodrugs have been developed to help reduce the GI side effects that occur when large doses of a drug are necessary to get only a small amount of absorption.

The primary chemical change that drugs undergo in the body takes place in the liver. The liver works like a chemical factory to make substances needed by the body and to break down chemicals that are foreign to the body. As the blood passes through the liver, some of the drug may move into the liver for breakdown while the remaining drug stays in the blood for circulation throughout the body. Once in the liver, the drug may break down completely and its elements are then used to make new substances. Or the drug may break down to a smaller, different chemical called a "metabolite." Metabolites are still too large after the initial breakdown, so they are deposited back into the blood for circulation throughout the body. Some metabolites have a pharmaceutical benefit just like the active drug. Others just continue through the bloodstream until they are reduced further by the liver and are finally small enough to reuse or eliminate from the body in other ways.

The longer a drug stays in the body, the less frequently doses need to be taken. Some drugs begin to break down in the liver before they ever reach the heart for further circulation. In this case, high doses are needed to compensate for the initial drug loss. Other drugs are never broken down in the liver. Most people should have their liver function tested periodically (at least once a year) while taking prescription drugs. People with liver disease may need to have drug doses adjusted to compensate for their poor liver function.

REMOVAL

If you think about all the ways that the body eliminates fluid and waste, you can imagine the many ways that a drug can be removed from the body. Sweat, tears, urine, semen, vaginal discharge, feces, and breast milk are all used. This is why some drugs can cause staining of the clothes, others change the color of the urine, and others are associated with birth defects even when used in men.

The primary organ for eliminating most drugs is the kidney. The kidneys work like a filter to collect chemical waste from the blood. The waste comes from our food, drinks, drugs, and supplements. Sometimes, even creams and eyedrops can put waste products into our bodies. Only waste that dissolves in water can be eliminated through the kidneys. Waste that does not dissolve in water must be further broken down or removed from the body in other ways.

As blood flows through the kidneys, some drugs move into the kidneys for filtering. But every drug that might be filtered out is not always removed. The collection of all different waste products in the kidneys may make the conditions less favorable for removing the drug. For example, when you drink grapefruit juice, the acidity of the urine changes and may interfere with the removal of some drugs. Because the kidneys process everything you eat and drink, they are a primary organ for drug interactions and side effects. Drugs that move into the kidneys for removal may be reabsorbed into the blood. This may cause higher blood levels of the drug than expected, putting the patient at risk for developing side effects or toxicity. Kidney function should be tested at least once a year while taking prescription drugs and may be needed more frequently depending on the drug.

Some drugs take hours to be removed from the body while others take months. This is why the effects and side effects for many drugs can continue long after the drug is no longer taken.

5

Taking Charge of Your Prescription

The slip of paper that you present to your pharmacy is called a prescription. The drug the pharmacy dispenses is also called a prescription. In order to take charge of your prescription, you need to understand the prescription process from start to finish.

The prescription process starts when the doctor creates the written prescription. Several decisions are made by the doctor without much input from the patient, such as what drug should be used, how many doses should be issued, the number of refills, and if a generic drug can be used. The doctor tells the patient how the prescription should be taken and what to watch for, but there are several questions that patients should think about asking that may help save them time and money.

The patient then takes the written prescription to his or her choice of pharmacy where the pharmacist makes several other decisions on behalf of the patient. Those decisions include applying insurance benefits, clarifying the written prescription if necessary, and selecting the product. The more information that can be supplied up front to your doctor and pharmacist, the more control you will have over your prescription.

READING A PRESCRIPTION

In order to know what questions to ask about a written prescription, you need to know the requirements. Minimum standards have been established for the written prescription; it must include the patient's name, date, drug name, instructions for use, quantity, the doctor's signature, and more (see Figure 1).

In general, a written prescription is valid for one year or less from the date originally written. However, all written prescriptions do not follow a single set of requirements. Although federal regulations have set up minimum standards, each state has the ability to create tighter regulations and controls. So a prescription in California may have different requirements than a prescription in Florida.

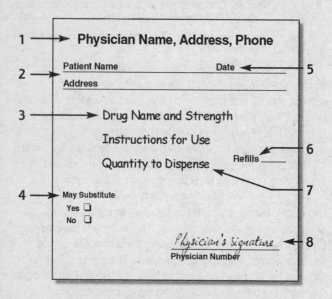

FIGURE 1: Eight Sections of the Basic Written Prescription

1. Doctor information
2. Patient information
3. Prescription
4. Substitution area
5. Date
6. Refills
7. Amount
8. Authorization

WHEN TO TALK TO YOUR DOCTOR

Two sections on the written prescription are related more to economics than to healthcare. First is the "Substitution" area (see Figure 2). This area is the place a doctor can authorize the use of a generic drug in place of a brand-name drug. If this area is not filled in correctly, the pharmacist must call the doctor for additional instructions. The "Substitution" may look like the example in Figure 2, but may have different terminology. The terminology may read "Generic OK" with yes/no checkboxes, or just a line that says "May Substitute," which must be acknowledged in writing. Since doctors must buy their own prescription pads, they usually select terminology they prefer while still meeting legal requirements. As a patient, if you want a generic drug, make sure your doctor has written something in the "Substitution" area of the written prescription.

Other areas of importance on the written prescription are the quantity dispensed and the refills (see Figure 3). Getting the optimum number of doses filled in a single prescription can mean more money saved. In order to determine the optimum number of doses, calculate the number of doses based on the expected length of treatment. Will you be taking the drug for a week, a

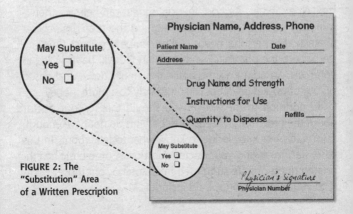

FIGURE 2: The "Substitution" Area of a Written Prescription

month, or a year? How many doses do you take a day? Is this the first time you are taking the drug and is it the right drug? Does the dose change over time? Once you have an estimate of the number of doses you will need, estimate the number of doses allowed by insurance. Does the insurance co-pay cover one month, two months, or three months? In some cases, such as older antibiotics and some pain medications, the cost of the drug may be lower than the co-pay. In this case, paying for the prescription out of pocket rather than through insurance may save you money.

In the case of pain medications, your doctor may prescribe more than you need just to make sure you do not run out. In that case, the ideal prescription quantity may be a lesser number of doses than the doctor would normally write. Ask instead for fewer doses and more refills. Also make sure you have the maximum number of allowable refills written on the prescription to avoid having to contact the doctor when you run out of the drug. For example, if you take a drug once a day and plan to continue treatment for a year, the optimal quantity would be 90 doses with three refills.

The optimal quantity for a prescription will also depend on the payment process. If paying out of pocket instead of through insurance, you may not want to have your money tied up in the medicine cabinet. A good financial model can help you determine the optimal quantity by weighing the prescription cost against other personal needs. But remember that each time you go back to the pharmacy, a dispensing fee will be included in your cost. So adjusting the optimal quantity downward based on out-of-pocket payment will ultimately cost more money.

In addition to the above, you should talk to your doctor about the prescription itself. Most patients do not have enough information or knowledge to know what to talk about. In this case, start by asking your doctor questions. Some basic health-related questions are suggested in Chapter 3, but those specific to your prescription should include:

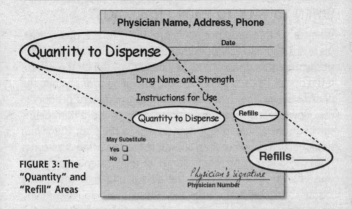

FIGURE 3: The "Quantity" and "Refill" Areas

- Are there nondrug alternatives that can be tried before starting a drug?
- Are there other drugs that can be used to treat my condition?
- How will my condition respond to the drug?
- How long will I have to take the drug?
- What will happen if I don't take the drug?
- What will happen if I don't change my diet or exercise?
- Am I prescribed a high dose that would be associated with more side effects?
- How many strengths of the drug are available?
- Is there a less expensive strength of the drug that could be used?
- Is there an extended-release form of the drug?

The answers to these questions will provide you the information needed to determine whether you are getting the most cost effective treatment, to calculate your optimal quantity, and to make sure you get a generic product. Use the drug summaries in Chapter 6 to help find products and cost comparisons.

WHEN TO TALK TO YOUR PHARMACIST

When a written prescription is presented to the pharmacist, there are not many changes that the pharmacist can make. Basically, the prescription must be filled as written by the doctor. If the doctor has authorized the use of a generic drug, then the pharmacist has the choice of selecting which generic product to use. However, generic substitution is different from therapeutic substitution. A therapeutic substitute is a different drug with similar activity and is not an allowable change without an order from the doctor. Any other change to the written prescription must also be authorized by the doctor and may result in a longer than expected wait at the pharmacy. So make sure you let your doctor know any special concerns or requests when the prescription is written.

The decisions made by the pharmacy include applying insurance, adjusting the fill quantity according to refills or drug shortages, selecting the exact product when multiple manufacturers make the same drug, and selecting the container. You should start at the pharmacy by asking the price of the prescription in advance. From that point, you will know whether you want to apply insurance or pay out of pocket. Ideally, the fill quantity and refills have been discussed with the doctor and adjustments are not needed at the pharmacy.

Next, ask if there are any limitations to the number of doses that you can get based on drug shortages. If yes, ask about waiving the pharmacy fee when picking up subsequent supplies. You can also question the choice of manufacturer although it may not be important. Some drugs have a slightly different effect when switching from one manufacturer to another, so it is important to stay on a supply from the same company. This type of information is highlighted in the drug summaries in Chapter 6 when pertinent.

Finally, the pharmacy will carry a supply of pill bottles that do not have the childproof lids. These are for arthritic patients and those with loss of strength, to make the containers easier to open. If you have special needs for your prescription, let the pharmacist know when the written prescription is dropped off.

Although the pharmacist has limited flexibility with filling your prescription, they are a great source of information and should be used for prescription support. Ask questions that can provide you with a greater sense of confidence in your prescription drug, such as:

- How common is this drug?

- Is this the most common strength used?

- How do people usually respond to treatment?

- Have you heard complaints from other customers about this drug?

- Will food, vitamins, or supplements interfere with the drug? If yes, which ones?

- Are there OTC drugs or other prescription drugs that should not be taken?

The answers to these questions along with any drug-information questions should guide you in taking prescription drug treatment effectively and safely.

REPORTING A PROBLEM

While there are state agencies that handle insurance disputes, no public program is set up to handle complaints over the price of prescription drugs. Instead, there are a few public programs for gathering information on medication errors, side effects, and other potential problems.

The FDA has set up a program called MedWatch for reporting problems and unexpected reactions to a drug (http://www.fda.gov/medwatch/). As a consumer, you have the right to file a report if you have a serious reaction or notice something wrong with your drug. Healthcare professionals can also file reports. The reports are used to generate safety alerts, recalls, withdrawals, and important labeling changes. MedWatch quickly shares this information via their website and e-mail service with healthcare professionals and the general public. If you do not have access to the Internet, ask your doctor or pharmacist for a MedWatch reporting form.

Another program for reporting a medical problem is called Speak Up. This program applies to nursing homes, clinics, and hospitals rather than to retail pharmacies. The intention is to prevent errors before they occur. So reporting of activities that do not look right, such as hand washing without soap or contamination of supplies, is encouraged. The Speak Up program was launched in March 2002 and is still gaining momentum. Consumers can download reporting forms from the Internet through the Joint Commission on Accreditation of Healthcare Organizations (JCAHO) website at http://www.jcaho.org.

If you have a problem with a retail pharmacy that you suspect of unethical or illegal practices, there is no formal reporting program established. Instead, each pharmacy is licensed through the state and would be held accountable to the State Board of Pharmacy. Check with your local government office for more information. U.S.-based Internet pharmacies are licensed through the National Association of Boards of Pharmacy.

DISCARDING OLD DRUGS

The medicine cabinet is filled with old prescription drugs, and they were so expensive that you do not want to throw them away. Someone might need them, right? If you agree, then you are not alone. Millions of people hold on to their old prescription drugs so they can avoid going to the doctor in the event they have the same problem again. I suppose it is similar to never cleaning out the closet and getting rid of old clothes. The clothes or drugs were once good and may still have a use.

This mindset is very dangerous. All drugs have an expiration date and they should be viewed more like food that can go bad when they expire rather than like clothes that only go out of style. Taking an old drug can do one of three things depending on how far it is past the expiration date:

1. Work as originally expected.

2. Not work effectively.

3. Not work and create side effects. •

Drugs are much like fruits or vegetables that undergo small changes of decomposition every day. The older the fruit or vegetable, the more rotten it can get. The older the drug, the less effective it can become. Drugs continue to decompose whether they are in tablet, capsule, cream, or liquid form. Drugs can even continue to decompose when frozen although cold will often slow the rate of decomposition.

The manufacturer labels every drug with an expiration date. The pharmacy that fills your prescription will often make a note of the expiration date on your record, but this information is not usually available on your prescription label. The pharmacist makes sure that the expiration date is long enough to cover you through the period of time that the drug is intended for use. So, if you get a three-month supply of a drug, you are only assured that the drug does not expire within those three months.

The storage place for your prescription drugs may influence the decomposition. Light, heat, and moisture usually contribute to a quicker decomposition process. So, if you keep your drugs on a shelf, near the light in your bathroom, the drug may be losing strength faster than expected. Find a cool (not necessarily cold), dark, dry place to store your prescription drugs to get the most out of their expiration dates.

The rule of thumb used to estimate the expiration of a prescription drug is one year from the date the prescription is filled. There are some exceptions to this rule. Tetracyclines produce dangerous byproducts when they decompose and can cause serious side effects. Fortovase (saquinavir) capsules are only stable for three months from the time of manufacturing and may not be effective if stored longer. Your pharmacist can provide specific information about your prescription drug.

Many people are faced with the dilemma of how to discard their unused drugs. Because of this, many pharmacies sponsor a "Clean Your Medicine Cabinet Day." Pharmacies are not allowed to reuse the old drugs but will make sure they are destroyed and discarded properly. Check with your local pharmacy to find out if they sponsor this type of program.

When discarding old drugs on your own, you should always think about destroying them so that children or animals cannot be harmed. The most common way to destroy oral drugs is to flush them down the toilet. However, local environmental regulations may restrict that type of activity. Check with your local government to determine if a restriction applies in your area. The drug may also cause trouble with your plumbing and may need to be crushed prior to flushing.

Creams and ointments should be emptied from their tube into an empty envelope and thrown in the garbage. Do not lick the envelope shut. The process of smearing the drug into the envelope makes it more difficult for a child or animal to accidentally eat a large quantity.

Drugs that are given by injection, such as insulin, should be discarded by removing the drug from the vial and flushing. Needles and syringes should be placed in a rigid plastic container, such as a plastic laundry detergent container, where they cannot cause harm by puncturing or infecting someone. Your pharmacy should provide additional information about discarding needles and syringes.

6

Prescription Drug Summaries

One of the goals in healthcare is to prevent illness from interfering with everyday life. There is a science around this concept called Quality of Life, complete with evaluation and measurement methods. When a doctor asks how you feel, he or she needs to hear how the signs and symptoms of your disease and treatment are affecting your lifestyle. For example, a taxi driver taking a drug that causes dizziness is at risk of not performing his or her job safely. If continued, the drug may cause the driver to lose the job or have an accident. Either of these events would cause a change to the quality of the person's life. This type of information should be communicated to the doctor. There may be another drug this person can use to treat the disease that does not cause as much dizziness.

All patients do not respond to prescription drugs in the same way. The response will vary a little from patient to patient. The different responses are caused by differences in weight, body type, genes, the disease stage, and hundreds of other characteristics that are not fully understood. The individual patient response explains why a drug will work for one patient and not another. For this reason, there are usually multiple drugs available to treat a single disease. Drugs are generally sorted to identify similarities between the reason for use, drug action, and chemical structure. The decision to prescribe one drug over another is often based on published clinical studies that suggest which drug is most effective. But the individual patient response means that only the patient can tell if the drug is right for him or her. And only the patient knows if the drug is causing undesirable side effects. It may be the wrong drug. Effectively communicating how you feel will let your doctor know if a change in treatment is needed.

Cost is also a factor when Quality of Life is evaluated. A person who cannot afford a drug may not take it as prescribed. The impact of this action could be detrimental to both the patient's health and cost of care. Discussing prescription drug costs with the doctor will help emphasize the financial aspects that need to be considered during treatment. Requesting a generic product should be done automatically.

This chapter will provide insight into prescription drugs sold through a pharmacy. A summary of practical information is written for each prescription drug that includes the availability of generic products, a cost comparison between products, side effects, and many other helpful comments. This information should be used as a guide to the lowest cost drugs and possible alternatives. Additionally, the drug summaries provide information that will help the patient to effectively communicate with the doctor when asked, "How do you feel?"

Remember that only a doctor can order prescription drugs. Asking questions and presenting your doctor with information will guide your doctor in determining the right drug for you. Ensuring that a drug is matched to the patient's modified lifestyle as well as to the disease can help doctors meet their goal to provide a better Quality of Life.

HOW TO USE THE DRUG SUMMARIES

There are nearly 500 drug summaries in this chapter. The drugs selected are sold through a pharmacy and are primarily taken by mouth. Drugs available without a presecription such as aspirin, are not included.

Each drug summary begins with the name of the active drug ingredient, which is also known as the generic name. Do not confuse the generic name with the availability of a generic product. Generic-product alternatives are identified later in the summary.

Following the generic name is the date the drug was first available for sale in the United States. This date applies to any form of the drug even if the original product is no longer sold. Drugs that have been on the market longer are more likely to have a generic-product alternative as well as competitive pricing. The date of availability also provides a sense of experience with patients. The longer a drug is available, the more patient experience is gathered to identify safety issues. Keep in mind that drug information may change over time. The drug summary information in this book is only current at the time of publication. Ask your doctor or pharmacist to update you on any changes related to your prescription drug.

Beneath the generic drug name are several sections, identified with various headers. The information is specific to the active drug ingredient no matter what other names are used to identify products. See the headers below for further explanation.

Commonly Used to Treat

This section provides a plain-language description of the most frequent reasons for prescribing the drug. The plain language does not identify specific disease information and should not be viewed as a clinical reference. For example, a drug may be indicated to treat closed angle glaucoma, but the plain-language description only specifies glaucoma. This section includes the main reasons a drug is used but not every reason. Many times, there is evidence that supports a drug use beyond the primary indications. Do not be alarmed if you are using the drug for a reason not included in this section. If you have concerns, you should discuss them with your doctor or pharmacist.

Drug Category

By comparing the information in this section to the Index of Drugs by Category and Class in Chapter 7, the user can find a listing of other similar drugs. The other drugs may be discussed with the doctor as possible alternatives when treatment is reviewed.

Products

Drugs are sold by many different companies, each of which sells its own unique products. Since drug products are sold under different names, this section will not only identify the drug alias names, but also include the strength and form of the products that contain the active drug ingredient. The products are sorted into three basic subsections based on the availability of a generic product as follows:

1. Brand-Name Products with no Generic Alternative

There is not a generic product available for every strength or form of an original brand-name drug. When the drug is relatively new, is used by few patients, or is priced competitively, a generic product is usually not developed. This section lists only those products, by brand names, that do not have a generic alternative. A cost-comparison symbol is provided next to each product as a gauge to the pricing. Use the Cost-Comparison Key on page 55 for an explanation of the symbols. If all the products sold are available as generic products, this section will drop off the drug summary. Note that there may be more than one brand-name product with the same strength. Although these are not generics, there may be a cost difference between products.

If there are no generic alternatives, this section will confirm that fact and briefly explain why a generic product is not available. A statement of the patent and/or exclusivity limitation by year (see Chapter 3 for a full explanation) is included. The year gives an idea of the earliest date a generic may be able to enter

the market. The year does not guarantee that a generic product
will be developed.

2. Brand-Name Products with Generic Alternatives

When generic products are available, they are identified in this
section. Products are grouped with the brand-name product listed first followed immediately below by the equivalent generic
product. The two products have the same active drug ingredient, same strength, same form, and the same effect on the
body. The generic product is preceded by the word "Generic." A
cost-comparison symbol is provided next to each product as a
gauge of the pricing. Since there are often several generic companies that make the same drug, the cost-comparison symbol
for the generic product represents the lowest cost alternative
even if more than one generic product is available. Use the Cost-
Comparison Key on page 55 for an explanation of the symbols.

If all the products sold are either brand-name products without a generic alternative, or generic products without a brand-
name alternative, this section will drop off the drug summary.

3. Products Available Only as Generics

Drugs that have been available for a long time may be sold
only as generic products. In this case, the company that first developed the drug has chosen to discontinue or sell the product,
leaving only generic products on the market. These products
are sold under either the generic name or one of the generic
product names listed in the next subsection (Other Generic
Product Names). A cost-comparison symbol is provided next to
each product as a gauge of the pricing. Since there are often
several generic companies that make the same drug, the cost
comparison symbol for the generic product represents the lowest cost alternative even if more than one generic product is
available. Use the Cost Comparison Key on page 55 for an explanation of the symbols. If there are no products available
only as generics, this section will drop off the drug summary.

In addition to the three subsections listed above, two others are included to provide a complete set of alias names and products made with the drug. They are described below.

4. *Other Generic Product Names*
A generic product may be identified by the generic name, but may also be sold under a brand name. This subsection identifies all the other names used for generic products. If you receive a prescription with one of the names in this section, it is a generic product. If generic products are sold only by the generic name, this section will drop off the drug summary.

5. *Combination Products That Contain This Drug*
Many times a patient must take more than one drug to treat a disease. Some of the common drug combinations are formulated into a single product. While the cost of combination drugs is often higher than products containing only one drug, they may be less expensive than the cost of two different drugs. A cross-reference of the active drug ingredients in these products is provided in the Index of Combination Drugs in Chapter 8. Review these products with your doctor if taking more than one drug. Much of the drug information in the summary will apply to combination drugs although dosing may differ. If there are no combination products, this section will drop off the drug summary.

Dosing and Food

This section presents the usual drug dosing, including when to take the drug in conjunction with food as well as what to do if a dose is forgotten. This section should NOT be used to change the dose of the drug or the interval at which it is taken without the consent of a doctor. Remember that the dose is specific to the diagnosis, not to the drug. Taking a higher drug dose is not necessarily more effective and is often associated with a greater risk of side effects. Follow the prescription instructions closely and try not to forget or skip any doses.

Drug dosing is often based on weight or body size, especially in children. You may see doses listed in "mg/kg" or "mg/m². Kilograms (kg) represent body weight. There are 2.2 pounds per kilogram, so a 22 pound infant weighs 10 kg. Meters squared (m²) is a measure of body surface area and requires special charts to estimate. Your doctor can estimate body surface area.

Foods that interfere with the absorption of the drug are highlighted in this section as well as any food that should be avoided entirely. Note that spices are not specified here but are included under Alcohol, Drug, Herb, and Supplement Interactions if any apply. Remember to take your prescription drug with a full glass of water to help the dose dissolve and make the drug more available for absorption. See Chapter 4 for additional details about drug absorbtion.

The decision to take a dose after it has been accidentally forgotten is based on the way the body handles the drug as well as the prescription schedule. The information provided on forgotten doses is based on usual dosing schedules. Never take two doses at the same time (double dosing) unless specifically instructed to do so by your doctor.

Alcohol, Drug, Herb, and Supplement Interactions

Interactions that occur when taking a drug with alcohol, other drugs, herbs, and supplements are explained in this section. Review the list and follow up with your doctor or pharmacist if you see anything on the list that you take. Herb and supplement interactions are identified with an explanation and recommendations for change. Drug interactions, which may include prescription drugs, OTC drugs such as vitamin and mineral supplements, and illegal street drugs, are grouped into three different categories with headings as follows:

1. *Taking this drug with any of the ones listed below may change the effect of either drug with the possibility of causing toxicity or decreasing effectiveness.*

The dose or interval of one of the drugs should be adjusted. Your doctor may have taken this into consideration when writing the prescription. Do not adjust your drug dose or interval without instructions from your doctor. Frequent monitoring may be needed. **Note that entire categories of drugs are identified in this section with a † symbol.** Individual drug names can be found in the Index of Drugs by Category and Class in Chapter 7.

2. *Severe reactions are possible when this drug is taken with those listed below:*

These drugs should not be taken while on the prescription drug. **Note that entire categories of drugs are identified in this section with a † symbol.** Individual drug names can be found in the Index of Drugs by Category and Class in Chapter 7.

3. *Increased effects or side effects are possible when this drug is taken with those listed below:*

The patient should be aware of the drugs listed here and report any unusual side effects to the doctor or nurse. **Note that categories of drugs are identified in this section with a † symbol.** Individual drug names can be found in the Index of Drugs by Category and Class in Chapter 7.

It is important to note that all drugs in this section are called by the generic name. If you do not know the generic drug name for a product you are taking, ask your pharmacist. The generic name is used most often as the standard for communications.

Allergic Reactions and Side Effects

A special warning about the risk of allergic reactions is identified at the beginning of this section. If you are allergic to a drug, do not take it. Allergy symptoms may begin with a rash, but may also start with flulike symptoms. If an allergic reaction is suspected, go to the nearest emergency room. Notifying the doctor of allergies to foods, dyes, and other chemicals may help identify a potential drug allergy in advance.

The risks concerning exposure to sunlight, if any, are fully explained next. The remainder of this section includes other side effects sorted according to their relative frequency: more common, less common, or rare. Less common side effects generally affect 1 percent or more of the patients taking the drug. In some cases, the more common side effects can be seen in 15 to 20 percent of patients. Side effects are seen more frequently in patients taking the drug in high doses or for a long period of time. Many side effects can last for over a month after the drug has been stopped. All side effects should be reported to the doctor since they may be a sign of more serious complications.

Also noted is the severity of side effects. **An asterisk (*) indicates a potentially serious reaction that should be reported to your doctor right away no matter how common or rare.** These effects may be an indication of toxicity or other complications related to the use of the drug. Side effects that occur very suddenly or with great severity should be reported to your doctor immediately and may require emergency care and discontinuation of the drug.

Precautions

This section of warnings includes information similar to that provided by the doctor and pharmacist when a prescription is started. The warnings are general and may vary depending on the individual patient and treatment. Any statements that cause concern about using the drug should be discussed with the doctor or pharmacist.

Pregnancy and Breast-Feeding

Safe use of drugs during pregnancy and breast-feeding is not routinely studied in humans because of ethical reasons. Animal studies are performed before the drug is approved, but the information does not provide conclusive answers for humans. The pregnancy precautions supplied in this section are based on a standard classifications system gathered from animal data. No such system exists for breast-feeding recommendations. Instead, breast-feeding recommendations represent the anticipated risk based on the published reports of adverse reactions in newborns. Always discuss breast-feeding and pregnancy with your doctor or pharmacist before taking a prescription drug.

Helpful Comments

This section contains a variety of tips and comments to supplement the drug information. These tips may be helpful to make the use of a prescription drug more acceptable.

COST-COMPARISON SYMBOLS

The price paid for prescription drugs will vary based on the pharmacy. This makes prescription price a poor means of comparison. Instead, each drug manufacturer publishes a price associated with their drug called the Average Wholesale Price (AWP). AWP is a standard means of price communication within healthcare. The cost-comparison symbols are based on AWP, which does not include the pharmacy fee. AWP should be used to compare the relative cost between products rather than the actual cost of a prescription. Remember that the cost of a single dose cannot be used to evaluate the overall cost of therapy. Comparisons should be made based on the number of doses per day or per week in order to be useful.

The cost comparison of products that are not in solid form is somewhat difficult. The symbol for oral liquids is based on 5 milliliters (ml) since that most closely compares to tablet and capsule doses. However, newer oral liquids are often concentrated, making the usual dose less than 5 ml. For that reason, the cost-comparison symbol does not compare directly to tablets and capsules. Eyedrops, ear drops, nasal sprays, topical solutions, and other liquid drugs are not dosed in regular 5 ml or 1 ml doses, making a casual glance at the cost-comparison symbol less helpful.

When the AWP is not readily available, the term "n/a" is listed on the drug summary. This often applies to products that are not frequently sold due to high pricing or uncommon doses. In some cases, the drug is new and the AWP is not yet established. Talk to your local pharmacist if you would like more recent information about the cost of drugs that contain the "n/a" symbol.

See "How to Compare Costs" on the following page.

COST-COMPARISON KEY		
SYMBOL	SOLID (EACH) OR LIQUIDS (PER 5 ML)	SEMI-SOLID (PER GRAM, ML, OR EACH)
(¢)	$0.10 or less	$0.50 or less
(¢¢)	$0.11 to $0.25	$0.51 to $1.00
(¢¢¢)	$0.26 to $0.50	$1.01 to $1.50
(¢¢¢¢)	$0.51 to $0.75	$1.51 to $2.00
(¢¢¢¢¢)	$0.76 to $1.00	$2.01 to $2.50
($)	$1.01 to $1.50	$2.51 to $3.00
($$)	$1.51 to $2.50	$3.01 to $3.50
($$$)	$2.51 to $5.00	$3.51 to $4.00
($$$$)	$5.01 to $10.00	$4.01 to $5.00
($$$$$)	Over $10.00	Over $5.00
(n/a)	Indicates that cost information is not available.	

- **Solid:** capsule, patch, suppository, tablet, vaginal tablet
- **Semi-Solid:** aerosol, cream, gel, lotion, ointment, powder, powder for oral suspension, topical solution, topical swab
- **Liquid:** concentrate, drops, elixir, oral solution, suspension, syrup

HOW TO COMPARE COSTS

Multiply the estimated drug cost by the number of doses per day to effectively compare the cost between products. For example, if a drug is taken four times a day with a cost-comparison symbol of (¢) and an extended-release product is available with a cost-comparison symbol of (¢¢¢), the extended-release product may be less expensive if taken only once a day.

The cost-comparison symbols used in this book represent the price paid by the pharmacy to purchase the drug (average whole-sale price published in 2002). The information should not be used to determine the actual cost of a prescription since prices may vary and the pharmacy fee is not included. Instead, the symbols provide a standardized reference for comparison between products.

ABACAVIR SULFATE

Available since December 1998

COMMONLY USED TO TREAT

HIV-1 infection

DRUG CATEGORY

antiretroviral
Class: nucleoside reverse transcriptase inhibitor (NsRTI)

PRODUCTS

Brand-Name Products with No Generic Alternative
Ziagen 300 mg tablet ($$$)
Ziagen 20 mg per ml oral solution ($$)
No generics available.
Multiple patents that begin to expire in 2009.
Combination Products That Contain This Drug
Trizivir tablet ($$$$$)

DOSING AND FOOD

Doses are taken 2 times a day.

This drug may be taken with or without food.

Adults: Up to 600 mg per day in divided doses.

Children age 3 months to 16 years: Up to 16 mg/kg (maximum 600 mg) per day in divided doses.

Forgotten doses: If you are scheduled to take the next dose within a few hours, do not take the forgotten dose. Otherwise take it as soon as you remember.

ALCOHOL, DRUG, HERB, AND SUPPLEMENT INTERACTIONS

Alcohol may increase some of the side effects from this drug, depending on the amount consumed. Ask your doctor about the risks caused by drinking alcohol with your condition.

There are currently no known drug, herb, or supplement interactions.

ALLERGIC REACTIONS AND SIDE EFFECTS

This drug is known to cause severe allergic reactions. Contact your doctor immediately if you start to feel ill, or develop a fever, skin rash, fatigue, nausea, vomiting, diarrhea, or abdominal pain.

MORE COMMON SIDE EFFECTS: Diarrhea*, loss of appetite, stomach upset, vomiting*

LESS COMMON SIDE EFFECTS: Headache, sleeping difficulty, tiredness

RARE SIDE EFFECTS: Breathing difficulty, fever*, itching*, stomach pain*, tiredness*

PRECAUTIONS

This drug is usually prescribed in combination with another antiretroviral drug. Ask your pharmacist about the type of drug interaction that may occur between antiretroviral drugs† to coordinate the administration times of multiple drugs.

PREGNANCY AND BREAST-FEEDING

Safety during pregnancy has not been established although the drug is known to harm animal fetuses.

Breast-feeding while taking this drug is not recommended.

HELPFUL COMMENTS

Your doctor or pharmacist should report each case of allergic reaction to the Abacavir Hypersensitivity Registry at 1-800-270-0425.

---

† See page 52.   * See page 53.

ACARBOSE

Available since September 1995

COMMONLY USED TO TREAT

High blood sugar, specifically type 2 diabetes that has not responded to other treatments

DRUG CATEGORY

antidiabetic
Class: alphaglucosidase inhibitor

PRODUCTS

Brand-Name Products with No Generic Alternative
Precose 25 mg tablet (¢¢¢¢)
Precose 50 mg tablet (¢¢¢¢)
Precose 100 mg tablet (¢¢¢¢)
No generics available.
Patent expires in 2007.

DOSING AND FOOD

Doses are taken 3 times a day.
The dose should always be taken with the first bite of each meal.
Adults: Up to 300 mg per day in divided doses.
This drug is rarely used in children under age 18.
Forgotten doses: If more than 2 hours have passed since the last meal, do not take the forgotten dose. Monitor your blood sugar closely if a dose is forgotten.

ALCOHOL, DRUG, HERB, AND SUPPLEMENT INTERACTIONS

Alcohol may increase some of the side effects from this drug, depending on the amount consumed. Alcohol may cause changes in your blood sugar. Ask your doctor about the risks caused by drinking alcohol with your condition.

Aloe, bilberry leaf, bitter melon, burdock, dandelion, fenugreek, garlic, ginkgo biloba, and ginseng may lower blood sugar and cause the need for a dose adjustment when taken with this drug. Tell your doctor if you are taking any of these supplements.

Taking this drug with any of the ones listed below may change the effect of either drug with the possibility of causing toxicity or decreasing effectiveness: activated charcoal, amylase, pancreatin

Increased effects or side effects are possible when this drug is taken with those listed below:

antidiabetics[t], calcium channel blockers[t], corticosteroids[t], diuretics[t], estrogens[t], isoniazid, nicotinic acid, oral contraceptives[t], phenothiazines[t], phenytoin, sympathomimetics[t], thyroid hormones[t]

ALLERGIC REACTIONS AND SIDE EFFECTS

You should tell your doctor about all your allergies and any unexplained symptoms you may have while taking this drug.

MORE COMMON SIDE EFFECTS: Bloated feeling, diarrhea, gas, stomach pain

RARE SIDE EFFECTS: Yellow eyes or skin*

PRECAUTIONS

A liver test should be run every 3 months while taking this drug.

This drug should not be used in people with diabetic ketoacidosis, cirrhosis, inflammatory bowel disease, colonic ulceration, partial intestinal obstruction, people prone to intestinal obstruction, or in people who have chronic intestinal disease with digestion or absorption problems.

Burns, diarrhea, fever, hormonal changes, infection, malnourishment, severe stress, uncontrolled thyroid disease, and vomiting may cause changes in blood sugar that may make this drug less effective.

PREGNANCY AND BREAST-FEEDING

Safety during pregnancy has not been established although there was no evidence of harm during studies in animals.

Breast-feeding while taking this drug is not recommended.

HELPFUL COMMENTS

Side effects usually develop in the first few weeks of treatment.

You may test the effects of this drug by measuring your blood sugar 1 hour after eating. If your blood sugar is still high, you may need a dose adjustment or a change in treatment.

This drug is usually taken with another antidiabetic.

If you do not treat high blood sugar, you may develop more serious problems such as heart failure, blood vessel disease, eye disease, or kidney disease.

---

[t] *See page 52.*   * *See page 53.*

ACEBUTOLOL

Available since December 1984

COMMONLY USED TO TREAT

High blood pressure, also known as hypertension
Irregular heartbeat, specifically ventricular arrhythmia
Chest pain, also known as angina

DRUG CATEGORY

antianginal
antiarrhythmic
antihypertensive
Class: beta blocker

PRODUCTS

Brand-Name Products with Generic Alternatives
Sectral 200 mg tablet ($)
   Generic: acebutolol 200 mg tablet (¢¢¢¢¢)
Sectral 400 mg tablet ($$)
   Generic: acebutolol 400 mg tablet ($)

DOSING AND FOOD

Doses are taken 1 to 2 times a day.
This drug may be taken with or without food.
Adults: Up to 2,400 mg per day in divided doses.
Adults over age 65 should not take more than 800 mg a day.
Lower doses are used in people with kidney disease.
This drug is rarely used in children.
Forgotten doses: Take the forgotten dose as soon as you remember unless
  it is within 3 to 4 hours of the next scheduled dose.

ALCOHOL, DRUG, HERB, AND SUPPLEMENT INTERACTIONS

Alcohol may increase some of the side effects from this drug, depending
  on the amount consumed. Ask your doctor about the risks caused by
  drinking alcohol with your condition.
Several OTC drugs used for appetite control, asthma, colds, cough, hay
  fever, or sinus problems may cause an increase in blood pressure when
  taken with this drug. Check with your pharmacist when selecting OTC
  products.

Taking this drug with any of the ones listed below may change the effect of either drug with the possibility of causing toxicity or decreasing effectiveness: aminophylline, anesthetics†, antidiabetics†, caffeine, calcium channel blockers†, carbonic anhydrase inhibitors†, clonidine, dyphylline, epinephrine, guanabenz, lidocaine, nonsteroidal antiinflammatories†, oxtriphylline, pilocarpine, reserpine, theophylline

Severe reactions are possible when this drug is taken with those listed below: allergy shots, beta blockers†, cocaine, monoamine oxidase inhibitors†

Increased effects or side effects are possible when this drug is taken with those listed below:
antihypertensives†

ALLERGIC REACTIONS AND SIDE EFFECTS

If you are allergic to any other beta blockers†, you may also be allergic to this drug.

This drug may exaggerate the reaction from your current allergies. Inform your doctor of any allergies that you have as well as the severity of the allergic reaction before starting this drug.

MORE COMMON SIDE EFFECTS: Dizziness, drowsiness, lightheadedness, sexual dysfunction, sleeping difficulty, tiredness, weakness

LESS COMMON SIDE EFFECTS: Anxiety, breathing difficulty*, cold hands*, cold feet*, constipation, depression*, diarrhea, frequent urination, itching, nausea, nervousness, numbness, shortness of breath*, slow heartbeat*, sore eyes, stomachache, stuffy nose, swelling, tingling, vivid dreams, vomiting, wheezing

RARE SIDE EFFECTS: Back pain*, bleeding*, bruising*, chest pain*, confusion*, dark urine*, dizziness*, fever*, hallucinations*, irregular heartbeat*, joint pain*, lightheadedness*, rash*, skin irritation*, sore throat*, yellow eyes or skin*

PRECAUTIONS

This drug should not be used in people with a heart rate that is routinely less than 60 beats per minute (bradycardia), or in people with heart block, heart failure, or cardiogenic shock.

People with asthma may not be able to take this drug.

You need to wait 2 weeks after stopping a monoamine oxidase inhibitor† before starting this drug.

Stopping this drug suddenly may cause chest pain or heart attack. If you wish to stop taking this drug, ask your doctor for specific instructions.

---

†See page 52.   *See page 53.

Be careful driving or handling equipment while taking this drug because the drug may cause drowsiness.

If you are diabetic, this drug may increase blood sugar levels or make the symptoms of low blood sugar less noticeable.

This drug may cause nondiabetics to develop type 2 diabetes.

If you have psoriasis or myasthenia gravis, this drug may make those conditions worse.

PREGNANCY AND BREAST-FEEDING

Safety during pregnancy has not been established although there is some evidence that infants have lower birth weights and changes in blood pressure and heart rate for the first 72 hours.

Breast-feeding while taking this drug is not recommended.

HELPFUL COMMENTS

This drug may make you more sensitive to cold temperatures.

It may take 1 to 2 months to notice the full effect of this drug.

If you do not treat high blood pressure, you may develop more serious problems such as heart failure, blood vessel disease, stroke, or kidney disease. Losing weight, exercising, eating more fruits and vegetables, and avoiding salty foods, such as lunchmeat and pickles, may help make drug treatment more successful.

ACETAZOLAMIDE

Available prior to 1982

COMMONLY USED TO TREAT

Fluid retention caused by drugs or heart failure
Increased pressure in the eye, also known as glaucoma
Mountain sickness
Periodic paralysis
Seizures, not all types

DRUG CATEGORY

altitude sickness agent
anticonvulsant
antiglaucoma drug
diuretic
Class: carbonic anhydrase inhibitor

PRODUCTS

Brand-Name Products with No Generic Alternative
Diamox Sequels 500 mg extended-release capsule ($)

Brand-Name with Generic Alternatives
Diamox 125 mg tablet (¢¢¢)
  Generic: acetazolamide 125 mg tablet (¢¢¢)
Diamox 250 mg tablet (¢¢¢¢)
  Generic: acetazolamide 250 mg tablet (¢¢¢)

DOSING AND FOOD

Doses are taken 1 to 6 times a day.

It is best to take this drug on an empty stomach, but taking this drug with
a little food may avoid the stomach upset that some people suffer.

Adults: Up to 1,000 mg per day in divided doses.

Children: Up to 30 mg/kg per day in divided doses.

Forgotten doses: If you are scheduled to take the next dose within a few
hours, do not take the forgotten dose. Otherwise take the forgotten dose
as soon as you remember.

ALCOHOL, DRUG, HERB, AND SUPPLEMENT INTERACTIONS

Alcohol may increase some of the side effects from this drug, depending
on the amount consumed. Ask your doctor about the risks caused by
drinking alcohol with your condition.

**Taking this drug with any of the ones listed below may change the effect of
either drug with the possibility of causing toxicity or decreasing effectiveness:**
amphetamines†, aspirin, flecainide, lithium, mecamylamine, methenamine,
phenobarbital, procainamide, quinidine

ALLERGIC REACTIONS AND SIDE EFFECTS

If you are allergic to any carbonic anhydrase inhibitors†, sulfonamides†, or
thiazide diuretics†, you may also be allergic to this drug.

This drug promotes the effect of sunlight on the body and may cause
severe sunburn and increased sensitivity of the eyes.

MORE COMMON SIDE EFFECTS: Diarrhea, loss of appetite, metallic taste,
nausea, numbness, tingling, tiredness*, urinary changes*, vomiting,
weakness*, weight loss

LESS COMMON SIDE EFFECTS: Back pain, bloody urine*, constipation, de-
pression*, dizziness, drowsiness, dry mouth*, headache, irregular heart-

---

† *See page 52.*   * *See page 53.*

beat*, irritability, loss of smell, mood swings, muscle cramps*, nausea*, nervousness, painful urination, taste changes, tiredness*, thirst*, vomiting*, weakness*, weak pulse*

RARE SIDE EFFECTS: Black stools*, bleeding*, bruising*, clumsiness*, confusion*, dark urine*, fever*, hives*, itching*, pale stools*, ringing in ears*, seizures*, skin rash*, sore throat*, trembling*, weakness*, yellow eyes or skin*

PRECAUTIONS

This drug should not be taken by people who have low sodium or potassium blood levels, or in people with kidney disease, liver disease, adrenal gland failure, or hyperchloremic acidosis.

Do not break or crush extended-release products.

This drug should not be used for long-term treatment of chronic noncongestive angle-closure glaucoma.

Be careful driving or handling equipment while taking this drug because the drug may cause drowsiness.

People with diabetes, gout, emphysema, and other respiratory diseases may not be able to take this drug.

PREGNANCY AND BREAST-FEEDING

Safety during pregnancy has not been established although the drug is known to harm animal fetuses.

Breast-feeding while taking this drug is not recommended.

HELPFUL COMMENTS

Your body may lose potassium while taking this drug, which may cause severe side effects. Potassium levels should be monitored periodically and may need to be supplemented while taking this drug. Foods high in potassium include meat, fish, apricots, avocados, bananas, melons, kiwi, lima beans, milk, oranges, potatoes, prunes, spinach, tomatoes, and squash.

Take the last dose of the day before 6 P.M. to reduce the chance of having to urinate during the night.

The effects of this drug do not continue after the drug is stopped. If you are taking the drug for seizures, talk to your doctor about a gradual decrease in dosage.

ACETOHEXAMIDE

Available since February 1987

COMMONLY USED TO TREAT

High blood sugar, specifically type 2 diabetes

DRUG CATEGORY

antidiabetic
Class: sulfonylurea: first generation

PRODUCTS

Products Only Available as Generics
acetohexamide 250 mg tablet (¢¢¢)
acetohexamide 500 mg tablet (¢¢¢)

DOSING AND FOOD

Doses are taken 1 to 2 times a day.
This drug should be taken just before a meal.
Adults: Up to 1,500 mg per day in divided doses.
This drug is rarely used in children.
People with kidney or liver disease may need lower doses.
Forgotten doses: If you are scheduled to take the next dose within a few
hours, do not take the forgotten dose. Otherwise take the forgotten dose
as soon as you remember.

ALCOHOL, DRUG, HERB, AND SUPPLEMENT INTERACTIONS

Alcohol should not be used while taking this drug. Small amounts of alcohol may cause redness in the face, arms, and neck that may be uncom-
fortable. Alcohol may also cause changes in blood sugar. Ask your doctor
about the risks caused by drinking alcohol with your condition.

Aloe, bilberry leaf, bitter melon, burdock, dandelion, fenugreek, garlic,
ginkgo biloba, and ginseng may lower blood sugar and cause the need
for a dose adjustment when taken with this drug. Tell your doctor if you
are taking any of these supplements.

Several OTC drugs used for asthma, colds, cough, hay fever, sleep aid, or sinus problems may seriously change the effects of this drug. Check with
your pharmacist when selecting OTC products.

---

†See page 52.   *See page 53.

Taking this drug with any of the ones listed below may change the effect of either drug with the possibility of causing toxicity or decreasing effectiveness: anticoagulants†, antihistamines†, aspirin, beta blockers†, chloramphenicol, cimetidine, corticosteroids†, cyclosporine, fluconazole, fluoroquinolones†, insulin, lithium, miconazole, probenecid, quinine, quinidine, ranitidine, salicylates†, sulfonamides†, thiazide diuretics†

Severe reactions are possible when this drug is taken with those listed below: guanethidine, monoamine oxidase inhibitors†, octreotide, pentamidine

ALLERGIC REACTIONS AND SIDE EFFECTS

If you are allergic to any sulfonylureas† or sulfonamides†, you may also be allergic to this drug. You should tell your doctor about all your allergies and any unexplained symptoms you may have while taking this drug.

This drug promotes the effect of sunlight on the body and may cause severe sunburn and increased sensitivity of the eyes.

MORE COMMON SIDE EFFECTS: Anxiety*, appetite changes, behavior change*, blurry vision*, chills*, confusion*, constipation, diarrhea, difficulty concentrating*, dizziness, drowsiness*, fast heartbeat*, frequent urination, gas, headache*, heartburn, hunger*, low blood sugar*, nausea*, nervousness*, nightmares*, shakiness*, sleep disorders*, slurry speech*, stomach pain, sweating*, taste changes, tiredness*, vomiting, weakness*, weight gain*

LESS COMMON SIDE EFFECTS: Seizures*, skin irritation*, unconsciousness*

RARE SIDE EFFECTS: Bleeding*, bruising*, chest pain*, coughing up blood*, dark urine*, excess sputum*, fever*, hives*, pale skin*, pale stools*, shortness of breath*, sore throat*, yellow eyes or skin*

PRECAUTIONS

The dose of this drug may need to change frequently if you have an uncontrolled thyroid condition.

You need to wait 2 weeks after stopping a monoamine oxidase inhibitor† before starting this drug.

People with underactive adrenal and pituitary glands may develop low blood sugar while taking this drug.

Weak or malnourished people may develop low blood sugar while taking this drug.

Burns, diarrhea, fever, hormonal changes, infection, malnourishment, severe stress, uncontrolled thyroid disease, and vomiting may cause changes in blood sugar that may make this drug less effective.

PREGNANCY AND BREAST-FEEDING

There is evidence that this drug may harm the fetus, but the drug may be necessary to the health of the mother.

Breast-feeding while taking this drug is not recommended.

HELPFUL COMMENTS

Blood sugar levels should be checked if you experience any side effects.

If you are a smoker and stop smoking while taking this drug, your dose may need to be reduced.

If you do not treat high blood sugar, you may develop more serious problems such as heart failure, blood vessel disease, eye disease, or kidney disease.

ACETYLCYSTEINE

Available for over 20 years

COMMONLY USED TO TREAT

Acetaminophen overdose
Thick mucus in the lungs

DRUG CATEGORY

mucolytic
Class: amino acid derivative

PRODUCTS

Brand-Name Products with Generic Alternatives
Mucomyst 10% inhalation solution ($$)
  Generic: acetylcysteine 10% inhalation solution ($)
Mucomyst 20% inhalation solution ($$)
  Generic: acetylcysteine 20% inhalation solution ($)
Other Generic Product Names
Mucosil

DOSING AND FOOD

Doses are taken 1 to 24 times a day.
This drug may be taken with or without food.
Adults and children: Up to 120 ml per day by inhalation, or 70 mg/kg orally in divided doses.

---

† See page 52.   * See page 53.

Forgotten doses: Take the forgotten dose as soon as you remember, then continue with the normal schedule.

ALCOHOL, DRUG, HERB, AND SUPPLEMENT INTERACTIONS

Alcohol may increase some of the side effects from this drug, depending on the amount consumed. Ask your doctor about the risks caused by drinking alcohol with your condition.

Taking this drug with any of the ones listed below may change the effect of either drug with the possibility of causing toxicity or decreasing effectiveness: activated charcoal

ALLERGIC REACTIONS AND SIDE EFFECTS

You should tell your doctor about all your allergies and any unexplained symptoms you may have while taking this drug.

LESS COMMON SIDE EFFECTS: Breathing difficulty, chest pain, clammy skin, congestion, fever, nausea, runny nose, sore mouth, vomiting, wheezing*

RARE SIDE EFFECTS: Skin rash*

PRECAUTIONS

If you have asthma, this drug may make that condition worse.

If you cannot cough up the mucus, it may have to be removed by suction.

This drug smells like rotten eggs, but the odor will go away soon after it is used. Make sure to rinse your mouth after the treatment to avoid nausea.

PREGNANCY AND BREAST-FEEDING

Safety during pregnancy has not been established although there was no evidence of harm during studies in animals.

It is not known if this drug passes into breast milk. Talk to your doctor about the risks associated with breast-feeding while taking this drug.

HELPFUL COMMENTS

Store the unused portion of each vial in the refrigerator for no longer than 96 hours.

Use plastic or stainless steel when measuring this drug since it may darken and tarnish other metals.

This drug may turn light purple, but is still acceptable for use.

N-acetylcysteine, also called NAC, is an antioxidant found in many dietary supplements.

ACITRETIN

Available since October 1996

COMMONLY USED TO TREAT

Skin irritation, specifically psoriasis

DRUG CATEGORY

antipsoriatic
Class: retinoid

PRODUCTS

Brand-Name Products with No Generic Alternative
Soriatane 10 mg capsule ($$$$)
Soriatane 25 mg capsule ($$$$$)
No generics available.
No patents, no exclusivity.

DOSING AND FOOD

Doses are taken once a day.
It is best to take this drug with food or milk.
Adults: Up to 75 mg per day.
Forgotten doses: If you are scheduled to take the next dose in less than 5 hours, do not take the forgotten dose. Otherwise take the forgotten dose as soon as you remember.

ALCOHOL, DRUG, HERB, AND SUPPLEMENT INTERACTIONS

Alcohol should not be used while taking this drug and for 2 months after the drug is stopped. Alcohol may cause changes to the drug making it stay in the body about 60 times longer than expected.

Taking this drug with any of the ones listed below may change the effect of either drug with the possibility of causing toxicity or decreasing effectiveness: cyclosporine, dantrolene, ethotoin, fosphenytoin, phenytoin, progestins

Severe reactions are possible when this drug is taken with those listed below: etretinate, isotretinoin, tetracycline, tretinoin

Increased side effects are possible when this drug is taken with those listed below: methotrexate, vitamin A

ALLERGIC REACTIONS AND SIDE EFFECTS

If you are allergic to etretinate, isotretinoin, tretinoin, or vitamin A, you

---

† See page 52.　　* See page 53.

may also be allergic to this drug. You should tell your doctor about all your allergies and any unexplained symptoms you may have while taking this drug.

This drug promotes the effect of sunlight on the body and may cause severe sunburn and increased sensitivity of the eyes.

MORE COMMON SIDE EFFECTS: Back pain*, dry eyes, earwax, hair loss, headache*, itching*, joint pain*, lip irritation, mouth irritation, nausea*, nosebleeds, runny nose, stiffness*, thirst, walking difficulty*, vomiting*

LESS COMMON SIDE EFFECTS: Blurry vision*, constipation, diarrhea, eye pain*, eye problems*, fatigue, loose fingernails*, sweating, watery eyes*

RARE SIDE EFFECTS: Abdominal pain*, cough*, dark urine*, drowsiness*, eyelid irritation*, hoarseness*, irritability*, itchy ears*, skin infection*, skin irritation*, skin odor*, skin ulcers*, speaking difficulty*, vaginal discharge*, vaginal irritation*, vision changes*, yellow eyes or skin*

PRECAUTIONS

Women of childbearing age must use 2 methods of birth control for 3 years after stopping this drug before becoming pregnant because of the high risk of developing birth defects.

The "mini pill" used to prevent pregnancy may not work while taking this drug. Another form of contraceptive is recommended.

A pregnancy test, run 1 week prior to starting this drug, is required for all women of childbearing age.

Do not donate blood while taking this drug and for 3 years after the drug is stopped.

If you have high cholesterol, high triglycerides, or diabetes, this drug may make those conditions worse.

People with a history of having too much vitamin A in their body may not be able to take this drug.

Drink plenty of fluids to avoid dehydration when sweating, such as in hot weather and during exercise.

Women of childbearing age must sign a consent form that explains the risk of birth defects before this drug can be prescribed.

PREGNANCY AND BREAST-FEEDING

This drug may cause birth defects and should not be used during pregnancy. Breast-feeding while taking this drug is not recommended.

HELPFUL COMMENTS

This drug can also be called by the generic names 13-cis acitretin, etretin, or isoetretin.

It takes about 3 weeks before the effects of this drug are noticed.
You may not be able to wear contact lenses while taking this drug because
  it may cause dry eyes and other eye irritation. Eye irritation caused by the
  sun may be reduced by wearing sunglasses when outside.

ACYCLOVIR

Available since January 1985

COMMONLY USED TO TREAT

Viral infections, especially herpes and chickenpox

DRUG CATEGORY

antiviral
Class: synthetic purine nucleoside

PRODUCTS

Brand-Name Products with No Generic Alternative
Zovirax 5% topical ointment ($$$$)
Brand-Name Products with Generic Alternatives
Zovirax 200 mg capsule ($)
  Generic: acyclovir 200 mg capsule (¢¢¢)
Zovirax 400 mg tablet ($$$)
  Generic: acyclovir 400 mg tablet (¢¢¢)
Zovirax 800 mg tablet ($$$$)
  Generic: acyclovir 800 mg tablet (¢¢¢¢)
Zovirax 200 mg/5 ml oral suspension ($)
  Generic: acyclovir 200 mg/5 ml oral suspension ($)

DOSING AND FOOD

Doses are taken 3 to 5 times a day.
This drug may be taken with or without food.
Adults and children over age 12: Up to 800 mg per day in divided doses.
Lower doses are used in people with kidney disease.
Children under age 12: Up to 80 mg/kg per day in divided doses.
Forgotten doses: If you are scheduled to take the next dose within a few
  hours, do not take the forgotten dose. Otherwise take the forgotten dose
  as soon as you remember.

ALCOHOL, DRUG, HERB, AND SUPPLEMENT INTERACTIONS

Alcohol may increase some of the side effects from this drug, depending on the amount consumed. Ask your doctor about the risks caused by drinking alcohol with your condition.

Taking this drug with any of the ones listed below may change the effect of either drug with the possibility of causing toxicity or decreasing effectiveness: probenecid

Severe reactions are possible when this drug is taken with those listed below: methotrexate

Increased side effects are possible when this drug is taken with those listed below: acetaminophen, antibiotics†, aspirin, carmustine, cisplatin, cyclosporine, deferoxamine, gold salts†, lithium, nonsteroidal antiinflammatories†, penicillamine, plicamycin, streptozocin, tiopronin, zidovudine

ALLERGIC REACTIONS AND SIDE EFFECTS

You should tell your doctor about all your allergies and any unexplained symptoms you may have while taking this drug.

MORE COMMON SIDE EFFECTS: General discomfort

LESS COMMON SIDE EFFECTS: Abdominal pain*, diarrhea, headache, loss of appetite*, nausea*, thirst*, tiredness, urinary changes*, vomiting*, weakness*

RARE SIDE EFFECTS: Agitation*, black stools*, bleeding*, bloody urine*, bluish coloring*, blurry vision*, breathing difficulty*, bruising*, chills*, clumsiness*, confusion*, cough*, dizziness*, drowsiness*, eye irritation*, fainting*, fast heartbeat*, fever*, hair loss*, hallucinations*, hives*, irritability*, itching*, mood swings*, mouth sores*, muscle cramps*, pale skin*, seizures*, shakiness*, skin irritation*, skin rash*, sore throat*, swallowing difficulty*, swelling*, tingling, trembling*, unconsciousness*, unsteadiness*, vision changes*, weakness*, yellow eyes or skin*

PRECAUTIONS

People with kidney disease or dehydration are at greater risk of developing side effects when taking this drug.

If you have a nervous condition, this drug may make that condition worse.

PREGNANCY AND BREAST-FEEDING

Safety during pregnancy has not been established although the drug is known to harm animal fetuses.

This drug passes into breast milk, but does not appear to harm the baby.

Talk to your doctor about the risks associated with breast-feeding while taking this drug.

HELPFUL COMMENTS

If your symptoms do not improve after a few days of treatment, you may need to ask your doctor about a change in treatment.

Do not stop treatment early if you start to feel better. It takes the full prescription for this drug to work completely.

This drug does not prevent the spread of a viral disease to others. Avoid sexual intercourse during an active genital infection.

It is best to start this drug at the first sign of infection, such as tingling, itching, or pain.

ADEFOVIR DIPIVOXIL

Available since September 2002

COMMONLY USED TO TREAT

Hepatitis B infection

DRUG CATEGORY

antiviral
Class: nucleoside analogue

PRODUCTS

Brand-Name Products with No Generic Alternative
Hepsera 10 mg tablet (n/a)
No generics available.
Multiple patents that begin to expire in 2006. Exclusivity until 2007.

DOSING AND FOOD

Doses are taken once a day to once a week.
This drug may be taken with or without food.
Adults: Up to 10 mg per day.
Lower doses are used in people with kidney disease.

Forgotten doses: If you are scheduled to take the next dose within a few hours, do not take the forgotten dose. Otherwise take the forgotten dose as soon as you remember and adjust the time for the next scheduled dose based on the number of days between doses.

ALCOHOL, DRUG, HERB, AND SUPPLEMENT INTERACTIONS

Alcohol may increase some of the side effects from this drug, depending on the amount consumed. Ask your doctor about the risks caused by drinking alcohol with your condition.

This drug is still relatively new. Check with your pharmacist for a current update on drug interactions.

Increased side effects are possible when this drug is taken with those listed below: abacavir, didanosine, lamivudine, stavudine, tenofovir, zalcitabine, zidovudine

ALLERGIC REACTIONS AND SIDE EFFECTS

You should tell your doctor about all your allergies and any unexplained symptoms you may have while taking this drug.

MORE COMMON SIDE EFFECTS: Abdominal pain*, headache, weakness*

LESS COMMON SIDE EFFECTS: Diarrhea, gas, indigestion, nausea*

RARE SIDE EFFECTS: Breathing difficulty*, chills*, cough, dark urine*, dizziness*, irregular heartbeat*, itching, lightheadedness*, loss of appetite*, rash, pale stools*, sore throat, stuffy nose, tiredness*, vomiting, yellow eyes or skin*

PRECAUTIONS

Liver function and kidney function should be tested periodically while taking this drug.

Regular blood tests are needed for several months after you stop taking this drug to ensure that the hepatitis infection does not get worse.

If you have an HIV infection and are not taking drug therapy, this drug may make the HIV drugs less effective when needed.

People who are overweight are more likely to develop serious side effects while taking this drug.

This drug is only effective in suppressing hepatitis and cannot cure or prevent the spread of the disease.

People with a history of kidney disease may not be able to take this drug.

PREGNANCY AND BREAST-FEEDING

Safety during pregnancy has not been established although the drug is known to harm animal fetuses.

Breast-feeding while taking this drug is not recommended.

HELPFUL COMMENTS

Do not stop treatment early if you start to feel better. It takes the full prescription for this drug to work completely.

ALBENDAZOLE

Available since June 1996

COMMONLY USED TO TREAT

Tapeworm infections

DRUG CATEGORY

antihelminic
Class: benzimidazole

PRODUCTS

Brand-Name Products with No Generic Alternative
Albenza 200 mg tablet ($)
No generics available.
Exclusivity until 2003.

DOSING AND FOOD

Doses are taken 2 times a day.
Taking this drug with fatty foods will help increase absorption of the drug.
  Be careful not to eat too much fatty food.
Adults: Up to 800 mg per day in divided doses.
Children: Up to 15 mg/kg per day in divided doses.
Forgotten doses: If you are scheduled to take the next dose within a few
  hours, do not take the forgotten dose. Otherwise take the forgotten dose
  as soon as you remember.

ALCOHOL, DRUG, HERB, AND SUPPLEMENT INTERACTIONS

Alcohol may increase some of the side effects from this drug, depending
  on the amount consumed. Ask your doctor about the risks caused by
  drinking alcohol with your condition.

**Taking this drug with any of the ones listed below may change the effect of
either drug with the possibility of causing toxicity or decreasing effectiveness:**
cimetidine, corticosteroids†, praziquantel

ALLERGIC REACTIONS AND SIDE EFFECTS

You should tell your doctor about all your allergies and any unexplained
  symptoms you may have while taking this drug.
LESS COMMON SIDE EFFECTS: Abdominal pain, diarrhea, dizziness,
  headache, nausea, vomiting

---

†See page 52.   *See page 53.

RARE SIDE EFFECTS: Fever*, hair loss, itching*, skin rash*, sore throat*, tiredness*, weakness*

PRECAUTIONS

Do not crush, break, or chew the tablets.

This drug may cause harm to your liver and requires regular testing and follow up with the doctor. Call your doctor right away if you begin to feel poorly, lose your appetite, have stomach pains, or notice a yellowing of the skin or eyes.

PREGNANCY AND BREAST-FEEDING

Safety during pregnancy has not been established although the drug is known to harm animal fetuses.

It is not known if this drug passes into breast milk. Talk to your doctor about the risks associated with breast-feeding while taking this drug.

HELPFUL COMMENTS

Do not stop treatment early if you start to feel better. It takes the full prescription for this drug to work completely.

ALBUTEROL

Available since May 1982

COMMONLY USED TO TREAT

Breathing difficulty, specifically asthma

DRUG CATEGORY

bronchodilator
Class: adrenergic

PRODUCTS

Brand-Name Products with No Generic Alternative
Accuneb 0.021% inhalation solution ($$$)
Accuneb 0.042% inhalation solution ($$$)
Proventil HFA inhaler ($$$$)
Ventolin HFA inhaler ($$$$)

Brand-Name Products with Generic Alternatives
Proventil inhaler (¢¢¢¢¢)
Ventolin inhaler (¢¢¢¢¢)

Generic: albuterol inhaler (¢¢¢¢¢)
Proventil 0.083% inhalation solution ($$$)
  Generic: albuterol 0.083% inhalation solution ($$)
Proventil 0.5% inhalation solution ($$$$)
  Generic: albuterol 0.5% inhalation solution ($$)
Proventil 2 mg /5 ml oral syrup (n/a)
  Generic: albuterol 2 mg /5 ml oral syrup (¢)
Proventil 2 mg tablet (¢¢¢¢)
  Generic: albuterol 2 mg tablet (¢)
Proventil 4 mg tablet (¢¢¢¢¢)
  Generic: albuterol 4 mg tablet (¢)
Proventil 4 mg extended-release tablet ($)
Volmax 4 mg extended-release tablet ($)
  Generic: albuterol 4 mg extended-release tablet (¢¢¢¢¢)
Volmax 8 mg extended-release tablet ($$)
  Generic: albuterol 8 mg extended-release tablet ($$)

Combination Products That Contain This Drug
Combivent aerosol inhaler ($$)
Duoneb inhalation solution (¢¢)

DOSING AND FOOD

Doses are taken 2 to 4 times a day.
This drug may be taken with or without food.
Adults: Up to 32 mg per day in divided doses.
Lower doses are used in adults over age 65.
Children age 6 to 14: Up to 24 mg per day in divided doses.
Children under age 6: Up to 6 mg per day in divided doses.
Forgotten doses: If you are scheduled to take the next dose within a few
  hours, do not take the forgotten dose. Otherwise take the forgotten dose
  as soon as you remember.

ALCOHOL, DRUG, HERB, AND SUPPLEMENT INTERACTIONS

Alcohol may increase some of the side effects from this drug, depending
  on the amount consumed. Ask your doctor about the risks caused by
  drinking alcohol with your condition.
Many OTC drugs used for appetite control, asthma, colds, cough, hay fever,
  pain, or sinus problems affect the central nervous system and may
  change the severity of side effects when taken with this drug. Check with
  your pharmacist for products to avoid.

---

† See page 52.   * See page 53.

Taking this drug with any of the ones listed below may change the effect of
either drug with the possibility of causing toxicity or decreasing effectiveness:
beta blockers†, monoamine oxidase inhibitors†, thyroid hormones†

Severe reactions are possible when this drug is taken with those listed below:
cocaine, digoxin, quinidine, sympathomimetics†, tricyclic antidepressants†

Increased side effects are possible when this drug is taken with those listed below:
amphetamines†

ALLERGIC REACTIONS AND SIDE EFFECTS

Allergies are rare but would have the following symptoms: Hoarseness,
large hivelike swellings on eyelids, face, genitals, hands or feet, lips,
throat, and tongue, sudden trouble in swallowing or breathing, tightness in throat.

Severe reactions reported in children have the following symptoms: Bleeding or crusting sores on lips, chest pain, chills, fever, general feeling of illness, muscle cramps or pain, nausea, painful eyes, painful sores, ulcers,
white spots in mouth or on lips, red or irritated eyes, skin rash, hives, sore
throat, vomiting.

MORE COMMON SIDE EFFECTS: Fast heartbeat*, headache, irregular heartbeat*, nervousness, tremor

LESS COMMON SIDE EFFECTS: Dizziness, shortness of breath*, sleeping difficulty, sweating,

RARE SIDE EFFECTS: Chest pain*, hives*, mental problems*, muscle
cramps*, muscle pain*, nausea*, seizures*, tiredness*, urinary trouble*,
vomiting*, weakness*

PRECAUTIONS

People with cardiovascular disease, high blood pressure, hyperthyroidism
or diabetes may not be able to take this drug.

Do not crush or break the extended-release tablets.

If you have a history of seizures, you may be at greater risk of developing a
seizure while taking this drug.

You need to wait 2 weeks after stopping a monoamine oxidase inhibitor†
before starting this drug.

If you are diabetic, you may need a change in the dose of your antidiabetic drug† or insulin, since this drug may cause changes in blood sugar.

PREGNANCY AND BREAST-FEEDING

Safety during pregnancy has not been established although the drug is
known to harm animal fetuses.

Breast-feeding while taking this drug is not recommended.

HELPFUL COMMENTS

If using more than one type of inhaler, you should wait about 15 minutes between drugs.

Children may get excited and nervous when given this drug.

ALENDRONATE SODIUM

Available since September 1995

COMMONLY USED TO TREAT

Bone disease, specifically Paget's disease
Bone loss, also known as osteoporosis

DRUG CATEGORY

antiosteoporotic
Class: osteoclast-mediated bone resorption inhibitor

PRODUCTS

Brand-Name Products with No Generic Alternative
Fosamax 5 mg tablet ($$)
Fosamax 10 mg tablet ($$)
Fosamax 35 mg tablet ($$$$$)
Fosamax 40 mg tablet ($$$$)
Fosamax 70 mg tablet ($$$$$)
No generics available.
Multiple patents that begin to expire in 2007.

DOSING AND FOOD

Doses are taken once a day to once a week.
This drug must be taken on an empty stomach, at least 30 minutes before eating breakfast.
Do not take this drug with any beverage except plain water.
Adults: Up to 40 mg per day.
This drug is not used in children.
Forgotten doses: Do not take a forgotten dose. Go back to your usual schedule with the next dose.

ALCOHOL, DRUG, HERB, AND SUPPLEMENT INTERACTIONS

Alcohol may increase some of the side effects from this drug, depending on the amount consumed. Ask your doctor about the risks caused by drinking alcohol with your condition.

Severe reactions are possible when this drug is taken with those listed below: aspirin, nonsteroidal antiinflammatories†

ALLERGIC REACTIONS AND SIDE EFFECTS

You should tell your doctor about all your allergies and any unexplained symptoms you may have while taking this drug.

MORE COMMON SIDE EFFECTS: Abdominal pain*

LESS COMMON SIDE EFFECTS: Bloating, constipation, diarrhea, gas, headache, heartburn*, muscle pain*, nausea, swallowing difficulty*

RARE SIDE EFFECTS: Skin rash*

PRECAUTIONS

People with digestion problems, esophagus problems, intestinal problems, kidney problems, or stomach problems may not be able to take this drug.

Do not lie down for 30 minutes after taking this drug.

Vitamin D deficiency or low calcium levels should be corrected before starting this drug.

PREGNANCY AND BREAST-FEEDING

Safety during pregnancy has not been established although the drug is known to harm animal fetuses.

Breast-feeding while taking this drug is not recommended.

HELPFUL COMMENTS

Wait at least 30 minutes after taking this drug before taking any other drug or supplement.

There is no evidence that hormone replacement therapy is effective when given with this drug.

ALLOPURINOL

Available for over 20 years

COMMONLY USED TO TREAT

Gout
High uric acid level
Kidney stones

DRUG CATEGORY

antigout
antihyperuricemic
Class: xanthine oxidase inhibitor

PRODUCTS

Brand-Name Products with Generic Alternatives
Zyloprim 100 mg tablet (¢¢¢)
  Generic: allopurinol 100 mg tablet (¢)
Zyloprim 300 mg tablet (¢¢¢¢¢)
  Generic: allopurinol 300 mg tablet (¢¢)

DOSING AND FOOD

Doses are taken 1 to 3 times a day.
It is best to take this drug on an empty stomach, but taking this drug with
  a little food may avoid the stomach upset that some people suffer.
Adults: Up to 800 mg per day in divided doses.
Children age 6 to 10: Up to 300 mg per day in divided doses.
Children under age 6: Up to 150 mg per day in divided doses.
Lower doses are used in people with kidney disease.
Forgotten doses: If you are scheduled to take the next dose within a few
  hours, do not take the forgotten dose. Otherwise take the forgotten dose
  as soon as you remember.

ALCOHOL, DRUG, HERB, AND SUPPLEMENT INTERACTIONS

Alcohol may decrease the effects of this drug.

Taking this drug with any of the ones listed below may change the effect of
either drug with the possibility of causing toxicity or decreasing effectiveness:
aminophylline, anticoagulants†, azathioprine, chlorpropamide, mercaptopurine, theophylline

---

† See page 52.   * See page 53.

Severe reactions are possible when this drug is taken with those listed below:
co-trimoxazole, cyclophosphamide, thiazide diuretics†

Increased side effects are possible when this drug is taken with those listed below:
amoxicillin, ampicillin

ALLERGIC REACTIONS AND SIDE EFFECTS

This drug should be discontinued immediately if you develop any unexplained skin rash or other signs of allergy. Call your doctor for instructions.

MORE COMMON SIDE EFFECTS: Hives*, itching*, skin rash*

LESS COMMON SIDE EFFECTS: Diarrhea, drowsiness, hair loss, headache,
indigestion, nausea, vomiting*, stomach pain

RARE SIDE EFFECTS: Black stools*, bleeding*, bloody urine*, breathing
difficulty*, bruising*, chest tightness*, chills*, eye irritation*, fever*, lip
sores*, loose fingernails*, mouth sores*, muscle pains*, nausea*, nosebleeds*, numbness*, pain*, rapid weight gain*, shortness of breath*, sore
throat*, swelling*, tingling*, tiredness*, urinary changes*, weakness*,
wheezing*, yellow eyes or skin*

PRECAUTIONS

People with congestive heart disease, diabetes, high blood pressure, or
kidney disease are at greater risk of developing severe allergic reactions
and other serious side effects that may be dose related.

Be careful driving or handling equipment while taking this drug because
the drug may cause drowsiness.

PREGNANCY AND BREAST-FEEDING

Safety during pregnancy has not been established although the drug is
known to harm animal fetuses.

Breast-feeding while taking this drug is not recommended.

HELPFUL COMMENTS

Try to drink 10 to 12 glasses of water each day while taking this drug unless your doctor has advised otherwise.

Changes in your diet may help prevent stones from forming again.

ALMOTRIPTAN MALATE

Available since May 2001

COMMONLY USED TO TREAT

Migraine headache

DRUG CATEGORY

antimigraine
Class: triptan

PRODUCTS

Brand-Name Products with No Generic Alternative
Axert 6.25 mg tablet ($$$$$)
Axert 12.5 mg tablet ($$$$$)
No generics available.
Patent expires in 2013.

DOSING AND FOOD

Doses are taken 1 to 2 times a day.
This drug may be taken with or without food. Do not drink grapefruit juice
   while taking this drug.
Adults: Up to 25 mg per day in divided doses.
Lower doses are used in people with kidney or liver disease.
This drug is not used in children.
Forgotten doses: This drug is only used when you have a headache. Do
   not take more than 2 doses in 24 hours. Make sure the doses are at least
   2 hours apart.

ALCOHOL, DRUG, HERB, AND SUPPLEMENT INTERACTIONS

Alcohol may make your headache worse. Ask your doctor about the risks
   caused by drinking alcohol with your condition.
Cheese, chocolate, citrus fruits, caffeine, and alcohol are all known to trigger migraine headaches.
Taking this drug with any of the ones listed below may change the effect of
either drug with the possibility of causing toxicity or decreasing effectiveness:
ergotamines†

Severe reactions are possible when this drug is taken with those listed below:
serotonin agonists†, SSRIs†

---

†*See page 52.*   **See page 53.*

Increased side effects are possible when this drug is taken with those listed below:
amiodarone, chloroquine, cimetidine, clarithromycin, cyclosporine, danazol, delavirdine, diltiazem, erythromycin, fluconazole, fluoxetine, fluphenazine, fluvoxamine, haloperidol, indinavir, isoniazid, itraconazole, ketoconazole, metronidazole, miconazole, nefazodone, nelfinavir, nicardipine, nifedipine, norfloxacin, omeprazole, paroxetine, perphenazine, prednisone, propafenone, propoxyphene, quinidine, quinine, refabutin, ritonavir, saquinavir, sertraline, thioridazine, troleandomycin, verapamil, zafirlukast

ALLERGIC REACTIONS AND SIDE EFFECTS

You should tell your doctor about all your allergies and any unexplained symptoms you may have while taking this drug.

This drug promotes the effect of sunlight on the body and may cause severe sunburn and increased sensitivity of the eyes.

MORE COMMON SIDE EFFECTS: Burning, dizziness, dry mouth, headache, nausea, numbness, sleepiness, tingling

LESS COMMON SIDE EFFECTS: Anxiety, back pain, belching, chest pain*, chills, cough, eye irritation*, fast heartbeat*, fatigue, flushing, hearing changes, heartburn, indigestion, itching*, muscle aches, neck pain*, nosebleeds, numbness, painful menstruation, palpitations*, restlessness, shivering, shortness of breath*, skin rash*, sleeping difficulty*, sore throat, spinning feeling, stuffy nose, taste changes, tight throat*, trembling, vomiting, warmth, weakness

RARE SIDE EFFECTS: Abdominal pain*, altered sense of smell, black stools*, chest pressure*, clumsiness, cough, depression, diarrhea*, difficulty concentrating, drooling, dry eyes, dry throat, earache*, eye movements, eye pain*, fainting*, fever*, heartburn*, hoarseness, loss of appetite*, loss of voice, muscle stiffness, nervousness, nightmares, pale skin*, rapid breathing*, ringing in ears, sneezing, stabbing pain, swallowing difficulty*, sweating*, swelling, thirst, tingling, vision changes*, weight loss*

PRECAUTIONS

People with chest pain, heart disease, high blood pressure, kidney disease, liver disease, or a history of stroke are at greater risk of developing serious side effects from this drug.

If you have cataracts, this drug may make that condition worse.

You need to wait 2 weeks after stopping a monoamine oxidase inhibitor† before starting this drug.

People with obesity, diabetes, and other risk factors for coronary artery disease should be carefully monitored while on this drug.

This drug may cause dry mouth, which is associated with a greater risk of cavities. Your dentist may recommend that you clean your teeth and mouth differently to avoid infection.

PREGNANCY AND BREAST-FEEDING

Safety during pregnancy has not been established although the drug is known to harm animal fetuses.
Breast-feeding while taking this drug is not recommended.

HELPFUL COMMENTS

For faster relief, this drug should be taken at the first sign of the visual aura associated with a migraine.

ALOSETRON HYDROCHLORIDE

Available since February 2000

COMMONLY USED TO TREAT

Diarrhea, pain, and other symptoms caused by irritable bowel syndrome (IBS)

DRUG CATEGORY

antispasmodic
Class: selective 5-HT3 receptor antagonist

PRODUCTS

Brand-Name Products with No Generic Alternative
Lotronex 1 mg tablet (n/a)
No generics available.
Multiple patents that begin to expire in 2010. Exclusivity until 2005.

DOSING AND FOOD

Doses are taken 1 to 2 times a day.
This drug may be taken with or without food.
Women: Up to 2 mg per day in divided doses.
Forgotten doses: If you are scheduled to take the next dose within a few hours, do not take the forgotten dose. Otherwise take the forgotten dose as soon as you remember.

---

† See page 52.   * See page 53.

ALCOHOL, DRUG, HERB, AND SUPPLEMENT INTERACTIONS

Alcohol may increase some of the side effects from this drug, depending on the amount consumed. Ask your doctor about the risks caused by drinking alcohol with your condition.

There may be additional drug interactions that have not yet been identified since this drug is relatively new. Check with your pharmacist for the current list of drug interactions.

ALLERGIC REACTIONS AND SIDE EFFECTS

You should tell your doctor about all your allergies and any unexplained symptoms you may have while taking this drug.

LESS COMMON SIDE EFFECTS: Constipation*

RARE SIDE EFFECTS: Breathing difficulty*, abdominal pain*, behavior changes*, diarrhea*, fever*, poor coordination*, rectal bleeding*, seizures, trembling*

PRECAUTIONS

This drug was temporarily removed from the market because of serious and sometimes fatal side effects, but it is available since June 2002 under restricted conditions. Not all doctors can prescribe the drug and patients must sign an agreement before using it.

Constipation may be the first sign of a more serious side effect from this drug and should be reported to the doctor right away.

Since this drug is still relatively new, ask your pharmacist about any additional precautions each time you get your prescription refilled.

Women should only use this drug if they have not responded to other treatments.

This drug is not used in men since it is not as effective as in women.

People with a history of constipation, intestinal obstruction, coagulation disorders, Crohn's disease, ulcerative colitis, or diverticulitis may not be able to take this drug.

This drug may easily reach toxic levels in the body. Dosing must be very exact and regular blood tests are needed to assure safety.

PREGNANCY AND BREAST-FEEDING

Safety during pregnancy has not been established although there was no evidence of harm during studies in animals.

It is not known if this drug passes into breast milk. Talk to your doctor about the risks associated with breast-feeding while taking this drug.

HELPFUL COMMENTS

If you have taken this drug for 4 weeks and have not responded, it is not likely that you will see any additional benefit by staying on the drug longer.

The symptoms of IBD may return in 1 to 2 weeks after stopping this drug.

ALPRAZOLAM

Available for over 20 years

COMMONLY USED TO TREAT

Nervous and panic disorders

DRUG CATEGORY

antitremor
antipanic
anxiolytic
sedative-hypnotic
Class: benzodiazepine

PRODUCTS

Brand-Name Products with No Generic Alternative
Xanax XR 0.5 mg extended-release tablet (n/a)
Xanax XR 1 mg extended-release tablet (n/a)
Xanax XR 2 mg extended-release tablet (n/a)
Xanax XR 3 mg extended-release tablet (n/a)
No generic extended-release products available.
Exclusivity until 2006.

Brand-Name Products with Generic Alternatives
Xanax 0.25 mg tablet ($)
  Generic: alprazolam 0.25 mg tablet (¢)
Xanax 0.5 mg tablet ($)
  Generic: alprazolam 0.5 mg tablet (¢)
Xanax 1 mg tablet ($$)
  Generic: alprazolam 1 mg tablet (¢)
Xanax 2 mg tablet ($$)
  Generic: alprazolam 2 mg tablet (¢¢)

Products Only Available as Generics
alprazolam intensol 1 mg/ml oral concentrate ($$$$)

---

† *See page 52.*   * *See page 53.*

DOSING AND FOOD

Doses are taken 1 to 3 times a day.

This drug may be taken with or without food.

Adults: Up to 4 mg per day in divided doses.

Lower doses are used in people over age 65 and in people with kidney or liver disease.

This drug is rarely used in children under age 18.

Forgotten doses: If you are scheduled to take the next dose within a few hours, do not take the forgotten dose. Otherwise take the forgotten dose as soon as you remember.

ALCOHOL, DRUG, HERB, AND SUPPLEMENT INTERACTIONS

Alcohol should not be used while taking this drug.

Catnip, kava, lady's slipper, lemon balm, passion flower, sassafras, skullcap, and valerian should not be used while taking this drug since they may cause an increased sedative effect.

Taking this drug with any of the ones listed below may change the effect of either drug with the possibility of causing toxicity or decreasing effectiveness: cimetidine, digoxin, disulfiram, fluvoxamine, haloperidol, itraconazole, ketoconazole, nefazodone, rifampin

Severe reactions are possible when this drug is taken with those listed below: antihistamines†, antidepressants†, anesthetics†, barbiturates†, monoamine oxidase inhibitors†, narcotics†, phenothiazines†

Increased side effects are possible when this drug is taken with those listed below: aminophylline, theophylline

ALLERGIC REACTIONS AND SIDE EFFECTS

You should tell your doctor about all your allergies and any unexplained symptoms you may have while taking this drug.

MORE COMMON SIDE EFFECTS: Clumsiness, dizziness, drowsiness, lightheadedness, slurry speech

LESS COMMON SIDE EFFECTS: Anxiety*, confusion*, constipation, depression*, diarrhea, difficulty urinating, dry mouth, headache, irregular heartbeat*, memory loss*, muscle spasm, nausea, sexual dysfunction, sleeping difficulty*, stomach cramps, thirst, trembling, vision changes, vomiting, watery mouth

RARE SIDE EFFECTS: Agitation*, behavior changes*, bleeding*, bruising*, chills*, delusions*, disorientation*, excitement*, eye movement*, fever*, hallucinations*, irritability*, low blood pressure*, mouth sores*, muscle weakness*, nervousness*, seizures*, skin irritation*, sleeping difficulty*, sore throat*, spastic movements*, tiredness*, weakness*, yellow eyes or skin*

PRECAUTIONS

This drug may be habit forming and will cause severe withdrawal symptoms if stopped abruptly. If you wish to stop taking this drug, ask your doctor for specific instructions.

Do not use kava while taking this drug since it may cause an increased risk of coma.

You need to wait 2 weeks after stopping a monoamine oxidase inhibitor† before starting this drug.

If you have asthma, bronchitis, difficulty swallowing , emphysema, glaucoma, hyperactivity, mental depression, mental illness, myasthenia gravis, porphyria, or sleep apnea, this drug may make those conditions worse.

Heavy smoking may cause this drug to be less effective.

Be careful driving or handling equipment while taking this drug because the drug may cause dizziness and drowsiness.

PREGNANCY AND BREAST-FEEDING

There is evidence that this drug may harm the fetus, but the drug may be necessary to the health of the mother.

Breast-feeding while taking this drug is not recommended.

HELPFUL COMMENTS

Dangling your legs over the side of the bed for a few minutes may help reduce dizziness when first waking up.

AMANTADINE HYDROCHLORIDE

Available for over 20 years

COMMONLY USED TO TREAT

The flu, also known as influenza A virus
Parkinson's disease

DRUG CATEGORY

antidyskinetic
antiviral

---

†See page 52.　　*See page 53.

Class: synthetic cyclic primary amine

PRODUCTS

Brand-Name Products with Generic Alternatives
Symmetrel 100 mg oral capsule ($)
  Generic: amantadine 100 mg oral capsule (¢¢¢)
Symmetrel 50 mg/5 ml oral syrup ($)
  Generic: amantadine 50 mg/5 ml oral syrup (¢¢¢¢)

DOSING AND FOOD

Doses are taken 1 to 2 times a day.
This drug may be taken with or without food but is best taken with food to reduce the stomach upset that some people suffer.

Adults and children over age 10: Up to 200 mg per day in divided doses.

Children age 1 to 9: Up to 8.8 mg/kg (maximum 150 mg) per day in divided doses.

Lower doses are used in people over age 65 and people with kidney disease.

Forgotten doses: If you are scheduled to take the next dose within a few hours, do not take the forgotten dose. Otherwise take the forgotten dose as soon as you remember.

ALCOHOL, DRUG, HERB, AND SUPPLEMENT INTERACTIONS

Alcohol should not be used while taking this drug. Lightheadedness, confusion, fainting, and low blood pressure may occur.

Using the supplement jimsonweed when taking this drug may increase the risk of side effects related to your heart.

Taking this drug with any of the ones listed below may change the effect of either drug with the possibility of causing toxicity or decreasing effectiveness: hydrochlorothiazide, quinine, quinidine, triamterene

Severe reactions are possible when this drug is taken with those listed below: CNS stimulants†

Increased side effects are possible when this drug is taken with those listed below: amphetamines†, antiasthmatic, anticholinergics†, antihistamines†, appetite suppressants, benztropine, caffeine, chlophedianol, cocaine, methylphenidate, nabilone, pemoline, trihexyphenidyl

ALLERGIC REACTIONS AND SIDE EFFECTS

You should tell your doctor about all your allergies and any unexplained symptoms you may have while taking this drug.

MORE COMMON SIDE EFFECTS: Agitation, anxiety, dizziness, headache, irritability, lightheadedness, loss of appetite, nausea, nervousness, nightmares, poor concentration, skin discoloration, sleeping difficulty

LESS COMMON SIDE EFFECTS: Blurry vision*, confusion*, constipation, diarrhea, drowsiness, dry mouth, fainting*, hallucinations*, headache, sexual dysfunction, swelling*, tiredness, urinary changes*, vomiting, weakness

RARE SIDE EFFECTS: Chills*, depression*, memory loss *, eye irritation*, eye swelling*, fever*, increased blood pressure*, lack of coordination*, mood swings*, muscle movement*, seizures*, shortness of breath*, skin rash*, slurry speech*, sore throat*, suicidal thoughts*, vision change*

PRECAUTIONS

This drug may increase the risk of seizures in people with epilepsy or other seizure disorders.

This drug may make heart disease or circulation problems worse.

If you are taking this drug for Parkinson's disease, do not stop taking the drug without talking to your doctor. The symptoms of the disease may get worse very quickly.

Be careful driving or handling equipment while taking this drug because it may cause dizziness and lightheadedness.

PREGNANCY AND BREAST-FEEDING

Safety during pregnancy has not been established although the drug is known to harm animal fetuses.

Breast-feeding while taking this drug is not recommended.

HELPFUL COMMENTS

If you get blotchy skin while taking this drug, it usually goes away in less than 3 months.

Avoid quick movements to minimize dizziness. Dangling your legs over the side of the bed for a few minutes may help reduce dizziness when first waking up.

If you notice a decrease in the effect of the drug after a few months, you may need a change in treatment.

---

† See page 52.　　 * See page 53.

AMILORIDE HYDROCHLORIDE

Available for over 20 years

COMMONLY USED TO TREAT

High blood pressure, also known as hypertension

DRUG CATEGORY

antihypertensive
antihypokalemic
Class: potassium-sparing diuretic

PRODUCTS

Brand-Name Products with Generic Alternatives
Midamor 5 mg tablet (¢¢¢¢)
   Generic: amiloride 5 mg tablet (¢¢¢)
Combination Products That Contain This Drug
Moduretic 5-50 tablet (¢¢¢¢)

DOSING AND FOOD

Doses are taken 1 to 2 times a day.
It is better to take this drug on an empty stomach, but taking this drug
   with food may avoid the stomach upset that some people suffer.
Adults: Up to 20 mg per day in divided doses.
Children: Up to 0.625 mg/kg per day in divided doses.
Forgotten doses: If you are scheduled to take the next dose within a few
   hours, do not take the forgotten dose. Otherwise take the forgotten dose
   as soon as you remember.

ALCOHOL, DRUG, HERB, AND SUPPLEMENT INTERACTIONS

Alcohol may increase some of the side effects from this drug, depending
   on the amount consumed. Talk to your doctor about the risks caused by
   drinking alcohol with your condition.
Licorice may interfere with the effects of this drug.

**Taking this drug with any of the ones listed below may change the effect of
either drug with the possibility of causing toxicity or decreasing effectiveness:**
antihypertensives[†], digoxin, lithium

Severe reactions are possible when this drug is taken with those listed below:
ACE inhibitors[†], cyclosporine, nonsteroidal antiinflammatories[†], potassium-containing drugs, potassium-sparing diuretics[†]

ALLERGIC REACTIONS AND SIDE EFFECTS

If you are allergic to spironolactone or triamterene, you may also be allergic to this drug. You should tell your doctor about all your allergies and any unexplained symptoms you may have while taking this drug.

LESS COMMON SIDE EFFECTS: Constipation, diarrhea, dizziness, headache, muscle cramps, nausea, sexual dysfunction, stomach cramps, vomiting

RARE SIDE EFFECTS: Itching*, shortness of breath*, skin rash*

PRECAUTIONS

This drug does not eliminate potassium from the body like other diuretics. Do not add extra potassium to your diet or use salt substitutes that contain potassium while taking this drug. Foods high in potassium include meat, fish, apricots, avocados, bananas, melons, kiwi, lima beans, milk, oranges, potatoes, prunes, spinach, tomatoes, and squash.

People with diabetes, kidney disease, or liver disease may have a greater risk of developing side effects while taking this drug.

Severe side effects may occur if you get dehydrated or have excess vomiting or diarrhea. Call your doctor before your symptoms get too bad.

PREGNANCY AND BREAST-FEEDING

Safety during pregnancy has not been established although there was no evidence of harm during studies in animals.

This drug passes into breast milk, but does not appear to harm the baby. Talk to your doctor about the risks associated with breast-feeding while taking this drug.

HELPFUL COMMENTS

Take the last dose of the day before 6 P.M. to reduce the chance of having to urinate during the night.

If you do not treat high blood pressure, you may develop more serious problems such as heart failure, blood vessel disease, stroke, or kidney disease. Losing weight, exercising, eating more fruits and vegetables, and avoiding salty foods, such as lunchmeat and pickles, may help make drug treatment more successful.

---

† *See page 52.*   * *See page 53.*

AMINOCAPROIC ACID

Available for over 20 years

COMMONLY USED TO TREAT

Excessive bleeding and hemorrhage

DRUG CATEGORY

hemostatic
Class: fibrinolysis inhibitor

PRODUCTS

Brand-Name Products with Generic Alternatives
Amicar 500 mg tablet ($$)
  Generic: aminocaproic acid 500 mg tablet ($$)
Amicar 1.25 mg/5 ml oral syrup ($$$$)
  Generic: aminocaproic acid 1.25 mg/5 ml oral syrup ($$$)

DOSING AND FOOD

Doses are taken 1 to 3 times a day.
This drug may be taken with or without food.
Adults: Up to 30 g per day in divided doses.
Children: Up to 18 g/m^2 per day in divided doses.
Forgotten doses: Take the forgotten dose as soon as you remember even if
  it is time for the next dose.

ALCOHOL, DRUG, HERB, AND SUPPLEMENT INTERACTIONS

Alcohol may increase some of the side effects from this drug, depending
  on the amount consumed. Ask your doctor about the risks caused by
  drinking alcohol with your condition.

**Taking this drug with any of the ones listed below may change the effect of
either drug with the possibility of causing toxicity or decreasing effectiveness:**
estrogens†

ALLERGIC REACTIONS AND SIDE EFFECTS

You should tell your doctor about all your allergies and any unexplained
  symptoms you may have while taking this drug.

LESS COMMON SIDE EFFECTS: Chest pain*, decreased urine*, dizziness*,
  headache*, lack of coordination*, muscle pain*, ringing in ears*, short-

ness of breath*, skin rash*, slurry speech*, stomach cramps*, stuffy nose*, swelling*, tiredness*, vision changes*, weakness*, weight gain*

PRECAUTIONS

The side effects from this drug may be increased if you have a history of blood clots, blood in the urine, color blindness, heart disease, kidney disease or liver disease.

Blood tests are routinely needed when taking this drug for a long time.

PREGNANCY AND BREAST-FEEDING

Safety during pregnancy has not been established although the drug is known to harm animal fetuses.

This drug may pass into breast milk, but does not appear to harm the baby. Talk to your doctor about the risks associated with breast-feeding while taking this drug.

HELPFUL COMMENTS

Avoid quick movements to minimize dizziness. Dangling your legs over the side of the bed for a few minutes may help reduce dizziness when first waking up.

AMINOPHYLLINE

Available for over 20 years

COMMONLY USED TO TREAT

Breathing difficulty

DRUG CATEGORY

bronchodilator
respiratory stimulant
Class: xanthine derivative

PRODUCTS

Brand-Name Products with No Generic Alternative
Truphylline 250 mg rectal suppository (n/a)
Truphylline 500 mg rectal suppository (n/a)

Products Only Available as Generics
aminophylline 100 mg tablet (¢)
aminophylline 200 mg tablet (¢)

† See page 52.   * See page 53.

aminophylline 105 mg/5 ml oral solution (¢¢)
aminophylline dye free 105 mg/5 ml oral solution (¢¢¢)

DOSING AND FOOD

Doses are taken 2 to 4 times a day.

This drug may be taken with or without food but is best taken with food to
   reduce the stomach upset that some people suffer.

Adults and children over age 16: Up to 13 mg/kg daily in divided doses.

Children age 12 to 16: Up to 18 mg/kg per day in divided doses.

Children age 9 to 12: Up to 20 mg/kg per day in divided doses.

Children age 1 to 9: Up to 24 mg/kg per day in divided doses.

Higher doses may be needed in people who smoke.

Lower doses are used in people with heart failure and liver disease.

Forgotten doses: If you are scheduled to take the next dose within a few
   hours, do not take the forgotten dose. Otherwise take the forgotten dose
   as soon as you remember.

ALCOHOL, DRUG, HERB, AND SUPPLEMENT INTERACTIONS

Alcohol may increase some of the side effects from this drug, depending
   on the amount consumed. Ask your doctor about the risks caused by
   drinking alcohol with your condition.

Many OTC drugs used for appetite control, asthma, colds, cough, hay
   fever, pain, or sinus problems affect the central nervous system and may
   interfere with this drug. Check with your pharmacist for products to
   avoid.

**Taking this drug with any of the ones listed below may change the effect of
either drug with the possibility of causing toxicity or decreasing effectiveness.**
allopurinol, aminoglutethimide, carbamazepine, cimetidine, erythromycin,
   lithium, moricizine, phenobarbital, phenytoin, propranolol, quinolones†,
   rifampin, troleandomycin

Increased side effects are possible when this drug is taken with those listed below:
ciprofloxacin, clarithromycin, enoxacin, fluvoxamine, mexiletine, pentoxifylline, propranolol, tacrine, thiabendazole, ticlopidine

ALLERGIC REACTIONS AND SIDE EFFECTS

You should tell your doctor about all your allergies and any unexplained
   symptoms you may have while taking this drug.

LESS COMMON SIDE EFFECTS: Fast heartbeat, headache, heartburn*, increased
   urination, nausea, nervousness, sleeping difficulty, trembling, vomiting*

RARE SIDE EFFECTS: Hives*, skin rash*, sloughing of skin*

PRECAUTIONS

Large quantities of chocolate, coffee, tea, and other caffeinated food or
  drink may trigger a toxic reaction from this drug.
Seizures and irregular heartbeat may be the first signs of toxicity. Call your
  doctor right away if these occur.

PREGNANCY AND BREAST-FEEDING

Safety during pregnancy has not been established although the drug is
  known to harm animal fetuses.
This drug passes into breast milk and may cause irritability, insomnia, and
  agitation in the baby.

HELPFUL COMMENTS

Tobacco and marijuana decrease the effectiveness of this drug. Do not
  change your smoking pattern while taking this drug without telling your
  doctor first.
If using a suppository, remove the foil and run under cold water before
  inserting.

AMIODARONE HYDROCHLORIDE

Available since August 1995

COMMONLY USED TO TREAT

Irregular heart rhythm

DRUG CATEGORY

antiarrhythmic
Class: benzofuran derivative

PRODUCTS

Brand-Name Products with Generic Alternatives
Cordarone 200 mg tablet ($$$)
  Generic: amiodarone 200 mg tablet ($$$)

Products Only Available as Generics
amiodarone 400 mg tablet ($$$)

Other Generic Product Names
Pacerone

---

† See page 52.   * See page 53.

DOSING AND FOOD

Doses are taken 1 to 3 times a day.

Take this drug with food to improve absorption.

Adults: Up to 600 mg per day in divided doses.

Children: Up to 2.5 mg/kg per day in divided doses.

Higher doses are used for the first few weeks.

Forgotten doses: If you are scheduled to take the next dose within a few hours, do not take the forgotten dose. Otherwise take the forgotten dose as soon as you remember.

ALCOHOL, DRUG, HERB, AND SUPPLEMENT INTERACTIONS

Alcohol may increase some of the side effects from this drug, depending on the amount consumed. Ask your doctor about the risks caused by drinking alcohol with your condition.

Do not use pennyroyal while taking this drug since it may lead to toxicity.

Taking this drug with any of the ones listed below may change the effect of either drug with the possibility of causing toxicity or decreasing effectiveness: cholestyramine, cyclosporine, digoxin, flecainide, lidocaine, phenytoin, procainamide, theophylline

Severe reactions are possible when this drug is taken with those listed below: amprenavir, anesthetics†, beta blockers†, calcium channel blockers†, disopyramide, phenothiazines†, pimozide, quinidine, ritonavir, sparfloxacin, tricyclic antidepressants†, warfarin

ALLERGIC REACTIONS AND SIDE EFFECTS

You should tell your doctor about all your allergies and any unexplained symptoms you may have while taking this drug.

This drug promotes the effect of sunlight on the body and may cause severe sunburn and increased sensitivity of the eyes.

MORE COMMON SIDE EFFECTS: Constipation, cough*, dizziness*, fainting*, fever*, headache, lightheadedness*, loss of appetite, nausea, numbness*, painful breathing*, shaky hands*, shortness of breath*, trembling*, trouble walking*, vomiting, weakness*

LESS COMMON SIDE EFFECTS: Blurry vision*, coldness*, dizziness, dry eyes*, facial flushing, irregular heartbeat*, metallic taste, nervousness*, scrotum pain*, sensitivity to heat*, sexual dysfunction, skin discoloration*, sleeping difficulty*, spastic movements*, sweating*, swelling*, tiredness*, weight change*

RARE SIDE EFFECTS: Skin rash*, yellow eyes or skin*

PRECAUTIONS

This drug may cause changes in thyroid function.

Do not use this drug if you are taking ritonavir.

This drug may cause severe side effects related to the lung, liver, and eye. Regular monitoring and testing is needed about every 6 months.

PREGNANCY AND BREAST-FEEDING

There is evidence that this drug may harm the fetus, but the drug may be necessary to the health of the mother.

Breast-feeding while taking this drug is not recommended.

HELPFUL COMMENTS

If your skin has changed color from being on this drug, it will take several months to return to the normal color after the drug is stopped.

Frequent use of lubricating eyedrops may reduce the possibility of visual disturbances.

AMITRIPTYLINE HYDROCHLORIDE

Available for over 20 years

COMMONLY USED TO TREAT

Depression
Bed-wetting
Anorexia and bulimia
Nerve pain

DRUG CATEGORY

antibulimic
antidepressant
antienuretic
antineuralgic
Class: tricyclic antidepressant

PRODUCTS

Brand-Name Products with No Generic Alternative
Endep 40 mg/ml oral concentrate (n/a)

Brand-Name Products with Generic Alternatives
Elavil 10 mg tablet (¢¢)
  Generic: amitriptyline hydrochloride 10 mg tablet (¢)

---

† See page 52.   * See page 53.

Elavil 25 mg tablet (¢¢)
　Generic: amitriptyline hydrochloride 25 mg tablet (¢)
Elavil 50 mg tablet (¢¢¢¢)
　Generic: amitriptyline hydrochloride 50 mg tablet (¢)
Elavil 75 mg tablet ($)
　Generic: amitriptyline hydrochloride 75 mg tablet (¢)
Elavil 100 mg tablet ($$)
　Generic: amitriptyline hydrochloride 100 mg tablet (¢)

Products Only Available as Generics
amitriptyline hydrochloride 150 mg tablet (¢¢)

Other Generic Product Names
Vanatrip

Combination Products That Contain This Drug
Limbitrol tablet ($)
Limbitrol DS tablet ($$)

DOSING AND FOOD

Doses are taken 1 to 4 times a day. Once daily doses are taken at bedtime.
Taking this drug with food or milk may avoid the stomach upset that some
　people suffer.

Adults: Up to 150 mg per day in divided doses.

Lower doses are used in teenagers and people over age 65.

This drug is not recommended for use in children under age 12.

Forgotten doses: If you have forgotten a bedtime dose, do not take the
　forgotten dose. Just go back to your usual schedule with the next dose. If
　you have forgotten a daytime dose and are scheduled to take the next
　dose within a few hours, do not take the forgotten dose. Otherwise take
　the forgotten dose as soon as you remember.

ALCOHOL, DRUG, HERB, AND SUPPLEMENT INTERACTIONS

Alcohol should not be used while taking this drug.

Evening primrose oil, SAMe, St. John's wort, and yohimbe may cause seri-
　ous reactions when taken with this drug. Tell your doctor if you are taking
　any of these supplements.

Several OTC drugs used for asthma, colds, cough, hay fever, sleep aid, or
　sinus problems may seriously change the effects of this drug. Check with
　your pharmacist when selecting OTC products.

**The effect of this drug or the ones listed below may be changed with either
drug with the possibility of causing toxicity or decreasing effectiveness:**
anesthetics, antipsychotics†, anxiolytics†, barbiturates†, beta blockers†,

cimetidine, clonidine, fluoxetine, guanabenz, guanadrel, guanethidine, haloperidol, methyldopa, methylphenidate, narcotics†, oral contraceptives, phenothiazines†, propoxyphene, reserpine

Severe reactions are possible when this drug is taken with those listed below: amphetamines†, anticholinergics†, antidyskinetics†, antihistamines†, antithyroid drugs†, anxiolytics†, appetite suppressants, barbiturates†, disopyramide, disulfiram, ephedrine, epinephrine, ethchlorvynol, isoproterenol, meperidine, metrizamide, monoamine oxidase inhibitors†, narcotics†, phenylephrine, pimozide, procainamide, quinidine, warfarin

Increased side effects are possible when this drug is taken with those listed below: alseroxylon, deserpidine, metoclopramide, metyrosine, pemoline, promethazine, rauwolfia serpentine, reserpine, trimeprazine

ALLERGIC REACTIONS AND SIDE EFFECTS

You should tell your doctor about all your allergies and any unexplained symptoms you may have while taking this drug.

This drug promotes the effect of sunlight on the body and may cause severe sunburn and increased sensitivity of the eyes.

MORE COMMON SIDE EFFECTS: Blurry vision*, dizziness, drowsiness, dry mouth, headache, increased appetite, irregular heartbeat*, seizures*, sweating, taste changes, tiredness, weakness*, weight gain

LESS COMMON SIDE EFFECTS: Confusion*, constipation*, diarrhea, expressionless face*, eye pain*, fainting*, hallucinations*, heartburn, loss of balance*, nausea, nervousness*, restlessness*, shakiness*, shuffling walk*, sleeping difficulty, stiffness*, swallowing difficulty*, trembling*, urinary difficulty*, vomiting

RARE SIDE EFFECTS: Anxiety*, breast enlargement*, fever*, hair loss, irritability*, muscle twitching*, ringing in ears*, skin rash*, sore throat*, swelling*, teeth or gum problems*, yellow eyes or skin*

PRECAUTIONS

If you have a history of asthma, blood disorders, seizures, enlarged prostates, glaucoma, heart disease, high blood pressure, urinary difficulty, schizophrenia, or manic depression, this drug may make those conditions worse.

You need to wait 2 weeks after stopping a monoamine oxidase inhibitor† before starting this drug.

Be careful driving or handling equipment while taking this drug because it may cause drowsiness and dizziness.

---

† See page 52.　　* See page 53.

Stopping this drug abruptly may result in withdrawal symptoms that include nausea, headache, and general discomfort.

This drug may cause dry mouth, which is associated with a greater risk of cavities and other dental problems. Your dentist may recommend that you clean your teeth and mouth differently to avoid infection.

PREGNANCY AND BREAST-FEEDING

Safety during pregnancy has not been established although the drug is known to harm animal fetuses. There have been reports of babies suffering from muscle spasms, heart problems, breathing difficulty, and urinary problems when the mother was taking this drug.

Breast-feeding while taking this drug is not recommended.

HELPFUL COMMENTS

Heavy smoking may decrease the effectiveness of this drug.

It may take 4 weeks for the full effect of this drug to be noticed.

Taking your bedtime dose in the early evening may avoid a hangover feeling in the morning.

Sucking on hard sugarless candy or chewing sugarless gum may help relieve dry mouth caused by this drug.

AMLODIPINE BESYLATE

Available since July 1992

COMMONLY USED TO TREAT

Chest pain, also known as angina

High blood pressure, also known as hypertension

DRUG CATEGORY

antianginal

antihypertensive

Class: calcium channel blocker

PRODUCTS

Brand-Name Products with No Generic Alternative

Norvasc 2.5 mg tablet ($)

Norvasc 5 mg tablet ($)

Norvasc 10 mg tablet ($$)

No generics available.

Multiple patents that begin to expire in 2006.

Combination Products That Contain This Drug

Lotrel 2.5-10 capsule ($$)

Lotrel 5-10 capsule ($$)

Lotrel 5-12 capsule ($$)

DOSING AND FOOD

Doses are taken once a day.

This drug may be taken with or without food.

Adults: Up to 10 mg per day.

Lower doses are used in people over 65, people with liver disease, or people taking other antihypertensive drugs.

This drug is rarely used in children.

Forgotten doses: If you are scheduled to take the next dose within a few hours, do not take the forgotten dose. Otherwise take the forgotten dose as soon as you remember.

ALCOHOL, DRUG, HERB, AND SUPPLEMENT INTERACTIONS

Alcohol may increase some of the side effects from this drug, depending on the amount consumed. Ask your doctor about the risks caused by drinking alcohol with your condition.

Several OTC drugs used for appetite control, asthma, colds, cough, hay fever, or sinus problems may cause an increase in blood pressure when taken with this drug. Check with your pharmacist when selecting OTC products.

Taking this drug with any of the ones listed below may change the effect of either drug with the possibility of causing toxicity or decreasing effectiveness: carbamazepine, cyclosporine, digoxin, procainamide, quinidine, rifampin

Severe reactions are possible when this drug is taken with those listed below: beta blockers†

ALLERGIC REACTIONS AND SIDE EFFECTS

You should tell your doctor about all your allergies and any unexplained symptoms you may have while taking this drug.

MORE COMMON SIDE EFFECTS: Headache, fluid retention, swelling*

LESS COMMON SIDE EFFECTS: Breathing difficulty*, constipation, cough*, diarrhea, dizziness, dry mouth, flushing, irregular heartbeat*, nausea, skin rash*, shortness of breath*, tiredness, weakness, wheezing*

RARE SIDE EFFECTS: Chest pain*, fainting*, tender gums*

---

†See page 52.   * See page 53.

PRECAUTIONS

Learn how to measure your heart rate and call your doctor if it falls below 60 beats per minute.

People with heart failure or liver disease may not be able to use this drug.

This drug may cause dry mouth, which is associated with a greater risk of cavities and other dental problems. Your dentist may recommend that you clean your teeth and mouth differently to avoid infection.

PREGNANCY AND BREAST-FEEDING

Safety during pregnancy has not been established although the drug is known to harm animal fetuses.

Breast-feeding while taking this drug is not recommended.

HELPFUL COMMENTS

Sucking on hard sugarless candy or chewing sugarless gum may help relieve dry mouth caused by this drug.

It takes 7 to 14 days before the full effects of this drug are noticed.

If you do not treat high blood pressure, you may develop more serious problems such as heart failure, blood vessel disease, stroke, or kidney disease. Losing weight, exercising, eating more fruits and vegetables, and avoiding salty foods, such as lunchmeat and pickles, may help make drug treatment more successful.

AMOXAPINE

Available since May 1989

COMMONLY USED TO TREAT

Depression

DRUG CATEGORY

antidepressant
Class: tricyclic antidepressant

PRODUCTS

Products Only Available as Generics
amoxapine 25 mg tablet (¢¢¢¢)
amoxapine 50 mg tablet (¢¢¢¢¢)
amoxapine 100 mg tablet ($$)
amoxapine 150 mg tablet ($$$)

DOSING AND FOOD

Doses are taken 1 to 3 times a day.

Taking this drug with food or milk may avoid the stomach upset that some people suffer.

Adults: Up to 400 mg per day in divided doses.

Lower doses are used in people over age 65.

This drug is not recommended for use in children under age 16.

Forgotten doses: If you are scheduled to take the next dose within a few hours, do not take the forgotten dose. Otherwise take the forgotten dose as soon as you remember.

ALCOHOL, DRUG, HERB, AND SUPPLEMENT INTERACTIONS

Alcohol should not be used while taking this drug.

Evening primrose oil, SAMe, St. John's wort, and yohimbe may cause serious reactions when taken with this drug. Tell your doctor if you are taking any of these supplements.

Several OTC drugs used for asthma, colds, cough, hay fever, sleep aid, or sinus problems may seriously change the effects of this drug. Check with your pharmacist when selecting OTC products.

The effect of this drug or the ones listed below may be changed with either drug with the possibility of causing toxicity or decreasing effectiveness:
antipsychotics†, anxiolytics†, beta blockers†, cimetidine, clonidine, fluoxetine, guanabenz, guanadrel, guanethidine, haloperidol, methyldopa, methylphenidate, narcotics†, oral contraceptives, phenothiazines†, propoxyphene, reserpine

Severe reactions are possible when this drug is taken with those listed below:
amphetamines†, anesthetics, anticholinergics†, antidyskinetics†, antihistamines†, antithyroid drugs†, appetite suppressants, barbiturates†, disopyramide, disulfiram, ephedrine, epinephrine, ethchlorvynol, isoproterenol, meperidine, metrizamide, monoamine oxidase inhibitors†, narcotics†, phenylephrine, pimozide, procainamide, quinidine, warfarin

Increased side effects are possible when this drug is taken with those listed below:
alseroxylon, deserpidine, metoclopramide, metyrosine, pemoline, pimozide, promethazine, rauwolfia serpentine, reserpine, trimeprazine

ALLERGIC REACTIONS AND SIDE EFFECTS

You should tell your doctor about all your allergies and any unexplained symptoms you may have while taking this drug.

This drug promotes the effect of sunlight on the body and may cause severe sunburn and increased sensitivity of the eyes.

---

† See page 52.   * See page 53.

MORE COMMON SIDE EFFECTS: Blurry vision*, constipation*, dizziness, drowsiness, dry mouth, headache, increased appetite, irregular heartbeat*, nausea, seizures*, sweating, sexual dysfunction, taste changes, tiredness, urinary changes*, weakness*, weight gain

LESS COMMON SIDE EFFECTS: Chewing motion, confusion*, diarrhea, expressionless face*, eye pain*, fainting*, hallucinations*, heartburn, lip smacking, loss of balance*, nervousness*, puffy cheeks, restlessness*, shakiness*, shuffling walk*, sleeping difficulty, stiffness*, swallowing difficulty*, tongue movements, trembling*, vomiting

RARE SIDE EFFECTS: Anxiety*, breast enlargement*, hair loss, irritability*, muscle twitching*, ringing in ears*, skin rash*, sore throat*, fever*, swelling*, teeth or gum problems*, yellow eyes or skin*

PRECAUTIONS

You need to wait 2 weeks after stopping a monoamine oxidase inhibitor† before starting this drug.

Stopping this drug abruptly may result in withdrawal symptoms that include nausea, headache, and general discomfort.

If you have a history of asthma, blood disorders, seizures, enlarged prostate, glaucoma, heart disease, high blood pressure, urinary difficulty, schizophrenia or manic depression, this drug may make those conditions worse.

Be careful driving or handling equipment while taking this drug because it may cause drowsiness and dizziness.

This drug may cause dry mouth, which is associated with a greater risk of cavities. Your dentist may recommend that you clean your teeth and mouth differently to avoid infection.

PREGNANCY AND BREAST-FEEDING

Safety during pregnancy has not been established although the drug is known to harm animal fetuses.

Breast-feeding while taking this drug is not recommended.

HELPFUL COMMENTS

Heavy smoking may decrease the effectiveness of this drug.

It may take 2 weeks for the effect of this drug to be noticed and up to 6 weeks before the full effects are seen.

Sucking on hard sugarless candy or chewing sugarless gum may help relieve dry mouth caused by this drug.

AMOXICILLIN

Available for over 20 years

COMMONLY USED TO TREAT

Infection

DRUG CATEGORY

antibiotic
Class: aminopenicillin

PRODUCTS

Brand-Name Products with Generic Alternatives
Amoxil 125 mg chewable tablet (¢¢)
  Generic: amoxicillin 125 mg chewable tablet (¢¢)
Amoxil 200 mg chewable tablet (¢¢¢¢)
  Generic: amoxicillin 200 mg chewable tablet (¢¢¢)
Amoxil 250 mg chewable tablet (¢¢¢)
  Generic: amoxicillin 250 mg chewable tablet (¢¢)
Amoxil 400 mg chewable tablet (¢¢¢¢)
  Generic: amoxicillin 400 mg chewable tablet (¢¢¢¢)
Amoxil 250 mg capsule (¢¢)
  Generic: amoxicillin 250 mg capsule (¢)
Amoxil 500 mg capsule (¢¢¢)
  Generic: amoxicillin 500 mg capsule (¢¢)
Amoxil 500 mg tablet (¢¢¢¢)
  Generic: amoxicillin 500 mg tablet (¢¢¢)
Amoxil 875 mg tablet (¢¢¢¢¢)
  Generic: amoxicillin 875 mg tablet (¢¢¢¢¢)
Amoxil 50 mg/5 ml oral suspension (¢¢¢¢)
  Generic: amoxicillin 50 mg/5 ml oral suspension (¢¢¢¢)
Amoxil 125 mg/5 ml oral suspension (¢¢)
  Generic: amoxicillin 125 mg/5 ml oral suspension (¢¢)
Amoxil 200 mg/5 ml oral suspension (¢¢)
  Generic: amoxicillin 200 mg/5 ml oral suspension (¢¢¢)
Amoxil 250 mg/5 ml oral suspension (¢¢¢)
  Generic: amoxicillin 250 mg/5 ml oral suspension (¢)
Amoxil 400 mg/5 ml oral suspension (¢¢¢¢)
  Generic: amoxicillin 400 mg/5 ml oral suspension (¢¢¢¢)

---

†See page 52.   *See page 53.

Other Generic Product Names
Amoxicot, Larotid, Moxilin, Trimox, Wymox

Combination Products That Contain This Drug
Prevpac extended-release capsule ($$$$$)
Augmentin (wide variety)

DOSING AND FOOD

Doses are taken 3 times a day.

Taking this drug with food may avoid the stomach upset that some people suffer.

Adults: Up to 3 g per day in divided doses.

Children age 6 to 9: Up to 80 mg/kg per day in divided doses.

Children under age 6: Up to 50 mg/kg per day in divided doses.

Neonates and children up to 12 weeks: Up to 30 mg/kg per day in divided doses.

Lower doses may be used in people with kidney disease.

Forgotten doses: If you are scheduled to take the next dose within a few hours, do not take the forgotten dose. Otherwise take the forgotten dose as soon as you remember.

ALCOHOL, DRUG, HERB, AND SUPPLEMENT INTERACTIONS

Alcohol may increase some of the side effects from this drug, depending on the amount consumed. Ask your doctor about the risks caused by drinking alcohol with your condition.

Taking this drug with any of the ones listed below may change the effect of either drug with the possibility of causing toxicity or decreasing effectiveness: chloramphenicol, clavulanate, erythromycins†, methotrexate, oral contraceptives, probenecid, sulfonamides†, tetracyclines†

Severe reactions are possible when this drug is taken with those listed below: allopurinol

ALLERGIC REACTIONS AND SIDE EFFECTS

If you are allergic to any penicillins† or cephalosporins†, you may also be allergic to this drug. You should tell your doctor about all your allergies and any unexplained symptoms you may have while taking this drug.

MORE COMMON SIDE EFFECTS: Diarrhea*, headache, mouth sores*, vaginal discharge, vaginal itching

LESS COMMON SIDE EFFECTS: Fainting*, fever*, hives*, irregular breathing*, itching*, joint pain*, lightheadedness*, scaly skin*, shortness of breath*, skin rash*, swelling*.

RARE SIDE EFFECTS: Abdominal pain*, bleeding*, bruising*, depression*, nausea*, seizures*, sore throat*, stomach cramps*, urinary changes*, vomiting*, yellow eyes or skin*

PRECAUTIONS

If you have phenylketonuria, do not use the chewable tablets since they contain aspartame.

Oral contraceptives may not work properly when taken with this drug. You need to use a barrier contraceptive, such as a condom, or other nonhormonal contraceptive to prevent pregnancy.

If you have a history of stomach or intestinal disease, you may be at greater risk of developing colitis while taking this drug. Tell your doctor if you get severe or watery diarrhea.

PREGNANCY AND BREAST-FEEDING

Safety during pregnancy has not been established although there was no evidence of harm during studies in animals.

This drug passes into breast milk. Allergic reactions, diarrhea, fungal infections, and skin rash have been reported in babies.

HELPFUL COMMENTS

This drug is routinely taken with clavulanate potassium in the combination drug Augmentin for greater effectiveness.

Infant drops may be added to formula, milk, fruit juice, or soft drinks, but make sure the child drinks the entire quantity of the beverage to get the full dose.

Chewable tablets should be chewed completely and followed by a glass of water.

Contact your doctor if your symptoms do not improve after a couple of days.

Do not stop treatment early if you start to feel better. It takes the full prescription for this drug to work completely.

AMPICILLIN/AMPICILLIN TRIHYDRATE

Available for over 20 years

COMMONLY USED TO TREAT

Infection

DRUG CATEGORY

antibiotic
Class: aminopenicillin

PRODUCTS

Brand-Name Products with No Generic Alternative
Omnipen 400 mg tablet (n/a)

Brand-Name Products with Generic Alternatives
Omnipen 250 mg capsule (n/a)
  Generic: ampicillin 250 mg capsule (¢¢)
Omnipen 500 mg capsule (n/a)
  Generic: ampicillin 500 mg capsule (¢¢)
Omnipen 100 mg/ml oral suspension (n/a)
  Generic: principen 100 mg/ml oral suspension (n/a)
Omnipen 125 mg/5 ml oral suspension (n/a)
  Generic: ampicillin 125 mg/5 ml oral suspension (¢¢)
Omnipen 250 mg/5 ml oral suspension (n/a)
  Generic: ampicillin 250 mg/5 ml oral suspension (¢¢)

Other Generic Product Names
Marcillin, Omnipen, Principen, Totacillin

DOSING AND FOOD

Doses are taken 4 times a day.
Taking this drug with food may avoid the stomach upset some people suffer.
Adults: Up to 3.5 g per day in divided doses.
Children under 40 kg: Up to 100 mg/kg per day in divided doses.
Lower doses may be used in people with kidney disease.
Forgotten doses: If you are scheduled to take the next dose within a few
  hours, do not take the forgotten dose. Otherwise take the forgotten dose
  as soon as you remember.

ALCOHOL, DRUG, HERB, AND SUPPLEMENT INTERACTIONS

Alcohol may increase some of the side effects from this drug, depending

on the amount consumed. Ask your doctor about the risks caused by drinking alcohol with your condition.

Taking this drug with any of the ones listed below may change the effect of either drug with the possibility of causing toxicity or decreasing effectiveness: chloramphenicol, clavulanate, erythromycins†, methotrexate, oral contraceptives, probenecid, sulfonamides†, tetracyclines†

Severe reactions are possible when this drug is taken with those listed below: allopurinol

ALLERGIC REACTIONS AND SIDE EFFECTS

If you are allergic to any penicillins† or cephalosporins†, you may also be allergic to this drug. You should tell your doctor about all your allergies and any unexplained symptoms you may have while taking this drug.

MORE COMMON SIDE EFFECTS: Diarrhea*, headache, mouth sores, vaginal discharge, vaginal itching

LESS COMMON SIDE EFFECTS: Fainting*, fever*, hives*, irregular breathing*, itching*, joint pain*, lightheadedness*, scaly skin*, shortness of breath*, skin rash*, swelling*

RARE SIDE EFFECTS: Abdominal pain*, bleeding*, bruising*, depression*, nausea*, seizures*, sore throat*, stomach cramps*, urine changes*, vomiting*, yellow eyes or skin*

PRECAUTIONS

If you have a history of stomach or intestinal disease, you may be at greater risk of developing colitis while taking this drug. Tell your doctor if you get severe or watery diarrhea.

If you have mononucleosis, this drug may cause a severe skin rash.

Oral contraceptives may not work properly when taken with this drug. You need to use a barrier contraceptive, such as a condom, or other nonhormonal contraceptive to prevent pregnancy.

PREGNANCY AND BREAST-FEEDING

Safety during pregnancy has not been established although there was no evidence of harm during studies in animals.

This drug passes into breast milk. Allergic reactions, diarrhea, fungal infections, and skin rash have been reported in babies.

HELPFUL COMMENTS

Contact your doctor if symptoms do not improve after a couple of days.

Do not stop treatment early if you start to feel better. It takes the full prescription for this drug to work completely.

---

† See page 52.   * See page 53.

AMPRENAVIR

Available since April 1999

COMMONLY USED TO TREAT

HIV infection

DRUG CATEGORY

antiretroviral
Class: protease inhibitor (PI)

PRODUCTS

Brand-Name Products with No Generic Alternative
Agenerase 50 mg capsule (¢¢¢)
Agenerase 150 mg capsule ($)
Agenerase 15 mg/ml oral solution (¢¢¢¢)
No generics available.
Multiple patents that begin to expire in 2013. Exclusivity until 2004.

DOSING AND FOOD

Doses are taken 2 to 3 times a day.

This drug may be taken with or without food. Stay away from high-fat foods since they may decrease the absorption of this drug.

CAPSULE PRODUCT

Adults and children over age 17: Up to 2,400 mg daily in divided doses.

Children age 4 to 16: Up to 45 mg/kg (maximum 2,400 mg) per day in divided doses.

ORAL SOLUTION PRODUCT

Adults and children over age 17: Up to 2,800 mg per day in divided doses.

Children age 4 to 16: Up to 51 mg/kg (maximum 2,800 mg) per day in divided doses.

Lower doses may be needed in people with kidney disease.

Forgotten doses: If more than 4 hours have passed since the forgotten dose, do not take the dose. Otherwise take the forgotten dose as soon as you remember.

ALCOHOL, DRUG, HERB, AND SUPPLEMENT INTERACTIONS

Alcohol may increase some of the side effects from this drug, depending on the amount consumed. Ask your doctor about the risks caused by drinking alcohol with your condition.

St. John's wort may noticeably interfere with the effects of this drug and should not be used at any time during treatment.

Serious side effects may occur if taking disulfiram or metronidazole with the oral solution.

Taking this drug with any of the ones listed below may change the effect of either drug with the possibility of causing toxicity or decreasing effectiveness: amiodarone, astemizole, atorvastatin, bepridil, carbamazepine, clozapine, lovastatin, oral contraceptives, phenobarbital, phenytoin, pravastatin, quinidine, rifabutin, rifampin, simvastatin, tricyclic antidepressants†, warfarin

Severe reactions are possible when this drug is taken with those listed below: dihydroergotamine, ergonovine, ergotamine, flecainide, methylergonovine, midazolam, pimozide, propafenone, triazolam

Increased side effects are possible when this drug is taken with those listed below: sildenafil

ALLERGIC REACTIONS AND SIDE EFFECTS

If you are allergic to any sulfonamides†, you may also be allergic to this drug. You should tell your doctor about all your allergies and any unexplained symptoms you may have while taking this drug.

MORE COMMON SIDE EFFECTS: Abdominal pain, diarrhea, dry skin*, fatigue*, hunger*, itching*, nausea, skin rash*, thirst*, urination*, vomiting

LESS COMMON SIDE EFFECTS: Depression*, mood swings*, prickling*, taste changes

RARE SIDE EFFECTS: Fever*, hunchback*, skin irritation*, weight loss*

PRECAUTIONS

The dose of oral solution is different from the dose of the capsule products and cannot be substituted without a new prescription.

Children under age 4 should not use the oral solution product since it contains an inactive ingredient that may be harmful.

Do not take vitamin E supplements while taking this drug since the capsules contain a form of vitamin E that exceeds the daily requirements.

This drug is usually prescribed in combination with another antiretroviral drug. Ask your pharmacist about the type of drug interaction that may occur between antiretroviral drugs† to coordinate the administration times of multiple drugs.

People with kidney or liver disease may not be able to take this drug.

---

†See page 52.   *See page 53.

If you have diabetes or hemophilia, this drug may make those conditions worse.

This drug does not prevent transmission of the virus.

If you are also taking the antiretroviral drug didanosine, you need to take the dose at least 1 hour before or after this drug to avoid an interaction.

Skin rash that develops while taking this drug may become life threatening and should be reported immediately to your doctor.

PREGNANCY AND BREAST-FEEDING

Safety during pregnancy has not been established although the drug is known to harm animal fetuses.

Breast-feeding while taking this drug is not recommended.

HELPFUL COMMENTS

Oral contraceptives may not work properly when taken with this drug. You need to use a barrier contraceptive, such as a condom, or other nonhormonal contraceptive to prevent pregnancy.

If you need to take an antacid, take it either 2 hours before or after taking this drug.

Do not measure doses of the oral solution with anything but a measuring cup intended for use with prescription drugs. Slight inaccuracy from other measuring spoons may result in over- or under-dosing.

ANAGRELIDE HYDROCHLORIDE

Available since March 1997

COMMONLY USED TO TREAT

People at risk of developing blood clots

DRUG CATEGORY

antiplatelet
Class: megakaryocyte disrupter

PRODUCTS

Brand-Name Products with No Generic Alternative
Agrylin 0.5 mg capsule ($$$$)
Agrylin 1 mg capsule ($$$$$)
No generics available.
No patents. Exclusivity until 2004.

DOSING AND FOOD

Doses are taken 2 to 4 times a day.

This drug may be taken with or without food.

Adults: Up to 10 mg per day in divided doses.

Forgotten doses: If you are scheduled to take the next dose within a few hours, do not take the forgotten dose. Otherwise take the forgotten dose as soon as you remember.

ALCOHOL, DRUG, HERB, AND SUPPLEMENT INTERACTIONS

Alcohol may increase some of the side effects from this drug, depending on the amount consumed. Ask your doctor about the risks caused by drinking alcohol with your condition.

Taking this drug with any of the ones listed below may change the effect of either drug with the possibility of causing toxicity or decreasing effectiveness: sucralfate

ALLERGIC REACTIONS AND SIDE EFFECTS

You should tell your doctor about all your allergies and any unexplained symptoms you may have while taking this drug.

This drug promotes the effect of sunlight on the body and may cause severe sunburn and increased sensitivity of the eyes.

MORE COMMON SIDE EFFECTS: Abdominal pain*, bloating, diarrhea, dizziness*, gas, heartburn, irregular heartbeat*

LESS COMMON SIDE EFFECTS: Anxiety*, back pain, bleeding*, bloody urine*, blurry vision*, breathing difficulty*, bruising*, chest pain*, chills, cold sores, confusion, constipation, depression, fainting*, fever, flushing*, hair loss, headache*, increased heart rate*, itching, joint pain, leg cramps, loss of appetite, muscle pain, nausea*, nervousness, numbness*, ringing in ears, sensitivity to light, shortness of breath*, skin rash, sleep disorders, sleepiness, stuffy nose, sweating*, swelling*, tingling*, tiredness*, urinary changes*, vomiting*, weakness*

PRECAUTIONS

People with heart disease, kidney disease, or liver disease may be at greater risk of developing side effects while taking this drug.

This drug may cause unwanted effects on the heart and may even cause a heart attack. Get emergency medical help if you develop pain in the chest, arm, jaw, back, or neck or have other symptoms of a heart attack, such as anxiety, nausea, shortness of breath, or sweating.

---

†See page 52.　　*See page 53.

Be careful driving or handling equipment while taking this drug because it may cause dizziness.

Stopping this drug suddenly may cause an increased risk of developing a blood clot. If you wish to stop taking this drug, ask your doctor for specific instructions.

PREGNANCY AND BREAST-FEEDING

Safety during pregnancy has not been established although the drug is known to harm animal fetuses.

Breast-feeding while taking this drug is not recommended.

HELPFUL COMMENTS

If your hair begins to thin while taking this drug, it should return to normal once the drug is stopped.

Avoid quick movements to minimize dizziness.

Eye irritation caused by the sun may be reduced by wearing sunglasses when outside.

It takes 7 to 14 days for the effects of this drug to be noticed.

ANASTROZOLE

Available since December 1995

COMMONLY USED TO TREAT

Breast cancer

DRUG CATEGORY

antineoplastic
Class: aromatase inhibitor

PRODUCTS

Brand-Name Products with No Generic Alternative
Arimidex 1 mg tablet ($$$$)
No generics available.
Patent expires in 2009.

DOSING AND FOOD

Doses are taken once a day.
It is best to take this drug on an empty stomach.

Adults: Up to 1 mg per day.

This drug is not used in children.

Forgotten doses: Do not take a forgotten dose. Just go back to your usual schedule with the next dose.

ALCOHOL, DRUG, HERB, AND SUPPLEMENT INTERACTIONS

Alcohol may increase some of the side effects from this drug, depending on the amount consumed. Ask your doctor about the risks caused by drinking alcohol with your condition.

There are currently no known drug, herb, or supplement interactions. Ask your pharmacist for the latest update on interactions.

ALLERGIC REACTIONS AND SIDE EFFECTS

You should tell your doctor about all your allergies and any unexplained symptoms you may have while taking this drug.

MORE COMMON SIDE EFFECTS: Appetite change, back pain, body aches, bone pain*, chest pain*, congestion, constipation, cough*, diarrhea, dizziness*, dry mouth, dry throat, fever*, flushing, headache*, hoarseness*, hot flashes, mood swings, nausea, runny nose, shortness of breath*, skin rash, skin redness, stomachache, swallowing difficulty, sweating, swelling*, swollen glands, voice changes, vomiting, warmth, weakness

LESS COMMON SIDE EFFECTS: Anxiety, bluish coloring*, breathing difficulty, chest tightness*, chills*, confusion, difficulty urinating*, drowsiness, increased blood pressure*, itching, loss of hair, nervousness, numbness, runny nose, shivering, shortness of breath*, sleeping difficulty, sore throat*, tingling, tiredness*, vaginal bleeding*, vaginal dryness, weight gain, wheezing

PRECAUTIONS

Call your doctor immediately if you have chest pain, shortness of breath, or swelling in the feet or legs.

PREGNANCY AND BREAST-FEEDING

There is evidence that this drug may cause miscarriage, fetal death, low birth weight, or bone deformation. It is not recommended during pregnancy.

Breast-feeding while taking this drug is not recommended.

HELPFUL COMMENTS

It is very important to continue taking this drug as ordered by the doctor even if the side effects make you feel ill.

† See page 52.   * See page 53.

ARIPIPRAZOLE

Available since November 2002

COMMONLY USED TO TREAT

Mental disorders, specifically schizophrenia

DRUG CATEGORY

antipsychotic
Class: unclassified

PRODUCTS

Brand-Name Products with No Generic Alternative
Abilify 2 mg tablet (n/a)
Abilify 5 mg tablet (n/a)
Abilify 10 mg tablet (n/a)
Abilify 15 mg tablet (n/a)
Abilify 20 mg tablet (n/a)
Abilify 30 mg tablet (n/a)
No generics available.
Multiple patents that begin to expire in 2005. Exclusivity until 2007.

DOSING AND FOOD

Doses are taken once a day.
This drug may be taken with or without food. Do not drink grapefruit juice
while taking this drug.
Adults: Up to 30 mg per day.
Forgotten doses: If you are scheduled to take the next dose within 5
hours, do not take the forgotten dose. Otherwise take the forgotten dose
as soon as you remember.

ALCOHOL, DRUG, HERB, AND SUPPLEMENT INTERACTIONS

Alcohol should not be used while taking this drug.
Many OTC drugs used for appetite control, asthma, colds, cough, hay
fever, pain, or sinus problems affect the central nervous system and may
interfere with this drug. Check with your pharmacist for products to avoid.

**Taking this drug with any of the ones listed below may change the effect of
either drug with the possibility of causing toxicity or decreasing effectiveness:**
amiodarone, barbiturates, carbamazepine, chloroquine, cimetidine,

clarithromycin, corticosteroids†, cyclosporine, danazol, delavirdine, diltiazem, erythromycin, fluconazole, fluoxetine, fluphenazine, fluvoxamine, griseofulvin, haloperidol, indinavir, isoniazid, itraconazole, ketoconazole, metronidazole, miconazole, nafcillin, nefazodone, nelfinavir, nicardipine, nifedipine, norfloxacin, omeprazole, paroxetine, perphenazine, phenytoin, prednisone, primidone, propafenone, propoxyphene, quinidine, quinine, rifabutin, rifampin, ritonavir, saquinavir, sertraline, thioridazine, troglitazone, troleandomycin, verapamil, zafirlukast

ALLERGIC REACTIONS AND SIDE EFFECTS

You should tell your doctor about all your allergies and any unexplained symptoms you may have while taking this drug.

This drug may cause your eyes to be more sensitive to sunlight, but there are no special risks associated with sunburn while taking this drug.

MORE COMMON SIDE EFFECTS: Congestion, cough, depression, drowsiness, dry skin, falling, itching, muscle cramps, nervousness, suicidal thoughts*, sweating*, weight gain

LESS COMMON SIDE EFFECTS: Anxiety, bone pain, constipation, dizziness*, fainting*, headache, increase in appetite, lightheadedness*, mouth sores, nausea, shortness of breath*, sleep disorders, spastic movements*, swallowing difficulty, swelling, tongue movements*, tooth problems, vomiting, weakness

RARE SIDE EFFECTS: Behavior changes*, bloating, blood pressure changes*, blurry vision, chest pain, chills*, deafness*, fever*, irregular heartbeat*, neck pain, rash, runny nose, seizures*, shakiness, stiffness*

PRECAUTIONS

People with heart disease, low blood pressure or head injury may not be able to take this drug.

Be careful driving or handling equipment while taking this drug because the drug may cause drowsiness.

You are more likely to overheat when taking this drug and should avoid exercising in hot weather and using a sauna or hot tub.

This drug may cause changes to your gums and mouth. Your dentist may recommend that you clean your teeth and mouth differently to avoid infection.

Stopping this drug suddenly may cause serious side effects. If you wish to stop taking this drug, ask your doctor for specific instructions.

---

† See page 52.   * See page 53.

PREGNANCY AND BREAST-FEEDING

Safety during pregnancy has not been established although the drug is known to harm animal fetuses.

Breast-feeding while taking this drug is not recommended.

HELPFUL COMMENTS

It takes about 2 weeks for the full effects of this drug to be noticed.

Avoid quick movements to minimize dizziness. Dangling your legs over the side of the bed for a few minutes may help reduce dizziness when first waking up.

Eye irritation caused by the sun may be reduced by wearing sunglasses when outside.

ATENOLOL

Available for over 20 years

COMMONLY USED TO TREAT

Chest pain, also known as angina
Heart attack
High blood pressure, also known as hypertension
Irregular heartbeat, also known as arrhythmias

DRUG CATEGORY

antianginal
antiarrhythmic
antihypertensive
vascular headache prophylactic
Class: beta blocker

PRODUCTS

Brand-Name Products with Generic Alternatives
Tenormin 25 mg tablet ($)
　Generic: atenolol 25 mg tablet (¢)
Tenormin 50 mg tablet ($)
　Generic: atenolol 50 mg tablet (¢)
Tenormin 100 mg tablet ($$)
　Generic: atenolol 100 mg tablet (¢)

Combination Products That Contain This Drug
Tenoretic 50 tablet ($)
Tenoretic 100 tablet ($$)

DOSING AND FOOD

Doses are taken 1 to 2 times a day.

This drug may be taken with or without food.

Adults: Up to 200 mg per day.

Lower doses are used in people with kidney disease.

This drug is rarely used in children.

Forgotten doses: Take the forgotten dose as soon as you remember unless it is within 3 to 4 hours of the next scheduled dose.

ALCOHOL, DRUG, HERB, AND SUPPLEMENT INTERACTIONS

Alcohol may increase some of the side effects from this drug, depending on the amount consumed. Ask your doctor about the risks caused by drinking alcohol with your condition.

Several OTC drugs used for appetite control, asthma, colds, cough, hay fever, or sinus problems may cause an increase in blood pressure when taken with this drug. Check with your pharmacist when selecting OTC products.

Taking this drug with any of the ones listed below may change the effect of either drug with the possibility of causing toxicity or decreasing effectiveness:
aminophylline, antidiabetics[†], caffeine, calcium channel blockers[†], carbonic anhydrase inhibitors[†], clonidine, dyphylline, epinephrine, anesthetics[†], guanabenz, lidocaine, nonsteroidal antiinflammatories[†], oxtriphylline, pilocarpine, reserpine, theophylline

Severe reactions are possible when this drug is taken with those listed below:
beta blockers[†], cocaine, monoamine oxidase inhibitors[†]

Increased effects or side effects are possible when this drug is taken with those listed below:
antihypertensives[†]

ALLERGIC REACTIONS AND SIDE EFFECTS

If you are allergic to any other beta blockers[†], you may also be allergic to this drug.

This drug may exaggerate the reaction from your current allergies. Inform your doctor of any allergies that you have as well as the severity of the allergic reaction before starting this drug.

[†] See page 52.   * See page 53.

MORE COMMON SIDE EFFECTS: Dizziness*, drowsiness, lightheadedness*, sexual dysfunction, sleeping difficulty, tiredness, weakness

LESS COMMON SIDE EFFECTS: Anxiety, breathing difficulty*, cold hands or feet*, constipation, depression*, diarrhea, itching, nausea, nervousness, numbness, shortness of breath*, slow heartbeat*, sore eyes, stomachache, stuffy nose, swelling, tingling, vivid dreams, vomiting, wheezing

RARE SIDE EFFECTS: Back pain*, bleeding*, bruising*, chest pain*, confusion*, fever*, hallucinations*, irregular heartbeat*, joint pain*, skin irritation*, sore throat*

PRECAUTIONS

People with asthma, heart disease, or a heart rate that is routinely less than 60 beats per minute (bradycardia) may not be able to take this drug.

Stopping this drug suddenly may cause chest pain or heart attack. If you wish to stop taking this drug, ask your doctor for specific instructions.

If you are diabetic, this drug may increase blood sugar levels or make the symptoms of low blood sugar less noticeable.

You need to wait 2 weeks after stopping a monoamine oxidase inhibitor† before starting this drug.

Be careful driving or handling equipment while taking this drug because the drug may cause drowsiness.

This drug may cause nondiabetics to develop type 2 diabetes.

If you have psoriasis or myasthenia gravis, this drug may make those conditions worse.

PREGNANCY AND BREAST-FEEDING

Safety during pregnancy has not been established although the drug is known to harm animal fetuses.

Breast-feeding while taking this drug is not recommended.

HELPFUL COMMENTS

This drug may make you more sensitive to cold temperatures.

It may take 7 to 14 days for the full effects of this drug to be noticed.

If you do not treat high blood pressure, you may develop more serious problems such as heart failure, blood vessel disease, stroke, or kidney disease. Losing weight, exercising, eating more fruits and vegetables, and avoiding salty foods, such as lunchmeat and pickles, may help make drug treatment more successful.

ATOMOXETINE HYDROCHLORIDE

Available since November 2002

COMMONLY USED TO TREAT

Hyperactivity in children and adults, specifically attention deficit/hyperactivity disorder (ADHD)

DRUG CATEGORY

behavioral agent
Class: norepinephrine reuptake inhibitor

PRODUCTS

Brand-Name Products with No Generic Alternative
Strattera 5 mg capsule (n/a)
Strattera 10 mg capsule (n/a)
Strattera 18 mg capsule (n/a)
Strattera 25 mg capsule (n/a)
Strattera 40 mg capsule (n/a)
Strattera 60 mg capsule (n/a)
No generics available.
Patents expire in 2015. Exclusivity until 2008.

DOSING AND FOOD

Doses are taken 1 to 2 times a day.
This drug may be taken with or without food. Do not drink grapefruit juice while taking this drug.
Adults: Up to 150 mg per day in divided doses.
Children over 70 kg: Up to 100 mg per day in divided doses.
Children up to 70 kg: Up to 1.4 mg/kg (maximum 100 mg) per day in divided doses.
Forgotten doses: If you are scheduled to take the next dose within a few hours, do not take the forgotten dose. Otherwise take the forgotten dose as soon as you remember.

ALCOHOL, DRUG, HERB, AND SUPPLEMENT INTERACTIONS

Alcohol may increase some of the side effects from this drug, depending on the amount consumed. Ask your doctor about the risks caused by drinking alcohol with your condition.

---

† See page 52.   * See page 53.

Taking this drug with any of the ones listed below may change the effect of either drug with the possibility of causing toxicity or decreasing effectiveness: clarithromycin, cyclosporine, danazol, delavirdine, diltiazem, erythromycin, fluconazole, fluoxetine, fluvoxamine, indinavir, isoniazid, itraconazole, ketoconazole, metronidazole, miconazole, nefazodone, nelfinavir, nicardipine, nifedipine, norfloxacin, omeprazole, prednisone, quinidine, quinine, rifabutin, ritonavir, saquinavir, sertraline, troleandomycin, verapamil, zafirlukast

Severe reactions are possible when this drug is taken with those listed below: albuterol, monoamine oxidase inhibitors†

ALLERGIC REACTIONS AND SIDE EFFECTS

You should tell your doctor about all your allergies and any unexplained symptoms you may have while taking this drug.

MORE COMMON SIDE EFFECTS: Abdominal pain, constipation, dizziness, dry mouth, heartburn, loss of appetite, mood swings, nausea, sexual dysfunction, sleep disorders, sleepiness, urinary changes*, vomiting

LESS COMMON SIDE EFFECTS: Cough, headache, irritability

RARE SIDE EFFECTS: Crying, diarrhea, ear pain, gas, hot flashes, irregular heartbeat, runny nose, skin irritation*, sweating, swelling*, tiredness, weight loss

PRECAUTIONS

You need to wait 2 weeks after stopping a monoamine oxidase inhibitor† before starting this drug.

People with glaucoma, heart disease, or high blood pressure may not be able to take this drug.

This drug may cause you to grow at a slower rate or lose 1–2 inches in height.

Be careful driving or handling equipment while taking this drug because it may cause dizziness.

This drug may cause dry mouth, which is associated with a greater risk of cavities. Your dentist may recommend that you clean your teeth and mouth differently to avoid infection.

PREGNANCY AND BREAST-FEEDING

Safety during pregnancy has not been established although the drug is known to harm animal fetuses.

It is not known if this drug passes into breast milk. Talk to your doctor about the risks associated with breast-feeding while taking this drug.

HELPFUL COMMENTS

Sucking on hard sugarless candy or chewing sugarless gum may help relieve dry mouth caused by this drug.

Avoid quick movements to minimize dizziness. Dangling your legs over the side of the bed for a few minutes may help reduce dizziness when first waking up.

ATORVASTATIN CALCIUM

Available since December 1996

COMMONLY USED TO TREAT

High blood cholesterol and lipids, also known as hyperlipidemia

DRUG CATEGORY

antilipemic
Class: HMG CoA reductase inhibitor (statin)

PRODUCTS

Brand-Name Products with No Generic Alternative
Lipitor 10 mg tablet ($$)
Lipitor 20 mg tablet ($$$)
Lipitor 40 mg tablet ($$$)
Lipitor 80 mg tablet ($$$)
No generics available.
Multiple patents that begin to expire in 2009.

DOSING AND FOOD

Doses are taken once a day.

This drug may be taken with or without food. Do not drink grapefruit juice while taking this drug.

Adults and children over age 9: Up to 80 mg per day.

Forgotten doses: If you are scheduled to take the next dose within a few hours, do not take the forgotten dose. Otherwise take the forgotten dose as soon as you remember.

ALCOHOL, DRUG, HERB, AND SUPPLEMENT INTERACTIONS

Alcohol should not be used while taking this drug.

Red yeast rice, banned from sale in the U.S. since 2001, contains a nutrient

---

similar to this class of drugs and may cause toxicity if used while taking this drug.

Taking this drug with any of the ones listed below may change the effect of either drug with the possibility of causing toxicity or decreasing effectiveness: antacids, digoxin, oral contraceptives

Severe reactions are possible when this drug is taken with those listed below: azole antifungals†, clofibrate, cyclosporine, erythromycin, fenofibrate, fibric acid derivatives†, gemfibrozil, immunosuppressants†, niacin

Increased side effects are possible when this drug is taken with those listed below: acetaminophen, amiodarone, anabolic steroids†, androgens†, antibiotics†, antithyroid drugs†, carbamazepine, carmustine, chloroquine, dantrolene, daunorubicin, disulfiram, divalproex, etetinate, gold salts†, hydroxy-chloroquine, isoniazid, mercaptopurine, methotrexate, naltrexone, phe-nothiazines†, phenytoin, plicamycin, valproic acid

ALLERGIC REACTIONS AND SIDE EFFECTS

If you are allergic to any HMG-CoA reductase inhibitors†, you may also be allergic to this drug. You should tell your doctor about all your allergies and any unexplained symptoms you may have while taking this drug.

MORE COMMON SIDE EFFECTS: Constipation, diarrhea, dizziness, gas, headache, heartburn, nausea, skin rash, stomachache

LESS COMMON SIDE EFFECTS: Fever*, muscle cramps*, stomach pain*, tired-ness*, weakness*

RARE SIDE EFFECTS: Sexual dysfunction, sleeping difficulty

PRECAUTIONS

People with liver disease may not be able to take this drug.
Liver function should be tested every 1 to 6 months while taking this drug.

PREGNANCY AND BREAST-FEEDING

This drug may cause birth defects and should not be used during pregnancy. Breast-feeding while taking this drug is not recommended.

HELPFUL COMMENTS

You need to continue with a low-cholesterol diet even after this drug is started.

ATOVAQUONE

Available since November 1992

COMMONLY USED TO TREAT

Pneumonia, specifically *Pneumocystis carinii* pneumonia (PCP)

DRUG CATEGORY

antiprotozoal
Class: hydroxynapthalenedione

PRODUCTS

Brand-Name Products with No Generic Alternative
Mepron 250 mg tablet (n/a)
Mepron 750 mg/5 ml oral suspension ($$$$$)
No generics available.
Multiple patents that begin to expire in 2009.
Combination Products That Contain This Drug
Malarone tablet ($$$)
Malarone Pediatric tablet ($$)

DOSING AND FOOD

Doses are taken 1 to 3 times a day.
Taking this drug with fatty foods will help increase absorption of the drug.
  Be careful not to eat too much fatty food.
Adults and teenagers: Up to 2,250 mg per day in divided doses.
Forgotten doses: If you are scheduled to take the next dose within a few
  hours, do not take the forgotten dose. Otherwise take the forgotten dose
  as soon as you remember.

ALCOHOL, DRUG, HERB, AND SUPPLEMENT INTERACTIONS

Alcohol may increase some of the side effects from this drug, depending
  on the amount consumed. Ask your doctor about the risks caused by
  drinking alcohol with your condition.
**Taking this drug with any of the ones listed below may change the effect of
either drug with the possibility of causing toxicity or decreasing effectiveness:**
metoclopramide, rifampin, tetracycline

ALLERGIC REACTIONS AND SIDE EFFECTS

You should tell your doctor about all your allergies and any unexplained
  symptoms you may have while taking this drug.

† See page 52.   * See page 53.

MORE COMMON SIDE EFFECTS: Cough, diarrhea, fever*, headache, nausea, skin rash*, sleeping difficulty, vomiting

PRECAUTIONS

If you have stomach or intestinal problems, this drug may be less effective.

PREGNANCY AND BREAST-FEEDING

Safety during pregnancy has not been established although the drug is known to harm animal fetuses.
Breast-feeding while taking this drug is not recommended.

HELPFUL COMMENTS

If you vomit within 1 hour of taking your dose, you may take the dose again. Ask your doctor for addition instruction.

AURANOFIN

Available since May 1985

COMMONLY USED TO TREAT

Arthritis

DRUG CATEGORY

antirheumatic
Class: gold salt

PRODUCTS

Brand-Name Products with No Generic Alternative
Ridura 3 mg oral capsules ($$$)
No generics available.
No patents, no exclusivity.

DOSING AND FOOD

Doses are taken 1 to 3 times a day.
This drug may be taken with or without food.
Adults: Up to 9 mg per day in divided doses.
This drug is rarely used in children.
Forgotten doses: If you are scheduled to take the next dose within a few hours, do not take the forgotten dose. Otherwise take the forgotten dose as soon as you remember.

ALCOHOL, DRUG, HERB, AND SUPPLEMENT INTERACTIONS

Alcohol may increase some of the side effects from this drug, depending on the amount consumed. Ask your doctor about the risks caused by drinking alcohol with your condition.

Taking this drug with any of the ones listed below may change the effect of either drug with the possibility of causing toxicity or decreasing effectiveness: nonsteroidal antiinflammatories†

Increased side effects are possible when this drug is taken with those listed below: penacillamine

ALLERGIC REACTIONS AND SIDE EFFECTS

You should tell your doctor about all your allergies and any unexplained symptoms you may have while taking this drug.

This drug promotes the effect of sunlight on the body and may cause severe sunburn and increased sensitivity of the eyes.

MORE COMMON SIDE EFFECTS: Bloating, diarrhea, gas, indigestion, itching*, loss of appetite, nausea, skin rash*, mouth sores*, stomach cramps*, vomiting*

LESS COMMON SIDE EFFECTS: Constipation, hives*, metallic taste* tongue irritation*, urinary changes*

RARE SIDE EFFECTS: Back pain*, black stools*, bleeding*, breathing difficulty*, bruising*, chest tightness*, confusion*, cough*, dark urine*, eye irritation*, fever*, hair loss*, hallucinations*, heartburn*, hoarseness*, lung irritation*, nausea*, nose irritation*, numbness*, pale stools*, poor coordination*, seizures*, shortness of breath*, skin irritation*, sore throat*, stomach pain*, swallowing difficulty*, swelling*, tingling*, tiredness*, vaginal irritation*, vision changes*, vomiting*, weakness*, wheezing*, yellow eyes or skin*

PRECAUTIONS

People with necrotizing enterocolitis, pulmonary fibrosis, exfoliative dermatitis, bone marrow aplasia, severe hematologic disorders, or those people who have had toxicity from heavy metals may not be able to take this drug.

This drug causes changes in your blood that put you at greater risk of getting an infection. Be careful not to cut yourself or get bruised. Tell your doctor if you develop signs of infection, such as fever or sore throat. Your dentist may recommend that you clean your teeth and mouth differently to avoid infection.

---

† See page 52.   * See page 53.

People with blood disease, colitis, kidney disease, lupus erythematosus, Sjögren's syndrome, or skin disease are at greater risk of developing side effects while taking this drug.

PREGNANCY AND BREAST-FEEDING

Safety during pregnancy has not been established although the drug is known to harm animal fetuses.

Breast-feeding while taking this drug is not recommended.

HELPFUL COMMENTS

It may take 3 months for the effects of this drug to be noticed.

AZATADINE MALEATE

Available for over 20 years

COMMONLY USED TO TREAT

Allergies
Hay fever

DRUG CATEGORY

antihistamine
Class: H1 receptor blocker: piperidine

PRODUCTS

Brand-Name Products with No Generic Alternative
Optimine 1 mg tablet ($)
No generics available.
No patents, no exclusivity.
Combination Products That Contain This Drug
Trinalin extended-release tablet ($)

DOSING AND FOOD

Doses are taken 2 to 3 times a day.
This drug may be taken with or without food.
Adults: Up to 6 mg per day in divided doses.
Children over age 12: Up to 2 mg per day in divided doses.
Forgotten doses: If you are scheduled to take the next dose within a few hours, do not take the forgotten dose. Otherwise take the forgotten dose as soon as you remember.

ALCOHOL, DRUG, HERB, AND SUPPLEMENT INTERACTIONS

Alcohol may increase some of the side effects from this drug, depending on the amount consumed. Ask your doctor about the risks caused by drinking alcohol with your condition.

Severe reactions are possible when this drug is taken with those listed below: monoamine oxidase inhibitors†

Increased side effects are possible when this drug is taken with those listed below: anticholinergics†, benzodiazepines†, tricyclic antidepressants†

ALLERGIC REACTIONS AND SIDE EFFECTS

You should tell your doctor about all your allergies and any unexplained symptoms you may have while taking this drug.

This drug promotes the effect of sunlight on the body and may cause severe sunburn and increased sensitivity of the eyes.

MORE COMMON SIDE EFFECTS: Appetite changes, drowsiness, dry mouth, headache*, nausea, stomachache, weight gain

LESS COMMON SIDE EFFECTS: Belching, bleeding*, blurry vision, bruising*, clumsiness, confusion, congestion, constipation, cough, diarrhea*, dizziness*, early menstruation, excitement, fatigue, fever*, heartburn, hoarseness, indigestion, irregular heartbeat, irritability, joint pain, menstrual pain, muscle cramps, nausea, nervousness, pain, restlessness, ringing in ears, runny nose, skin rash*, sore throat*, sour stomach, stiffness, sweating, swollen glands, tiredness*, tremor, unsteadiness, urinary changes, vision changes, vomiting, weakness*

RARE SIDE EFFECTS: Abdominal pain*, breathing difficulty*, chest tightness*, chills*, dark urine*, flushing*, hallucinations*, hives*, itching*, lightheadedness*, pale stools*, seizures*, shortness of breath*, sleep disorders*, swallowing difficulty*, swelling*, tingling, wheezing*

PRECAUTIONS

You need to wait 2 weeks after stopping a monoamine oxidase inhibitor† before starting this drug.

This drug may cause dry mouth, which is associated with a greater risk of cavities. Your dentist may recommend that you clean your teeth and mouth differently to avoid infection.

Be careful driving or handling equipment while taking this drug because the drug may cause drowsiness.

People with glaucoma, ulcers, asthma, enlarged prostate, bladder prob-

---

†See page 52.   *See page 53.

lems, high thyroid levels, or high blood pressure may not be able to take this drug.

This drug may interfere with skin tests used to diagnose allergies and should be stopped for at least 4 days before the test.

PREGNANCY AND BREAST-FEEDING

Safety during pregnancy has not been established although there was no evidence of harm during studies in animals.

Breast-feeding while taking this drug is not recommended.

HELPFUL COMMENTS

Take your dose of this drug with a full glass of water.

Sucking on hard sugarless candy or chewing sugarless gum may help relieve dry mouth caused by this drug.

Several antihistamines are sold without a prescription by the following generic names: brompheniramine, chlorpheniramine, clemastine, diphenhydramine, doxylamine, loratadine. Ask your pharmacist about specific products that contain these drugs.

AZATHIOPRINE

Available for over 20 years

COMMONLY USED TO TREAT

Arthritis, specifically refractory rheumatoid arthritis
Kidney transplant recipients at risk of organ rejection

DRUG CATEGORY

immunosuppressant
antirheumatic
Class: purine antagonist

PRODUCTS

Brand-Name Products with Generic Alternatives
Imuran 50 mg tablet ($$)
  Generic: azathioprine 50 mg tablet ($)

DOSING AND FOOD

Doses are taken 1 to 2 times a day.

Taking this drug with a little food may avoid the stomach upset that some
people suffer.

Adults and children: Up to 5 mg/kg per day in divided doses.

Forgotten doses: If you are taking more than one dose per day, take the
forgotten dose as soon as you remember, then continue with the normal
schedule. If you take only one dose per day, do not take the forgotten dose.

ALCOHOL, DRUG, HERB, AND SUPPLEMENT INTERACTIONS

Alcohol may increase some of the side effects from this drug, depending
on the amount consumed. Ask your doctor about the risks caused by
drinking alcohol with your condition.

**Taking this drug with any of the ones listed below may change the effect of
either drug with the possibility of causing toxicity or decreasing effectiveness:**
allopurinol, chlorambucil, corticosteroids†, cyclophosphamide, cyclosporine, mercaptopurine, methotrexate, muromonab-CD3, pancuronium,
tubocurarine

Severe reactions are possible when this drug is taken with those listed below:
ACE inhibitors†

ALLERGIC REACTIONS AND SIDE EFFECTS

You should tell your doctor about all your allergies and any unexplained
symptoms you may have while taking this drug.

MORE COMMON SIDE EFFECTS: Back pain*, cough*, fever* chills*, hoarseness*, tiredness*, urinary changes*, weakness*

LESS COMMON SIDE EFFECTS: Black stools*, bleeding*, bloody urine*, bruising*, skin irritation*

RARE SIDE EFFECTS: Diarrhea*, fast heartbeat*, joint pain*, mouth sores*,
muscle pain*, nausea*, shortness of breath*, skin irritation*, stomachache*,
swelling*, vomiting*

PRECAUTIONS

Liver function should be tested regularly while taking this drug.

This drug causes changes in your blood that put you at greater risk of getting an infection. Be careful not to cut yourself or get bruised. Tell your
doctor if you develop signs of infection, such as fever or sore throat. Your
dentist may recommend that you clean your teeth and mouth differently
to avoid infection.

---

†*See page 52.*   **See page 53.*

PREGNANCY AND BREAST-FEEDING

There is evidence that this drug may harm the fetus, but the drug may be necessary to the health of the mother.

Breast-feeding while taking this drug is not recommended.

HELPFUL COMMENTS

It may take as long as 12 weeks of treatment with this drug to notice an improvement in arthritis pain.

If you are using a nonsteroidal antiinflammatory† drug to treat arthritis, you do not need to stop that drug when this drug is started.

AZITHROMYCIN DIHYDRATE

Available since November 1991

COMMONLY USED TO TREAT

Infection

DRUG CATEGORY

antibiotic
Class: macrolide

PRODUCTS

Brand-Name Products with No Generic Alternative
Zithromax 250 mg capsule ($$$$)
Zithromax 250 mg tablet ($$$$)
Zithromax 500 mg tablet (n/a)
Zithromax 600 mg tablet ($$$$$)
Zithromax 100 mg/5 ml oral suspension ($$$$)
Zithromax 200 mg/5 ml oral suspension ($$$)
No generics available.
No patents, no exclusivity.

DOSING AND FOOD

Doses are taken once a day.
This drug should always be taken on an empty stomach, 1 hour before meals or 2 hours after meals.
Adults: Up to 2 g per day.
Children: Up to 20 mg/kg (maximum 1 g) per day.

Forgotten doses: If you are scheduled to take the next dose within a few hours, do not take the forgotten dose. Otherwise take the forgotten dose as soon as you remember.

ALCOHOL, DRUG, HERB, AND SUPPLEMENT INTERACTIONS

Alcohol may increase some of the side effects from this drug, depending on the amount consumed. Ask your doctor about the risks caused by drinking alcohol with your condition.

Taking this drug with any of the ones listed below may change the effect of either drug with the possibility of causing toxicity or decreasing effectiveness: antacids, barbiturates†, carbamazepine, cyclosporine, dihydroergotamine, ergotamine, phenytoin, theophylline, triazolam, warfarin

ALLERGIC REACTIONS AND SIDE EFFECTS

If you are allergic to erythromycin or other macrolides†, you may also be allergic to this drug. You should tell your doctor about all your allergies and any unexplained symptoms you may have while taking this drug.

Less Common Side Effects: Diarrhea*, nausea, stomach pain*

Rare Side Effects: Abdominal tenderness*, breathing difficulty*, dizziness, fever*, headache, joint pain*, skin rash*, swelling*

PRECAUTIONS

People with liver disease may be at greater risk of developing side effects while taking this drug.

PREGNANCY AND BREAST-FEEDING

Safety during pregnancy has not been established although there was no evidence of harm during studies in animals.

It is not known if this drug passes into breast milk. Talk to your doctor about the risks associated with breast-feeding while taking this drug.

HELPFUL COMMENTS

Contact your doctor if your symptoms do not improve after a couple of days.

Do not stop treatment early if you start to feel better. It takes the full prescription for this drug to work completely.

If you need to take an antacid, take it either 2 hours before or after taking this drug.

---

† See page 52.   * See page 53.

BACAMPICILLIN HYDROCHLORIDE

Available for over 20 years

COMMONLY USED TO TREAT

Infection

DRUG CATEGORY

antibiotic
Class: aminopenicillin

PRODUCTS

Brand-Name Products with No Generic Alternative
Spectrobid 400 mg tablet (n/a)
Spectrobid 125 mg/5 ml oral suspension (n/a)
No generics available.
No patents, no exclusivity.

DOSING AND FOOD

Doses are taken 2 times a day.
This drug works best if taken on an empty stomach with a full glass of water, but taking it with food may avoid the stomach upset that some people suffer.
Adults: Up to 800 mg per day in divided doses.
Children over 25 kg: Up to 50 mg/kg per day in divided doses.
Forgotten doses: If you are scheduled to take the next dose within a few hours, do not take the forgotten dose. Otherwise take the forgotten dose as soon as you remember.

ALCOHOL, DRUG, HERB, AND SUPPLEMENT INTERACTIONS

Alcohol may increase some of the side effects from this drug, depending on the amount consumed. Ask your doctor about the risks caused by drinking alcohol with your condition.

Taking this drug with any of the ones listed below may change the effect of either drug with the possibility of causing toxicity or decreasing effectiveness: chloramphenicol, clavulanate, erythromycins†, methotrexate, oral contraceptives, probenecid, sulfonamides†, tetracyclines†

Severe reactions are possible when this drug is taken with those listed below: allopurinol

ALLERGIC REACTIONS AND SIDE EFFECTS

If you are allergic to any penicillins† or cephalosporins†, you may also be allergic to this drug. You should tell your doctor about all your allergies and any unexplained symptoms you may have while taking this drug.

MORE COMMON SIDE EFFECTS: Headache, diarrhea*, mouth sores, vaginal discharge, vaginal itching

LESS COMMON SIDE EFFECTS: Fainting*, fever*, hives*, irregular breathing*, itching*, joint pain*, lightheadedness*, scaly skin*, shortness of breath*, skin rash*, swelling*

RARE SIDE EFFECTS: Abdominal pain*, bleeding*, bruising*, depression*, nausea*, seizures*, sore throat*, stomach cramps*, urinary changes*, vomiting*, yellow eyes or skin*

PRECAUTIONS

If you have a history of stomach or intestinal disease, you may be at greater risk of developing colitis while taking this drug. Tell your doctor if you get watery or severe diarrhea.

Oral contraceptives may not work properly when taken with this drug. You need to use a barrier contraceptive, such as a condom, or other nonhormonal contraceptive to prevent pregnancy.

If you have mononucleosis, this drug may cause a severe skin rash.

PREGNANCY AND BREAST-FEEDING

Safety during pregnancy has not been established although there was no evidence of harm during studies in animals.

This drug passes into breast milk. Allergic reactions, diarrhea, fungal infections, and skin rash have been reported in babies.

HELPFUL COMMENTS

Contact your doctor if your symptoms do not improve after a couple of days.

Do not stop treatment early if you start to feel better. It takes the full prescription for this drug to work completely.

This drug is converted to ampicillin once it is in the body.

---

† *See page 52.*   * *See page 53.*

BACLOFEN

Available since June 1992

COMMONLY USED TO TREAT

Muscle spasms

DRUG CATEGORY

skeletal muscle relaxant
Class: chlorophenyl derivative

PRODUCTS

Products Only Available as Generics
baclofen 10 mg tablet (¢¢¢)
baclofen 20 mg tablet (¢¢¢¢)

DOSING AND FOOD

Doses are taken 3 to 4 times a day.
This drug may be taken with or without food.

Adults: Up to 80 mg per day in divided doses.

Lower doses are used in people over age 65.

This drug is not recommended for children under age 12.

Forgotten doses: If you are scheduled to take the next dose within a few
  hours, do not take the forgotten dose. Otherwise take the forgotten dose
  as soon as you remember.

ALCOHOL, DRUG, HERB, AND SUPPLEMENT INTERACTIONS

Alcohol should not be used while taking this drug.
Several OTC drugs used for asthma, colds, cough, hay fever, sleep aid, or sinus problems may increase the risk of side effects when taken with this
  drug. Check with your pharmacist when selecting OTC products.

**Taking this drug with any of the ones listed below may change the effect of
either drug with the possibility of causing toxicity or decreasing effectiveness:**
antidiabetics†, antipsychotics†, anxiolytics†, anesthetics, insulin, narcotics†

Severe reactions are possible when this drug is taken with those listed below:
amitriptyline, amoxapine, clomipramine, desipramine, doxepin, imipramine,
  monoamine oxidase inhibitors†, nortriptyline, protriptyline, trimipramine

ALLERGIC REACTIONS AND SIDE EFFECTS

You should tell your doctor about all your allergies and any unexplained symptoms you may have while taking this drug.

MORE COMMON SIDE EFFECTS: Confusion, dizziness, drowsiness, lightheadedness, nausea, weakness

LESS COMMON SIDE EFFECTS: Bloody urine*, chest pain*, clumsiness, constipation, depression*, diarrhea, excitement, fainting*, hallucinations*, headache, irregular heartbeat*, itching, joint pain, loss of appetite, low blood pressure, muscle pain, muscle stiffness, numbness, poor coordination, ringing in ears*, sexual dysfunction, skin rash*, sleeping difficulty, slurry speech, stomach pain, stuffy nose, swelling, tingling, tiredness, urinary changes*, weight gain

PRECAUTIONS

This drug may cause severe withdrawal symptoms if stopped abruptly. If you wish to stop taking this drug, ask your doctor for specific instructions.

Be careful driving or handling equipment while taking this drug because the drug may cause drowsiness.

You need to wait 2 weeks after stopping a monoamine oxidase inhibitor† before starting this drug.

If you are a diabetic, you may need a change in the dose of your antidiabetic drug† or insulin, since this drug may cause changes in blood sugar.

People with epilepsy, kidney disease, emotional problems, or brain disease may be at greater risk of developing side effects while taking this drug.

PREGNANCY AND BREAST-FEEDING

Safety during pregnancy has not been established although the drug is known to harm animal fetuses.

This drug passes into breast milk, but does not appear to harm the baby. Talk to your doctor about the risks associated with breast-feeding while taking this drug.

HELPFUL COMMENTS

It takes about 2 weeks of incrementally lower doses to stop this drug without developing withdrawal symptoms.

---

† See page 52.   * See page 53.

BALSALAZIDE DISODIUM

Available since July 2000

COMMONLY USED TO TREAT

Inflammation in the bowel, specifically ulcerative colitis

DRUG CATEGORY

antiinflammatory
Class: nonsteroidal antiinflammatory: salicylate

PRODUCTS

Brand-Name Products with No Generic Alternative
Colazal 750 mg capsule (¢¢¢¢¢)
No generics available.
Market exclusivity until July 2005.

DOSING AND FOOD

Doses are taken 3 times a day.
This drug may be taken with or without food.
Adults: Up to 6.75 g per day in divided doses.
Forgotten doses: If you are scheduled to take the next dose within a few
hours, do not take the forgotten dose. Otherwise take the forgotten dose
as soon as you remember.

ALCOHOL, DRUG, HERB, AND SUPPLEMENT INTERACTIONS

Alcohol may increase some of the side effects from this drug, depending
on the amount consumed. Ask your doctor about the risks caused by
drinking alcohol with your condition.

**Taking this drug with any of the ones listed below may change the effect of
either drug with the possibility of causing toxicity or decreasing effectiveness:**
antibiotics†

ALLERGIC REACTIONS AND SIDE EFFECTS

If you are allergic to aspirin, you should not take this drug. You should tell
your doctor about all your allergies and any unexplained symptoms you
may have while taking this drug.
MORE COMMON SIDE EFFECTS: Diarrhea, stomachache
LESS COMMON SIDE EFFECTS: Back pain*, bloody urine*, constipation,

cough, dry mouth, fever, gas, heartburn, joint pain, loss of appetite, muscle pain, painful urination, sleeping difficulty, stuffy nose*, tiredness*, weakness*, yellow eyes or skin*

PRECAUTIONS

If you have pyloric stenosis, you may see an initial delay in the effects of this drug or a longer effectiveness.

People with liver or kidney disease may not be able to take this drug.

PREGNANCY AND BREAST-FEEDING

Safety during pregnancy has not been established although there was no evidence of harm during studies in animals.

It is not known if this drug passes into breast milk. Talk to your doctor about the risks associated with breast-feeding while taking this drug.

HELPFUL COMMENTS

This drug is usually only taken for 8 weeks and not beyond 12 weeks.

Make sure to swallow the capsules whole rather than breaking or opening.

Call your doctor if your symptoms become worse while taking this drug.

BENAZEPRIL HYDROCHLORIDE

Available since June 1991

COMMONLY USED TO TREAT

High blood pressure, also known as hypertension

DRUG CATEGORY

antihypertensive
Class: ACE inhibitor

PRODUCTS

Brand-Name Products with No Generic Alternative
Lotensin 5 mg tablet (¢¢¢¢¢)
Lotensin 10 mg tablet (¢¢¢¢¢)
Lotensin 20 mg tablet (¢¢¢¢¢)
Lotensin 40 mg tablet (¢¢¢¢¢)
No generics available.
Patent expires in 2003.

---

† See page 52. *See page 53.

Combination Products That Contain This Drug
Lotensin HCT tablet (¢¢¢¢¢)
Lotrel capsule ($$)

DOSING AND FOOD

Doses are taken 1 to 2 times a day.

This drug may be taken with or without food.

Adults: Up to 40 mg per day in divided doses.

Lower doses may be needed in people with kidney disease.

Forgotten doses: If you are scheduled to take the next dose within a few hours, do not take the forgotten dose. Otherwise take the forgotten dose as soon as you remember.

ALCOHOL, DRUG, HERB, AND SUPPLEMENT INTERACTIONS

Alcohol may cause your blood pressure to rise, making this drug less effective. Ask your doctor about the risks caused by drinking alcohol with your condition.

Licorice may interfere with the effects of this drug.

Capsaicin and other foods or supplements, including hot peppers, sweet peppers, paprika, and chili powder, derived from the capsicum family of plants may increase the risk of developing a cough and should not be taken with this drug.

Taking this drug with any of the ones listed below may change the effect of either drug with the possibility of causing toxicity or decreasing effectiveness: antihypertensives†, digoxin, diuretics†, lithium

Severe reactions are possible when this drug is taken with those listed below: allopurinol, potassium supplements, salt substitutes

ALLERGIC REACTIONS AND SIDE EFFECTS

If you are allergic to other ACE inhibitors†, you may also be allergic to this drug. You should tell your doctor about all your allergies and any unexplained symptoms you may have while taking this drug.

MORE COMMON SIDE EFFECTS: Dry cough, headache

LESS COMMON SIDE EFFECTS: Diarrhea, dizziness*, fainting*, fever*, joint pain*, lightheadedness*, loss of taste, nausea*, skin rash*, tiredness

RARE SIDE EFFECTS: Abdominal pain*, breathing difficulty*, chest pain*, chills*, confusion*, hoarseness*, irregular heartbeat*, itching*, nausea*, nervousness*, numbness*, stomach pain*, swallowing difficulty*, swelling*, vomiting*, weakness*, yellow eyes or skin*

PRECAUTIONS

Do not use potassium-containing products, including salt substitutes, while taking this drug.

Diuretics† should be stopped 2 to 3 days prior to starting this drug. If not possible to stop the diuretic, the dose of this drug should be lowered.

Drink plenty of fluids to avoid dehydration when sweating, such as in hot weather and during exercise.

Be careful driving or handling equipment while taking this drug because the drug may cause drowsiness.

People with systemic lupus erythematosus may be at greater risk of developing blood problems while taking this drug.

PREGNANCY AND BREAST-FEEDING

Safety during pregnancy has not been established although the drug is known to harm animal fetuses.

Breast-feeding while taking this drug is not recommended.

HELPFUL COMMENTS

A persistent dry cough may appear while taking this drug, but it will go away when the drug is stopped.

It may take several weeks for the full effect of this drug to be noticed.

Avoid quick movements to minimize dizziness. Dangling your legs over the side of the bed for a few minutes may help reduce dizziness when first waking up.

If you do not treat high blood pressure, you may develop more serious problems such as heart failure, blood vessel disease, stroke, or kidney disease. Losing weight, exercising, eating more fruits and vegetables, and avoiding salty foods, such as lunchmeat and pickles, may help make drug treatment more successful.

BENDROFLUMETHIAZIDE

Available for over 20 years

COMMONLY USED TO TREAT

Fluid retention, also known as edema

Frequent urination in people with diabetes

High blood pressure, also known as hypertension

---

† See page 52.   * See page 53.

DRUG CATEGORY

antihypertensive
Class: thiazide diuretic

PRODUCTS

Brand-Name Products with No Generic Alternative
Naturetin 5 mg tablet ($)
No generics available.
No patents, no exclusivity.
Combination Products That Contain This Drug
Corzide 40/5 tablet ($$)
Corzide 80/5 tablet ($$)

DOSING AND FOOD

Doses are taken 1 to 2 times a day, but may be taken as little as 3 times a week.
Adults: Up to 20 mg per day in divided doses.
Children: Up to 400 mcg/kg per day in divided doses.
This drug should be taken with food to reduce the stomach upset that many people suffer. Avoid food with excess salt.
Forgotten doses: If you are scheduled to take the next dose within a few hours, do not take the forgotten dose. Otherwise take the forgotten dose as soon as you remember.

ALCOHOL, DRUG, HERB, AND SUPPLEMENT INTERACTIONS

Alcohol may cause your blood pressure to rise, making this drug less effective. Ask your doctor about the risks caused by drinking alcohol with your condition.
Licorice root may increase potassium loss and should not be used while taking this drug.
Several OTC drugs used for appetite control, asthma, colds, cough, hay fever, or sinus problems may cause an increase in blood pressure when taken with this drug. Check with your pharmacist when selecting OTC products.

Taking this drug with any of the ones listed below may change the effect of either drug with the possibility of causing toxicity or decreasing effectiveness: antidiabetics†, cholestyramine, colestipol, digoxin, insulin, lithium

ALLERGIC REACTIONS AND SIDE EFFECTS

If you are allergic to acetazolamide, bumetanide, dichlorphenamide, furosemide, methazolamide, sulfonamides†, or thiazide diuretics†, you may also be allergic to this drug. You should tell your doctor about all your allergies and any unexplained symptoms you may have while taking this drug.

This drug promotes the effect of sunlight on the body and may cause severe sunburn and increased sensitivity of the eyes.

LESS COMMON SIDE EFFECTS: Diarrhea*, dizziness, lightheadedness, loss of appetite, sexual dysfunction, stomach upset

RARE SIDE EFFECTS: Back pain*, black stools*, bleeding*, bloody urine*, breathing difficulty*, bruising*, chest pain*, chills*, confusion*, cough*, fatigue*, fever*, hives*, headache*, hoarseness*, irregular heartbeat*, joint pain*, leg pain*, muscle cramps*, nausea*, numbness*, painful urination*, shortness of breath*, skin rash*, stomach pain*, swelling*, weakness*, vomiting*, yellow eyes or skin*.

PRECAUTIONS

This drug may cause your blood sugar level to rise and may lead to type 2 diabetes.

Your body may lose potassium while taking this drug, which may cause severe side effects. Potassium levels should be monitored periodically and may need to be supplemented while taking this drug. Eat food rich in potassium, such as apricots, bananas, citrus fruit, dates, and tomatoes, if you are not taking a potassium supplement or potassium-sparing diuretic.†

People with kidney disease may not be able to take this drug.

This drug may increase the uric acid levels in the body putting people with a prior history of gout at greater risk of developing side effects.

If you have lupus erythematosus or pancreatitis, this drug may make those conditions worse.

Nicotine in cigarettes may increase blood pressure, making this drug less effective.

This drug may cause an increase in the levels of cholesterol or triglyceride in the blood.

PREGNANCY AND BREAST-FEEDING

Safety during pregnancy has not been established although the drug is known to harm animal fetuses.

Breast-feeding while taking this drug is not recommended.

---

† See page 52.   * See page 53.

HELPFUL COMMENTS

Take your last dose of the day no later than 6 P.M. to avoid urination during the night.

Avoid quick movements to minimize dizziness. Dangling your legs over the side of the bed for a few minutes may help reduce dizziness when first waking up.

Record your weight twice a day, when first getting up in the morning and after the drug causes urination. A weight gain or loss of more than 2 pounds per day should be reported to your doctor.

The blood-pressure-lowering effects of this drug will last about 1 week after it is stopped.

If you do not treat high blood pressure, you may develop more serious problems such as heart failure, blood vessel disease, stroke, or kidney disease. Losing weight, exercising, eating more fruits and vegetables, and avoiding salty foods, such as lunchmeat and pickles, may help make drug treatment more successful.

BENZTROPINE MESYLATE

Available for over 20 years

COMMONLY USED TO TREAT

Irregular muscle tremors or jerking movement

DRUG CATEGORY

antidyskinetic
Class: anticholinergic

PRODUCTS

Products Only Available as Generics
benztropine mesylate 0.5 mg tablet (¢¢)
benztropine mesylate 1 mg tablet (¢¢)
benztropine mesylate 2 mg tablet (¢¢)

DOSING AND FOOD

Doses are taken 1 to 2 times a day.
This drug should be taken after meals to avoid stomach upset.
Adults: Up to 6 mg per day in divided doses.
Lower doses are used in children.
This drug is rarely used in children under age 3.

Forgotten doses: If you are scheduled to take the next dose within a few hours, do not take the forgotten dose. Otherwise take the forgotten dose as soon as you remember.

ALCOHOL, DRUG, HERB, AND SUPPLEMENT INTERACTIONS

Alcohol should not be used while taking this drug.

Many OTC drugs used for appetite control, asthma, colds, cough, hay fever, pain, or sinus problems affect the central nervous system and may change the effects or side effects of this drug. Check with your pharmacist for products to avoid.

Taking this drug with any of the ones listed below may change the effect of either drug with the possibility of causing toxicity or decreasing effectiveness: antacids, antidiarrhealst, haloperidol, phenothiazinest

Increased side effects are possible when this drug is taken with those listed below: amantadine, anesthetics, anticholinergicst, antihistaminest, anxiolyticst, barbituratest, narcoticst, tricyclic antidepressantst

ALLERGIC REACTIONS AND SIDE EFFECTS

If you are allergic to other anticholinergict drugs, you may also be allergic to this drug. You should tell your doctor about all your allergies and any unexplained symptoms you may have while taking this drug.

This drug may cause your eyes to be more sensitive to sunlight, but there are no special risks associated with sunburn while taking this drug.

MORE COMMON SIDE EFFECTS: Blurry vision, constipation, decreased sweating, difficulty urinating, drowsiness, dry mouth*, nausea, sensitivity to light, vomiting

LESS COMMON SIDE EFFECTS: Dizziness, headache, lightheadedness, memory loss, muscle cramps, nervousness, numbness, sore mouth, stomachache, weakness

RARE SIDE EFFECTS: Confusion*, eye pain*, skin rash*

PRECAUTIONS

This drug may cause withdrawal symptoms if stopped suddenly. If you wish to stop taking this drug, ask your doctor for specific instructions.

People with glaucoma may not be able to take this drug.

Be careful driving or handling equipment while taking this drug because the drug may cause drowsiness.

This drug may cause dry mouth, which is associated with a greater risk of cavities. Your dentist may recommend that you clean your teeth and mouth differently to avoid infection.

---

† See page 52.   * See page 53.

This drug makes you sweat less, putting you at greater risk of developing heatstroke. Avoid exercising in hot weather and using hot tubs or saunas.

PREGNANCY AND BREAST-FEEDING

Safety during pregnancy has not been established although the drug is known to harm animal fetuses.

Breast-feeding while taking this drug is not recommended.

HELPFUL COMMENTS

It takes 2 to 3 days before the effects of this drug are noticed.

If you are taking the drug once a day and have too many side effects, talk to your doctor about twice-a-day dosing.

You may only need to take this drug for a couple of weeks if you are using it to treat the side effects caused by another drug.

If you need to take an antacid, take it either 2 hours before or after taking this drug.

Sucking on hard sugarless candy or chewing sugarless gum may help relieve dry mouth caused by this drug.

BEPRIDIL HYDROCHLORIDE

Available since December 1990

COMMONLY USED TO TREAT

Chest pain, also known as angina

DRUG CATEGORY

antianginal
Class: calcium channel blocker

PRODUCTS

Brand-Name Products with No Generic Alternative
Vascor 200 mg tablet ($$$)
Vascor 300 mg tablet ($$$)
No generics available.
No patents, no exclusivity.

DOSING AND FOOD

Doses are taken once a day.

This drug should be taken with food to reduce the stomach upset that many people suffer.

Adults: Up to 400 mg per day.

This drug is not used in children under age 18.

Forgotten doses: If you are scheduled to take the next dose within a few hours, do not take the forgotten dose. Otherwise take the forgotten dose as soon as you remember.

ALCOHOL, DRUG, HERB, AND SUPPLEMENT INTERACTIONS

Alcohol may increase some of the side effects from this drug, depending on the amount consumed. Ask your doctor about the risks caused by drinking alcohol with your condition.

Taking this drug with any of the ones listed below may change the effect of either drug with the possibility of causing toxicity or decreasing effectiveness: digoxin

Severe reactions are possible when this drug is taken with those listed below: acetazolamide, beta blockers†, corticosteroids†, dichlorphenamide, diuretics†, methazolamide, procainamide, quinidine, tricyclic antidepressants†

ALLERGIC REACTIONS AND SIDE EFFECTS

If you are allergic to other calcium channel blockers†, you may also be allergic to this drug. You should tell your doctor about all your allergies and any unexplained symptoms you may have while taking this drug.

MORE COMMON SIDE EFFECTS: Nausea

LESS COMMON SIDE EFFECTS: Breathing difficulty*, constipation, cough*, diarrhea, dizziness, flushing, headache, irregular heartbeat*, leg swelling*, skin rash*, tiredness, weakness, wheezing*

RARE SIDE EFFECTS: Chest pain*, fainting*, swollen gums*

PRECAUTIONS

This drug may cause a serious change in heart rate, heartbeat, or heart rhythm. Tell your doctor immediately if you notice any symptoms.

The level of potassium in your body is critical for the safe use of this drug and should be monitored regularly.

This drug causes changes in your blood that put you at greater risk of getting an infection. Be careful not to cut yourself or get bruised. Tell your doctor if you develop signs of infection, such as fever or sore throat. Your dentist may recommend that you clean your teeth and mouth differently to avoid infection.

†*See page 52.*   ** See page 53.*

PREGNANCY AND BREAST-FEEDING

Safety during pregnancy has not been established although the drug is known to harm animal fetuses.

Breast-feeding while taking this drug is not recommended.

HELPFUL COMMENTS

This drug is only used in people who have not responded to other antianginal† drugs.

Learn how to measure your heart rate and call your doctor if it falls below 50 beats per minute.

BETAINE ANHYDROUS

Available since October 1996

COMMONLY USED TO TREAT

High levels of homocysteine in the body.

DRUG CATEGORY

antihomocystinuric
Class: glycine derivative

PRODUCTS

Brand-Name Products with No Generic Alternative
Cystadane powder for oral solution (¢¢)
No generics available.
Exclusivity until 2003.

DOSING AND FOOD

Doses are taken 2 times a day.
It is best to take this drug with food.
Adults: Up to 6 grams per day in divided doses.
Lower doses are used in children.
Forgotten doses: If you are scheduled to take the next dose within a few hours, do not take the forgotten dose. Otherwise take the forgotten dose as soon as you remember.

ALCOHOL, DRUG, HERB, AND SUPPLEMENT INTERACTIONS

Alcohol may increase some of the side effects from this drug, depending

on the amount consumed. Ask your doctor about the risks caused by drinking alcohol with your condition.

No drug interactions have been reported.

ALLERGIC REACTIONS AND SIDE EFFECTS

You should tell your doctor about all your allergies and any unexplained symptoms you may have while taking this drug.

LESS COMMON SIDE EFFECTS: Diarrhea, nausea, stomachache

PRECAUTIONS

If the powder changes color in solution or does not dissolve completely, it may be an indication that the drug has gone bad. Make sure the cap is always on tight to protect the drug from moisture.

PREGNANCY AND BREAST-FEEDING

Safety during pregnancy has not been established although the drug is known to harm animal fetuses.

It is not known if this drug passes into breast milk. Talk to your doctor about the risks associated with breast-feeding while taking this drug.

HELPFUL COMMENTS

This drug should be completely dissolved in $1/2$ cup of juice, milk, or water. Do not mix doses in advance.

One level scoop is equal to 1 gram of drug.

BETAMETHASONE

Available for over 20 years

COMMONLY USED TO TREAT

Allergic reactions
Severe inflammation

DRUG CATEGORY

antiinflammatory
immunosuppressant
Class: glucocorticoid

PRODUCTS

Brand-Name Products with No Generic Alternative
Celestone 0.6 mg/5 ml oral syrup ($$)

---

† *See page 52.*   * *See page 53.*

Celestone 0.6 mg tablet ($$)
Diprolene AF 0.05% topical cream (¢¢¢¢)
Diprolene 0.05% topical gel (¢¢¢¢)
Diprolene 0.05% topical lotion (¢¢¢)
Luxiq 0.12% topical foam (¢¢)

Brand-Name Products with Generic Alternatives
Diprosone 0.05% topical cream (¢¢¢)
  Generic: betamethasone diproprionate 0.05% topical cream (¢)
Diprosone 0.05% topical lotion (¢¢¢)
  Generic: betamethasone diproprionate 0.05% topical lotion (¢)
Diprosone 0.05% topical ointment (¢¢¢)
  Generic: betamethasone diproprionate 0.05% topical ointment (¢)
Diprolene 0.05% topical ointment (¢¢¢¢)
  Generic: betamethasone diproprionate augmented 0.05% topical oint-
  ment (¢¢¢)

Products Only Available as Generics
betamethasone valerate 0.1% topic cream (¢)
betamethasone valerate 0.1% topical lotion (¢)
betamethasone valerate 0.1% topical ointment (¢)

Other Generic Product Names
Alphatrex, Betaderm, Betamethacot, Betatrex, Beta-Val, Celestone, Del-Beta,
  Dermabet, Maxivate, Valnac

Combination Products That Contain This Drug
Lotrisone lotion (¢¢¢)
Lotrisone cream (¢¢¢)

DOSING AND FOOD

Doses are taken 1 to 4 times a day.
The oral form of this drug should be taken with food.
Adults: Up to 7.2 mg per day in divided doses.
Children: Up to 0.25 mg/kg per day in divided doses.
Topical preparations should be applied in a thin layer.
Forgotten doses: Determining when to take a forgotten dose will depend
  on your prescription schedule. If you remember the forgotten dose within
  a few hours of when it was due, you may take the dose immediately and
  continue with your regular schedule. If you are tapering the drug to avoid
  withdrawal symptoms, you may need to evaluate the time since the last
  dose and the interval between the next doses. A complete change in sched-
  ule may be needed. Talk to your doctor or pharmacist for more help.

ALCOHOL, DRUG, HERB, AND SUPPLEMENT INTERACTIONS

Alcohol may increase the risk of side effects from this drug, especially stomach problems. Ask your doctor about the risks caused by drinking alcohol with your condition.

Taking this drug with any of the ones listed below may change the effect of either drug with the possibility of causing toxicity or decreasing effectiveness: aminoglutethimide, antacids, anticoagulants†, antidiabetics†, barbiturates†, carbamazepine, cholestyramine, colestipol, diuretics†, estrogens†, griseofulvin, insulin, isoniazid, mitotane, phenylbutazone, phenytoin, primidone, rifampin, salicylates†, somatrem, somatropin

Severe reactions are possible when this drug is taken with those listed below: aspirin, amphotericin B, cardiac glycosides†, immunizations, nonsteroidal antiinflammatories†, ritodrine

ALLERGIC REACTIONS AND SIDE EFFECTS

If you are allergic to any corticosteroids†, you may also be allergic to this drug. You should tell your doctor about all your allergies and any unexplained symptoms you may have while taking this drug.

This drug may cause your eyes to be more sensitive to sunlight, but there are no special risks associated with sunburn while taking this drug.

MORE COMMON SIDE EFFECTS: Increased appetite, indigestion, nervousness, restlessness

LESS COMMON SIDE EFFECTS: Acne*, bloody stools*, bruising*, dizziness, eye pain*, flushing, frequent urination*, hair growth*, headache*, hiccups, irregular heartbeat*, lightheadedness, menstrual problems*, muscle cramps*, nausea*, red eyes*, rounding of the face*, skin discoloration, skin irritation*, sleeping difficulty*, spinning sensation, stomach pain*, stunted growth*, sweating, swelling*, tearing of eyes*, thirst*, tiredness*, vision changes*, vomiting*, weakness*, weight gain*, wounds that will not heal*

RARE SIDE EFFECTS: Confusion*, depression*, excitement*, hallucinations*, hives*, mood swings*, restlessness*, skin rash*

PRECAUTIONS

This drug may cause severe and possibly fatal withdrawal symptoms if stopped abruptly. If you wish to stop taking this drug, ask your doctor for specific instructions.

The topical form of this drug is absorbed through the skin and may be associated with the same warnings as the oral product if it is used for a long time, on a large area of skin, or on broken or irritated skin.

† See page 52.   * See page 53.

This drug may cause an increase in blood sugar or cholesterol level, calcium loss, and/or retention of fluid.

Avoid contact with anyone who has the chickenpox, measles, or other communicable disease since it may be easier to catch the infection while taking this drug.

Exposure to skin tests, immunizations, and people who have received immunizations may put you at a greater risk of developing the disease when you are taking this drug.

PREGNANCY AND BREAST-FEEDING

Safety during pregnancy has not been established although the drug is known to harm animal fetuses.

This drug passes into breast milk and may cause growth problems in the baby. The risk is related to the dose and route of the drug. Small amounts of the drug are absorbed into the body from topical products.

HELPFUL COMMENTS

If you need to take an antacid, take it either 2 hours before or after taking this drug.

When using topical foam, it should be sprayed on a clean surface rather than into the hand to make sure the strength of the drug is not decreased.

If you are using the drug topically and develop skin irritation, broken skin, or infection, the drug may need to be stopped.

BETAXOLOL HYDROCHLORIDE

Available since August 1985

COMMONLY USED TO TREAT

High blood pressure, also known as hypertension
Increased pressure in the eye, also known as glaucoma

DRUG CATEGORY

antihypertensive
Class: beta blocker

PRODUCTS

Brand-Name Products with Generic Alternatives
Kerlone 10 mg tablet ($)

Generic: betaxolol hydrochloride 10 mg tablet (¢¢¢¢¢)
Kerlone 20 mg tablet ($$)
   Generic: betaxolol hydrochloride 20 mg tablet ($)
Betoptic S 0.25% ophthalmic suspension ($$$$$)
   Generic: betaxolol hydrochloride 0.25% ophthalmic suspension ($$$$$)

DOSING AND FOOD

Doses are taken 1 to 2 times a day.

This drug may be taken with or without food.

Adults: Up to 40 mg per day in divided doses.

Lower doses are used in children, people with kidney disease, and people over age 65.

Eyedrops: Usually 1 to 2 eyedrops are used per dose.

Forgotten doses: Take the forgotten dose as soon as you remember unless it is within 8 hours of the next scheduled dose.

ALCOHOL, DRUG, HERB, AND SUPPLEMENT INTERACTIONS

Alcohol may increase some of the side effects from this drug, depending on the amount consumed. Ask your doctor about the risks caused by drinking alcohol with your condition.

Several OTC drugs used for appetite control, asthma, colds, cough, hay fever, or sinus problems may cause an increase in blood pressure when taken with this drug. Check with your pharmacist when selecting OTC products.

Taking this drug with any of the ones listed below may change the effect of either drug with the possibility of causing toxicity or decreasing effectiveness:
aminophylline, anesthetics[†], antidiabetics[†], caffeine, calcium channel blockers[†], carbonic anhydrase inhibitors[†], clonidine, dyphylline, epinephrine, guanabenz, lidocaine, nonsteroidal antiinflammatories[†], oxtriphylline, pilocarpine, reserpine, theophylline

Severe reactions are possible when this drug is taken with those listed below:
allergy shots, beta blockers[†], cocaine, monoamine oxidase inhibitors[†]

Increased effects or side effects are possible when this drug is taken with those listed below:
antihypertensives[†]

ALLERGIC REACTIONS AND SIDE EFFECTS

If you are allergic to any other beta blockers[†], you may also be allergic to this drug.

[†] See page 52.   [*] See page 53.

This drug may exaggerate the reaction from your current allergies. Inform your doctor of any allergies that you have as well as the severity of the allergic reaction before starting this drug.

If using the eyedrops, your eyes may be more sensitive to sunlight.

MORE COMMON SIDE EFFECTS: Dizziness, drowsiness, lightheadedness*, sexual dysfunction, sleeping difficulty, tiredness, weakness

LESS COMMON SIDE EFFECTS: Anxiety, breathing difficulty*, cold hands and feet*, constipation, depression*, diarrhea, irregular heartbeat*, itching, nausea, nervousness, numbness, shortness of breath*, sore eyes, stomachache, stuffy nose, swelling, tingling, vivid dreams, vomiting, wheezing

RARE SIDE EFFECTS: Back pain*, bleeding*, bruising*, chest pain*, confusion*, dizziness*, fever*, hallucinations*, joint pain*, rash*, scaly skin*, sore throat*

PRECAUTIONS

People with asthma, heart disease, or a heart rate that is routinely less than 60 beats per minute (bradycardia) may not be able to take this drug.

Stopping this drug suddenly may cause chest pain or heart attack. If you wish to stop taking this drug, ask your doctor for specific instructions.

Be careful driving or handling equipment while taking this drug because the drug may cause drowsiness.

You need to wait 2 weeks after stopping a monoamine oxidase inhibitor† before starting this drug.

If you are diabetic, this drug may increase blood sugar levels or make the symptoms of low blood sugar less noticeable.

This drug may cause nondiabetics to develop type 2 diabetes.

If you have psoriasis or myasthenia gravis, this drug may make those conditions worse.

PREGNANCY AND BREAST-FEEDING

Safety during pregnancy has not been established although the drug is known to harm animal fetuses.

This drug passes into breast milk in an amount adequate to have an effect on the baby.

HELPFUL COMMENTS

It takes 7 to14 days for the full effect of this drug to be noticed.

Make sure you shake the ophthalmic suspension before use.

This drug may make you more sensitive to cold temperatures.

If you do not treat high blood pressure, you may develop more serious problems such as heart failure, blood vessel disease, stroke, or kidney disease. Losing weight, exercising, eating more fruits and vegetables, and avoiding salty foods, such as lunchmeat and pickles, may help make drug treatment more successful.

BETHANECHOL CHLORIDE

Available since May 1984

COMMONLY USED TO TREAT

Bladder problems

DRUG CATEGORY

urinary tract stimulant
Class: cholinergic agonist

PRODUCTS

Brand-Name Products with No Generic Alternative
Urecholine 5 mg tablet (¢¢¢¢)
Urecholine 10 mg tablet ($)
Urecholine 25 mg tablet ($$)
Urecholine 50 mg tablet ($$$)
No generics available.
No patents, no exclusivity.

DOSING AND FOOD

Doses are taken 2 to 4 times a day.
This drug should be taken on an empty stomach.
Adults: Up to 400 mg per day in divided doses.
Children: Up to 0.6 mg/kg per day in divided doses.
This drug is rarely used in children.
Forgotten doses: If more than 2 hours have passed since the forgotten dose, do not take the forgotten dose. Take your next dose at the scheduled time.

ALCOHOL, DRUG, HERB, AND SUPPLEMENT INTERACTIONS

Alcohol may increase some of the side effects from this drug, depending on the amount consumed. Ask your doctor about the risks caused by drinking alcohol with your condition.

---

† See page 52.   * See page 53.

Taking this drug with any of the ones listed below may change the effect of either drug with the possibility of causing toxicity or decreasing effectiveness: procainamide, quinidine

Severe reactions are possible when this drug is taken with those listed below: cholinergics†, cholinesterase inhibitors†, ganglionic blockers†

ALLERGIC REACTIONS AND SIDE EFFECTS

You should tell your doctor about all your allergies and any unexplained symptoms you may have while taking this drug.

MORE COMMON SIDE EFFECTS: Abdominal cramps, diarrhea

LESS COMMON SIDE EFFECTS: Belching, dizziness, fainting, frequent urination, headache, insomnia, lightheadedness, nausea, nervousness, salivation, seizures, skin irritation, vision changes, vomiting

RARE SIDE EFFECTS: Chest tightness*, shortness of breath*, wheezing*

PRECAUTIONS

If you have asthma, epilepsy, heart disease, intestinal blockage, low blood pressure, Parkinson's disease, stomach problems, or urination difficulty , this drug may make those conditions worse.

This drug may cause blood pressure to lower.

PREGNANCY AND BREAST-FEEDING

Safety during pregnancy has not been established although the drug is known to harm animal fetuses.

Breast-feeding while taking this drug is not recommended.

HELPFUL COMMENTS

Avoid quick movements to minimize dizziness. Dangling your legs over the side of the bed for a few minutes may help reduce dizziness when first waking up.

BEXAROTENE

Available since December 1999

COMMONLY USED TO PREVENT

Skin tumor growth

DRUG CATEGORY

antineoplastic

Class: retinoid

PRODUCTS

Brand-Name Products with No Generic Alternative
Targretin 75 mg capsule ($$$$$)
Targretin 1% topical gel ($$$$$)
No generics available.
Multiple patents that begin to expire in 2012.

DOSING AND FOOD

Doses are taken once a day.

Taking this drug with fatty foods will help increase absorption of the drug. Be careful not to eat too much fatty food. Grapefruit and grapefruit juice may cause erratic response to this drug and should be avoided. Do not eat raw oysters or other raw shellfish at any time while taking this drug.

Adults: Up to 400 mg/m^2 per day.

Lower doses are used in people with liver disease.

This drug is rarely used in children.

The topical gel should be applied in a thick layer making sure not to get the drug on the unaffected area.

Forgotten doses: If more than 12 hours have passed since the forgotten dose, do not take the dose. Otherwise take the forgotten dose as soon as you remember.

ALCOHOL, DRUG, HERB, AND SUPPLEMENT INTERACTIONS

Alcohol may increase the risk of liver damage from this drug. Ask your doctor about the risks caused by drinking alcohol with your condition.

Taking this drug with any of the ones listed below may change the effect of either drug with the possibility of causing toxicity or decreasing effectiveness: acetohexamide, chlorpropamide, erythromycin, glipizide, gemfibrozil, glimepiride, glyburide, insulin, itraconazole, ketoconazole, phenobarbital, phenytoin, pioglitazone, rifampin, rosiglitazone, tamoxifen, tolazamide, tolbutamide

Severe reactions are possible when this drug is taken with those listed below: acyclovir, alpha interferons, amphotericin B, analgesics†, antibiotics†, anticonvulsants†, antidiabetics†, antineoplastics†, antipsychotics†, antithyroid drugs†, azathioprine, captopril, chloramphenicol, colchicine, cyclophosphamide, enalapril, flecainide, flucytosine, ganciclovir, gold salts†, imipenem, lisinopril, maprotiline, penicillamine, pimozide, pro-

---

†*See page 52.* **See page 53.*

cainamide, promethazine, ramipril, sulfasalazine, tiopronin, tocainide, tricyclic antidepressants†, trimeprazine, zidovudine.

Increased side effects are possible when this drug is taken with those listed below: vitamin A

ALLERGIC REACTIONS AND SIDE EFFECTS

If you are allergic to other vitamin A preparations, you may also be allergic to this drug. You should tell your doctor about all your allergies and any unexplained symptoms you may have while taking this drug.

This drug promotes the effect of sunlight on the body and may cause severe sunburn and increased sensitivity of the eyes.

MORE COMMON SIDE EFFECTS: Abdominal pain, back pain*, chills*, cough*, diarrhea, difficulty urinating*, dry skin, fever*, hair loss, headache, hoarseness*, loss of appetite, mouth sores*, nausea, skin changes*, skin rash*, sleep disorders, swelling*, tiredness*, vomiting, weakness*, weight gain*

LESS COMMON SIDE EFFECTS: Shortness of breath*, yellow eyes or skin*

PRECAUTIONS

This drug may increase lipid and cholesterol levels and should not be used in people with pancreatitis, excessive alcohol use, uncontrolled hyperlipidemia, uncontrolled diabetes, or biliary tract disease.

Avoid contact with anyone who has the chickenpox, measles, or other communicable disease since it may be easier to catch the infection while taking this drug.

Exposure to skin tests, immunizations, and people who have received immunizations may put you at a greater risk of developing the disease when you are taking this drug.

If using this drug on your skin, do not use DEET-containing insect repellant.

This drug causes changes in your blood that put you at greater risk of getting an infection. Be careful not to cut yourself or get bruised. Tell your doctor if you develop signs of infection, such as fever or sore throat. Your dentist may recommend that you clean your teeth and mouth differently to avoid infection.

Do not get this drug in the mouth, eyes, nose, vagina, or rectum.

Capsules should not be crushed, opened, or broken.

PREGNANCY AND BREAST-FEEDING

This drug may cause birth defects and should not be used during pregnancy.

Men taking the drug should use a condom during intercourse. After stopping the drug, a condom should be used during intercourse for 1 month. Women of childbearing age are not usually given more than a 1-month supply of this drug and are required to have a monthly pregnancy test.

Breast-feeding while taking this drug is not recommended.

HELPFUL COMMENTS

The dose of this drug is usually adjusted after 8 weeks if the desired effect is not noticed.

Touching the insides of your nose or eyes may increase the risk of infection unless your hands have just been washed.

Wash your hands right after applying the topical gel.

BICALUTAMIDE

Available since October 1995

COMMONLY USED TO TREAT

Prostate cancer

DRUG CATEGORY

antineoplastic
Class: nonsteroidal antiandrogen

PRODUCTS

Brand-Name Products with No Generic Alternative
Casodex 50 mg tablet ($$$$$)
No generics available.
Patent expires in 2008.

DOSING AND FOOD

Doses are taken once a day.

This drug may be taken with or without food.

Men: Up to 50 mg per day.

Forgotten doses: If you are scheduled to take the next dose in less than 8 hours, do not take the forgotten dose. Otherwise take the forgotten dose as soon as you remember. If you vomit shortly after taking a dose, call your doctor to find out if the dose should be repeated.

ALCOHOL, DRUG, HERB, AND SUPPLEMENT INTERACTIONS

Alcohol may increase some of the side effects from this drug, depending

†*See page 52.*   **See page 53.*

on the amount consumed. Ask your doctor about the risks caused by drinking alcohol with your condition.

Taking this drug with any of the ones listed below may change the effect of either drug with the possibility of causing toxicity or decreasing effectiveness: anticoagulants†

ALLERGIC REACTIONS AND SIDE EFFECTS

If you are allergic to flutamide, or nilutamide, you may also be allergic to this drug. You should tell your doctor about all your allergies and any un-explained symptoms you may have while taking this drug.

MORE COMMON SIDE EFFECTS: Breast tenderness, breast swelling, chest tightness*, constipation, cough*, diarrhea, dizziness*, fever*, headache, hoarseness*, loss of appetite, loss of color vision, nausea, runny nose*, sexual dysfunction, sleep disorders, sneezing*, sore throat*, urinary difficulty, wheezing*

LESS COMMON SIDE EFFECTS: Bloating, bloody stools*, breathing difficulty*, chest pain*, confusion, depression*, drowsiness, dry mouth, gas, indigestion, itching*, nervousness, numbness*, pain*, shortness of breath*, skin rash*, swelling*, tingling*, tiredness*, vomiting, weakness*

RARE SIDE EFFECTS: Abdominal pain*, bleeding*, bruising*, dark urine*, skin irritation*, yellow eyes or skin*

PRECAUTIONS

People with liver disease may not be able to take this drug.

Be careful driving or handling equipment while taking this drug because it may cause dizziness.

PREGNANCY AND BREAST-FEEDING

This drug should not be used in women but, if necessary, should not be used during pregnancy. This drug may interfere with the normal development of a male fetus.

Breast-feeding while taking this drug is not recommended.

HELPFUL COMMENTS

This drug is usually given in combination with another hormone drug.

It is very important to continue taking this drug as ordered by the doctor even if the side effects make you feel ill.

Avoid quick movements to minimize dizziness. Dangling your legs over the side of the bed for a few minutes may help reduce dizziness when first waking up.

BIPERIDEN HYDROCHLORIDE

Available for over 20 years

COMMONLY USED TO TREAT

Irregular muscle tremors or jerking movement

DRUG CATEGORY

antidyskinetic
Class: anticholinergic

PRODUCTS

Brand-Name Products with No Generic Alternative
Akineton 2 mg tablet (¢¢¢)
No generics available.
No patents, no exclusivity.

DOSING AND FOOD

Doses are taken 1 to 4 times a day.
This drug should be taken with food to reduce the stomach upset that
  many people suffer.
Adults: Up to 16 mg per day in divided doses.
This drug is rarely used in children.
Forgotten doses: If you are scheduled to take the next dose within a few
  hours, do not take the forgotten dose. Otherwise take the forgotten dose
  as soon as you remember.

ALCOHOL, DRUG, HERB, AND SUPPLEMENT INTERACTIONS

Alcohol should not be used while taking this drug.
Many OTC drugs used for appetite control, asthma, colds, cough, hay
  fever, pain, or sinus problems affect the central nervous system and may
  change the effects or side effects of this drug. Check with your pharmacist for products to avoid.

**Taking this drug with any of the ones listed below may change the effect of
either drug with the possibility of causing toxicity or decreasing effectiveness:**
antacids, antidiarrheals, haloperidol, phenothiazines[†]

Increased side effects are possible when this drug is taken with those listed below:
amantadine, anesthetics, anticholinergics[†], antihistamines[†], anxiolytics[†],
  barbiturates[†], narcotics[†], tricyclic antidepressants[†]

[†]*See page 52.*   *See page 53.*

ALLERGIC REACTIONS AND SIDE EFFECTS

If you are allergic to other anticholinergics†, you may also be allergic to this drug. You should tell your doctor about all your allergies and any unexplained symptoms you may have while taking this drug.

This drug may cause your eyes to be more sensitive to sunlight, but there are no special risks associated with sunburn while taking this drug.

MORE COMMON SIDE EFFECTS: Blurry vision, constipation, decreased sweating, difficulty urinating, drowsiness, dry mouth*, nausea, sensitivity to light, vomiting

LESS COMMON SIDE EFFECTS: Dizziness, headache, lightheadedness, memory loss, muscle cramps, nervousness, numbness, sore mouth, stomachache, weakness

RARE SIDE EFFECTS: Confusion*, eye pain*, skin rash*

PRECAUTIONS

This drug may cause withdrawal symptoms if stopped suddenly. If you wish to stop taking this drug, ask your doctor for specific instructions.

People with glaucoma may not be able to take this drug.

Be careful driving or handling equipment while taking this drug because the drug may cause drowsiness.

This drug may cause dry mouth, which is associated with a greater risk of cavities. Your dentist may recommend that you clean your teeth and mouth differently to avoid infection.

This drug makes you sweat less, putting you at greater risk of developing heatstroke. Avoid exercising in hot weather and using hot tubs or saunas.

PREGNANCY AND BREAST-FEEDING

Safety during pregnancy has not been established although the drug is known to harm animal fetuses.

Breast-feeding while taking this drug is not recommended.

HELPFUL COMMENTS

You may only need to take this drug for a couple of weeks if you are using it to treat the side effects caused by another drug.

If you need to take an antacid, take it either 2 hours before or after taking this drug.

Sucking on hard sugarless candy or chewing sugarless gum may help relieve dry mouth caused by this drug.

BISOPROLOL FUMARATE

Available since July 1992

COMMONLY USED TO TREAT

High blood pressure, also known as hypertension

DRUG CATEGORY

antihypertensive
Class: beta blocker

PRODUCTS

Brand-Name Products with Generic Alternatives
Zebeta 5 mg tablet ($)
  Generic: bisoprolol fumarate 5 mg tablet ($)
Zebeta 10 mg tablet ($)
  Generic: bisoprolol fumarate 10 mg tablet ($)
Combination Products That Contain This Drug
Ziac tablet ($)

DOSING AND FOOD

Doses are given once a day.
This drug may be taken with or without food.
Adults: Up to 20 mg per day.
Lower doses are used in people with kidney disease, liver disease, and heart failure.
This drug is rarely used in children.
Forgotten doses: If you are scheduled to take the next dose within 8 hours, do not take the forgotten dose. Otherwise take the forgotten dose as soon as you remember.

ALCOHOL, DRUG, HERB, AND SUPPLEMENT INTERACTIONS

Alcohol may increase some of the side effects from this drug, depending on the amount consumed. Ask your doctor about the risks caused by drinking alcohol with your condition.
Several OTC drugs used for appetite control, asthma, colds, cough, hay fever, or sinus problems may cause an increase in blood pressure when taken with this drug. Check with your pharmacist when selecting OTC products.

---

† See page 52.   * See page 53.

Taking this drug with any of the ones listed below may change the effect of either drug with the possibility of causing toxicity or decreasing effectiveness: aminophylline, anesthetics, antidiabetics†, caffeine, calcium channel blockers†, carbonic anhydrase inhibitors†, clonidine, dyphylline, epinephrine, guanabenz, lidocaine, nonsteroidal antiinflammatories†, oxtriphylline, pilocarpine, reserpine, theophylline

Severe reactions are possible when this drug is taken with those listed below: allergy shots, beta blockers†, cocaine, monoamine oxidase inhibitors

Increased effects or side effects are possible when this drug is taken with those listed below:
antihypertensives†

ALLERGIC REACTIONS AND SIDE EFFECTS

If you are allergic to any other beta blockers†, you may also be allergic to this drug.

This drug may exaggerate the reaction from your current allergies. Inform your doctor of any allergies that you have as well as the severity of the allergic reaction before starting this drug.

MORE COMMON SIDE EFFECTS: Dizziness, drowsiness, lightheadedness*, sexual dysfunction, sleeping difficulty, tiredness, weakness

LESS COMMON SIDE EFFECTS: Anxiety, breathing difficulty*, cold hands and feet*, constipation, depression*, diarrhea, itching, nausea, nervousness, numbness, shortness of breath*, slow heartbeat*, sore eyes, stomachache, stuffy nose, swelling, tingling, vivid dreams, vomiting, wheezing

RARE SIDE EFFECTS: Back pain*, bleeding*, bruising*, chest pain*, confusion*, dark urine*, dizziness*, fever*, hallucinations*, irregular heartbeat*, joint pain*, rash*, scaly skin*, sore throat*, yellow eyes or skin*

PRECAUTIONS

People with asthma, heart disease, or a heart rate that is routinely less than 60 beats per minute (bradycardia) may not be able to take this drug.

Stopping this drug suddenly may cause chest pain or heart attack. If you wish to stop taking this drug, ask your doctor for specific instructions.

Be careful driving or handling equipment while taking this drug because the drug may cause drowsiness.

You need to wait 2 weeks after stopping a monoamine oxidase inhibitor† before starting this drug.

If you are diabetic, this drug may increase blood sugar levels or make the symptoms of low blood sugar less noticeable.

This drug may cause nondiabetics to develop type 2 diabetes.

If you have psoriasis or myasthenia gravis, this drug may make those conditions worse.

PREGNANCY AND BREAST-FEEDING

Safety during pregnancy has not been established although the drug is known to harm animal fetuses.

It is not known if this drug passes into breast milk. Talk to your doctor about the risks associated with breast-feeding while taking this drug.

HELPFUL COMMENTS

This drug may make you more sensitive to cold temperatures.

If you do not treat high blood pressure, you may develop more serious problems such as heart failure, blood vessel disease, stroke, or kidney disease. Losing weight, exercising, eating more fruits and vegetables, and avoiding salty foods, such as lunchmeat and pickles, may help make drug treatment more successful.

BOSENTAN

Available since November 2001

COMMONLY USED TO TREAT

High blood pressure that affects the lungs

DRUG CATEGORY

antihypertensive
Class: endothelin receptor antagonist

PRODUCTS

Brand-Name Products with No Generic Alternative
Tracleer 62.5 mg tablet ($$$$$)
Tracleer 125 mg tablet ($$$$$)
No generics available.
Exclusivity until 2006.

DOSING AND FOOD

Doses are taken 2 times a day.
This drug may be taken with or without food.
Adults: Up to 250 mg per day in divided doses.

---

† See page 52.   * See page 53.

Lower doses are used in adults weighing less than 88 pounds.

Forgotten doses: If you are scheduled to take the next dose within a few hours, do not take the forgotten dose. Otherwise take the forgotten dose as soon as you remember.

ALCOHOL, DRUG, HERB, AND SUPPLEMENT INTERACTIONS

Alcohol may increase the risk of liver damage from this drug. Ask your doctor about the risks caused by drinking alcohol with your condition.

Taking this drug with any of the ones listed below may change the effect of either drug with the possibility of causing toxicity or decreasing effectiveness: cyclosporine, hormone-based contraceptives, statins†

Severe reactions are possible when this drug is taken with those listed below: glyburide

ALLERGIC REACTIONS AND SIDE EFFECTS

You should tell your doctor about all your allergies and any unexplained symptoms you may have while taking this drug.

MORE COMMON SIDE EFFECTS: Blurry vision*, chills*, confusion*, dark urine*, dizziness*, faintness*, fever*, irregular heartbeat*, lightheadedness*, loss of appetite*, muscle aches, nausea*, pale stools*, runny nose, sore throat, stomach pain*, sweating*, swelling*, tiredness*, vomiting*, weakness*, yellow eyes or skin*

LESS COMMON SIDE EFFECTS: Belching, heartburn, indigestion, itching, sour stomach, stomachache

RARE SIDE EFFECTS: Headache*

PRECAUTIONS

People with liver disease may not be able to take this drug.

Blood tests should be drawn about every 3 months to ensure the safe use of this drug.

To avoid the rapid return of symptoms caused by your condition, this drug should be stopped slowly over 3 to 7 days. If you wish to stop taking this drug, ask your doctor for specific instructions.

Since this drug is still relatively new, ask your pharmacist about any additional precautions each time you get your prescription refilled.

PREGNANCY AND BREAST-FEEDING

This drug may cause birth defects and should not be used during pregnancy. Breast-feeding while taking this drug is not recommended.

HELPFUL COMMENTS

Hormonal contraceptives, including oral, implanted, and injectable forms, may not work properly when taking this drug. You need to use a barrier contraceptive, such as a condom, or other nonhormonal contraceptive to prevent pregnancy.

Monthly pregnancy tests are recommended while taking this drug.

BROMOCRIPTINE MESYLATE

Available for over 20 years

COMMONLY USED TO TREAT

Overactive pituitary gland
Parkinson's disease
Unusual bone growth in adults, also known as acromegaly
Women after pregnancy to stop the production of milk

DRUG CATEGORY

antidyskinetic
growth hormone suppressant
lactation inhibitor
Class: ergot alkaloid

PRODUCTS

Brand-Name Products with Generic Alternatives
Parlodel 5 mg capsule ($$$)
Brand-Name Products with Generic Alternatives
Parlodel 2.5 mg tablet ($$)
 Generic: bromocriptine mesylate 2.5 mg tablet ($$)

DOSING AND FOOD

Doses are given 1 to 6 times a day.
This drug should be taken with food to reduce the stomach upset that many people suffer.
Adults: Up to 100 mg per day in divided doses.
This drug should not be used in children under age 15.
Forgotten doses: If you are scheduled to take the next dose within 4 hours, do not take the forgotten dose. Otherwise take the forgotten dose as soon as you remember.

---

† See page 52.   * See page 53.

ALCOHOL, DRUG, HERB, AND SUPPLEMENT INTERACTIONS

Alcohol may increase some of the side effects from this drug, depending on the amount consumed. Ask your doctor about the risks caused by drinking alcohol with your condition.

Taking this drug with any of the ones listed below may change the effect of either drug with the possibility of causing toxicity or decreasing effectiveness: amitriptyline, antihypertensives†, butyrophenones, ergot alkaloids†, erythromycin, imipramine, methyldopa, oral contraceptives, phenothiazines†, reserpine, risperidone, ritonavir

ALLERGIC REACTIONS AND SIDE EFFECTS

You should tell your doctor about all your allergies and any unexplained symptoms you may have while taking this drug.

MORE COMMON SIDE EFFECTS: Dizziness, lightheadedness, nausea

LESS COMMON SIDE EFFECTS: Confusion*, constipation, depression, diarrhea, drowsiness, dry mouth, hallucinations*, leg cramps, spastic movements*, stomach pain*, stuffy nose, tingling, tiredness, vomiting*

RARE SIDE EFFECTS: Back pain*, black stools*, bloody vomit*, chest pain*, fainting*, fast heartbeat*, headache*, increased urination*, loss of appetite*, nervousness*, runny nose*, seizures*, shortness of breath*, sweating*, vision changes, weakness*

PRECAUTIONS

Be careful driving or handling equipment while taking this drug because the drug may cause drowsiness.

Drowsiness is common after the first dose of this drug. Make sure you are in a place where you may lie down when taking the first dose. About 1% of people have an irregular heartbeat for 15 to 60 minutes after the first dose. This reaction is not common with the next dose.

If you have a history of mental illness, this drug may make your condition worse.

PREGNANCY AND BREAST-FEEDING

Safety during pregnancy has not been established although there was no evidence of harm during studies in animals.

Breast-feeding while taking this drug is not recommended.

HELPFUL COMMENTS

It may take 6 to 8 weeks for breast milk to stop and menses to begin.

Sucking on hard sugarless candy or chewing sugarless gum may help relieve dry mouth caused by this drug.

If you do not wish to get pregnant, it is important to use a nonhormonal
form of contraception such as a condom or spermicide.

BUDESONIDE

Available since February 1994

COMMONLY USED TO TREAT

Breathing difficulty, specifically asthma
Inflammation of the nasal membranes, also known as rhinitis
Intestinal inflammation, specifically Crohn's disease

DRUG CATEGORY

antiinflammatory
Class: corticosteroid

PRODUCTS

Brand-Name Products with No Generic Alternative
Pulmicort Turbohaler powder for inhalation (¢¢¢¢)
Rhinocort Aqua 0.032 mg nasal aerosol ($$$$$)
Rhinocort 0.032 mg nasal spray ($$$$$)
Entocort EC 3 mg extended-release capsule ($$)
Pulmicort Respules 0.25 mg/2 ml suspension for inhalation ($$$$$)
Pulmicort Respules 0.5 mg/2 ml suspension for inhalation ($$$$$)
No generics available.
Multiple patents that began expiring in 2002.

DOSING AND FOOD

ORAL PRODUCTS
Doses are taken once a day.
This drug should be taken before breakfast.
Adults: Up to 9 mg per day.
The oral form of this drug is rarely used in children.
Lower doses are used in people with liver disease.
Forgotten doses: If you are scheduled to take the next dose within a few
hours, do not take the forgotten dose. Otherwise take the forgotten dose
as soon as you remember.

---

† See page 52.   * See page 53.

NASAL AEROSOL

Doses are taken 1 to 2 times a day.

Adults and children over age 12: Up to 4 sprays per day.

Children age 6 to 12: Up to 2 sprays per day.

NASAL SPRAY

Doses are taken 1 to 2 times a day.

Adults and children over age 6: Up to 4 sprays per day.

POWDER FOR INHALATION

Doses are taken 1 to 2 times a day.

Adults: Up to 8 inhalations.

Children: Up to 4 inhalations.

SUSPENSION FOR INHALATION

Doses are taken 1 to 2 times a day.

Children age 12 months to 8 years: Up to 1 mg per day.

ALCOHOL, DRUG, HERB, AND SUPPLEMENT INTERACTIONS

Alcohol may increase the risk of side effects from this drug, especially stomach problems. Ask your doctor about the risks caused by drinking alcohol with your condition.

Taking this drug with any of the ones listed below may change the effect of either drug with the possibility of causing toxicity or decreasing effectiveness: aminoglutethimide, antacids, anticoagulants†, antidiabetics†, barbiturates†, carbamazepine, cholestyramine, colestipol, diuretics†, estrogens†, griseofulvin, insulin, isoniazid, mitotane, phenylbutazone, phenytoin, primidone, rifampin, salicylates†, somatrem, somatropin

Severe reactions are possible when this drug is taken with those listed below: aspirin, amphotericin B, cardiac glycosides†, immunizations, nonsteroidal antiinflammatories†, ritodrine

ALLERGIC REACTIONS AND SIDE EFFECTS

If you are allergic to any corticosteroids†, you may also be allergic to this drug. You should tell your doctor about all your allergies and any unexplained symptoms you may have while taking this drug.

MORE COMMON SIDE EFFECTS: Headache, head growth, infection, nausea

LESS COMMON SIDE EFFECTS: Acne*, bloody stools*, breathing difficulty*, bruising*, dizziness, eye pain*, flushing, frequent urination*, hair growth*, hiccups, irregular heartbeat*, lightheadedness, menstrual problems*, muscle cramps*, red eyes*, skin discoloration, skin irritation*, sleeping difficulty*, spinning sensation, stomach pain*, stunted growth*, sweating, swelling*, tearing of eyes*, thirst*, tiredness*, vision changes*, vomiting*, weakness*, weight gain*, wounds that will not heal*

RARE SIDE EFFECTS: Confusion*, depression*, excitement*, hallucinations*, hives*, mood swings*, restlessness*, skin rash*

PRECAUTIONS

Avoid contact with anyone who has the chickenpox, measles, or other communicable disease since it may be easier to catch the infection while taking this drug.

Exposure to skin tests, immunizations, and people who have received immunizations may put you at a greater risk of developing the disease when you are taking this drug.

This drug may cause an increase in blood sugar or cholesterol level, calcium loss, and/or retention of fluid.

If you have osteoporosis, psychosis, heart disease, high blood pressure, glaucoma, kidney disease, or kidney stones, this drug may make those conditions worse.

Do not open, crush, or chew the extended-release capsules.

This drug may cause withdrawal symptoms if stopped suddenly. If you wish to stop taking this drug, ask your doctor for specific instructions.

A small amount of the inhaled drug is absorbed into the blood and may be associated with some of the same side effects as the oral product.

Children using this drug may have slow growth rates and should be checked regularly.

Handling and storage of inhalation products (both oral and nasal) are important to maintain the drug's effectiveness. Make sure to follow the instructions provided or ask your pharmacist about proper storage.

PREGNANCY AND BREAST-FEEDING

Safety during pregnancy has not been established although the drug is known to harm animal fetuses.

Breast-feeding while taking this drug while taking the oral form of this drug is not recommended.

HELPFUL COMMENTS

If you need to take an antacid, take it either 2 hours before or after taking this drug.

Your pharmacist may provide instructions for the use of your inhaler.

The oral form of this drug is usually given for only 8 weeks.

If you are already taking prednisolone for Crohn's disease, do not stop it

---

†See page 52.   *See page 53.

abruptly. The doctor should lower your dose gradually over at least 1 week to avoid withdrawal symptoms.

It may take 1 to 2 weeks or longer before seeing the effects of the inhaled drug.

You will see the nasal spray begin to work in about 10 hours.

BUMETANIDE

Available since February 1983

COMMONLY USED TO TREAT

Fluid retention, also known as edema
High blood pressure, also known as hypertension
High calcium levels, also known as hypercalcemia

DRUG CATEGORY

antihypercalcemic
antihypertensive
Class: loop diuretic

PRODUCTS

Brand-Name Products with Generic Alternatives
Bumex 0.5 mg tablet (¢¢¢)
  Generic: bumetanide 0.5 mg tablet (¢¢)
Bumex 1 mg tablet (¢¢¢¢)
  Generic: bumetanide 1 mg tablet (¢¢¢)
Bumex 2 mg tablet (¢¢¢¢¢)
  Generic: bumetanide 2 mg tablet (¢¢¢)

DOSING AND FOOD

Doses are given 1 to 3 times a day.

It is better to take this drug on an empty stomach, but taking this drug with food or milk may avoid the stomach upset that some people suffer.

Adults: Up to 10 mg per day in divided doses.

Children: Up to 0.1 mg/kg per day.

Forgotten doses: If you are scheduled to take the next dose within a few hours, do not take the forgotten dose. Otherwise take the forgotten dose as soon as you remember.

ALCOHOL, DRUG, HERB, AND SUPPLEMENT INTERACTIONS

Alcohol may increase some of the side effects from this drug, depending

on the amount consumed. Ask your doctor about the risks caused by
drinking alcohol with your condition.

Several OTC drugs used for appetite control, asthma, colds, cough, hay fever,
or sinus problems may cause an increase in blood pressure when taken
with this drug. Check with your pharmacist when selecting OTC products.

Dandelion and licorice root may both interfere with this drug.

**Taking this drug with any of the ones listed below may change the effect of
either drug with the possibility of causing toxicity or decreasing effectiveness:**
amiloride, amphotericin B, antihypertensives†, corticosteroids†, diuretics†,
indomethacin, lithium, probenecid, spironolactone, triamterene

ALLERGIC REACTIONS AND SIDE EFFECTS

You should tell your doctor about all your allergies and any unexplained
symptoms you may have while taking this drug.

MORE COMMON SIDE EFFECTS: Dizziness, lightheadedness

LESS COMMON SIDE EFFECTS: Blurry vision, chest pain, diarrhea, headache,
loss of appetite, premature ejaculation, sexual dysfunction, stomach
cramps

RARE SIDE EFFECTS: Back pain*, black stools*, bleeding*, bloody urine,
bruising*, chills*, cough*, dry mouth*, fever*, hearing loss*, hives*,
hoarseness*, irregular heartbeat*, joint pain*, mood swings*, muscle
cramps*, nausea*, painful urination*, ringing in ears*, skin rash*, stomach pain*, thirst*, tiredness*, vomiting*, weak pulse*, weakness*, yellow
eyes or skin*

PRECAUTIONS

If you are diabetic, you may need a change in the dose of your antidiabetic
drug or insulin, since this drug may cause changes in blood sugar.

Your body may lose potassium while taking this drug, which may cause severe side effects. Potassium levels should be monitored periodically and
may need to be supplemented while taking this drug. Eat food rich in potassium, such as apricots, bananas, citrus fruit, dates, and tomatoes, if you
are not taking a potassium supplement or potassium-sparing diuretic†

If you have gout, hearing problems, or pancreatitis, this drug may make
those conditions worse.

Be careful driving or handling equipment while taking this drug because
the drug may cause drowsiness.

Drink plenty of fluids to avoid dehydration when sweating, such as in hot
weather and during exercise.

†See page 52.   *See page 53.

PREGNANCY AND BREAST-FEEDING

Safety during pregnancy has not been established although the drug is known to harm animal fetuses.

Breast-feeding while taking this drug is not recommended.

HELPFUL COMMENTS

This drug will cause you to urinate. The effect should start about 30 minutes after taking the dose and will peak at about 2 hours.

This drug should be taken in the morning to reduce the chance of having to urinate during the night.

Short-term changes in your weight are a direct indication of how much fluid you are retaining. Weigh yourself daily to monitor your condition.

If you do not treat high blood pressure, you may develop more serious problems such as heart failure, blood vessel disease, stroke, or kidney disease. Losing weight, exercising, eating more fruits and vegetables, and avoiding salty foods, such as lunchmeat and pickles, may help make drug treatment more successful.

BUPROPION HYDROCHLORIDE

Available since December 1985

COMMONLY USED TO TREAT

Mental depression
People trying to stop smoking

DRUG CATEGORY

antidepressant
smoking cessation aid
Class: aminoketone

PRODUCTS

Brand-Name Products with No Generic Alternative
Wellbutrin SR 100 mg extended-release tablet ($$)
Wellbutrin SR 150 mg extended-release tablet ($$)
Wellbutrin SR 200 mg extended-release tablet (n/a)
Wellbutrin SR 50 mg extended-release tablet (n/a)
Zyban 150 mg extended-release tablet ($$)
Products with Generic Alternatives
Wellbutrin 75 mg tablet (¢¢¢¢¢)

Generic: bupropion hydrochloride 75 mg tablet (¢¢¢¢¢)
Wellbutrin 100 mg tablet ($)
   Generic: bupropion hydrochloride 100 mg tablet (¢¢¢¢¢)

DOSING AND FOOD

Doses are taken 1 to 3 times a day.

This drug should be taken with food to reduce the stomach upset that many people suffer.

Adults: Up to 450 mg per day in divided doses.

Lower doses are used in people with kidney disease, liver disease, and heart failure.

This drug is not used in children.

Forgotten doses: Do not take a forgotten dose. Just go back to your usual schedule with the next dose.

ALCOHOL, DRUG, HERB, AND SUPPLEMENT INTERACTIONS

Alcohol should not be used while taking this drug because it increases the risk of seizures.

Taking this drug with any of the ones listed below may change the effect of either drug with the possibility of causing toxicity or decreasing effectiveness: carbamazepine, cimetidine, orphenadrine, phenobarbital, phenylzine, phenytoin

Severe reactions are possible when this drug is taken with those listed below: alcohol, antidepressants†, antipsychotics†, benzodiazepines, corticosteroids†, fluoxetine, levodopa, lithium, maprotiline, monoamine oxidase inhibitors†, phenothiazines†, ritonavir, theophylline, trazodone

ALLERGIC REACTIONS AND SIDE EFFECTS

You should tell your doctor about all your allergies and any unexplained symptoms you may have while taking this drug.

This drug promotes the effect of sunlight on the body and may cause severe sunburn and increased sensitivity of the eyes.

MORE COMMON SIDE EFFECTS: Abdominal pain, agitation*, anxiety*, constipation, decreased appetite, dizziness, dry mouth, nausea, seizures*, shaking, sleep disturbances, sweating, trembling, vomiting, weight loss

LESS COMMON SIDE EFFECTS: Blurry vision, drowsiness, frequent urination, headache*, hives*, irregular heartbeat, itching*, muscle pain, ringing in ears*, skin rash*, sore throat, taste changes

---

†See page 52.   * See page 53.

RARE SIDE EFFECTS: Confusion*, denial*, fainting*, hallucinations*, poor concentration*

PRECAUTIONS

Do not open, crush, break, or chew the extended-release products.

The risk of seizures is increased in people with anorexia, brain tumors, bulimia, drug abuse, head injury, mental retardation, and a history of seizure disorders.

If you have high blood pressure, bipolar disease, or other emotional illness, this drug may make those conditions worse.

If taking the extended-release products, there should be at least 8 hours between each dose of this drug to minimize the risk of seizures.

If taking the regular-release products, there should be at least 4 hours between each dose of this drug to minimize the risk of seizures.

You need to wait 2 weeks after stopping a monoamine oxidase inhibitor† before starting this drug.

Be careful driving or handling equipment while taking this drug because the drug may cause drowsiness.

This drug may cause dry mouth, which is associated with a greater risk of cavities. Your dentist may recommend that you clean your teeth and mouth differently to avoid infection.

PREGNANCY AND BREAST-FEEDING

Safety during pregnancy has not been established although there was no evidence of harm during studies in animals.

Breast-feeding while taking this drug is not recommended.

HELPFUL COMMENTS

If taking this drug to help stop smoking, it should be started 1 week before you stop.

If this drug has not helped you stop smoking after 2 weeks of treatment (1 week after you stop smoking), then it should be stopped. If you do notice an effect, the drug is usually continued for 7 to 12 weeks.

It will take several weeks before you notice the effects of this drug on your depression.

If taking this drug for depression, you should continue treatment for at least 6 months to prevent relapse.

BUSPIRONE HYDROCHLORIDE

Available since September 1986

COMMONLY USED TO TREAT

Nervousness, also known as anxiety

DRUG CATEGORY

anxiolytic
Class: azaspirodemayedione derivative

PRODUCTS

Brand-Name Products with Generic Alternatives
BuSpar 5 mg tablet (¢¢¢¢¢)
  Generic: buspirone hydrochloride 5 mg tablet (¢¢¢¢¢)
BuSpar 10 mg tablet ($$)
  Generic: buspirone hydrochloride 10 mg tablet ($)
BuSpar 15 mg tablet ($$)
  Generic: buspirone hydrochloride 15 mg tablet ($$)
BuSpar 30 mg tablet ($$$)
  Generic: buspirone hydrochloride 30 mg tablet ($$$)
Products Only Available as Generics
buspirone hydrochloride 7.5 mg tablet ($)

DOSING AND FOOD

Doses are taken 2 to 3 times a day.
It is best to take this drug with food or milk. Do not take this drug with
  grapefruit juice.
Adults: Up to 60 mg per day in divided doses.
Lower doses are used in people with kidney disease or liver disease.
This drug is not used in children.
Forgotten doses: If you are scheduled to take the next dose within a few
  hours, do not take the forgotten dose. Otherwise take the forgotten dose
  as soon as you remember.

ALCOHOL, DRUG, HERB, AND SUPPLEMENT INTERACTIONS

Alcohol should not be used while taking this drug.

**Taking this drug with any of the ones listed below may change the effect of
either drug with the possibility of causing toxicity or decreasing effectiveness:**
digoxin, erythromycin, haloperidol, itraconazole

†See page 52.   * See page 53.

Severe reactions are possible when this drug is taken with those listed below: monoamine oxidase inhibitors†

Increased side effects are possible when this drug is taken with those listed below: anesthetics, antihistamines†, anxiolytics†, barbiturates†, narcotics†, tricyclic antidepressants†

ALLERGIC REACTIONS AND SIDE EFFECTS

You should tell your doctor about all your allergies and any unexplained symptoms you may have while taking this drug.

MORE COMMON SIDE EFFECTS: Dizziness, excitement, headache, lightheadedness, nausea, nervousness, restlessness

LESS COMMON SIDE EFFECTS: Blurry vision, cramps, diarrhea, drowsiness, dry mouth, nightmares, muscle pain, poor concentration, ringing in ears, sleeping difficulty, stiffness, sweating, tiredness, vivid dreams, weakness

RARE SIDE EFFECTS: Chest pain*, confusion*, depression*, fast heartbeat*, fever*, hives*, numbness*, pain*, skin rash*, sore throat*, spastic movements*, stiffness*, tingling*, weakness*

PRECAUTIONS

Be careful driving or handling equipment while taking this drug because the drug may cause drowsiness.

You need to wait 2 weeks after stopping a monoamine oxidase inhibitor† before starting this drug.

PREGNANCY AND BREAST-FEEDING

Safety during pregnancy has not been established although there was no evidence of harm during studies in animals.

Breast-feeding while taking this drug is not recommended.

HELPFUL COMMENTS

Some people begin to see the effect of this drug in 7 to 10 days, while others do not see the effects for 3 to 4 weeks.

BUSULFAN

Available for over 20 years

COMMONLY USED TO TREAT

Changes in the bone marrow
Myelogenous leukemia

DRUG CATEGORY

antineoplastic
Class: alkylating agent

PRODUCTS

Brand-Name Products with No Generic Alternative
Myleran 2 mg tablet ($$)
No generics available.
No patents, no exclusivity.

DOSING AND FOOD

Doses are taken twice a week to once a day.
This drug may be taken with or without food. Do not eat raw oysters or
other raw shellfish at any time while taking this drug.
Adults: Up to 12 mg per day.
Children: Up to 0.12 mg/kg per day.
Forgotten doses: Do not take a forgotten dose. Just go back to your usual
schedule with the next dose. It is important to take this drug at the same
time each day.

ALCOHOL, DRUG, HERB, AND SUPPLEMENT INTERACTIONS

Alcohol may increase some of the side effects from this drug, depending
on the amount consumed. Ask your doctor about the risks caused by
drinking alcohol with your condition.

Taking this drug with any of the ones listed below may change the effect of
either drug with the possibility of causing toxicity or decreasing effectiveness:
acetaminophen, acyclovir, antibiotics†, anticonvulsants†, antidiabetics†, anti-
neoplastics†, antipsychotics†, antithyroid drugs†, auranofin, azathioprine,
captopril, carbamazepine, chloramphenicol, colchicine, cyclophosphamide,
enalapril, flecainide, flucytosine, ganciclovir, interferon, itraconazole, lisino-
pril, maprotiline, mercaptopurine, methotrexate, nonnarcotic antiinflamma-
tories†, penicillamine, pimozide, plicamycin, procainamide, promethazine,
ramipril, sulfasalazine, tocainide, tricyclic antidepressants†, trimeprazine,
zidovudine

Severe reactions are possible when this drug is taken with those listed below:
probenecid, sulfinpyrazone

Increased side effects are possible when this drug is taken with those listed below:
aspirin

---

† See page 52.   * See page 53.

ALLERGIC REACTIONS AND SIDE EFFECTS

You should tell your doctor about all your allergies and any unexplained symptoms you may have while taking this drug.

MORE COMMON SIDE EFFECTS: Abdominal pain*, anxiety, back pain*, black stools*, bleeding*, bloody urine*, bruising*, chills*, cough*, diarrhea, fatigue, fever*, headache, hoarseness*, irregular menstruation, loss of appetite, muscle pain, nausea, painful urination*, skin irritation*, skin rash*, sleeping difficulty, swelling*, vomiting, weight loss

LESS COMMON SIDE EFFECTS: Bloody nose, chest pain*, confusion, constipation, decreased blood pressure*, depression, dizziness*, dry mouth, irregular breathing*, itching, joint pain*, lightheadedness*, rapid heartbeat*, runny nose, skin discoloration, sneezing, sore throat, stuffy nose, sweating*, swelling*, tingling*

RARE SIDE EFFECTS: Bloody vomit*, blurry vision*, heartburn*, swallowing difficulty*

PRECAUTIONS

If you have gout, kidney stones, or a history of seizures, this drug may make those conditions worse.

Avoid contact with anyone who has the chickenpox, measles, or other communicable disease since it may be easier to catch the infection while taking this drug.

Exposure to skin tests, immunizations, and people who have received immunizations may put you at a greater risk of developing the disease when you are taking this drug.

This drug causes changes in your blood that put you at greater risk of getting an infection. Be careful not to cut yourself or get bruised. Tell your doctor if you develop signs of infection, such as fever or sore throat. Your dentist may recommend that you clean your teeth and mouth differently to avoid infection.

PREGNANCY AND BREAST-FEEDING

There is evidence that this drug may harm the fetus, but the drug may be necessary to the health of the mother.

Breast-feeding while taking this drug is not recommended.

HELPFUL COMMENTS

Drinking extra water while taking this drug may help prevent kidney problems.

This drug may cause vomiting soon after taking a dose. Check with your doctor to find out if you should repeat the dose if you vomit.

Touching these tablets may cause skin irritation. You should wash your hands immediately after taking the dose.

The effects of this drug are usually noticed after 2 weeks of treatment.

You may have side effects from this drug for 4 to 6 months after it is stopped.

BUTABARBITAL SODIUM

Available for over 20 years

COMMONLY USED TO TREAT

Sleeping difficulty, also known as insomnia

DRUG CATEGORY

sedative-hypnotic
Class: barbiturate

PRODUCTS

Brand-Name Products with No Generic Alternative
Butisol Sodium 50 mg tablet ($)
Butisol Sodium 30 mg/5 ml oral elixir ($$)

Brand-Name Products with Generic Alternatives
Butisol Sodium 30 mg tablet ($)
  Generic: butabarbital sodium 30 mg tablet (n/a)

Products Only Available as Generics
butabarbital sodium 16.2 mg tablet (n/a)
butabarbital sodium 32.4 mg tablet (n/a)

DOSING AND FOOD

Doses are taken 1 to 4 times a day.

It is best to take this drug on an empty stomach with a full glass of water at least 1 hour before meals or 2 hours after a meal.

Adults: Up to 120 mg per day in divided doses.

Children: Up to 6 mg/kg (maximum 100 mg) per day in divided doses.

Forgotten doses: Do not take a forgotten dose. Just go back to your usual schedule with the next dose.

---

† See page 52.   * See page 53.

ALCOHOL, DRUG, HERB, AND SUPPLEMENT INTERACTIONS

Alcohol should not be used while taking this drug.

Several OTC drugs used for appetite control, asthma, colds, cough, hay fever, pain, or sinus problems may seriously increase the side effects of this drug. Check with your pharmacist when selecting OTC products.

Taking this drug with any of the ones listed below may change the effect of either drug with the possibility of causing toxicity or decreasing effectiveness: anticoagulants†, carbamazepine, corticosteroids†, corticotropin, divalproex sodium, oral contraceptives, valproic acid

Increased side effects are possible when this drug is taken with those listed below: anesthetics, antihistamines†, anxiolytics†, barbiturates†, narcotics†, tricyclic antidepressants†

ALLERGIC REACTIONS AND SIDE EFFECTS

Allergic reactions are more likely to occur in people with a history of asthma or allergies to other drugs. You should tell your doctor about all your allergies and any unexplained symptoms you may have while taking this drug.

MORE COMMON SIDE EFFECTS: Clumsiness, dizziness, drowsiness, lightheadedness, unsteadiness

LESS COMMON SIDE EFFECTS: Anxiety, confusion*, constipation, depression*, excitement*, fainting, headache, irritability, nausea, nervousness, sleep disorders, vomiting

RARE SIDE EFFECTS: Bleeding*, bone pain*, bruising*, chest pain*, chest tightness*, fever*, hallucinations*, hives*, loss of appetite*, mouth sores*, muscle pain*, skin rash*, sore throat*, swelling*, tiredness*, weakness*, weight loss*, wheezing*, yellow eyes or skin*

PRECAUTIONS

Be careful driving or handling equipment while taking this drug because the drug may cause dizziness and drowsiness.

If you have anemia, asthma, high blood sugar, hyperactivity, depression, thyroid problems, liver disease, kidney disease, or porphyria, this drug may make those conditions worse.

This drug may be habit forming when taken for a long time. It should be stopped slowly to avoid withdrawal symptoms. It may take 2 weeks for the body to adjust after the drug is stopped.

PREGNANCY AND BREAST-FEEDING

There is evidence that this drug may harm the fetus, but the drug may be necessary to the health of the mother.

This drug passes into breast milk, and may cause drowsiness, slow heartbeat, and breathing difficulty in the baby.

HELPFUL COMMENTS

If used regularly for more than 2 weeks, this drug may lose the ability to make you sleep.

Oral contraceptives may not work properly when taken with this drug. You need to use a barrier contraceptive, such as a condom, or other nonhormonal contraceptive to prevent pregnancy.

This drug has a calming effect and is also used to treat anxiety.

You may need to increase the fiber in your diet since this drug may cause constipation.

This drug is often confused with butalbital, which is a different drug in the same category with similar effects.

CANDESARTAN CILEXETIL

Available since June 1998

COMMONLY USED TO TREAT

High blood pressure, also known as hypertension

DRUG CATEGORY

antihypertensive
Class: angiotensin II receptor antagonist

PRODUCTS

Brand-Name Products with No Generic Alternative
Atacand 4 mg tablet ($)
Atacand 8 mg tablet ($)
Atacand 16 mg tablet ($)
Atacand 32 mg tablet ($$)
No generics available.
Multiple patents that begin to expire in 2011.

Combination Products That Contain This Drug
Atacand HCT tablet ($$)

---

†*See page 52.* **See page 53.*

DOSING AND FOOD

Doses are taken 1 to 2 times a day.

This drug may be taken with or without food.

Adults: Up to 32 mg per day in divided doses.

This drug is rarely used in children.

Forgotten doses: If you are scheduled to take the next dose within a few hours, do not take the forgotten dose. Otherwise take the forgotten dose as soon as you remember.

ALCOHOL, DRUG, HERB, AND SUPPLEMENT INTERACTIONS

Alcohol may increase some of the side effects from this drug, depending on the amount consumed. Ask your doctor about the risks caused by drinking alcohol with your condition.

Several OTC drugs used for appetite control, asthma, colds, cough, hay fever, or sinus problems may cause an increase in blood pressure when taken with this drug. Check with your pharmacist when selecting OTC products.

Taking this drug with any of the ones listed below may change the effect of either drug with the possibility of causing toxicity or decreasing effectiveness: diuretics†

ALLERGIC REACTIONS AND SIDE EFFECTS

You should tell your doctor about all your allergies and any unexplained symptoms you may have while taking this drug.

Less Common Side Effects: Back pain*, congestion, cough, ear pain, fever*, headache, sneezing, sore throat, stuffy nose

Rare Side Effects: Bleeding gums, chills*, cough*, dizziness*, fainting*, hoarseness*, joint pain*, lightheadedness*, nosebleeds*, painful urination*, swelling*

PRECAUTIONS

If you are dehydrated, the blood-pressurer-lowering effect of this drug may be increased. Drink plenty of fluids to avoid dehydration when sweating, such as in hot weather and during exercise.

Be careful driving or handling equipment while taking this drug because the drug may cause drowsiness.

If you have kidney disease, this drug may make that condition worse.

PREGNANCY AND BREAST-FEEDING

There is evidence that this drug may harm the fetus, but the drug may be
  necessary to the health of the mother.
Breast-feeding while taking this drug is not recommended.

HELPFUL COMMENTS

It may take 4 to 6 weeks before the full effects of this drug are noticed.
If you do not treat high blood pressure, you may develop more serious
  problems such as heart failure, blood vessel disease, stroke, or kidney
  disease. Losing weight, exercising, eating more fruits and vegetables,
  and avoiding salty foods, such as lunchmeat and pickles, may help make
  drug treatment more successful.

CAPECITABINE

Available since April 1998

COMMONLY USED TO TREAT

Breast cancer
Colorectal cancer

DRUG CATEGORY

antineoplastic
Class: antimetabolite

PRODUCTS

Brand-Name Products with No Generic Alternative
Xeloda 150 mg tablet ($$$)
Xeloda 500 mg tablet ($$$$)
No generics available.
Multiple patents that begin to expire in 2011.

DOSING AND FOOD

Doses are taken twice a day.
This drug should be taken with a full glass of water within 30 minutes of
  finishing breakfast and dinner. Do not eat raw oysters or other raw shell-
  fish at any time while taking this drug.
Adults: Up to 2,500 mg/m^2 per day in divided doses.
Lower doses are used in children and people with kidney disease.

---

† See page 52.   * See page 53.

Forgotten doses: Do not take a forgotten dose. Just go back to your usual schedule with the next dose.

ALCOHOL, DRUG, HERB, AND SUPPLEMENT INTERACTIONS

Alcohol may increase some of the side effects from this drug, depending on the amount consumed. Ask your doctor about the risks caused by drinking alcohol with your condition.

Taking this drug with any of the ones listed below may change the effect of either drug with the possibility of causing toxicity or decreasing effectiveness: amphotericin B, antacids, antithyroid drugs†, azathioprine, chloramphenicol, colchicine, flucytosine, ganciclovir, interferon, leucovorin, plicamycin, zidovudine

Severe reactions are possible when this drug is taken with those listed below: anticoagulants†, folic acid

ALLERGIC REACTIONS AND SIDE EFFECTS

If you are allergic to 5-fluorouracil, you may also be allergic to this drug. You should tell your doctor about all your allergies and any unexplained symptoms you may have while taking this drug.

This drug promotes the effect of sunlight on the body and may cause severe sunburn and increased sensitivity of the eyes.

MORE COMMON SIDE EFFECTS: Changes to the bottoms of feet*, changes to the palms of hands*, constipation*, diarrhea*, loss of appetite, mouth sores*, nausea*, stomachache*, vomiting*

LESS COMMON SIDE EFFECTS: Blood pressure changes*, clumsiness*, dark urine*, dizziness, headache, heartburn, insomnia, itching*, muscle pain, nosebleeds*, pale stools*, poor coordination*, skin rash*, sore eyes, swollen glands*, unsteadiness*

RARE SIDE EFFECTS: Abdominal pain*, back pain*, bleeding*, bloody stools*, bloody urine*, bloody vomit*, breathing diffiulty*, bruising*, chest pain*, chest tightness*, chills*, cough*, difficulty urinating*, fever*, hoarseness*, irregular heartbeat*, shortness of breath*, skin irritation*, sneezing*, sore throat*, stomach cramps*, stuffy nose*, swallowing difficulty*, swelling*, tiredness*, weakness*, wheezing*, white spots in mouth*, yellow eyes or skin*

PRECAUTIONS

Avoid contact with anyone who has the chickenpox, measles, or other communicable disease since it may be easier to catch the infection while taking this drug.

Exposure to skin tests, immunizations, and people who have received immunizations may put you at a greater risk of developing the disease when you are taking this drug.

This drug may cause changes to the blood resulting in an increased risk of blood-clotting problems.

Touching these tablets may cause skin irritation. You should wash your hands immediately after taking the dose.

This drug causes changes in your blood that put you at greater risk of getting an infection. Be careful not to cut yourself or get bruised. Tell your doctor if you develop signs of infection, such as fever or sore throat. Your dentist may recommend that you clean your teeth and mouth differently to avoid infection.

PREGNANCY AND BREAST-FEEDING

There is evidence that this drug may harm the fetus, but the drug may be necessary to the health of the mother.

Breast-feeding while taking this drug is not recommended.

HELPFUL COMMENTS

This drug is usually taken for 2 weeks followed by 1 week without the drug. The 3-week cycles are then repeated.

This drug is converted by the body to 5-fluorouracil, another cancer drug.

If you need to take an antacid, take it either 2 hours before or after taking this drug.

It is very important to continue taking this drug as ordered by the doctor even if the side effects make you feel ill.

CAPTOPRIL

Available for over 20 years

COMMONLY USED TO TREAT

High blood pressure, also known as hypertension

DRUG CATEGORY

antihypertensive
Class: ACE inhibitor

---

†See page 52.   *See page 53.

PRODUCTS

Brand-Name Products with Generic Alternatives
Capoten 12.5 mg tablet (¢¢¢¢¢)
  Generic: captopril 12.5 mg tablet (¢¢)
Capoten 25 mg tablet ($)
  Generic: captopril 25 mg tablet (¢)
Capoten 50 mg tablet ($$)
  Generic: captopril 50 mg tablet (¢)
Capoten 100 mg tablet ($$)
  Generic: captopril 100 mg tablet ($)
Combination Products That Contain This Drug
Capozide tablet ($) to ($$)

DOSING AND FOOD

Doses are taken 2 to 3 times a day.
It is best to take this drug on an empty stomach at least 1 hour before meals.
Adults: Up to 450 mg per day in divided doses.
Lower doses are used in people with kidney disease and people over age 65.
Forgotten doses: If you are scheduled to take the next dose within a few
  hours, do not take the forgotten dose. Otherwise take the forgotten dose
  as soon as you remember.

ALCOHOL, DRUG, HERB, AND SUPPLEMENT INTERACTIONS

Alcohol may cause your blood pressure to rise, making this drug less effective. Ask your doctor about the risks caused by drinking alcohol with
  your condition.
Black catechu should not be used with this drug because of an increased
  risk of lowering the blood pressure too much.
Licorice may interfere with the effects of this drug.
Capsaicin increases the risk of developing a cough and should not be taken
  at the same time as this drug.
Several OTC drugs used for appetite control, asthma, colds, cough, hay fever,
  or sinus problems may cause an increase in blood pressure when taken
  with this drug. Check with your pharmacist when selecting OTC products.
**Taking this drug with any of the ones listed below may change the effect of
either drug with the possibility of causing toxicity or decreasing effectiveness:**
antacids, antidiabetics†, antihypertensives†, digoxin, diuretics†, insulin,
  lithium, nonsteroidal antiinflammatories†, potassium supplements, salt
  substitutes

ALLERGIC REACTIONS AND SIDE EFFECTS

If you are allergic to any ACE inhibitors†, you may also be allergic to this drug. You should tell your doctor about all your allergies and any unexplained symptoms you may have while taking this drug.

MORE COMMON SIDE EFFECTS: Dry cough, headache

LESS COMMON SIDE EFFECTS: Diarrhea, dizziness*, fainting*, fever*, joint pain*, lightheadedness*, loss of taste, nausea*, skin rash*, tiredness

RARE SIDE EFFECTS: Abdominal pain*, breathing difficulty*, chest pain*, chills*, confusion*, hoarseness*, irregular heartbeat*, itching*, nausea*, nervousness*, numbness*, stomach pain*, swallowing difficulty*, swelling*, vomiting*, weakness*, yellow eyes or skin*

PRECAUTIONS

Be careful driving or handling equipment while taking this drug because the drug may cause drowsiness.

People with systemic lupus erythematosus may be at greater risk of developing blood problems while taking this drug.

Do not use potassium-containing products, including salt substitutes, while taking this drug.

Diuretics† should be stopped 2 to 3 days prior to starting this drug. If it is not possible to stop the diuretic, the dose of this drug should be lowered.

Drink plenty of fluids to avoid dehydration when sweating, such as in hot weather and during exercise.

PREGNANCY AND BREAST-FEEDING

Safety during pregnancy has not been established although the drug is known to harm animal fetuses.

Breast-feeding while taking this drug is not recommended.

HELPFUL COMMENTS

It may take several weeks before the full effects of this drug are noticed.

A persistent dry cough may appear while taking this drug, but it will go away when the drug is stopped.

If you need to take an antacid, take it either 2 hours before or after taking this drug.

Avoid quick movements to minimize dizziness. Dangling your legs over the side of the bed for a few minutes may help reduce dizziness when first waking up.

If you do not treat high blood pressure, you may develop more serious

---

† See page 52.   * See page 53.

problems such as heart failure, blood vessel disease, stroke, or kidney disease. Losing weight, exercising, eating more fruits and vegetables, and avoiding salty foods, such as lunchmeat and pickles, may help make drug treatment more successful.

CARBAMAZEPINE

Available for over 20 years

COMMONLY USED TO TREAT

Explosive outbursts
Pain in the nerves, also known as neuralgia
Seizures, also known as convulsions

DRUG CATEGORY

anticonvulsant
antineuralgic
Class: iminostilbene derivative

PRODUCTS

Brand-Name Products with No Generic Alternative
Carbatrol 100 mg extended-release capsule (n/a)
Carbatrol 200 mg extended-release capsule (¢¢¢¢)
Carbatrol 300 mg extended-release capsule (¢¢¢¢)
Tegretol-XR 100 mg extended-release capsule (¢¢)
Tegretol-XR 200 mg extended-release capsule (¢¢¢¢)
Tegretol-XR 400 mg extended-release capsule ($)
No generic extended-release product available.
Multiple patents that begin to expire in 2007.

Brand-Name Products with Generic Alternatives
Tegretol 200 mg tablet (¢¢¢¢)
  Generic: carbamazepine 200 mg tablet (¢¢)
Tegretol 100 mg chewable tablet (¢¢¢)
  Generic: carbamazepine 100 mg chewable tablet (¢¢)
Tegretol 100 mg/5 ml oral suspension (¢¢¢)
  Generic: carbamazepine 100 mg/5 ml oral suspension (¢¢¢)

Products Only Available as Generics
carbamazepine 200 mg chewable tablet (n/a)

Other Generic Product Names
Epitol

DOSING AND FOOD

Doses are taken 2 to 4 times a day. Extended-release products are taken twice a day.

It is best to take this drug with food.

Adults: Up to 1,600 mg per day in divided doses.

Children over age 15: Up to 1,200 mg per day in divided doses.

Children under age 6: Up to 35 mg/kg per day in divided doses.

Forgotten doses: If you are scheduled to take the next dose within a few hours, do not take the forgotten dose. Otherwise take the forgotten dose as soon as you remember.

ALCOHOL, DRUG, HERB, AND SUPPLEMENT INTERACTIONS

Alcohol may decrease the effects of this drug and should not be used.

Plantain and psyllium seed interfere with the absorption of this drug.

Many OTC drugs used for appetite control, asthma, colds, cough, hay fever, pain, or sinus problems affect the central nervous system and may interfere with this drug. Check with your pharmacist for products to avoid.

Taking this drug with any of the ones listed below may change the effect of either drug with the possibility of causing toxicity or decreasing effectiveness: anticonvulsants†, cimetidine, corticosteroids†, danazol, diltiazem, doxycycline, estrogens†, felbamate, fluoxetine, fluvoxamine, haloperidol, isoniazid, itraconazole, ketoconazole, macrolides†, oral contraceptives, phenobarbital, phenytoin, primidone, propoxyphene, quinidine, risperidone, theophylline, tricyclic antidepressants†, valproic acid, verapamil, warfarin

Severe reactions are possible when this drug is taken with those listed below: lithium, monoamine oxidase inhibitors†

ALLERGIC REACTIONS AND SIDE EFFECTS

You should tell your doctor about all your allergies and any unexplained symptoms you may have while taking this drug.

This drug promotes the effect of sunlight on the body and may cause severe sunburn and increased sensitivity of the eyes.

MORE COMMON SIDE EFFECTS: Clumsiness, dizziness, drowsiness, eye movements*, lightheadedness, nausea*, unsteadiness, vision changes*, vomiting

LESS COMMON SIDE EFFECTS: Agitation*, behavior changes*, confusion*, constipation, diarrhea*, drowsiness*, dry mouth, hair loss, headache*, hives*, hostility*, itching*, joint aches, loss of appetite, mouth irritation,

---

† See page 52.   * See page 53.

muscle aches, sexual dysfunction, skin rash*, stomach pain, sweating, vomiting*

RARE SIDE EFFECTS: Back pain*, black stools*, bleeding*, bloody urine*, bone pain*, breathing difficulty*, bruising*, chest pain*, chest tightness, chills*, cough*, dark urine*, depression*, fainting*, fever*, hallucinations*, hoarseness*, irregular heartbeat*, mood swings*, mouth sores*, muscle cramps*, nervousness*, nosebleeds*, numbness*, pale stools*, restlessness*, rigidity*, ringing in ears*, shortness of breath*, skin irritation*, slurry speech*, sore throat*, stomach cramps*, swelling*, swollen glands*, tingling*, tiredness*, trembling*, uncontrolled body movements*, urinary changes*, weakness*, weight gain*, wheezing*, yellow eyes or skin*

PRECAUTIONS

Carbatrol extended-release products are specially formulated so the capsules may be opened and the contents sprinkled over food. Do not crush, break, or chew the pellets inside the extended-release products.

Be careful driving or handling equipment while taking this drug because the drug may cause drowsiness.

If you have anemia, behavioral disorders, glaucoma, heart disease, or difficulty urinating, this drug may make those conditions worse.

You need to wait 2 weeks after stopping a monoamine oxidase inhibitor† before starting this drug.

The effects of this drug do not continue after the drug is stopped. If you are taking the drug for seizures, talk to your doctor about a gradual decrease in dosage.

PREGNANCY AND BREAST-FEEDING

There is evidence that this drug may harm the fetus, but the drug may be necessary to the health of the mother.

Breast-feeding while taking this drug is not recommended.

HELPFUL COMMENTS

Oral contraceptives may not work properly when taken with this drug. You need to use a barrier contraceptive, such as a condom, or other nonhormonal contraceptive to prevent pregnancy.

Children are more likely to have behavior changes than adults. People over age 65 are more likely to develop confusion and agitation.

CARBENICILLIN INDANYL SODIUM

Available for over 20 years

COMMONLY USED TO TREAT

Infection

DRUG CATEGORY

antibiotic
Class: extended spectrum penicillin

PRODUCTS

Brand-Name Products with No Generic Alternative
Geocillin 382 mg tablet ($$)
No generics available.
No patents, no exclusivity.

DOSING AND FOOD

Doses are taken 4 times a day.
This drug works best if taken on an empty stomach with a full glass of water, but taking it with food may avoid the stomach upset that some people suffer.
Adults: Up to 4 g per day in divided doses.
Lower doses may be used in children.
Forgotten doses: If you are scheduled to take the next dose within a few hours, do not take the forgotten dose. Otherwise take the forgotten dose as soon as you remember.

ALCOHOL, DRUG, HERB, AND SUPPLEMENT INTERACTIONS

Alcohol may increase some of the side effects from this drug, depending on the amount consumed. Ask your doctor about the risks caused by drinking alcohol with your condition.

Taking this drug with any of the ones listed below may change the effect of either drug with the possibility of causing toxicity or decreasing effectiveness: chloramphenicol, erythromycins†, methotrexate, probenecid, sulfonamides†, tetracyclines†

Severe reactions are possible when this drug is taken with those listed below: anticoagulants†, dipyridamole, divalproex, heparin, nonnarcotic anti-inflammatories†, pentoxifylline, plicamycin, sulfinpyrazone, valproic acid

---

† *See page 52.*   * *See page 53.*

ALLERGIC REACTIONS AND SIDE EFFECTS

If you are allergic to any penicillins† or cephalosporins†, you may also be allergic to this drug. You should tell your doctor about all your allergies and any unexplained symptoms you may have while taking this drug.

MORE COMMON SIDE EFFECTS: Headache, diarrhea*, mouth sores*, vaginal discharge, vaginal itching

LESS COMMON SIDE EFFECTS: Fainting*, fever*, hives*, irregular breathing*, itching*, joint pain*, lightheadedness*, scaly skin*, shortness of breath*, skin rash*, swelling*

RARE SIDE EFFECTS: Abdominal pain*, bleeding*, bruising*, decreased urine output, depression*, nausea*, seizures*, sore throat*, stomach cramps*, vomiting*, yellow eyes or skin*

PRECAUTIONS

If you have a history of stomach or intestinal disease, you may be at greater risk of developing colitis while taking this drug. Tell your doctor if you get severe or watery diarrhea.

PREGNANCY AND BREAST-FEEDING

Safety during pregnancy has not been established although there was no evidence of harm during studies in animals.

This drug passes into breast milk. Allergic reactions, diarrhea, fungal infections, and skin rash have been reported in babies.

HELPFUL COMMENTS

Contact your doctor if your symptoms do not improve after a couple of days. Do not stop treatment early if you start to feel better. It takes the full prescription for this drug to work completely.

CARISOPRODOL

Available for over 20 years

COMMONLY USED TO TREAT

Muscle stiffness and pain caused by injury

DRUG CATEGORY

skeletal muscle relaxant
Class: carbamate

PRODUCTS

Brand-Name Products with Generic Alternatives
Soma 350 mg tablet ($$$)
  Generic: carisoprodol 350 mg tablet (¢¢)
Combination Products That Contain This Drug
Soma Compound tablet ($$$)
Soma Compound with Codeine tablet ($$$)

DOSING AND FOOD

Doses are taken 4 times a day.

This drug should be taken with food to reduce the stomach upset that many people suffer.

Adults: Up to 1,400 mg per day in divided doses.

Children age 5 to age 12: Up to 25 mg/kg per day in divided doses.

Forgotten doses: If you are scheduled to take the next dose within a few hours, do not take the forgotten dose. Otherwise take the forgotten dose as soon as you remember.

ALCOHOL, DRUG, HERB, AND SUPPLEMENT INTERACTIONS

Alcohol should not be used while taking this drug.

Several OTC drugs used for appetite control, asthma, colds, cough, hay fever, pain, or sinus problems may seriously increase the effects of this drug. Check with your pharmacist when selecting OTC products.

Increased side effects are possible when this drug is taken with those listed below: anesthetics, antihistamines†, anxiolytics†, barbiturates†, monoamine oxidase inhibitors†, narcotics†, tricyclic antidepressants†

ALLERGIC REACTIONS AND SIDE EFFECTS

If you are allergic to meprobamate or any other skeletal muscle relaxant†, you may also be allergic to this drug. Allergic reactions to this drug happen occasionally and are usually noticed within the first 4 doses. You should tell your doctor about all your allergies and any unexplained symptoms you may have while taking this drug.

MORE COMMON SIDE EFFECTS: Blurry vision, dizziness, drowsiness, lightheadedness, vision changes

LESS COMMON SIDE EFFECTS: Burning eyes*, chest tightness*, clumsiness, confusion, constipation, depression*, diarrhea, excitement, fainting*, fast heartbeat*, fever*, headache, heartburn, hiccups, hives*, irritability, itch-

---

† See page 52.   * See page 53.

ing*, nausea, nervousness, red face, restlessness, shortness of breath*, skin rash*, stomach cramps, stuffy nose*, vomiting, weakness*

RARE SIDE EFFECTS: Back pain*, black stools*, bleeding*, bloody urine*, bruising*, cough*, difficulty urinating*, hoarseness*, irregular breathing*, mouth sores*, muscle cramps*, sore throat*, swollen eyes*, swollen glands*, tiredness*, weakness*, yellow eyes or skin*

PRECAUTIONS

Be careful driving or handling equipment while taking this drug because the drug may cause drowsiness.

People with porphyria may not be able to take this drug.

This drug may cause withdrawal symptoms if stopped suddenly after long-term use. If you wish to stop taking this drug, ask your doctor for specific instructions.

PREGNANCY AND BREAST-FEEDING

Safety during pregnancy has not been established although there was no evidence of harm during studies in animals.

Breast-feeding while taking this drug is not recommended.

HELPFUL COMMENTS

Avoid quick movements to minimize dizziness. Dangling your legs over the side of the bed for a few minutes may help reduce dizziness when first waking up.

CARTEOLOL HYDROCHLORIDE

Available since December 1988

COMMONLY USED TO TREAT

Chest pain, also known as angina
High blood pressure, also known as hypertension
Pressure in the eye, also known as glaucoma

DRUG CATEGORY

antianginal
antihypertensive
Class: beta blocker

PRODUCTS

Brand-Name Products with No Generic Alternative
Cartrol 2.5 mg tablet ($)
Cartrol 5 mg tablet ($)
Brand-Name Products with Generic Alternatives
Ocupress 1% ophthalmic solution ($$$$$)
  Generic: carteolol hydrochloride 1% ophthalmic solution ($$$$$)

DOSING AND FOOD

Oral doses are taken once a day.
This drug may be taken with or without food.
Adults: Up to 10 mg per day.
Doses are taken every 2 to 3 days in people with kidney disease.
This drug is rarely used in children.
Eyedrops: Usually 1 eyedrop is used per dose.
Forgotten doses: If you are scheduled to take the next dose within 8 hours, do not take the forgotten dose. Otherwise take the forgotten dose as soon as you remember.

ALCOHOL, DRUG, HERB, AND SUPPLEMENT INTERACTIONS

Alcohol may increase some of the side effects from this drug, depending on the amount consumed. Ask your doctor about the risks caused by drinking alcohol with your condition.

Several OTC drugs used for appetite control, asthma, colds, cough, hay fever, or sinus problems may cause an increase in blood pressure when taken with this drug. Check with your pharmacist when selecting OTC products.

Taking this drug with any of the ones listed below may change the effect of either drug with the possibility of causing toxicity or decreasing effectiveness:
adrenergic blockers†, aminophylline, anesthetics†, antidiabetics†, caffeine, calcium channel blockers†, carbonic anhydrase inhibitors†, clonidine, dyphylline, epinephrine, guanabenz, insulin, lidocaine, nonsteroidal antiinflammatories†, oxtriphylline, pilocarpine, reserpine, theophylline

Severe reactions are possible when this drug is taken with those listed below:
allergy shots, beta blockers†, cocaine, digoxin, monoamine oxidase inhibitors†

Increased effects or side effects are possible when this drug is taken with those listed below:
antihypertensives†

---

† See page 52.   * See page 53.

ALLERGIC REACTIONS AND SIDE EFFECTS

If you are allergic to any other beta blockers†, you may also be allergic to this drug.

This drug may exaggerate the reaction from your current allergies. Inform your doctor of any allergies that you have as well as the severity of the allergic reaction before starting this drug.

When used as eyedrops, this drug may cause your eyes to be more sensitive to sunlight.

MORE COMMON SIDE EFFECTS: Dizziness, drowsiness, lightheadedness*, sexual dysfunction, sleeping difficulty, tiredness, weakness

LESS COMMON SIDE EFFECTS: Anxiety, breathing difficulty*, cold hands and feet*, constipation, depression*, diarrhea, frequent urination, itching, nausea, nervousness, numbness, shortness of breath*, slow heartbeat*, sore eyes, stomachache, stuffy nose, swelling, tingling, vivid dreams, vomiting, wheezing

RARE SIDE EFFECTS: Back pain*, bleeding*, bruising*, chest pain*, confusion*, dizziness*, fever*, hallucinations*, irregular heartbeat*, joint pain*, rash*, scaly skin*, sore throat*

PRECAUTIONS

People with asthma, heart disease, or a heart rate that is routinely less than 60 beats per minute (bradycardia) may not be able to take this drug.

You need to wait 2 weeks after stopping a monoamine oxidase inhibitor† before starting this drug.

Stopping this drug suddenly may cause chest pain or heart attack. If you wish to stop taking this drug, ask your doctor for specific instructions.

Be careful driving or handling equipment while taking this drug because the drug may cause drowsiness.

If you are diabetic, this drug may increase blood sugar levels or make the symptoms of low blood sugar less noticeable.

This drug may cause nondiabetics to develop type 2 diabetes.

If you have psoriasis or myasthenia gravis, this drug may make those conditions worse.

PREGNANCY AND BREAST-FEEDING

Safety during pregnancy has not been established although the drug is known to harm animal fetuses.

It is not known if this drug passes into breast milk. Talk to your doctor about the risks associated with breast-feeding while taking this drug.

HELPFUL COMMENTS

This drug may make you more sensitive to cold temperatures.

If you do not treat high blood pressure, you may develop more serious problems such as heart failure, blood vessel disease, stroke, or kidney disease. Losing weight, exercising, eating more fruits and vegetables, and avoiding salty foods, such as lunchmeat and pickles, may help make drug treatment more successful.

CARVEDILOL

Available since September 1995

COMMONLY USED TO TREAT

High blood pressure, also known as hypertension

DRUG CATEGORY

antihypertensive
Class: beta bocker

PRODUCTS

Brand-Name Products with No Generic Alternative
Coreg 3.125 mg tablet ($$)
Coreg 6.25 mg tablet ($$)
Coreg 12.5 mg tablet ($$)
Coreg 25 mg tablet ($$)
No generics available.
Multiple patents that begin to expire in 2007.

DOSING AND FOOD

Doses are taken twice a day.
This drug should be taken with food.
Adults: Up to 50 mg per day in divided doses.
Lower doses are used in people over age 65.
This drug is rarely used in children.
Forgotten doses: If you are scheduled to take the next dose within 4 hours, do not take the forgotten dose. Otherwise take the forgotten dose as soon as you remember.

---

† See page 52.　　* See page 53.

ALCOHOL, DRUG, HERB, AND SUPPLEMENT INTERACTIONS

Alcohol may increase some of the side effects from this drug, depending on the amount consumed. Ask your doctor about the risks caused by drinking alcohol with your condition.

Several OTC drugs used for appetite control, asthma, colds, cough, hay fever, or sinus problems may cause an increase in blood pressure when taken with this drug. Check with your pharmacist when selecting OTC products.

Taking this drug with any of the ones listed below may change the effect of either drug with the possibility of causing toxicity or decreasing effectiveness:
adrenergic blockers†, aminophylline, anesthetics, antidiabetics†, caffeine, calcium channel blockers†, carbonic anhydrase inhibitors†, cimetidine, clonidine, digoxin, dyphylline, epinephrine, guanabenz, insulin, lidocaine, nonsteroidal antiinflammatories†, oxtriphylline, pilocarpine, reserpine, rifampin, theophylline

Severe reactions are possible when this drug is taken with those listed below:
allergy shots, beta blockers†, cocaine, digoxin, monoamine oxidase inhibitors†

Increased effects or side effects are possible when this drug is taken with those listed below:
antihypertensives†

ALLERGIC REACTIONS AND SIDE EFFECTS

If you are allergic to any other beta blockers†, you may also be allergic to this drug.

This drug may exaggerate the reaction from your current allergies. Inform your doctor of any allergies that you have as well as the severity of the allergic reaction before starting this drug.

MORE COMMON SIDE EFFECTS: Dizziness, drowsiness, lightheadedness*, sexual dysfunction, sleeping difficulty, tiredness, weakness

LESS COMMON SIDE EFFECTS: Anxiety, breathing difficulty*, cold hands and feet*, constipation, depression*, diarrhea, dry eyes, frequent urination, itching, nausea, nervousness, numbness, shortness of breath*, slow heartbeat*, stomachache, stuffy nose, swelling, tingling, vivid dreams, vomiting, wheezing

RARE SIDE EFFECTS: Back pain*, bleeding*, bruising*, chest pain*, confusion*, dizziness*, fever*, hallucinations*, irregular heartbeat*, joint pain*, rash*, scaly skin*, sore throat*

PRECAUTIONS

People with asthma, heart disease, or a heart rate that is routinely less than 60 beats per minute (bradycardia) may not be able to take this drug.

You need to wait 2 weeks after stopping a monoamine oxidase inhibitor† before starting this drug.

Stopping this drug suddenly may cause chest pain or heart attack. If you wish to stop taking this drug, ask your doctor for specific instructions.

Be careful driving or handling equipment while taking this drug because the drug may cause drowsiness.

If you are diabetic, this drug may increase blood sugar levels or make the symptoms of low blood sugar less noticeable.

This drug may cause nondiabetics to develop type 2 diabetes.

If you have psoriasis or myasthenia gravis, this drug may make those conditions worse.

PREGNANCY AND BREAST-FEEDING

Safety during pregnancy has not been established although the drug is known to harm animal fetuses.

It is not known if this drug passes into breast milk. Talk to your doctor about the risks associated with breast-feeding while taking this drug.

HELPFUL COMMENTS

This drug may make you more sensitive to cold temperatures.

The dose is usually adjusted after 7 to 14 days if the desired effects are not seen.

If you do not treat high blood pressure, you may develop more serious problems such as heart failure, blood vessel disease, stroke, or kidney disease. Losing weight, exercising, eating more fruits and vegetables, and avoiding salty foods, such as lunchmeat and pickles, may help make drug treatment more successful.

You may need to use a lubricating eyedrop while taking this drug since it may reduce the formation of tears.

CEFACLOR

Available for over 20 years

COMMONLY USED TO TREAT

Infection

---

† See page 52.   * See page 53.

DRUG CATEGORY

antibiotic
Class: second generation cephalosporin

PRODUCTS

Brand-Name Products with Generic Alternatives
Ceclor 250 mg capsule ($$)
  Generic: cefaclor 250 mg capsule (¢¢¢¢)
Ceclor 500 mg capsule ($$)
  Generic: cefaclor 500 mg capsule ($)
Ceclor CD 500 mg extended-release tablet ($$$)
  Generic: cefaclor CD 500 mg extended-release tablet ($$$)
Ceclor 125 mg /5 ml oral suspension (¢¢¢¢¢)
  Generic: cefaclor 125 mg /5 ml oral suspension (¢¢¢)
Ceclor 187 mg/5 ml oral suspension ($$)
  Generic: cefaclor 187 mg/5 ml oral suspension ($)
Ceclor 250 mg/5 ml oral suspension ($$)
  Generic: cefaclor 250 mg/5 ml oral suspension (¢¢¢¢¢)
Ceclor 375 mg/5 ml oral suspension ($$$)
  Generic: cefaclor 375 mg/5 ml oral suspension ($$$)
Products Only Available as Generics
cefaclor 375 mg extended-release tablet (n/a)

DOSING AND FOOD

Doses are taken 2 to 3 times a day. Extended-release products are taken twice a day.

It is best to take this drug on an empty stomach, but taking this drug with a little food may avoid the stomach upset that some people suffer. Extended-release products are better absorbed when taken with food.

Adults: Up to 4 g per day in divided doses.

Children: Up to 20 mg/kg (maximum 1 gram) per day in divided doses.

Lower doses are used in people with kidney disease.

Forgotten doses: If you are scheduled to take the next dose within a few hours, do not take the forgotten dose. Otherwise take the forgotten dose as soon as you remember.

ALCOHOL, DRUG, HERB, AND SUPPLEMENT INTERACTIONS

Alcohol may increase some of the side effects from this drug, depending on the amount consumed. Ask your doctor about the risks caused by drinking alcohol with your condition.

Taking this drug with any of the ones listed below may change the effect of either drug with the possibility of causing toxicity or decreasing effectiveness: antacids, chloramphenicol, probenecid

Severe reactions are possible when this drug is taken with those listed below: aminoglycosides†, colistin, loop diuretics†, polymyxin B, vancomycin

Increased side effects are possible when this drug is taken with those listed below: alcohol, anticoagulants†, carbenicillin, dipyridamole, divalproex, heparin, pentoxifylline, plicamycin, sulfinpyrazone, ticarcillin, valproic acid

ALLERGIC REACTIONS AND SIDE EFFECTS

If you are allergic to other cephalosporins† or penicillins†, you may also be allergic to this drug. You should tell your doctor about all your allergies and any unexplained symptoms you may have while taking this drug.

MORE COMMON SIDE EFFECTS: Diarrhea*, headache, mouth sores, stomach cramps, vaginal discharge*, vaginal itching*

LESS COMMON SIDE EFFECTS: Abdominal tenderness*, bleeding*, bruising*, fever*

RARE SIDE EFFECTS: Breathing difficulty*, decreased urine output*, hearing loss*, itching*, joint pain*, loss of appetite*, nausea*, seizures*, skin irritation*, swelling*, tiredness*, vomiting*, weakness*, yellow eyes or skin*

PRECAUTIONS

Do not open, crush, break, or chew the extended-release products.
If you have a history of colitis, this drug may make that condition worse.
Severe diarrhea may be caused by this drug and should be reported to the doctor. Mild diarrhea may be treated with OTC drugs.
This drug may interfere with several diagnostic tests including some urine glucose tests. Diabetics should use glucose oxidase tests or glucose enzyme test strips.

PREGNANCY AND BREAST-FEEDING

Safety during pregnancy has not been established although there was no evidence of harm during studies in animals.
This drug passes into breast milk. The effect on the baby is not fully known.

HELPFUL COMMENTS

Contact your doctor if your symptoms do not improve after a couple of days.
If you need to take an antacid, take it either 2 hours before or after taking this drug.

† See page 52.   * See page 53.

Do not stop treatment early if you start to feel better. It takes the full prescription for this drug to work completely.

Oral suspensions should be discarded 14 days after mixing.

CEFADROXIL

Available for over 20 years

COMMONLY USED TO TREAT

Infection

DRUG CATEGORY

antibiotic
Class: first generation cephalosporin

PRODUCTS

Brand-Name Products with No Generic Alternative
Duricef 125 mg/5 ml oral suspension (n/a)
Duricef 250 mg/5 ml oral suspension ($$)
Duricef 500 mg/5 ml oral suspension ($$)
Brand-Name Products with Generic Alternatives
Duricef 500 mg capsule ($$$)
  Generic: cefadroxil 500 mg capsule ($$$)
Duricef 1,000 mg tablet ($$$$)
  Generic: cefadroxil 1,000 mg tablet ($$$$)

DOSING AND FOOD

Doses are taken 1 to 2 times a day.
It is best to take this drug on an empty stomach, but taking this drug with a little food may avoid the stomach upset that some people suffer.
Adults: Up to 2,000 mg per day in divided doses.
Children: Up to 3 mg/kg per day in divided doses.
Lower doses are used in people with kidney disease.
Forgotten doses: If you are scheduled to take the next dose within a few hours, do not take the forgotten dose. Otherwise take the forgotten dose as soon as you remember.

ALCOHOL, DRUG, HERB, AND SUPPLEMENT INTERACTIONS

Alcohol may increase some of the side effects from this drug, depending on the amount consumed. Ask your doctor about the risks caused by drinking alcohol with your condition.

Taking this drug with any of the ones listed below may change the effect of either drug with the possibility of causing toxicity or decreasing effectiveness: antacids, chloramphenicol, erythromycin, probenecid, tetracycline

Severe reactions are possible when this drug is taken with those listed below: aminoglycosides†, colistin, loop diuretics†, polymyxin B, vancomycin

Increased side effects are possible when this drug is taken with those listed below: alcohol, anticoagulants†, carbenicillin, dipyridamole, divalproex, heparin, pentoxifylline, plicamycin, sulfinpyrazone, ticarcillin, valproic acid

ALLERGIC REACTIONS AND SIDE EFFECTS

If you are allergic to other cephalosporins† or penicillins†, you may also be allergic to this drug. You should tell your doctor about all your allergies and any unexplained symptoms you may have while taking this drug.

MORE COMMON SIDE EFFECTS: Bleeding*, bruising*, diarrhea*, fever*, seizures*, skin irritation*

LESS COMMON SIDE EFFECTS: Abdominal tenderness*, headache, mouth sores, stomach cramps, vaginal discharge*, vaginal itching

RARE SIDE EFFECTS: Breathing difficulty*, decreased urine output*, hearing loss*, itching*, joint pain*, loss of appetite*, nausea*, swelling*, tiredness*, vomiting*, weakness*, yellow eyes or skin*

PRECAUTIONS

Severe diarrhea may be caused by this drug and should be reported to the doctor. Mild diarrhea may be treated with OTC drugs.
If you have a history of colitis, this drug may make that condition worse.
This drug may interfere with several diagnostic tests including some urine glucose tests. Diabetics should use glucose oxidase tests or glucose enzyme test strips.

PREGNANCY AND BREAST-FEEDING

Safety during pregnancy has not been established although there was no evidence of harm during studies in animals.
It is not known if this drug passes into breast milk. Talk to your doctor about the risks associated with breast-feeding while taking this drug.

HELPFUL COMMENTS

Contact your doctor if your symptoms do not improve after a couple of days.
If you need to take an antacid, take it either 2 hours before or after taking this drug.

---

† See page 52.   * See page 53.

Do not stop treatment early if you start to feel better. It takes the full prescription for this drug to work completely.

CEFDINIR

Available since December 1997

COMMONLY USED TO TREAT

Infection

DRUG CATEGORY

antibiotic
Class: third generation cephalosporin

PRODUCTS

Brand-Name Products with No Generic Alternative
Omnicef 300 mg capsule ($$$)
Omnicef 125 mg/5 ml oral suspension ($$$)
No generics available.
No patents, no exclusivity.

DOSING AND FOOD

Doses are taken 1 to 2 times a day.
It is best to take this drug on an empty stomach, but taking this drug with
   a little food may avoid the stomach upset that some people suffer.
Adults: Up to 600 mg per day in divided doses.
Children: Up to 14 mg/kg (maximum 600 mg) per day in divided doses.
Lower doses are used in people with kidney disease.
Forgotten doses: If you are scheduled to take the next dose within a few
   hours, do not take the forgotten dose. Otherwise take the forgotten dose
   as soon as you remember.

ALCOHOL, DRUG, HERB, AND SUPPLEMENT INTERACTIONS

Alcohol may increase some of the side effects from this drug, depending
   on the amount consumed. Ask your doctor about the risks caused by
   drinking alcohol with your condition.

**Taking this drug with any of the ones listed below may change the effect of
either drug with the possibility of causing toxicity or decreasing effectiveness:**
antacids, chloramphenicol, iron supplements, probenecid

Severe reactions are possible when this drug is taken with those listed below: aminoglycosides†, colistin, loop diuretics†, polymyxin B, vancomycin

Increased side effects are possible when this drug is taken with those listed below: alcohol, anticoagulants†, carbenicillin, dipyridamole, divalproex, heparin, pentoxifylline, plicamycin, sulfinpyrazone, ticarcillin, valproic acid

ALLERGIC REACTIONS AND SIDE EFFECTS

If you are allergic to other cephalosporins† or penicillins†, you may also be allergic to this drug. You should tell your doctor about all your allergies and any unexplained symptoms you may have while taking this drug.

MORE COMMON SIDE EFFECTS: Diarrhea*

LESS COMMON SIDE EFFECTS: Abdominal pain*, headache, nausea*, skin irritation*, vaginal discharge*, vaginal itching*, vomiting*

RARE SIDE EFFECTS: Bleeding*, breathing difficulty*, bruising*, decreased urine output*, fever*, hearing loss*, itching*, joint pain*, loss of appetite*, mouth sores, seizures*, swelling*, tiredness*, weakness*, yellow eyes or skin*

PRECAUTIONS

If you have a history of colitis, this drug may make that condition worse.

Severe diarrhea may be caused by this drug and should be reported to the doctor. Mild diarrhea may be treated with OTC drugs.

This drug may interfere with several diagnostic tests including some urine glucose tests. Diabetics should use glucose oxidase tests or glucose enzyme test strips.

PREGNANCY AND BREAST-FEEDING

Safety during pregnancy has not been established although there was no evidence of harm during studies in animals.

This drug passes into breast milk. Talk to your doctor about the risks associated with breast-feeding while taking this drug.

HELPFUL COMMENTS

Contact your doctor if your symptoms do not improve after a couple of days.

If you need to take an antacid or iron supplement, take it either 2 hours before or after taking this drug.

Do not stop treatment early if you start to feel better. It takes the full prescription for this drug to work completely.

---

† See page 52.　　* See page 53.

CEFDITOREN PIVOXIL

Available since August 2001

COMMONLY USED TO TREAT

Infection

DRUG CATEGORY

antibiotic
Class: third generation cephalosporin

PRODUCTS

Brand-Name Products with No Generic Alternative
Spectracef 200 mg tablet ($$)
No generics available.
Multiple patents that begin to expire in 2006.

DOSING AND FOOD

Doses are taken 2 times a day.
Taking this drug with fatty foods will help increase absorption of the drug.
  Be careful not to eat too much fatty food.
Adults: Up to 800 mg per day in divided doses.
This drug is not used in people under age 12.
Lower doses may be used in people with kidney disease.
Forgotten doses: If you are scheduled to take the next dose within a few
  hours, do not take the forgotten dose. Otherwise take the forgotten dose
  as soon as you remember.

ALCOHOL, DRUG, HERB, AND SUPPLEMENT INTERACTIONS

Alcohol may increase some of the side effects from this drug, depending
  on the amount consumed. Ask your doctor about the risks caused by
  drinking alcohol with your condition.

Taking this drug with any of the ones listed below may change the effect of
either drug with the possibility of causing toxicity or decreasing effectiveness:
antacids, chloramphenicol, cimetidine, erythromycin, famotidine,
  probenecid, ranitidine, tetracycline

Severe reactions are possible when this drug is taken with those listed below:
aminoglycosides†, colistin, loop diuretics†, polymyxin B, vancomycin

Increased side effects are possible when this drug is taken with those listed below: alcohol, anticoagulants†, carbenicillin, dipyridamole, divalproex, heparin, pentoxifylline, plicamycin, sulfinpyrazone, ticarcillin, valproic acid

ALLERGIC REACTIONS AND SIDE EFFECTS

If you are allergic to other cephalosporins†, milk, or penicillins†, you may also be allergic to this drug. You should tell your doctor about all your allergies and any unexplained symptoms you may have while taking this drug.

More Common Side Effects: Diarrhea*, nausea*, vaginal discharge*, vaginal itching*

Less Common Side Effects: Abdominal tenderness*, bleeding*, bruising*, fever*, headache, stomach cramps

Rare Side Effects: Breathing difficulty*, decreased urine output*, gas*, hearing loss*, itching*, joint pain*, loss of appetite*, mouth sores, seizures*, skin irritation*, stomach cramps, swelling*, tiredness*, vomiting*, weakness*, yellow eyes or skin*

PRECAUTIONS

If you have a history of colitis, this drug may make that condition worse.

Some people experience decreased carnitine levels while taking this drug. Tell your doctor if you are taking carnitine supplements.

Severe diarrhea may be caused by this drug and should be reported to the doctor. Mild diarrhea may be treated with OTC drugs.

This drug may interfere with several diagnostic tests including some urine glucose tests. Diabetics should use glucose oxidase tests or glucose enzyme test strips.

PREGNANCY AND BREAST-FEEDING

Safety during pregnancy has not been established although there was no evidence of harm during studies in animals.

Breast-feeding while taking this drug is not recommended.

HELPFUL COMMENTS

Contact your doctor if your symptoms do not improve after a couple of days.

If you need to take an antacid, take it either 2 hours before or after taking this drug.

Do not stop treatment early if you start to feel better. It takes the full prescription for this drug to work completely.

†See page 52.   *See page 53.

CEFPODOXIME PROXETIL

Available since August 1992

COMMONLY USED TO TREAT

Infection

DRUG CATEGORY

antibiotic
Class: third generation cephalosporin

PRODUCTS

Brand-Name Products with No Generic Alternative
Vantin 100 mg tablet ($$$)
Vantin 200 mg tablet ($$$)
Brand-Name Products with Generic Alternatives
Vantin 50 mg/5 ml oral suspension ($$)
  Generic: cefpodoxime 50 mg/5 ml oral suspension (n/a)
Vantin 100 mg/5 ml oral suspension ($$$)
  Generic: cefpodoxime 100 mg/5 ml oral suspension (n/a)

DOSING AND FOOD

Doses are taken twice a day.
It is best to take this drug with food or milk.
Adults: Up to 800 mg per day in divided doses.
Children age 2 months to 12 years: Up to 10 mg/kg (maximum 400 mg)
  per day in divided doses.
Lower doses are used in people with kidney disease.
Forgotten doses: If you are scheduled to take the next dose within a few
  hours, do not take the forgotten dose. Otherwise take the forgotten dose
  as soon as you remember.

ALCOHOL, DRUG, HERB, AND SUPPLEMENT INTERACTIONS

Alcohol may increase some of the side effects from this drug, depending
  on the amount consumed. Ask your doctor about the risks caused by
  drinking alcohol with your condition.

Taking this drug with any of the ones listed below may change the effect of
either drug with the possibility of causing toxicity or decreasing effectiveness:
antacids, chloramphenicol, cimetidine, erythromycin, famotidine, probenecid, ranitidine, tetracycline

Severe reactions are possible when this drug is taken with those listed below: aminoglycosides†, colistin, loop diuretics†, polymyxin B, vancomycin

Increased side effects are possible when this drug is taken with those listed below: alcohol, anticoagulants†, carbenicillin, dipyridamole, divalproex, heparin, pentoxifylline, plicamycin, sulfinpyrazone, ticarcillin, valproic acid

ALLERGIC REACTIONS AND SIDE EFFECTS

If you are allergic to other cephalosporins† or penicillins†, you may also be allergic to this drug. You should tell your doctor about all your allergies and any unexplained symptoms you may have while taking this drug.

MORE COMMON SIDE EFFECTS: Breathing difficulty*, diarrhea*, swelling*, weakness*

LESS COMMON SIDE EFFECTS: Abdominal pain*, fever*, headache, mouth sores, nausea*, skin irritation*, stomach cramps, vaginal discharge, vaginal itching, vomiting*

RARE SIDE EFFECTS: Bleeding*, bruising*, decreased urine output*, hearing loss*, itching*, joint pain*, loss of appetite*, seizures*, tiredness*, yellow eyes or skin*

PRECAUTIONS

If you have a history of colitis, this drug may make that condition worse.

Severe diarrhea may be caused by this drug and should be reported to the doctor. Mild diarrhea may be treated with OTC drugs.

This drug may interfere with several diagnostic tests including some urine glucose tests. Diabetics should use glucose oxidase tests or glucose enzyme test strips.

PREGNANCY AND BREAST-FEEDING

Safety during pregnancy has not been established although there was no evidence of harm during studies in animals.

Breast-feeding while taking this drug is not recommended.

HELPFUL COMMENTS

Contact your doctor if your symptoms do not improve after a couple of days.

If you need to take an antacid, take it either 2 hours before or after taking this drug.

Do not stop treatment early if you start to feel better. It takes the full prescription for this drug to work completely.

Oral suspensions should be discarded 14 days after mixing.

---

† See page 52.   * See page 53.

CEFPROZIL

Available since December 1991

COMMONLY USED TO TREAT

Infection

DRUG CATEGORY

antibiotic
Class: second generation cephalosporin

PRODUCTS

Brand-Name Products with No Generic Alternative
Cefzil 250 mg tablet ($$$)
Cefzil 500 mg tablet ($$$$)
Cefzil 125 mg/5 ml oral suspension ($$)
Cefzil 250 mg/5 ml oral suspension ($$$)
No generics available.
No patents, no exclusivity.

DOSING AND FOOD

Doses are taken 1 to 2 times a day.
It is best to take this drug on an empty stomach, but taking this drug with
  a little food may avoid the stomach upset that some people suffer.

Adults: Up to 1 g per day in divided doses.

Children: Up to 20 mg/kg per day in divided doses.

Lower doses may be used in people with kidney disease.

Forgotten doses: If you are scheduled to take the next dose within a few
  hours, do not take the forgotten dose. Otherwise take the forgotten dose
  as soon as you remember.

ALCOHOL, DRUG, HERB, AND SUPPLEMENT INTERACTIONS

Alcohol may increase some of the side effects from this drug, depending
  on the amount consumed. Ask your doctor about the risks caused by
  drinking alcohol with your condition.

**Taking this drug with any of the ones listed below may change the effect of
either drug with the possibility of causing toxicity or decreasing effectiveness:**
chloramphenicol, erythromycin, probenecid, tetracycline

Severe reactions are possible when this drug is taken with those listed below: aminoglycosides†, colistin, loop diuretics†, polymyxin B, vancomycin

Increased side effects are possible when this drug is taken with those listed below: alcohol, anticoagulants†, carbenicillin, dipyridamole, divalproex, heparin, pentoxifylline, plicamycin, sulfinpyrazone, ticarcillin, valproic acid

ALLERGIC REACTIONS AND SIDE EFFECTS

If you are allergic to other cephalosporins† or penicillins†, you may also be allergic to this drug. You should tell your doctor about all your allergies and any unexplained symptoms you may have while taking this drug.

MORE COMMON SIDE EFFECTS: Bleeding*, breathing difficulty*, bruising*, diarrhea*, headache, mouth sores, nausea*, stomach cramps, swelling*

LESS COMMON SIDE EFFECTS: Abdominal pain*, dizziness, fever*, vaginal discharge, vaginal itching

RARE SIDE EFFECTS: Decreased urine output*, hearing loss*, itching*, joint pain*, loss of appetite*, seizures*, skin irritation*, tiredness*, vomiting*, weakness*, yellow eyes or skin*

PRECAUTIONS

If you have a history of colitis, this drug may make that condition worse.

Severe diarrhea may be caused by this drug and should be reported to the doctor. Mild diarrhea may be treated with OTC drugs.

People with phenylketonuria should not use the oral suspension since it contains phenylalanine.

This drug may interfere with several diagnostic tests including some urine glucose tests. Diabetics should use glucose oxidase tests or glucose enzyme test strips.

PREGNANCY AND BREAST-FEEDING

Safety during pregnancy has not been established although there was no evidence of harm during studies in animals.

Breast-feeding while taking this drug is not recommended.

HELPFUL COMMENTS

Contact your doctor if your symptoms do not improve after a couple of days. Do not stop treatment early if you start to feel better. It takes the full prescription for this drug to work completely.

---

† See page 52.   * See page 53.

CEFTIBUTEN DIHYDRATE

Available since December 1995

COMMONLY USED TO TREAT

Infection

DRUG CATEGORY

antibiotic
Class: third generation cephalosporin

PRODUCTS

Brand-Name Products with No Generic Alternative
Cedax 400 mg capsule ($$$$)
Cedax 90 mg/5 ml oral suspension ($$$)
Cedax 180 mg/5 ml oral suspension (n/a)
No generics available.
No patents, no exclusivity.

DOSING AND FOOD

Doses are taken once a day.
It is best to take this drug on an empty stomach either 2 hours before or 1
  hour after a meal.
Adults: Up to 400 mg per day.
Children under age 12: Up to 9 mg/kg (maximum 400 mg) per day.
Lower doses are used in people with kidney disease.
Forgotten doses: If you are scheduled to take the next dose within a few
  hours, do not take the forgotten dose. Otherwise take the forgotten dose
  as soon as you remember.

ALCOHOL, DRUG, HERB, AND SUPPLEMENT INTERACTIONS

Alcohol may increase some of the side effects from this drug, depending
  on the amount consumed. Ask your doctor about the risks caused by
  drinking alcohol with your condition.

Taking this drug with any of the ones listed below may change the effect of
either drug with the possibility of causing toxicity or decreasing effectiveness:
antacids, chloramphenicol, erythromycin, probenecid, tetracycline

Severe reactions are possible when this drug is taken with those listed below:
aminoglycosides†, colistin, loop diuretics†, polymyxin B, vancomycin

Increased side effects are possible when this drug is taken with those listed below: alcohol, anticoagulants†, carbenicillin, dipyridamole, divalproex, heparin, pentoxifylline, plicamycin, sulfinpyrazone, ticarcillin, valproic acid

ALLERGIC REACTIONS AND SIDE EFFECTS

If you are allergic to other cephalosporins† or penicillins†, you may also be allergic to this drug. You should tell your doctor about all your allergies and any unexplained symptoms you may have while taking this drug.

LESS COMMON SIDE EFFECTS: Abdominal pain*, bleeding*, bruising*, diarrhea*, fever*, headache, mouth sores, stomach cramps, vaginal discharge*, vaginal itching*

RARE SIDE EFFECTS: Breathing difficulty*, decreased urine output*, hearing loss*, itching*, joint pain*, loss of appetite*, nausea*, seizures*, skin irritation*, swelling*, tiredness*, vomiting*, weakness*, yellow eyes or skin*

PRECAUTIONS

If you have a history of colitis, this drug may make that condition worse.

Severe diarrhea may be caused by this drug and should be reported to the doctor. Mild diarrhea may be treated with OTC drugs.

This drug may interfere with several diagnostic tests including some urine glucose tests. Diabetics should use glucose oxidase tests or glucose enzyme test strips.

PREGNANCY AND BREAST-FEEDING

Safety during pregnancy has not been established although there was no evidence of harm during studies in animals.

It is not known if this drug passes into breast milk. Talk to your doctor about the risks associated with breast-feeding while taking this drug.

HELPFUL COMMENTS

Contact your doctor if your symptoms do not improve after a couple of days.

If you need to take an antacid, take it either 2 hours before or after taking this drug.

Do not stop treatment early if you start to feel better. It takes the full prescription for this drug to work completely.

Oral suspensions should be discarded 14 days after mixing.

---

† See page 52.   * See page 53.

CEFUROXIME AXETIL

Available since October 1983

COMMONLY USED TO TREAT

Infection

DRUG CATEGORY

antibiotic
Class: second generation cephalosporin

PRODUCTS

Brand-Name Products with No Generic Alternative
Ceftin 125 mg /5 ml oral suspension ($$)
Ceftin 250 mg/5 ml oral suspension ($$$)
Brand-Name Products with Generic Alternatives
Ceftin 125 mg tablet ($$)
   Generic: cefuroxime axetil 125 mg tablet (n/a)
Ceftin 250 mg tablet ($$$)
   Generic: cefuroxime axetil 250 mg tablet (n/a)
Ceftin 500 mg tablet ($$$$)
   Generic: cefuroxime axetil 500 mg tablet (n/a)

DOSING AND FOOD

Doses are taken twice a day.
It is best to take this drug with food or milk.
Adults: Up to 1 g per day in divided doses.
Children age 3 months to 12 years: Up to 20 mg/kg (maximum 500 mg)
   per day in divided doses.
The dose of oral suspension is different from the dose of the tablet form of
   this drug and should not be automatically substituted.
Lower doses are used in people with kidney disease.
Forgotten doses: If you are scheduled to take the next dose within a few
   hours, do not take the forgotten dose. Otherwise take the forgotten dose
   as soon as you remember.

ALCOHOL, DRUG, HERB, AND SUPPLEMENT INTERACTIONS

Alcohol may increase some of the side effects from this drug, depending
   on the amount consumed. Ask your doctor about the risks caused by
   drinking alcohol with your condition.

Taking this drug with any of the ones listed below may change the effect of either drug with the possibility of causing toxicity or decreasing effectiveness: chloramphenicol, erythromycin, probenecid, tetracycline

Severe reactions are possible when this drug is taken with those listed below: aminoglycosides†, colistin, loop diuretics†, polymyxin B, vancomycin

Increased side effects are possible when this drug is taken with those listed below: alcohol, anticoagulants†, carbenicillin, dipyridamole, divalproex, heparin, pentoxifylline, plicamycin, sulfinpyrazone, ticarcillin, valproic acid

ALLERGIC REACTIONS AND SIDE EFFECTS

If you are allergic to other cephalosporins† or penicillins†, you may also be allergic to this drug. You should tell your doctor about all your allergies and any unexplained symptoms you may have while taking this drug.

MORE COMMON SIDE EFFECTS: Breathing difficulty*, diarrhea*, skin irritation*, swelling*, vomiting*

LESS COMMON SIDE EFFECTS: Abdominal pain*, bleeding*, bruising*, fever*, headache, mouth sores, stomach cramps

RARE SIDE EFFECTS: Decreased urine output*, hearing loss*, itching*, joint pain*, loss of appetite*, nausea*, seizures*, tiredness*, vaginal discharge*, vaginal itching*, weakness*, yellow eyes or skin*

PRECAUTIONS

If you have a history of colitis, this drug may make that condition worse.

Severe diarrhea may be caused by this drug and should be reported to the doctor. Mild diarrhea may be treated with OTC drugs.

This drug may interfere with several diagnostic tests including some urine glucose tests. Diabetics should use glucose oxidase tests or glucose enzyme test strips.

PREGNANCY AND BREAST-FEEDING

Safety during pregnancy has not been established although there was no evidence of harm during studies in animals.

It is not known if this drug passes into breast milk. Talk to your doctor about the risks associated with breast-feeding while taking this drug.

HELPFUL COMMENTS

Contact your doctor if your symptoms do not improve after a couple of days.

Do not stop treatment early if you start to feel better. It takes the full prescription for this drug to work completely.

Oral suspensions should be discarded 10 days after mixing.

---

† See page 52.   * See page 53.

CELECOXIB

Available since December 1998

COMMONLY USED TO TREAT

Arthritis
Fever
Pain

DRUG CATEGORY

analgesic
antiinflammatory
antipyretic
Class: nonsteroidal antiinflammatory: COX-2 inhibitor

PRODUCTS

Brand-Name Products with No Generic Alternative
Celebrex 100 mg capsule ($$)
Celebrex 200 mg capsule ($$$)
Celebrex 400 mg capsule (n/a)
No generics available.
Multiple patents that begin to expire in 2013.

DOSING AND FOOD

Doses are taken 1 to 2 times a day.
It is best to take this drug with food or milk.
Adults: Up to 800 mg per day in divided doses.
Lower doses are used in children and in people with liver disease.
Forgotten doses: If you are scheduled to take the next dose within a few
hours, do not take the forgotten dose. Otherwise take the forgotten dose
as soon as you remember.

ALCOHOL, DRUG, HERB, AND SUPPLEMENT INTERACTIONS

Alcohol should not be used while taking this drug because of the increased
risk of intestinal bleeding.
Dong quai, feverfew, garlic, ginger, horse chestnut, red clover, and St.
John's wort may increase the risk of side effects from this drug, some of
which may be severe.

Taking this drug with any of the ones listed below may change the effect of
either drug with the possibility of causing toxicity or decreasing effectiveness:
ACE inhibitors†, antacids, fluconazole, furosemide, lithium

Severe reactions are possible when this drug is taken with those listed below: warfarin

Increased side effects are possible when this drug is taken with those listed below: aspirin, fluconazole, nonsteroidal antiinflammatories†

ALLERGIC REACTIONS AND SIDE EFFECTS

If you are allergic to aspirin, nonsteroidal antiinflammatories†, or sulfonamides†, you may also be allergic to this drug. This drug may cause severe allergic reactions, but this does not occur often. You should tell your doctor about all your allergies and any unexplained symptoms you may have while taking this drug.

MORE COMMON SIDE EFFECTS: Back pain, cough*, dizziness*, fever*, headache*, heartburn, nausea*, skin rash*, sleep disorders, sneezing*, sore throat, stomach pain, stuffy nose, swelling*

LESS COMMON SIDE EFFECTS: Anxiety, blurry vision, constipation, depression, diarrhea, dry mouth, gas, irregular heartbeat*, joint pain, loss of energy, muscle pain, nervousness, ringing in ears, sleepiness, swallowing difficulty, sweating, taste changes, tingling, vomiting*

RARE SIDE EFFECTS: Bloody stools*, bloody vomit*, burning sensation*, breathing difficulty*, chills*, congestion*, decreased urine output*, diarrhea*, drowsiness*, fatigue*, loss of appetite*, muscle pain*, shortness of breath*, thirst*, tiredness*, weakness*, weight gain*, wheezing*

PRECAUTIONS

If you have anemia, asthma, high blood pressure, ulcers, or bleeding disorders, this drug may make those conditions worse.

People who use tobacco or alcohol have an increased risk of developing side effects.

Drink plenty of fluids to avoid dehydration when sweating, such as in hot weather and during exercise.

PREGNANCY AND BREAST-FEEDING

Safety during pregnancy has not been established although the drug is known to harm animal fetuses.

Breast-feeding while taking this drug is not recommended.

HELPFUL COMMENTS

If you need to take an antacid, take it either 2 hours before or after taking this drug.

It may take several days before the full effects of this drug are noticed.

† See page 52.   * See page 53.

CEPHALEXIN HYDROCHLORIDE

Available for over 20 years

COMMONLY USED TO TREAT

Infection

DRUG CATEGORY

antibiotic
Class: first generation cephalosporin

PRODUCTS

Brand-Name Products with No Generic Alternative
Keftab 500 mg tablet ($$$)
Keflex 100 mg/ml oral suspension (n/a)

Brand-Name Products with Generic Alternatives
Keflex 250 mg capsule ($$)
  Generic: cephalexin 250 mg capsule (¢¢)
Keflex 500 mg capsule ($$$)
  Generic: cephalexin 500 mg capsule (¢¢¢)
Keflex 125 mg/5 ml oral suspension (n/a)
  Generic: cephalexin 125 mg/5 ml oral suspension (¢¢¢)
Keflex 250 mg/5 ml oral suspension (n/a)
  Generic: cephalexin 250 mg/5 ml oral suspension (¢¢¢¢¢)
Keflet 250 mg tablet (n/a)
  Generic: cephalexin 250 mg tablet (¢¢¢¢)

Products Only Available as Generics
cephalexin 500 mg tablet ($)

Other Generic Product Names
Bio-Cef

DOSING AND FOOD

Doses are taken 2 to 4 times a day.
It is best to take this drug on an empty stomach, but taking this drug with
  a little food may avoid the stomach upset that some people suffer.
Adults: Up to 4,000 mg per day in divided doses.
Children: Up to 100 mg/kg per day in divided doses.
Lower doses are used in people with kidney disease.
Forgotten doses: If you are scheduled to take the next dose within a few

hours, do not take the forgotten dose. Otherwise take the forgotten dose as soon as you remember.

ALCOHOL, DRUG, HERB, AND SUPPLEMENT INTERACTIONS

Alcohol may increase some of the side effects from this drug, depending on the amount consumed. Ask your doctor about the risks caused by drinking alcohol with your condition.

Taking this drug with any of the ones listed below may change the effect of either drug with the possibility of causing toxicity or decreasing effectiveness: chloramphenicol, erythromycin, probenecid, tetracycline

Severe reactions are possible when this drug is taken with those listed below: aminoglycosides†, colistin, loop diuretics†, polymyxin B, vancomycin

Increased side effects are possible when this drug is taken with those listed below: alcohol, anticoagulants†, carbenicillin, dipyridamole, divalproex, heparin, pentoxifylline, plicamycin, sulfinpyrazone, ticarcillin, valproic acid

ALLERGIC REACTIONS AND SIDE EFFECTS

If you are allergic to other cephalosporins† or penicillins†, you may also be allergic to this drug. You should tell your doctor about all your allergies and any unexplained symptoms you may have while taking this drug.

MORE COMMON SIDE EFFECTS: Bleeding*, breathing difficulty*, bruising*, diarrhea*, loss of appetite*, nausea*, skin irritation*, swelling*

LESS COMMON SIDE EFFECTS: Abdominal pain*, fever*, headache, mouth sores, stomach cramps, vaginal discharge, vaginal itching

RARE SIDE EFFECTS: Decreased urine output*, hearing loss*, itching*, joint pain*, seizures*, tiredness*, vomiting*, weakness*, yellow eyes or skin*

PRECAUTIONS

If you have a history of colitis, this drug may make that condition worse.

Severe diarrhea may be caused by this drug and should be reported to the doctor. Mild diarrhea may be treated with OTC drugs.

This drug may interfere with several diagnostic tests including some urine glucose tests. Diabetics should use glucose oxidase tests or glucose enzyme test strips.

PREGNANCY AND BREAST-FEEDING

Safety during pregnancy has not been established although there was no evidence of harm during studies in animals.

It is not known if this drug passes into breast milk. Talk to your doctor about the risks associated with breast-feeding while taking this drug.

† See page 52.   * See page 53.

HELPFUL COMMENTS

Contact your doctor if your symptoms do not improve after a couple of days.
Do not stop treatment early if you start to feel better. It takes the full prescription for this drug to work completely.
Oral suspensions should be discarded 14 days after mixing.

CEPHRADINE

Available for over 20 years

COMMONLY USED TO TREAT

Infection

DRUG CATEGORY

antibiotic
Class: first generation cephalosporin

PRODUCTS

Brand-Name Products with Generic Alternatives
Velocef 250 mg capsule (¢¢¢¢¢)
　Generic: cephradine 250 mg capsule (¢¢¢¢)
Velocef 500 mg capsule ($$)
　Generic: cephradine 500 mg capsule ($$)
Velosef 125 mg/5 ml oral suspension (n/a)
　Generic: cephradine 125 mg/5 ml oral suspension (n/a)
Velosef 250 mg/5 ml oral suspension (¢¢¢¢¢)
　Generic: cephradine 250 mg/5 ml oral suspension (n/a)
Other Generic Product Names
Anspor

DOSING AND FOOD

Doses are taken 2 to 4 times a day.
It is best to take this drug on an empty stomach, but taking this drug with a little food may avoid the stomach upset that some people suffer.
Adults: Up to 4,000 mg per day in divided doses.
Children over 9 months: Up to 100 mg/kg (maximum 4,000 mg) per day in divided doses.
Lower doses are used in people with kidney disease.
Forgotten doses: If you are scheduled to take the next dose within a few

hours, do not take the forgotten dose. Otherwise take the forgotten dose as soon as you remember.

ALCOHOL, DRUG, HERB, AND SUPPLEMENT INTERACTIONS

Alcohol may increase some of the side effects from this drug, depending on the amount consumed. Ask your doctor about the risks caused by drinking alcohol with your condition.

Taking this drug with any of the ones listed below may change the effect of either drug with the possibility of causing toxicity or decreasing effectiveness: chloramphenicol, erythromycin, probenecid, tetracycline

Severe reactions are possible when this drug is taken with those listed below: aminoglycosides†, colistin, loop diuretics†, polymyxin B, vancomycin

Increased side effects are possible when this drug is taken with those listed below: alcohol, anticoagulants†, carbenicillin, dipyridamole, divalproex, heparin, pentoxifylline, plicamycin, sulfinpyrazone, ticarcillin, valproic acid

ALLERGIC REACTIONS AND SIDE EFFECTS

If you are allergic to other cephalosporins† or penicillins†, you may also be allergic to this drug. You should tell your doctor about all your allergies and any unexplained symptoms you may have while taking this drug.

MORE COMMON SIDE EFFECTS: Bleeding*, breathing difficulty*, bruising*, diarrhea*, loss of appetite*, skin irritation*, swelling*

LESS COMMON SIDE EFFECTS: Abdominal tenderness*, fever*, headache, mouth sores, stomach cramps, vaginal discharge*, vaginal itching

RARE SIDE EFFECTS: Decreased urine output*, hearing loss*, itching*, joint pain*, nausea*, seizures*, tiredness*, vomiting*, weakness*, yellow eyes or skin*

PRECAUTIONS

If you have a history of colitis, this drug may make that condition worse.
Severe diarrhea may be caused by this drug and should be reported to the doctor. Mild diarrhea may be treated with OTC drugs.
This drug may interfere with several diagnostic tests including some urine glucose tests. Diabetics should use glucose oxidase tests or glucose enzyme test strips.

PREGNANCY AND BREAST-FEEDING

Safety during pregnancy has not been established although there was no evidence of harm during studies in animals.

---

†See page 52.   *See page 53.

It is not known if this drug passes into breast milk. Talk to your doctor about the risks associated with breast-feeding while taking this drug.

HELPFUL COMMENTS

Contact your doctor if your symptoms do not improve after a couple of days. Do not stop treatment early if you start to feel better. It takes the full prescription for this drug to work completely.

Oral suspensions should be discarded 14 days after mixing

CETIRIZINE HYDROCHLORIDE

Available since December 1995

COMMONLY USED TO TREAT

Allergies
Breathing difficulty
Rash or hives that keep coming back, also known as chronic urticaria

DRUG CATEGORY

antiasthmatic
antihistamine
Class: H1 receptor blocker: piperazine

PRODUCTS

Brand-Name Products with No Generic Alternative
Zyrtec 5 mg tablet ($$)
Zyrtec 10 mg tablet ($$)
Zytec 5 mg/5 ml oral syrup ($)
No generics available.
Multiple patents that begin to expire in 2007.
Combination Products That Contain This Drug
Zyrtec-D extended-release tablet ($)

DOSING AND FOOD

Doses are taken once a day.
This drug may be taken with or without food.
Adults and children over age 6: Up to 10 mg per day.
Children age 2 to 6: Up to 5 mg per day.
Lower doses may be used in people with kidney disease or liver disease.
Forgotten doses: This drug should be taken no more often than once

every 24 hours. If you have forgotten a dose and are having symptoms, take the dose right away and reschedule the next dose for 24 hours later.

ALCOHOL, DRUG, HERB, AND SUPPLEMENT INTERACTIONS

Alcohol may increase some of the side effects from this drug, depending on the amount consumed. Ask your doctor about the risks caused by drinking alcohol with your condition.

Several OTC drugs used for appetite control, asthma, colds, cough, hay fever, pain, or sinus problems may seriously increase the effects of this drug. Check with your pharmacist when selecting OTC products.

Taking this drug with any of the ones listed below may change the effect of either drug with the possibility of causing toxicity or decreasing effectiveness: anticholinergics†, theophylline

Severe reactions are possible when this drug is taken with those listed below: monoamine oxidase inhibitors†

Increased side effects are possible when this drug is taken with those listed below: alcohol, anesthetics, antihistamines†, anxiolytics†, barbiturates†, narcotics†, tricyclic antidepressants†

ALLERGIC REACTIONS AND SIDE EFFECTS

If you are allergic to other antihistamines†, especially hydroxyzine, you may also be allergic to this drug. You should tell your doctor about all your allergies and any unexplained symptoms you may have while taking this drug.

This drug promotes the effect of sunlight on the body and may cause severe sunburn and increased sensitivity of the eyes.

MORE COMMON SIDE EFFECTS: Drowsiness, dry mouth, headache*, increased appetite, nausea, stomachache, thick mucus, weight gain

LESS COMMON SIDE EFFECTS: Belching, bleeding*, body aches, bruising*, clumsiness, confusion, congestion, constipation, cough*, diarrhea*, difficulty urinating, excitement, fatigue, fever*, heartburn, hoarseness, indigestion, irregular heartbeat*, irritability, joint pain, menstrual changes, muscle cramps, nervousness, nightmares, restlessness, ringing in ears, runny nose, skin rash, sore throat*, stiffness, sweating, swollen glands, swollen joints, tremor, vision changes, vomiting

RARE SIDE EFFECTS: Abdominal pain*, chest tightness*, chills*, dark urine*, dizziness*, facial swelling*, fever*, hives*, itching*, pale stools*, seizures*, shortness of breath*, skin irritation*, swallowing difficulty*, tingling*, tiredness*, weakness*, wheezing*

---

† See page 52.   * See page 53.

PRECAUTIONS

This drug should not be used to treat an asthma attack.

If you have glaucoma, enlarged prostate, or difficulty urinating, this drug may make those conditions worse.

This drug may interfere with skin tests used to diagnose allergies and should be stopped for at least 4 days before the test.

Be careful driving or handling equipment while taking this drug because the drug may cause drowsiness.

This drug may cause dry mouth, which is associated with a greater risk of cavities. Your dentist may recommend that you clean your teeth and mouth differently to avoid infection.

PREGNANCY AND BREAST-FEEDING

Safety during pregnancy has not been established although there was no evidence of harm during studies in animals.

Breast-feeding while taking this drug is not recommended.

HELPFUL COMMENTS

Sucking on hard sugarless candy or chewing sugarless gum may help relieve dry mouth caused by this drug.

Several antihistamines are sold without a prescription by the following generic names: brompheniramine, chlorpheniramine, clemastine, diphenhydramine, doxylamine, loratadine. Ask your pharmacist about specific products that contain these drugs.

CEVIMELINE HYDROCHLORIDE

Available since January 2000

COMMONLY USED TO TREAT

Dry mouth caused by disease

DRUG CATEGORY

prosecretory
Class: cholinergic agonist

PRODUCTS

Brand-Name Products with No Generic Alternative
Evoxac 30 mg capsule ($)
No generics available.

Multiple patents that begin to expire in 2006.

DOSING AND FOOD

Doses are taken 3 times a day.

It is best to take this drug on an empty stomach. Do not drink grapefruit juice while taking this drug.

Adults: Up to 30 mg per day in divided doses.

This drug is rarely used in children.

Forgotten doses: If you are scheduled to take the next dose within a few hours, do not take the forgotten dose. Otherwise take the forgotten dose as soon as you remember.

ALCOHOL, DRUG, HERB, AND SUPPLEMENT INTERACTIONS

Alcohol may increase some of the side effects from this drug, depending on the amount consumed. Ask your doctor about the risks caused by drinking alcohol with your condition.

Many OTC drugs used for appetite control, asthma, colds, cough, hay fever, pain, or sinus problems affect the central nervous system and may interfere with this drug. Check with your pharmacist for products to avoid.

Taking this drug with any of the ones listed below may change the effect of either drug with the possibility of causing toxicity or decreasing effectiveness: amiodarone, anticholinergics†, beta blockers†, chloroquine, cholinergics†, cimetidine, clarithromycin, cyclosporine, danazol, delaviridine, diltiazem, erythromycin, fluconazole, fluoxetine, fluphenazine, fluvoxamine, haloperidol, indinavir, isoniazid, itraconazole, ketoconazole, metronidazole, miconazole, nefazodone, nelfinavir, nicardipine, nifedipine, norfloxacin, omeprazole, paroxetine, perphenazine, prednisone, propafenone, propoxyphene, quinidine, quinine, rifabutin, ritonavir, saquinavir, sertraline, thioridazine, troleonadomycin, verapamil, zafirlukast

ALLERGIC REACTIONS AND SIDE EFFECTS

You should tell your doctor about all your allergies and any unexplained symptoms you may have while taking this drug.

MORE COMMON SIDE EFFECTS: Excessive sweating*, nausea, stuffy nose

LESS COMMON SIDE EFFECTS: Abdominal pain, back pain*, belching, bleeding, bloody nose, bone pain, breathing problems*, bruising, chest pain*, chest tightness, chills, clammy skin*, cloudy urine*, confusion*, constipation, cough*, depression, diarrhea*, dizziness*, dry mouth, earache*, eye irritation*, face pain, fast heartbeat*, fever, headache*, heartburn, hic-

---

† See page 52.   * See page 53.

cups, insomnia, itching*, joint pain, leg cramps, loss of appetite, migraine headache, mood swings, mouth sores*, muscle aches, nausea*, painful urination*, ringing in ears*, scaly skin*, shortness of breath*, skin irritation*, stiffness*, stomach cramps*, sweating*, swelling*, tiredness, toothache, trembling*, vaginal itch*, vision changes*, vomiting, watery eyes*, watery mouth, weak pulse*, weakness, weight changes*

RARE SIDE EFFECTS: Chest pain*, crying, bruising*, fainting*, lightheadedness*

PRECAUTIONS

Be careful driving or handling equipment while taking this drug because the drug may cause dizziness.
Visual disturbance may interfere with driving, especially at night.

PREGNANCY AND BREAST-FEEDING

Safety during pregnancy has not been established although the drug is known to harm animal fetuses.
It is not known if this drug passes into breast milk. Talk to your doctor about the risks associated with breast-feeding while taking this drug.

HELPFUL COMMENTS

Drink plenty of fluids to avoid dehydration especially in hot weather and during exercise.

CHLORAMBUCIL

Available for over 20 years

COMMONLY USED TO TREAT

Cancer of the blood and lymph system
Immune disorders

DRUG CATEGORY

antineoplastic
immunosuppressant
Class: alkylating agent: nitrogen mustard

PRODUCTS

Brand-Name Products with No Generic Alternative
Leukeran 2 mg tablet ($$)

No generics available.
No patents, no exclusivity.

DOSING AND FOOD

Doses are taken once a day.

This drug may be taken with or without food. Do not eat raw oysters or other raw shellfish at any time while taking this drug.

Adults: Up to 200 mcg/kg per day.

Forgotten doses: If more than a few hours have passed since the forgotten dose, do not take the dose unless otherwise directed by your doctor.

ALCOHOL, DRUG, HERB, AND SUPPLEMENT INTERACTIONS

Alcohol may increase some of the side effects from this drug, depending on the amount consumed. Ask your doctor about the risks caused by drinking alcohol with your condition.

Taking this drug with any of the ones listed below may change the effect of either drug with the possibility of causing toxicity or decreasing effectiveness: amphotericin B, antithyroid drugs†, azathioprine, chloramphenicol, colchicine, corticosteroids†, cyclophosphamide, cyclosporine, cytarabine, flucytosine, ganciclovir, interferon, mercaptopurine, muromonab-CD3, plicamycin, probenecid, sulfinpyrazone, tacrolimus, zidovudine

Severe reactions are possible when this drug is taken with those listed below: anticoagulants†, aspirin

ALLERGIC REACTIONS AND SIDE EFFECTS

You should tell your doctor about all your allergies and any unexplained symptoms you may have while taking this drug.

MORE COMMON SIDE EFFECTS: Back pain*, black stools*, bleeding*, bloody urine*, bruising*, chills*, cough*, difficulty urinating*, fever*, hoarseness*, seizures*, skin irritation*

LESS COMMON SIDE EFFECTS: Hives*, itching*, joint pain*, menstrual changes, mouth sores*, nausea, skin rash*, swelling*, vomiting

RARE SIDE EFFECTS: Agitation*, blisters*, confusion*, cough*, hallucinations*, muscle twitches*, paralysis*, shortness of breath*, tremors*, weakness*, yellow eyes or skin*

PRECAUTIONS

Avoid contact with anyone who has the chickenpox, measles, or other communicable disease since it may be easier to catch the infection while taking this drug.

† See page 52.   * See page 53.

Exposure to skin tests, immunizations, and people who have received immunizations may put you at a greater risk of developing the disease when you are taking this drug.

This drug may cause changes to the blood resulting in an increased risk of blood-clotting problems.

This drug causes changes in your blood that put you at greater risk of getting an infection. Be careful not to cut yourself or get bruised. Tell your doctor if you develop signs of infection, such as fever or sore throat. Your dentist may recommend that you clean your teeth and mouth differently to avoid infection.

Touching these tablets may cause skin irritation. You should wash your hands immediately after taking the dose.

PREGNANCY AND BREAST-FEEDING

There is evidence that this drug may harm the fetus, but the drug may be necessary to the health of the mother.

Breast-feeding while taking this drug is not recommended.

HELPFUL COMMENTS

Side effects may continue for up to a month after the drug is stopped.

If you have tried this drug in the past and it did not work, it should not be tried again.

It is very important to continue taking this drug as ordered by the doctor even if the side effects make you feel ill.

If you have difficulty swallowing, crush the tablets and mix them with a little bit of jelly or jam. Take the dose right after mixing. Do not mix doses in advance.

If you vomit shortly after taking this drug, call your doctor to find out if you should repeat the dose.

CHLORDIAZEPOXIDE HYDROCHLORIDE

Available for over 20 years

COMMONLY USED TO TREAT

Alcohol withdrawal
Anxiety and tension

DRUG CATEGORY

antitremor
anxiolytic

sedative-hypnotic
Class: benzodiazepine

PRODUCTS

Brand-Name Products with Generic Alternatives
Librium 5 mg capsule (¢)
  Generic: chlordiazepoxide 5 mg capsule (¢¢¢¢)
Librium 10 mg capsule (¢)
  Generic: chlordiazepoxide 10 mg capsule (¢¢¢¢¢)
Librium 25 mg capsule (¢)
  Generic: chlordiazepoxide 25 mg capsule ($$)
Combination Products That Contain This Drug
Limitrol tablet ($)
Limbitrol DS tablet ($$)

DOSING AND FOOD

Doses are taken 2 to 4 times a day.
This drug may be taken with or without food.
Adults: Up to 300 mg per day in divided doses.
Children over age 6 and adults over age 65: Up to 40 mg per day in divided doses.
Forgotten doses: If you are scheduled to take the next dose within a few hours, do not take the forgotten dose. Otherwise take the forgotten dose as soon as you remember.

ALCOHOL, DRUG, HERB, AND SUPPLEMENT INTERACTIONS

Alcohol should not be used while taking this drug.
Catnip, kava, lady's slipper, lemon balm, passion flower, sassafras, skullcap, and valerian should not be used while taking this drug since they may cause an increase is the sedative effect.

Taking this drug with any of the ones listed below may change the effect of either drug with the possibility of causing toxicity or decreasing effectiveness: cimetidine, digoxin, disulfiram, fluvoxamine, haloperidol, itraconazole, ketoconazole, levodopa, nefazodone, oral contraceptives, rifampin

Severe reactions are possible when this drug is taken with those listed below: anesthetics[†], antidepressants[†], antihistamines[†], barbiturates[†], monoamine oxidase inhibitors[†], narcotics[†], phenothiazines[†]

Increased side effects are possible when this drug is taken with those listed below: aminophylline, theophylline

[†] See page 52.   * See page 53.

ALLERGIC REACTIONS AND SIDE EFFECTS

If you are allergic to any benzodiazepines†, you may also be allergic to this drug. You should tell your doctor about all your allergies and any unexplained symptoms you may have while taking this drug.

MORE COMMON SIDE EFFECTS: Clumsiness, dizziness, drowsiness, lightheadedness, slurry speech

LESS COMMON SIDE EFFECTS: Anxiety*, confusion*, constipation, depression*, diarrhea, difficulty urinating, dry mouth, headache, irregular heartbeat*, memory loss*, muscle spasm, nausea, sexual dysfunction, stomach cramps, thirst, trembling, vision changes, vomiting, watery mouth

RARE SIDE EFFECTS: Agitation*, behavior changes*, bleeding*, bruising*, chills*, delusions*, disorientation*, excitement*, eye movement*, fever*, hallucinations*, irritability*, low blood pressure*, mouth sores*, nervousness*, seizures*, skin irritation*, sleeping difficulty*, sore throat*, spastic movements*, tiredness*, weakness*, yellow eyes or skin*

PRECAUTIONS

This drug may be habit forming and will cause severe withdrawal symptoms if stopped abruptly. If you wish to stop taking this drug, ask your doctor for specific instructions.

You need to wait 2 weeks after stopping a monoamine oxidase inhibitor† before starting this drug.

If you have difficulty swallowing, emphysema, asthma, bronchitis, glaucoma, hyperactivity, mental depression, mental illness, myasthenia gravis, porphyria, or sleep apnea, this drug may make those conditions worse.

Heavy smoking may cause this drug to be less effective.

Be careful driving or handling equipment while taking this drug because it may cause dizziness and drowsiness.

PREGNANCY AND BREAST-FEEDING

There is evidence that this drug may harm the fetus, but the drug may be necessary to the health of the mother.

Breast-feeding while taking this drug is not recommended.

HELPFUL COMMENTS

This drug may cause a false positive pregnancy test depending on the test method.

Dangling your legs over the side of the bed for a few minutes may help reduce dizziness when first waking up.

CHLOROQUINE PHOSPHATE

Available for over 20 years

COMMONLY USED TO TREAT

Amebic infections
Lupus erythematosus
Malaria

DRUG CATEGORY

amebicide
antiinflammatory
antimalarial
Class: 4-amino-quinoline

PRODUCTS

Brand-Name Products with Generic Alternatives
Aralen 500 mg (300 mg base) tablet ($$$$)
  Generic: chloroquine phosphate 500 mg (300 mg base) tablet ($$$)
Products Only Available as Generics
chloroquine phosphate 250 mg (150 mg base) tablet (¢¢¢)

DOSING AND FOOD

Doses are taken once a day to once a week.
It is best to take this drug with food or milk.
Dosing varies widely depending on the reason for use.
Adults: Up to 250 mg per day although higher doses are used initially.
Children: Up to 10 mg/kg per day although higher doses are used initially.
Forgotten doses: Taking a forgotten dose will depend on the prescription
  schedule. If it is closer to the next scheduled dose than the forgotten
  dose, do not take the forgotten dose. Instead go back to your usual
  schedule with the next dose.

ALCOHOL, DRUG, HERB, AND SUPPLEMENT INTERACTIONS

Alcohol may increase some of the side effects from this drug, depending
  on the amount consumed. Ask your doctor about the risks caused by
  drinking alcohol with your condition.
OTC drugs used to treat diarrhea may contain an ingredient that can inter-
  fere with the effects of this drug. Ask your pharmacist for help when se-
  lecting an OTC product.

---

† See page 52.   * See page 53.

Taking this drug with any of the ones listed below may change the effect of either drug with the possibility of causing toxicity or decreasing effectiveness: antacids, cimetidine, kaolin, rabies vaccine

Severe reactions are possible when this drug is taken with those listed below: mefloquine

ALLERGIC REACTIONS AND SIDE EFFECTS

If you are allergic to hydroxychloroquine, you may also be allergic to this drug. You should tell your doctor about all your allergies and any unexplained symptoms you may have while taking this drug.

This drug promotes the effect of sunlight on the body and may cause severe sunburn and increased sensitivity of the eyes.

MORE COMMON SIDE EFFECTS: Diarrhea, headache*, itching, loss of appetite, nausea, seizures*, stomach cramps, vomiting

LESS COMMON SIDE EFFECTS: Eye pain*, hair color change, hair loss, loss of vision*, skin discoloration, skin rash*, vision changes*

RARE SIDE EFFECTS: Back pain*, black stools*, bleeding*, bloody urine*, bruising*, chills*, cough*, difficulty urinating*, drowsiness*, excitability*, fever*, hearing loss*, hoarseness*, lightheadedness*, mental changes*, mood swings*, ringing in ears*, sore throat*, tiredness*, weakness*

PRECAUTIONS

If you have psoriasis or porphyria, this drug may make the condition worse.

Children are very sensitive to this drug, and may be at greater risk of developing side effects.

If you have glucose-6-phosphate dehydrogenase deficiency, this drug may cause serious side effects.

Regular eye examinations are needed while taking this drug.

PREGNANCY AND BREAST-FEEDING

Safety during pregnancy has not been established although the drug is known to harm animal fetuses.

This drug passes into breast milk, but does not appear to harm the baby. The amount of drug in the breast milk is not enough to prevent the baby from getting malaria. Talk to your doctor about the risks associated with breast-feeding while taking this drug.

HELPFUL COMMENTS

This drug works best when doses are taken on a strict schedule at the same time of day.

If using this drug to prevent malaria, you should also use a DEET-containing mosquito repellent and use other precautions when traveling.

CHLOROTHIAZIDE

Available for over 20 years

COMMONLY USED TO TREAT

Fluid retention, also known as edema
Frequent urination in people with diabetes
High blood pressure, also known as hypertension

DRUG CATEGORY

antihypertensive
Class: thiazide diuretic

PRODUCTS

Brand-Name Products with No Generic Alternative
Diuril 250 mg/5 ml oral suspension (¢¢¢)
Brand-Name Products with Generic Alternatives
Diuril 250 mg tablet (¢¢)
  Generic: chlorothiazide 250 mg tablet (¢)
Diuril 500 mg tablet (¢¢¢)
  Generic: chlorothiazide 500 mg tablet (¢)
Combination Products That Contain This Drug
Diupres tablet (n/a)

DOSING AND FOOD

Doses are taken 1 to 4 times a day.
It is best to take this drug on an empty stomach, but taking this drug with a little food may avoid the stomach upset that some people suffer. Avoid food with excess salt.
Adults: Up to 1,000 mg per day in divided doses.
Lower doses are used in children.
Forgotten doses: If you are scheduled to take the next dose within a few hours, do not take the forgotten dose. Otherwise take the forgotten dose as soon as you remember.

ALCOHOL, DRUG, HERB, AND SUPPLEMENT INTERACTIONS

Alcohol may cause your blood pressure to rise, making this drug less effec-

---

† See page 52.   * See page 53.

tive. Ask your doctor about the risks caused by drinking alcohol with your condition.

Licorice root may increase potassium loss and should not be used while taking this drug.

Several OTC drugs used for appetite control, asthma, colds, cough, hay fever, or sinus problems may cause an increase in blood pressure when taken with this drug. Check with your pharmacist when selecting OTC products.

Taking this drug with any of the ones listed below may change the effect of either drug with the possibility of causing toxicity or decreasing effectiveness: antidiabetics†, cholestyramine, colestipol, digoxin, insulin, lithium

ALLERGIC REACTIONS AND SIDE EFFECTS

If you are allergic to acetazolamide, bumetanide, dichlorphenamide, furosemide, methazolamide, sulfonamides†, or thiazide diuretics†, you may also be allergic to this drug. You should tell your doctor about all your allergies and any unexplained symptoms you may have while taking this drug.

This drug promotes the effect of sunlight on the body and may cause severe sunburn and increased sensitivity of the eyes.

LESS COMMON SIDE EFFECTS: Diarrhea*, dizziness, lightheadedness, loss of appetite, sexual dysfunction, stomach upset

RARE SIDE EFFECTS: Back pain*, black stools*, bleeding*, bloody urine*, breathing difficulty*, bruising*, chest pain*, chills*, confusion*, cough*, fatigue*, fever*, hives*, headache*, hoarseness*, irregular heartbeat*, joint pain*, leg pain*, muscle cramps*, nausea*, numbness*, painful urination*, shortness of breath*, skin rash*, stomach pain*, swelling*, vomiting*, weakness*, yellow eyes or skin*

PRECAUTIONS

This drug may cause your blood sugar level to rise and may lead to type 2 diabetes.

Your body may lose potassium while taking this drug, which may cause severe side effects. Potassium levels should be monitored periodically and may need to be supplemented while taking this drug. Eat food rich in potassium, such as apricots, bananas, citrus fruit, dates, and tomatoes, if you are not taking a potassium supplement or potassium-sparing diuretic†.

People with kidney disease may not be able to take this drug.

This drug may increase the level of uric acid in the body, which may lead to gout or kidney stones.

If you have lupus erythematosus or pancreatitis, this drug may make those conditions worse.

Nicotine in cigarettes may increase blood pressure, making this drug less effective.

This drug may cause an increase in the levels of cholesterol or triglyceride in the blood.

PREGNANCY AND BREAST-FEEDING

Safety during pregnancy has not been established although the drug is known to harm animal fetuses.

Breast-feeding while taking this drug is not recommended.

HELPFUL COMMENTS

Take your last dose of the day no later than 6 P.M. to avoid urination during the night.

Avoid quick movements to minimize dizziness. Dangling your legs over the side of the bed for a few minutes may help reduce dizziness when first waking up.

Record your weight twice a day, when first getting up in the morning and after the drug causes urination. A weight gain or loss of more than 2 pounds per day should be reported to your doctor.

The antihypertensive effects of this drug will last about 1 week after it is stopped.

If you do not treat high blood pressure, you may develop more serious problems such as heart failure, blood vessel disease, stroke, or kidney disease. Losing weight, exercising, eating more fruits and vegetables, and avoiding salty foods, such as lunchmeat and pickles, may help make drug treatment more successful.

CHLORPROMAZINE HYDROCHLORIDE

Available for over 20 years

COMMONLY USED TO TREAT

Mental disturbances, also known as psychosis
Nausea and vomiting

DRUG CATEGORY

antiemetic
antipsychotic
Class: phenothiazine: aliphatic derivative

† See page 52.   * See page 53.

PRODUCTS

Brand-Name Products with No Generic Alternative
Thorazine 200 mg extended-release capsule (n/a)
Thorazine 300 mg extended-release capsule (n/a)
Thorazine 25 mg rectal suppository ($$$)
Thorazine 100 mg rectal suppository ($$$$)

Brand-Name Products with Generic Alternatives
Thorazine 10 mg tablet (¢¢¢)
  Generic: chlorpromazine hydrochloride 10 mg tablet (¢)
Thorazine 25 mg tablet (¢¢¢¢)
  Generic: chlorpromazine hydrochloride 25 mg tablet (¢)
Thorazine 50 mg tablet (¢¢¢¢¢)
  Generic: chlorpromazine hydrochloride 50 mg tablet (¢)
Thorazine 100 mg tablet ($)
  Generic: chlorpromazine hydrochloride 100 mg tablet (¢)
Thorazine 200 mg tablet ($)
  Generic: chlorpromazine hydrochloride 200 mg tablet (¢)
Thorazine 10 mg/5 ml oral syrup ($)
  Generic: chlorpromazine hydrochloride 10 mg/5 ml oral syrup (n/a)
Thorazine 30 mg/ml oral concentration (n/a)
  Generic: chlorpromazine hydrochloride 30 mg/ml oral concentrate (¢¢)
Thorazine 100 mg/ml oral concentration (n/a)
  Generic: chlorpromazine hydrochloride 100 mg/ml oral concentrate (¢¢¢)

Other Generic Product Names
Sonazine

DOSING AND FOOD

Doses are taken 2 to 6 times a day. Extended-release or suppository products are taken 2 to 3 times a day.

Taking this drug with food or a full glass of milk or water may avoid the stomach upset that some people suffer.

Adults: Up to 800 mg by mouth per day in divided doses.

Children over 6 months: Up to 3.3 mg/kg by mouth per day in divided doses.

Lower doses are used in people over age 65.

Forgotten doses: If you are scheduled to take the next dose within a few hours, do not take the forgotten dose. Otherwise take the forgotten dose as soon as you remember.

ALCOHOL, DRUG, HERB, AND SUPPLEMENT INTERACTIONS

Alcohol should not be used while taking this drug.

Do not use caffeine or kava while taking this drug since the drug effects may be decreased and severe reactions may occur.

Several OTC drugs used for appetite control, asthma, colds, cough, hay fever, pain, or sinus problems may seriously increase the effects and side effects of this drug. Check with your pharmacist when selecting OTC products.

Taking this drug with any of the ones listed below may change the effect of either drug with the possibility of causing toxicity or decreasing effectiveness: antihypertensives†, caffeine, beta blockers†, levodopa, lithium, warfarin

Severe reactions are possible when this drug is taken with those listed below: alcohol, amantadine, anesthetics, antiarrhythmics†, anticholinergics†, antihistamines†, antithyroid drugs†, anxiolytics†, astemizole, bromocriptine, cisapride, barbiturates†, deferoxamine, disopyramide, diuretics, epinephrine, erythromycin, levobunolol, lithium, metipranolol, nabilone, narcotics†, pentamidine, probucol, procainamide, promethazine, propylthiouracil, quinidine, sympathomimetics†, tricyclic antidepressants†

Increased side effects are possible when this drug is taken with those listed below: antipsychotics†, metoclopramide, metyrosine, pemoline, pimozide, rauwolfia alkaloids†, trimeprazine

ALLERGIC REACTIONS AND SIDE EFFECTS

If you are allergic to any phenothiazines†, you may also be allergic to this drug. You should tell your doctor about all your allergies and any unexplained symptoms you may have while taking this drug.

This drug promotes the effect of sunlight on the body and may cause severe sunburn and increased sensitivity of the eyes.

MORE COMMON SIDE EFFECTS: Breathing difficulty*, chewing action*, congestion, constipation, decreased sweating*, dizziness, drowsiness, dry mouth, eye stare*, eyelid movement*, fainting*, lip smacking*, loss of balance*, muscle spasms*, muscle stiffness*, puffy cheeks*, restlessness*, shuffling walk*, tongue movements*, trembling*, twitching*, vision changes*

LESS COMMON SIDE EFFECTS: Breast-milk secretion, breast swelling, dark urine*, menstrual changes, rough tongue, sexual dysfunction, skin rash*, urinary difficulty*, watery mouth, weight gain

RARE SIDE EFFECTS: Abdominal pain*, aching muscles, agitation*, bleeding*, blood pressure change*, bruising*, chest pain*, chills*, clumsiness*,

†See page 52. *See page 53.

coma*, confusion*, diarrhea*, dreams*, drooling*, excitement*, fast heartbeat*, fever*, hair loss*, headache*, irregular heartbeat*, itching*, joint pain*, loss of bladder control*, mouth sores*, muscle stiffness*, nausea*, penile erection*, red hands*, seizures*, shivering*, skin discoloration*, sleep disorders*, sore throat*, speaking difficulty*, sweating*, tiredness*, vomiting*, weakness*, yellow eyes or skin*

PRECAUTIONS

Do not open, crush, break, or chew the extended-release products.

If you have a history of enlarged prostate, glaucoma, ulcers, seizures, heart disease, urinary difficulty, or Parkinson's disease, this drug may make those conditions worse.

This drug may decrease the cough reflex, putting people with lung disease at greater risk of developing pneumonia.

Heavy smoking may cause this drug to be less effective.

This drug may cause false results from several diagnostic tests including pregnancy tests and should be stopped for at least 4 days before the test.

This drug should not be stopped suddenly, due to an increased risk of side effects. If you wish to stop taking this drug, ask your doctor for specific instructions.

Be careful driving or handling equipment while taking this drug because it may cause dizziness and drowsiness.

You are more likely to overheat when taking this drug and should avoid exercising in hot weather and using a sauna or hot tub.

This drug may make you more sensitive to cold temperatures.

Touching the liquid form of this drug may cause skin irritation. Make sure you do not spill the liquid, and wash your hands immediately after taking the dose.

This drug may cause dry mouth, which is associated with a greater risk of cavities. Your dentist may recommend that you clean your teeth and mouth differently to avoid infection.

PREGNANCY AND BREAST-FEEDING

Safety during pregnancy has not been established although the drug is known to harm animal fetuses.

Breast-feeding while taking this drug is not recommended.

HELPFUL COMMENTS

If using a suppository, remove the foil and run under cold water before inserting.

If you need to take an antacid, take it either 2 hours before or after taking this drug.

Sucking on hard sugarless candy or chewing sugarless gum may help relieve dry mouth caused by this drug.

The liquid form of this drug should be mixed in $1/4$ to $1/2$ cup of applesauce, carbonated beverage, fruit juice, milk, pudding, soup, tomato juice, or water just before taking the dose.

CHLORPROPAMIDE

Available for over 20 years

COMMONLY USED TO TREAT

High blood sugar, specifically type 2 diabetes

DRUG CATEGORY

antidiabetic
antidiuretic
Class: sulfonylurea: first generation

PRODUCTS

Brand-Name Products with Generic Alternatives
Diabinese 100 mg tablet (¢¢¢)
  Generic: chlorpropamide 100 mg tablet (¢)
Diabinese 250 mg tablet (¢¢¢¢¢)
  Generic: chlorpropamide 250 mg tablet (¢)

DOSING AND FOOD

Doses are taken 1 to 2 times a day.

It is best to take this drug just before meals starting with the first meal of the day.

Adults: Up to 750 mg per day in divided doses.

Lower doses may be used in people over age 65 and in people with kidney or liver disease.

Forgotten doses: If you are scheduled to take the next dose within a few hours, do not take the forgotten dose. Otherwise take the forgotten dose as soon as you remember.

†See page 52.   *See page 53.

ALCOHOL, DRUG, HERB, AND SUPPLEMENT INTERACTIONS

Alcohol should not be used while taking this drug since the combination may cause a severe reaction.

Aloe, bilberry leaf, bitter melon, burdock, dandelion, fenugreek, garlic, ginkgo biloba, and ginseng may lower blood sugar and cause the need for a dose adjustment when taken with this drug. Tell your doctor if you are taking any of these supplements.

Several OTC drugs used for asthma, colds, cough, hay fever, sleep aid, or sinus problems may seriously change the effects of this drug. Check with your pharmacist when selecting OTC products.

Taking this drug with any of the ones listed below may change the effect of either drug with the possibility of causing toxicity or decreasing effectiveness: anticoagulants†, antihistamines†, aspirin, beta blockers†, chloramphenicol, cimetidine, corticosteroids†, cyclosporine, fluconazole, fluoro-quinolones†, insulin, lithium, miconazole, probenecid, quinine, quinidine, ranitidine, salicylates†, sulfonamides†, thiazide diuretics†

Severe reactions are possible when this drug is taken with those listed below: guanethidine, monoamine oxidase inhibitors†, octreotide, pentamidine

ALLERGIC REACTIONS AND SIDE EFFECTS

If you are allergic to any sulfonylureas† or sulfonamides†, you may also be allergic to this drug. You should tell your doctor about all your allergies and any unexplained symptoms you may have while taking this drug.

This drug promotes the effect of sunlight on the body and may cause severe sunburn and increased sensitivity of the eyes.

MORE COMMON SIDE EFFECTS: Anxiety*, appetite changes, behavior change*, blurry vision*, chills*, confusion*, constipation, diarrhea, difficulty concentrating*, dizziness, drowsiness*, fast heartbeat*, frequent urination, gas, headache*, heartburn, hunger*, low blood sugar*, nausea*, nervousness*, nightmares*, shakiness*, sleep disorders*, slurry speech*, stomach pain, sweating*, taste changes, tiredness*, vomiting, weakness*, weight gain*

LESS COMMON SIDE EFFECTS: Seizures*, skin irritation*, unconsciousness*

RARE SIDE EFFECTS: Bleeding*, bruising*, chest pain*, coughing up blood*, dark urine*, depression*, excess sputum*, fever*, hives*, pale skin*, pale stools*, shortness of breath*, sore throat*, swelling*, yellow eyes or skin*

PRECAUTIONS

Burns, diarrhea, fever, hormonal changes, infection, malnourishment, severe stress, uncontrolled thyroid disease, and vomiting may cause changes in blood sugar that may make this drug less effective.

You need to wait 2 weeks after stopping a monoamine oxidase inhibitor† before starting this drug.

This drug is not effective in treating type 1 diabetes.

Some people who take this drug may retain water, putting people with high blood pressure or heart disease at risk of complications.

PREGNANCY AND BREAST-FEEDING

Safety during pregnancy has not been established although the drug is known to harm animal fetuses.

Breast-feeding while taking this drug is not recommended.

HELPFUL COMMENTS

Blood sugar level should be checked if you experience any side effects.

If you are a smoker and stop smoking while taking this drug, your dose may need to be reduced.

This drug stays in the body for about a week after each dose.

If you do not treat high blood sugar, you may develop more serious problems such as heart failure, blood vessel disease, eye disease, or kidney disease.

CHLORTHALIDONE

Available for over 20 years

COMMONLY USED TO TREAT

Fluid retention, also known as edema
Frequent urination in people with diabetes
High blood pressure, also known as hypertension

DRUG CATEGORY

antihypertensive
Class: thiazidelike diuretic

PRODUCTS

Brand-Name Products with No Generic Alternative
Thalitone 15 mg tablet (¢¢¢¢¢)

Brand-Name Products with Generic Alternatives
Hygroton 25 mg tablet (n/a)

---

†See page 52.   * See page 53.

Generic: chlorthalidone 25 mg tablet (¢)
Hygroton 50 mg tablet (n/a)
Generic: chlorthalidone 50 mg tablet (¢)
Combination Products That Contain This Drug
Tenoretic tablet ($) to ($$)
Clorpres tablet (n/a)

DOSING AND FOOD

Doses are usually taken once a day but may be taken as little as 3 times a
week.
Taking this drug with a little food may avoid the stomach upset that some
people suffer. Avoid food with excess salt.
Adults: Up to 100 mg per day.
Lower doses may be used in children
Forgotten doses: If you are scheduled to take the next dose within a few
hours, do not take the forgotten dose. Otherwise take the forgotten dose
as soon as you remember.

ALCOHOL, DRUG, HERB, AND SUPPLEMENT INTERACTIONS

Alcohol may cause your blood pressure to rise, making this drug less effective. Ask your doctor about the risks caused by drinking alcohol with
your condition.
Licorice root may increase potassium loss and should not be used while
taking this drug.
Several OTC drugs used for appetite control, asthma, colds, cough, hay
fever, or sinus problems may cause an increase in blood pressure when
taken with this drug. Check with your pharmacist when selecting OTC
products.
**Taking this drug with any of the ones listed below may change the effect of
either drug with the possibility of causing toxicity or decreasing effectiveness:**
antidiabetics†, cholestyramine, colestipol, digoxin, insulin, lithium

ALLERGIC REACTIONS AND SIDE EFFECTS

If you are allergic to acetazolamide, bumetanide, dichlorphenamide,
furosemide, methazolamide, sulfonamides†, or thiazide diuretics†, you
may also be allergic to this drug. You should tell your doctor about all
your allergies and any unexplained symptoms you may have while taking this drug.

This drug promotes the effect of sunlight on the body and may cause severe sunburn and increased sensitivity of the eyes.

LESS COMMON SIDE EFFECTS: Diarrhea*, dizziness, lightheadedness, loss of appetite, sexual dysfunction, stomach upset

RARE SIDE EFFECTS: Back pain*, black stools*, bleeding*, bloody urine*, breathing difficulty*, bruising*, burning sensation*, chest pain*, chills*, confusion*, cough*, fatigue*, fever*, headache*, hives*, hoarseness*, irregular heartbeat*, joint pain*, leg pain*, muscle cramps*, nausea*, numbness*, painful urination*, shortness of breath*, skin rash*, stomach pain*, swelling*, vomiting*, weakness*, yellow eyes or skin*

PRECAUTIONS

This drug may cause your blood sugar level to rise and may lead to type 2 diabetes.

Your body may lose potassium while taking this drug, which may cause severe side effects. Potassium levels should be monitored periodically and may need to be supplemented while taking this drug. Eat food rich in potassium, such as apricots, bananas, citrus fruit, dates, and tomatoes, if you are not taking a potassium supplement or potassium-sparing diuretic†.

People with kidney disease may not be able to take this drug.

This drug may increase the level of uric acid in the body, which may lead to gout or kidney stones.

If you have lupus erythematosus or pancreatitis, this drug may make those conditions worse.

Nicotine in cigarettes may increase blood pressure, making this drug less effective.

This drug may cause an increase in the levels of cholesterol or triglyceride in the blood.

PREGNANCY AND BREAST-FEEDING

Safety during pregnancy has not been established although the drug is known to harm animal fetuses.

Breast-feeding while taking this drug is not recommended.

HELPFUL COMMENTS

Take your last dose of the day no later than 6 P.M. to avoid urination during the night.

Avoid quick movements to minimize dizziness. Dangling your legs over the side of the bed for a few minutes may help reduce dizziness when first waking up.

† See page 52.   * See page 53.

Record your weight twice a day, when first getting up in the morning and after the drug causes urination. A weight gain or loss of more than 2 pounds per day should be reported to your doctor.

The antihypertensive effects of this drug will last about 1 week after it is stopped.

If you do not treat high blood pressure, you may develop more serious problems such as heart failure, blood vessel disease, stroke, or kidney disease. Losing weight, exercising, eating more fruits and vegetables, and avoiding salty foods, such as lunchmeat and pickles, may help make drug treatment more successful.

CHLORZOXAZONE

Available for over 20 years

COMMONLY USED TO TREAT

Muscle stiffness and pain caused by injury

DRUG CATEGORY

skeletal muscle relaxant
Class: benzoxazole derivative

PRODUCTS

Brand-Name Products with Generic Alternatives
Parafon Forte DSC 500 mg tablet ($)
  Generic: chlorzoxazone 500 mg tablet (¢¢)
Products Only Available as Generics
chlorzoxazone 250 mg tablet (¢¢)
Other Generic Product Names
Strifon Forte DSC

DOSING AND FOOD

Doses are taken 3 to 4 times a day.
Taking this drug with a little food may avoid the stomach upset that some people suffer.
Adults: Up to 3,000 mg per day in divided doses.
Children: Up to 20 mg/kg per day in divided doses.
Forgotten doses: If more than 1 hour has passed since the forgotten dose, do not take the dose. Just go back to your usual schedule with the next dose.

ALCOHOL, DRUG, HERB, AND SUPPLEMENT INTERACTIONS

Alcohol should not be used while taking this drug.

Do not eat watercress while using this drug since it may increase the drug effect and lead to more side effects and possible toxicity.

Several OTC drugs used for appetite control, asthma, colds, cough, hay fever, pain, or sinus problems may seriously increase the effects of this drug. Check with your pharmacist when selecting OTC products.

Increased side effects are possible when this drug is taken with those listed below:
anesthetics, antihistamines†, anxiolytics†, barbiturates†, monoamine oxidase inhibitors†, narcotics†, tricyclic antidepressants†

ALLERGIC REACTIONS AND SIDE EFFECTS

If you are allergic to meprobamate or any other skeletal muscle relaxant†, you may also be allergic to this drug. You should tell your doctor about all your allergies and any unexplained symptoms you may have while taking this drug.

MORE COMMON SIDE EFFECTS: Dizziness, drowsiness, lightheadedness, shortness of breath*, swollen eyes*, swollen glands*

LESS COMMON SIDE EFFECTS: Chest tightness*, clumsiness, confusion, constipation, depression*, diarrhea, excitement, fainting*, fast heartbeat*, fever*, headache, heartburn, hiccups, hives*, irritability, itching*, muscle weakness, nausea, nervousness, restlessness, skin rash*, stomach cramps, stuffy nose*, vomiting

RARE SIDE EFFECTS: Back pain*, black stools*, bleeding*, bloody urine*, bruising*, cough*, difficulty urinating*, hoarseness*, irregular breathing*, mouth sores*, muscle cramps*, sore throat*, tiredness*, weakness*, yellow eyes or skin*

PRECAUTIONS

Be careful driving or handling equipment while taking this drug because it may cause dizziness and drowsiness.

Withdrawal symptoms may occur if this drug is stopped suddenly. If you wish to stop taking this drug, ask your doctor for specific instructions.

This drug may change the color of your urine to orange, red, or purple. The color change is not associated with harm and will return to normal once the drug is stopped.

---

† See page 52.   * See page 53.

PREGNANCY AND BREAST-FEEDING

Safety during pregnancy has not been established although the drug is known to harm animal fetuses.

This drug does not appear to harm the breast-fed baby. Talk to your doctor about the risks associated with breast-feeding while taking this drug.

HELPFUL COMMENTS

Avoid quick movements to minimize dizziness. Dangling your legs over the side of the bed for a few minutes may help reduce dizziness when first waking up.

This drug may be crushed and mixed with food, milk, or juice to make it easier to swallow.

CILOSTAZOL

Available since January 1999

COMMONLY USED TO TREAT

Leg pain caused by poor circulation, also know as intermittent claudication

DRUG CATEGORY

antiplatelet
Class: PDE III inhibitor

PRODUCTS

Brand-Name Products with No Generic Alternative
Pletal 50 mg tablet ($$)
Pletal 100 mg tablet ($$)
No generics available.
No patents. Exclusivity until 2004.

DOSING AND FOOD

Doses are taken 2 times a day.

It is best to take this drug on an empty stomach either $1/2$ hour before or 2 hours after breakfast and dinner. Do not drink grapefruit juice while taking this drug.

Adults: Up to 200 mg per day in divided doses.

Forgotten doses: If you are scheduled to take the next dose within a few hours, do not take the forgotten dose. Otherwise take the forgotten dose as soon as you remember.

ALCOHOL, DRUG, HERB, AND SUPPLEMENT INTERACTIONS

Alcohol may increase some of the side effects from this drug, depending on the amount consumed. Ask your doctor about the risks caused by drinking alcohol with your condition.

Taking this drug with any of the ones listed below may change the effect of either drug with the possibility of causing toxicity or decreasing effectiveness:

diltiazem, erythromycin, fluconazole, fluoxetine, fluvoxamine, itraconazole, ketoconazole, miconazole, nefazodone, omeprazole, paroxetine, sertraline

ALLERGIC REACTIONS AND SIDE EFFECTS

You should tell your doctor about all your allergies and any unexplained symptoms you may have while taking this drug.

MORE COMMON SIDE EFFECTS: Back pain, cough, dizziness, fever*, gas, headache, irregular heartbeat*, sore throat, stiff muscles, stuffy nose, swelling*

LESS COMMON SIDE EFFECTS: Black stools*, bleeding*, bone pain, bruising*, diarrhea*, fainting*, heartburn*, hives, nausea*, nosebleeds*, ringing in ears, stiff joints, stiff neck*, stomach pain*, swallowing difficulty

PRECAUTIONS

Tobacco products, such as cigarettes, may reduce the effectiveness of this drug and should be stopped.

People with heart disease may not be able to take this drug.

Since this drug is still relatively new, ask your pharmacist about any additional precautions each time you get your prescription refilled.

PREGNANCY AND BREAST-FEEDING

Safety during pregnancy has not been established although the drug is known to harm animal fetuses.

Breast-feeding while taking this drug is not recommended.

HELPFUL COMMENTS

It will take at least 2 weeks before the effects of this drug are noticed and up to 12 weeks before the full effects are noticed.

You may estimate how well this drug is working by measuring and comparing the distances that you can walk without pain.

---

†See page 52.   *See page 53.

CIMETIDINE

Available for over 20 years

COMMONLY USED TO TREAT

Stomach ulcers, specifically duodenal ulcers and gastric ulcers

DRUG CATEGORY

antiulcer
Class: H2 receptor antagonist

PRODUCTS

Brand-Name Products with Generic Alternatives
Tagamet 300 mg tablet ($)
  Generic: cimetidine 300 mg tablet (¢¢)
Tagamet 400 mg tablet ($$)
  Generic: cimetidine 400 mg tablet (¢¢)
Tagamet 800 mg tablet ($$$)
  Generic: cimetidine 800 mg tablet (¢¢¢)
Tagamet 300 mg/5 ml oral solution (n/a)
  Generic: cimetidine hydrochloride 300 mg/5 ml oral solution ($$)

DOSING AND FOOD

Doses are taken 1 to 4 times a day.
It is best to take this drug with food, milk, or within 1 hour before meals.
Adults: Up to 2,400 mg per day in divided doses.
Children: Up to 40 mg/kg per day in divided doses.
Lower doses are used in people with kidney or liver disease.
Forgotten doses: If you are scheduled to take the next dose within a few hours, do not take the forgotten dose. Otherwise take the forgotten dose as soon as you remember.

ALCOHOL, DRUG, HERB, AND SUPPLEMENT INTERACTIONS

Alcohol may increase some of the side effects from this drug, depending on the amount consumed. Ask your doctor about the risks caused by drinking alcohol with your condition.
Do not use guarana, pennyroyal, or yerba maté while taking this drug since the combination may lead to serious reactions.

Taking this drug with any of the ones listed below may change the effect of either drug with the possibility of causing toxicity or decreasing effectiveness: aminophylline, anticoagulants†, benzodiazepines†, beta blockers†, caffeine, carmustine, digoxin, disulfiram, flecainide, isoniazid, lidocaine, metoprolol, metronidazole, oral contraceptives, oxtriphylline, phenytoin, quinidine, theophylline, triamterene, tricyclic antidepressants†

ALLERGIC REACTIONS AND SIDE EFFECTS

If you are allergic to any H2 receptor antagonists†, you may also be allergic to this drug. You should tell your doctor about all your allergies and any unexplained symptoms you may have while taking this drug.

MORE COMMON SIDE EFFECTS: Diarrhea

LESS COMMON SIDE EFFECTS: Breast tenderness, constipation, dizziness*, drowsiness, dry mouth, hair loss, headache, ringing in ears, runny nose, sexual dysfunction, sleep disorders, sweating, urinary changes

RARE SIDE EFFECTS: Abdominal pain*, agitation*, anxiety*, back pain*, bleeding*, blisters*, breathing difficulty*, bruising*, chest tightness*, chills*, confusion*, cough*, dark urine*, depression*, fainting*, fever*, hallucinations*, hives*, irregular heartbeat*, itching*, joint pain*, leg pain*, loss of appetite*, mood swings*, muscle cramps*, nausea*, nervousness*, pain*, pale stools*, shallow breathing*, shortness of breath*, skin irritation*, sore eyes*, sore lips*, sore throat*, swallowing difficulty*, swelling*, tiredness*, vision changes*, vomiting*, weakness*, wheezing*, yellow eyes or skin*

PRECAUTIONS

Indomethacin, itraconazole, iron supplements, ketoconazole, and tetracyclines may interfere with the absorption of this drug. If you are taking one of these drugs, it should be taken at least 2 hours after this medicine.

This drug may cause false results from diagnostic skin tests.

This drug is available without a prescription in 200 mg tablets. The OTC product should not be taken for longer than 2 weeks unless recommended by your doctor.

Smoking may increase stomach acids, making your condition worse.

PREGNANCY AND BREAST-FEEDING

Safety during pregnancy has not been established although there was no evidence of harm during studies in animals.

Breast-feeding while taking this drug is not recommended.

---

† See page 52. * See page 53.

HELPFUL COMMENTS

Once-a-day doses should be taken at bedtime.

It takes several days before the effect of this drug is noticed.

If you need to take an antacid, take it either 2 hours before or after taking this drug.

CIPROFLOXACIN HYDROCHLORIDE

Available since April 1996

COMMONLY USED TO TREAT

Infection

DRUG CATEGORY

antibiotic

Class: fluoroquinolone

PRODUCTS

Brand-Name Products with No Generic Alternative

Cipro 100 mg tablet ($$$)

Cipro 250 mg tablet ($$$)

Cipro 500 mg tablet ($$$)

Cipro 750 mg tablet ($$$$)

Cipro 250 mg/5 ml oral suspension ($$$)

Cipro 500 mg/ 5 ml oral suspension ($$$)

Ciloxan 0.3% ophthalmic ointment ($$$$$)

Ciloxan 0.3% ophthalmic solution ($$$$$)

No generics available.

Multiple patents that begin to expire in 2003.

DOSING AND FOOD

Doses are taken twice a day.

It is best to take this drug on an empty stomach, 2 hours after a meal.

Adults: Up to 1,500 mg per day in divided doses.

Lower doses are used in people with kidney disease.

This drug is rarely used by mouth in children under age 18 because it may interfere with bone development. Eyedrops are used in children over age 12.

Eyedrops: 1 to 2 drops per dose, 1 to 60 times per day.

Forgotten doses: If you are scheduled to take the next dose within a few hours, do not take the forgotten dose. Otherwise take the forgotten dose as soon as you remember.

ALCOHOL, DRUG, HERB, AND SUPPLEMENT INTERACTIONS

Alcohol may increase some of the side effects from this drug, depending on the amount consumed. Ask your doctor about the risks caused by drinking alcohol with your condition.

The use of yerba maté while taking this drug may result in a toxic reaction.

Taking this drug with any of the ones listed below may change the effect of either drug with the possibility of causing toxicity or decreasing effectiveness: aminoglycosides†, antacids, beta lactams, caffeine, didanosine, iron, mineral supplements, phenytoin, probenecid, sucralfate, warfarin

Severe reactions are possible when this drug is taken with those listed below: aminophylline, oxtriphylline, theophylline

ALLERGIC REACTIONS AND SIDE EFFECTS

If you are allergic to any fluoroquinolones†, you may also be allergic to this drug. You should tell your doctor about all your allergies and any unexplained symptoms you may have while taking this drug.

This drug promotes the effect of sunlight on the body and may cause severe sunburn and increased sensitivity of the eyes.

More Common Side Effects: Diarrhea*, nausea, nervousness, rash, seizures*, skin irritation*, vomiting

Less Common Side Effects: Back pain, blisters*, difficulty urinating, dizziness, dreams, drowsiness, headache, lightheadedness, mouth sores, muscle pain, sleep disorders, stomachache, vaginal discharge, vaginal pain, taste changes, vision changes

Rare Side Effects: Abdominal pain*, agitation*, bloody urine*, confusion*, dark urine*, fever*, flushing*, hallucinations*, irregular heartbeat*, joint pain*, leg pain*, loss of appetite*, pale stools*, shakiness*, shortness of breath*, sweating*, swelling*, tiredness*, tremors*, weakness*, yellow eyes or skin*

PRECAUTIONS

Be careful driving or handling equipment while taking this drug because the drug may cause drowsiness.

If you have a history of tendinitis, this drug may make that condition worse.

If you are using eyedrops, many of the side effects and warnings do not ap-

†*See page 52.* *See page 53.*

ply. Watch for burning and irritation when the drops are used and report any rash, itching, swelling, or redness around the eye to your doctor.

PREGNANCY AND BREAST-FEEDING

Safety during pregnancy has not been established although the drug is known to harm animal fetuses.

Breast-feeding while taking this drug is not recommended.

HELPFUL COMMENTS

Contact your doctor if your symptoms do not improve after a couple of days.

Do not stop treatment early if you start to feel better. It takes the full prescription for this drug to work completely.

If you need to take an antacid, take it either 6 hours before or 2 hours after taking this drug.

Minerals, iron supplements, and caffeine may all reduce the effectiveness of this drug.

Drink a lot of water while taking this drug.

CITALOPRAM HYDROBROMIDE

Available since December 1999

COMMONLY USED TO TREAT

Depression

DRUG CATEGORY

antidepressant

Class: selective serotonin reuptake inhibitor (SSRI)

PRODUCTS

Brand-Name Products with No Generic Alternative

Celexa 10 mg tablet ($$)

Celexa 20 mg tablet ($$)

Celexa 40 mg tablet ($$)

Celexa 10 mg/5 ml oral solution ($$)

No generics available.

Exclusivity that begins to expire in 2003.

DOSING AND FOOD

Doses are taken once a day.

This drug may be taken with or without food.

Adults: Up to 40 mg per day.

Lower doses are used in people over age 65 and those with liver disease.

Forgotten doses: If more than 2 hours have passed since the forgotten dose, do not take the dose unless your doctor has instructed you differently.

ALCOHOL, DRUG, HERB, AND SUPPLEMENT INTERACTIONS

Alcohol should not be used while taking this drug.

St. John's wort should not be taken with this drug due to risk of toxicity. If you discontinue this drug, you need to wait at least 2 weeks before starting St. John's wort.

Several OTC drugs used for appetite control, asthma, colds, cough, hay fever, pain, or sinus problems may seriously increase the effects of this drug. Check with your pharmacist when selecting OTC products.

Taking this drug with any of the ones listed below may change the effect of either drug with the possibility of causing toxicity or decreasing effectiveness:
anesthetics, antihistamines†, anxiolytics†, barbiturates†, carbamazepine, imipramine, lithium, narcotics†, sumatriptan, tricyclic antidepressants†, warfarin

Severe reactions are possible when this drug is taken with those listed below:
monoamine oxidase inhibitors†

Increased side effects are possible when this drug is taken with those listed below:
bromocriptine, buspirone, dextromethorphan, fluoxetine, fluvoxamine, levodopa, lithium, LSD, marijuana, MDMA (ecstasy), meperidine, moclobemide, nefazodone, paroxetine, pentazocine, sertraline, tramadol, trazodone, triptans†, tryptophan, venlafaxine

ALLERGIC REACTIONS AND SIDE EFFECTS

You should tell your doctor about all your allergies and any unexplained symptoms you may have while taking this drug.

MORE COMMON SIDE EFFECTS: Dizziness*, drowsiness*, dry mouth, fast heartbeat*, nausea*, sexual dysfunction*, sleep disorders, sweating*, trembling*, vomiting*

LESS COMMON SIDE EFFECTS: Abdominal pain, agitation*, anxiety, blurry vision*, breathing difficulty*, confusion*, diarrhea, fever*, gas, headache, heartburn, increased salivation, increased urination*, itching*, joint pain,

---

†See page 52. *See page 53.

loss of appetite, memory loss*, menstrual changes*, muscle pain, runny
nose, shaking*, skin rash*, taste changes, tingling, tiredness, tooth grind-
ing, weakness, weight change, yawning

RARE SIDE EFFECTS: Behavior change*, black stools*, bleeding gums*,
bloating*, blue skin or lips*, breast enlargement*, breast-milk secretion*,
chills*, coma*, constipation*, cough*, dark urine*, drooling*, excitement*, eye irritation*, fainting*, hives*, hunger*, indigestion*, irregular
heartbeat*, lack of energy*, mood swings*, nervousness*, nosebleeds*,
painful urination*, penile erection*, poor coordination*, restlessness*,
seizures*, shivering*, sore throat*, stomach pain*, thirst*, twitching*, unconsciousness*

PRECAUTIONS

You need to wait 2 weeks after stopping a monoamine oxidase inhibitor†
before starting this drug.

If you have a history of mania or bipolar disease, this drug may cause those
conditions to return.

People with a history of seizures may be at greater risk of developing a
seizure while taking this drug.

Be careful driving or handling equipment while taking this drug because
the drug may cause drowsiness.

Discontinuing this drug may cause side effects which may be minimized by
gradually decreasing the dose over 2 weeks before stopping.

This drug may cause dry mouth, which is associated with a greater risk of
cavities. Your dentist may recommend that you clean your teeth and
mouth differently to avoid infection.

PREGNANCY AND BREAST-FEEDING

Safety during pregnancy has not been established although the drug is
known to harm animal fetuses.

Breast-feeding while taking this drug is not recommended. This drug passes into breast milk, and may cause drowsiness and weight loss in the
breast-fed baby.

HELPFUL COMMENTS

It may take 4 weeks before the effects of this drug are noticed.

CLARITHROMYCIN

Available since October 1991

COMMONLY USED TO TREAT

Infection

DRUG CATEGORY

antibiotic
Class: macrolide

PRODUCTS

Brand-Name Products with No Generic Alternative
Biaxin 250 mg tablet ($$$)
Biaxin 500 mg tablet ($$$)
Biaxin 125 mg/5 ml oral suspension ($$)
Biaxin 250 mg/5 ml oral suspension ($$$)
Biaxin XL 500 mg extended-release tablet ($$$)
No generics available.
No patents, no exclusivity.
Combination Products That Contain This Drug
Prevpac kit ($$$$$)

DOSING AND FOOD

Doses are taken twice a day. Extended-release products are taken once daily.
This drug may be taken with or without food. Extended-release products
  are better tolerated with food.
Adults: Up to 1,000 mg per day in divided doses.
Children: Up to 15 mg/kg per day in divided doses.
Lower doses are used in people with kidney disease.
Forgotten doses: If you are scheduled to take the next dose within a few
  hours, do not take the forgotten dose. Otherwise take the forgotten dose
  as soon as you remember.

ALCOHOL, DRUG, HERB, AND SUPPLEMENT INTERACTIONS

Alcohol may increase some of the side effects from this drug, depending
  on the amount consumed. Ask your doctor about the risks caused by
  drinking alcohol with your condition.

---

† *See page 52.*   * *See page 53.*

Taking this drug with any of the ones listed below may change the effect of either drug with the possibility of causing toxicity or decreasing effectiveness:

carbamazepine, cyclosporine, digoxin, dihydroergotamine, ergotamine, phenytoin, rifabutin, rifampin, theophylline, triazolam, warfarin, zidovudine

Increased side effects are possible when this drug is taken with those listed below:

anticoagulants†, cisapride, pimozide

ALLERGIC REACTIONS AND SIDE EFFECTS

If you are allergic to any macrolides†, or Erythromycin, you may also be allergic to this drug. You should tell your doctor about all your allergies and any unexplained symptoms you may have while taking this drug.

MORE COMMON SIDE EFFECTS: Diarrhea*, nausea*, taste changes

LESS COMMON SIDE EFFECTS: Back pain*, belching, bloating, chills*, cough*, fever*, gas, headache, heartburn, hoarseness*, indigestion, stomachache, urinary difficulty*

RARE SIDE EFFECTS: Abdominal pain*, bleeding*, bruising*, itching*, rash*, shortness of breath*, vomiting*, yellow eyes or skin*

PRECAUTIONS

Do not crush, break, or chew the extended-release products.
The oral suspensions do not require refrigeration and are no longer good after 14 days.

PREGNANCY AND BREAST-FEEDING

Safety during pregnancy has not been established although the drug is known to harm animal fetuses.
Breast-feeding while taking this drug is not recommended.

HELPFUL COMMENTS

Contact your doctor if your symptoms do not improve after a couple of days.
Do not stop treatment early if you start to feel better. It takes the full prescription for this drug to work completely.

CLINDAMYCIN HYDROCHLORIDE

Available for over 20 years

COMMONLY USED TO TREAT

Acne
Infection

DRUG CATEGORY

antibiotic
Class: lincosamide

PRODUCTS

Brand-Name Products with No Generic Alternative
Cleocin 75 mg/5 ml oral solution ($)
Cleocin 100 mg vaginal suppository ($$$$$)
Cleocin 2% vaginal cream (¢¢¢)

Brand-Name Products with Generic Alternatives
Cleocin HCL 75 mg capsule ($)
  Generic: clindamycin hydrochloride 75 mg capsule
Cleocin HCL 150 mg capsule ($$)
  Generic: clindamycin hydrochloride 150 mg capsule
Cleocin HCL 300 mg capsule ($$$)
  Generic: clindamycin hydrochloride 300 mg capsule
Cleocin 1% topical swab (¢¢)
  Generic: clindamycin phosphate 1% topical swab (¢¢)
Cleocin T 1% topical gel (¢¢¢)
  Generic: clindamycin phosphate 1% topical gel (¢¢)
Cleocin T 1% topical lotion (¢¢)
  Generic: clindamycin phosphate 1% topical lotion (n/a)
Cleocin T 1% topical solution (¢¢)
  Generic: clindamycin phosphate 1% topical solution (¢)

Other Generic Product Names
Clinda-Derm, Clindagel, Clindets

Other Products That Contain This Drug
Benzaclin topical gel (¢¢¢¢¢)
Duac topical gel (n/a)

DOSING AND FOOD

Oral doses are taken 3 to 4 times a day. Topical products are used twice a
  day. Vaginal products are used once a day at bedtime.

† *See page 52.*   * *See page 53.*

Oral products are best taken with food, milk, or a full glass of water to prevent irritation of the throat.

Adults: Up to 2,700 mg per day by mouth in divided doses.

Children over 1 month: Up to 20 mg/kg per day by mouth in divided doses.

Forgotten doses: If you are scheduled to take the next dose within a few hours, do not take the forgotten dose. Otherwise take the forgotten dose as soon as you remember.

ALCOHOL, DRUG, HERB, AND SUPPLEMENT INTERACTIONS

Alcohol may increase some of the side effects from this drug, depending on the amount consumed. Ask your doctor about the risks caused by drinking alcohol with your condition.

Cyclamate, an artificial sweetener, may decrease the absorption of this drug and should not be used when taking the oral form of this drug.

Several OTC drugs used for diarrhea may interfere with the effect of this drug. Check with your pharmacist before selecting a product.

Taking this drug with any of the ones listed below may change the effect of either drug with the possibility of causing toxicity or decreasing effectiveness: attapulgite, chloramphenicol, erythromycin, kaolin, neuromuscular blockers†

Increased side effects are possible when this drug is taken with those listed below: diphenoxylate, opiates†

ALLERGIC REACTIONS AND SIDE EFFECTS

If you are allergic to lincomycin or doxorubicin, you may also be allergic to this drug. You should tell your doctor about all your allergies and any unexplained symptoms you may have while taking this drug.

MORE COMMON SIDE EFFECTS: Abdominal pain*, diarrhea*, fever*, nausea, stomachache, vomiting

LESS COMMON SIDE EFFECTS: Bleeding*, bruising*, genital itch*, rectal itch*, skin rash*, sore throat*

PRECAUTIONS

Using this drug for acne in combination with another acne product may cause skin irritation and excessive dryness.

People with a history of stomach or intestinal disease may be at greater risk of developing side effects.

The oral solution should not be refrigerated and is no longer good after 14 days.

It is possible for the topical forms of this drug to be absorbed into the body and may produce the same side effects as oral products.

This drug is very irritating if it gets into your eye. Rinse your eye with a lot of cool tap water to reduce the pain.

If treating a vaginal infection, you need to use a barrier contraceptive, such as a condom, for 72 hours after the drug is stopped to prevent pregnancy.

Vaginal products may cause dizziness.

PREGNANCY AND BREAST-FEEDING

Safety in pregnancy has not been established although there was no evidence of harm during studies in animals.

This drug passes into breast milk, but does not appear to harm the baby.

HELPFUL COMMENTS

Contact your doctor if your symptoms do not improve after a couple of days when taking oral or vaginal products. Allow 6 weeks for acne treatment to notice the effects.

Do not stop the oral or vaginal treatment early if you start to feel better. It takes the full prescription for this drug to work completely.

The topical products should be applied in a wide area around the acne approximately 30 minutes after washing or shaving.

CLOFIBRATE

Available for over 20 years

COMMONLY USED TO TREAT

High blood lipids including cholesterol, also known as hyperlipidemia

DRUG CATEGORY

antilipemic
Class: fibric acid derivative

PRODUCTS

Brand-Name Products with Generic Alternatives
Atromid-S 500 mg capsule (n/a)
  Generic: Clofibrate 500 mg capsule (¢¢¢¢¢)

DOSING AND FOOD

Doses are taken 2 to 4 times a day.

Taking this drug with a little food may avoid the stomach upset that some people suffer.

Adults: Up to 2,000 mg per day in divided doses.

Lower doses are used in people with kidney disease.

Forgotten doses: If you are scheduled to take the next dose within a few hours, do not take the forgotten dose. Otherwise take the forgotten dose as soon as you remember.

ALCOHOL, DRUG, HERB, AND SUPPLEMENT INTERACTIONS

Alcohol may increase some of the side effects from this drug, depending on the amount consumed. Ask your doctor about the risks caused by drinking alcohol with your condition.

Taking this drug with any of the ones listed below may change the effect of either drug with the possibility of causing toxicity or decreasing effectiveness: anticoagulants†, cholestyramine, furosemide, sulfonylureas†

ALLERGIC REACTIONS AND SIDE EFFECTS

You should tell your doctor about all your allergies and any unexplained symptoms you may have while taking this drug.

MORE COMMON SIDE EFFECTS: Heartburn, increased appetite, irregular heartbeat*, nausea*, shortness of breath*, stomach pain*, vomiting*, weight gain

LESS COMMON SIDE EFFECTS: Diarrhea, gas, headache, mouth sores, muscle aches, sexual dysfunction, tiredness, weakness*

RARE SIDE EFFECTS: Back pain*, bloody urine*, chest pain*, chills*, cough*, fever*, hoarseness*, swelling*, urinary changes*

PRECAUTIONS

This drug may reduce the risk of heart attack.

If you have a history of stomach ulcers, intestinal ulcers, gallstones, or low thyroid levels, this drug may make those conditions worse.

This drug may increase the risk of cancer, liver disease, gallstones, and pancreatitis.

PREGNANCY AND BREAST-FEEDING

Safety during pregnancy has not been established although the drug is known to harm animal fetuses.

Breast-feeding while taking this drug is not recommended.

HELPFUL COMMENTS

If you are diabetic, you should check blood sugar levels regularly since this drug may interfere with many antidiabetic drugs.

CLOMIPHENE CITRATE

Available for over 20 years

COMMONLY USED TO TREAT

Infertility in women or men

DRUG CATEGORY

ovulation stimulant
Class: chlorotrianisene derivative

PRODUCTS

Brand-Name Products with Generic Alternatives
Clomid 50 mg tablet ($$$$)
  Generic: clomiphene citrate 50 mg tablet ($$$$)
Other Generic Product Names
Milophene, Serophene

DOSING AND FOOD

Doses are taken once a day.
This drug may be taken with or without food.
Women: Up to 250 mg per day.
Men: Up to 400 mg per day.
Forgotten doses: If you are scheduled to take the next dose within a few hours, do not take the forgotten dose. Otherwise take the forgotten dose as soon as you remember.

ALCOHOL, DRUG, HERB, AND SUPPLEMENT INTERACTIONS

Alcohol may increase some of the side effects from this drug, depending on the amount consumed. Ask your doctor about the risks caused by drinking alcohol with your condition.

ALLERGIC REACTIONS AND SIDE EFFECTS

You should tell your doctor about all your allergies and any unexplained symptoms you may have while taking this drug.
MORE COMMON SIDE EFFECTS: Bloating*, hot flashes, pelvic pain*, stomach pain*
LESS COMMON SIDE EFFECTS: Breast discomfort, depression, dizziness, headache, irregular menstruation, lightheadedness, nausea, nervous-

---

† See page 52.   * See page 53.

ness, restlessness, sleep disorders, tiredness, vision changes*, vomiting, yellow eyes or skin*

PRECAUTIONS

There is an increased risk of multiple pregnancies (twins and triplets) with higher doses.

Be careful driving or handling equipment while taking this drug because it may cause dizziness and vision changes.

If you have a history of blood clots, depression, ovarian cysts, endometriosis, or fibroid tumors, this drug may make those conditions worse.

PREGNANCY AND BREAST-FEEDING

This drug may cause birth defects and should not be used during pregnancy. This drug reduces milk production putting the baby at risk of malnutrition if breast-fed.

HELPFUL COMMENTS

It is helpful to measure body temperature daily to estimate the day of ovulation.

CLOMIPRAMINE HYDROCHLORIDE

Available since December 1989

COMMONLY USED TO TREAT

Obsessive-compulsive disorder (OCD)

DRUG CATEGORY

antibulemic
anticataplectic
antidepressant
antineuralgic
antipanic
Class: tricyclic antidepressant

PRODUCTS

Brand-Name Products with Generic Alternatives
Anafranil 25 mg capsule ($$)
  Generic: clomipramine hydrochloride 25 mg capsule (¢¢¢¢¢)
Anafranil 50 mg capsule ($$)

Generic: clomipramine hydrochloride 50 mg capsule ($)

Anafranil 75 mg capsule ($$$)

Generic: clomipramine hydrochloride 75 mg capsule ($)

DOSING AND FOOD

Doses are taken once a day, usually at bedtime. Twice-a-day dosing may be needed initially.

Taking this drug with food or milk may avoid the stomach upset that some people suffer. Do not eat grapefruit or drink grapefruit juice while taking this drug.

Adults: Up to 250 mg per day.

Children age 10 to 19: Up to 3 mg/kg (maximum 200 mg) per day.

Forgotten doses: If you have forgotten a bedtime dose, do not take the forgotten dose. Just go back to your usual schedule with the next dose. If you have forgotten a daytime dose and are scheduled to take the next dose within a few hours, do not take the forgotten dose. Otherwise take the forgotten dose as soon as you remember.

ALCOHOL, DRUG, HERB, AND SUPPLEMENT INTERACTIONS

Alcohol should not be used while taking this drug.

Evening primrose oil, SAMe, St. John's wort, and yohimbe may cause serious reactions when taken with this drug. Tell your doctor if you are taking any of these supplements.

Several OTC drugs used for asthma, colds, cough, hay fever, sleep aid, or sinus problems may seriously change the effects and side effects of this drug. Check with your pharmacist when selecting OTC products.

The effect of this drug or the ones listed below may be changed with either drug with the possibility of causing toxicity or decreasing effectiveness:
anesthetics, antipsychotics†, anxiolytics†, barbiturates†, beta blockers†, cimetidine, clonidine, fluoxetine, guanabenz, guanadrel, guanethidine, haloperidol, methyldopa, methylphenidate, narcotics†, oral contraceptives, phenothiazines†, propoxyphene, reserpine

Severe reactions are possible when this drug is taken with those listed below:
amphetamines†, anesthetics, anticholinergics†, antidyskinetics†, antihistamines†, antithyroid drugs†, anxiolytics†, appetite suppressants, barbiturates†, disopyramide, disulfiram, ephedrine, epinephrine, ethchlorvynol, isoproterenol, meperidine, metrizamide, monoamine oxidase inhibitors†, narcotics†, phenylephrine, pimozide, procainamide, quinidine, SSRIs†, tricyclic antidepressants†, warfarin

---

†See page 52.   *See page 53.

Increased side effects are possible when this drug is taken with those listed below: alseroxylon, deserpidine, metoclopramide, metyrosine, pemoline, pimozide, promethazine, rauwolfia serpentine, trimeprazine

ALLERGIC REACTIONS AND SIDE EFFECTS

If you are allergic to carbamazepine, maprotiline, trazodone, or any tricyclic antidepressants†, you may also be allergic to this drug. You should tell your doctor about all your allergies and any unexplained symptoms you may have while taking this drug.

This drug promotes the effect of sunlight on the body and may cause severe sunburn and increased sensitivity of the eyes.

MORE COMMON SIDE EFFECTS: Abdominal pain, blurry vision*, constipation*, dizziness, drowsiness, dry mouth, headache, heartburn, hoarseness, increased appetite, menstrual changes, nausea, runny nose, sexual dysfunction, taste changes, teeth or gum problems*, tiredness, trembling*, urinary changes*, weakness*, weight gain

LESS COMMON SIDE EFFECTS: Confusion*, diarrhea, expressionless face*, eye pain*, fainting*, hallucinations*, irregular heartbeat*, loss of balance*, nervousness*, restlessness*, shakiness*, shuffling walk*, sleeping difficulty*, stiffness*, swallowing difficulty*, sweating, vomiting

RARE SIDE EFFECTS: Anxiety*, breast enlargement*, fever*, hair loss, irritability*, muscle twitching*, ringing in ears*, seizures*, skin rash*, sore throat*, swelling*, yellow eyes or skin*

PRECAUTIONS

You need to wait 2 weeks after stopping a monoamine oxidase inhibitor† or SSRI† before starting this drug.

Be careful driving or handling equipment while taking this drug because it may cause drowsiness and dizziness.

Stopping this drug abruptly may result in withdrawal symptoms that include nausea, headache, and general discomfort. If you wish to stop this drug, ask your doctor for specific instructions.

If you have a history of asthma, blood disorders, seizures, enlarged prostate, glaucoma, heart disease, high blood pressure, urinary difficulty, schizophrenia, or manic depression, this drug may make those conditions worse.

This drug may cause dry mouth and other mouth problems, which are associated with a greater risk of cavities. Your dentist may recommend that you clean your teeth and mouth differently to avoid infection.

PREGNANCY AND BREAST-FEEDING

Safety during pregnancy has not been established although the drug is known to harm animal fetuses. There have been reports of babies suffering from muscle spasms, heart problems, breathing difficulty, and urinary problems when the mother was taking this drug.

Breast-feeding while taking this drug is not recommended.

HELPFUL COMMENTS

Heavy smoking may decrease the effectiveness of this drug.

You may need to take this drug for several weeks before you notice the effects.

Sucking on hard sugarless candy or chewing sugarless gum may help relieve dry mouth caused by this drug.

You may need to eat a high-fiber diet to avoid the constipation some people suffer.

CLONAZEPAM

Available for over 20 years

COMMONLY USED TO TREAT

Muscle twitches
Nerve pain
Seizures

DRUG CATEGORY

anticonvulsant
antipanic
sedative-hypnotic
Class: benzodiazepine

PRODUCTS

Brand-Name Products with Generic Alternatives
Klonopin 0.5 mg tablet (¢¢¢¢)
  Generic: clonazepam 0.5 mg tablet (¢)
Klonopin 1 mg tablet (¢¢¢¢¢)
  Generic: clonazepam 1 mg tablet (¢¢)
Klonopin 2 mg tablet ($)
  Generic: clonazepam 2 mg tablet (¢¢)

---

† See page 52.   * See page 53.

DOSING AND FOOD

Doses are taken 1 to 3 times a day.

This drug may be taken with or without food.

Adults: Up to 20 mg per day in divided doses.

Children: Up to 0.2 mg/kg per day in divided doses.

Doses are started low and gradually increased as needed.

Forgotten doses: If you are scheduled to take the next dose within a few hours, do not take the forgotten dose. Otherwise take the forgotten dose as soon as you remember.

ALCOHOL, DRUG, HERB, AND SUPPLEMENT INTERACTIONS

Alcohol should not be used while taking this drug.

Catnip, kava, lady's slipper, lemon balm, passion flower, sassafras, skullcap, and valerian should not be used while taking this drug due to an increased sedative effect.

Taking this drug with any of the ones listed below may change the effect of either drug with the possibility of causing toxicity or decreasing effectiveness: fluvoxamine, itraconazole, ketoconazole, nefazodone, ritonavir

Severe reactions are possible when this drug is taken with those listed below: anesthetics†, anticonvulsants†, antidepressants†, antihistamines†, barbiturates†, monoamine oxidase inhibitors†, narcotics†, phenothiazines†, valproic acid

ALLERGIC REACTIONS AND SIDE EFFECTS

If you are allergic to any benzodiazepines†, you may also be allergic to this drug. You should tell your doctor about all your allergies and any unexplained symptoms you may have while taking this drug.

MORE COMMON SIDE EFFECTS: Behavior changes*, dizziness, drowsiness, fever*, lightheadedness, shallow breathing*

LESS COMMON SIDE EFFECTS: Anxiety*, clumsiness, confusion*, constipation, depression*, diarrhea, difficulty urinating, dry mouth, headache, irregular heartbeat*, memory loss*, muscle spasm, nausea, sexual dysfunction, shortness of breath, slurry speech, stomach cramps, thirst, trembling, vision changes, vomiting, watery mouth

RARE SIDE EFFECTS: Agitation*, bleeding*, bruising*, chills*, delusions*, disorientation*, excitement*, eye movement*, hallucinations*, irritability*, low blood pressure*, mouth sores*, nervousness*, skin irritation*, sleeping difficulty*, sore throat*, tiredness*, weakness*, yellow eyes or skin*

PRECAUTIONS

This drug may be habit forming and may cause severe withdrawal symptoms if stopped abruptly. If you wish to stop taking this drug, ask your doctor for specific instructions.

If you have difficulty swallowing, emphysema, asthma, bronchitis, glaucoma, hyperactivity, mental depression, mental illness, myasthenia gravis, porphyria, or sleep apnea, this drug may make those conditions worse.

Be careful driving or handling equipment while taking this drug because the drug may cause dizziness and drowsiness.

PREGNANCY AND BREAST-FEEDING

Safety during pregnancy has not been established although the drug is known to harm animal fetuses.

Breast-feeding while taking this drug is not recommended.

HELPFUL COMMENTS

Dangling your legs over the side of the bed for a few minutes may help reduce dizziness when first waking up.

CLONIDINE HYDROCHLORIDE

Available for over 20 years

COMMONLY USED TO TREAT

Delayed growth in children
High blood pressure, also known as hypertension
Menstrual pain, also known as dysmenorrhea
Nerve pain, also known as neuralgia
Symptoms from nicotine and opiate withdrawal
Vascular headaches

DRUG CATEGORY

antihypertensive
Class: centrally acting antiadrenergic

PRODUCTS

Brand-Name Products with No Generic Alternative
Catapres-TTS-1 extended-release patch ($$$$$)
Catapres-TTS-2 extended-release patch ($$$$$)
Catapres-TTS-3 extended-release patch ($$$$$)

†See page 52.   *See page 53.

Brand-Name Products with Generic Alternatives
Catapres 0.1 mg tablet (¢¢¢¢¢)
  Generic: clonidine hydrochloride 0.1 mg tablet (¢¢)
Catapres 0.2 mg tablet ($)
  Generic: clonidine hydrochloride 0.2 mg tablet (¢¢)
Catapres 0.3 mg tablet ($$)
  Generic: clonidine hydrochloride 0.3 mg tablet (¢¢¢)

Combination Products That Contain This Drug
Clopres tablet (¢¢¢¢¢) to ($)

DOSING AND FOOD

Oral doses are taken 1 to 4 times a day. Patches are replaced weekly.
This drug may be taken with or without food.
The last dose of the day should be taken at bedtime.

Adults: Up to 2.4 mg per day in divided doses.

Children: Up to 0.15 mg/m^2 per day in divided doses.

Patches should be applied to a clean, dry area of skin on the upper arm or
  chest where there is little hair. Avoid areas of skin with cuts, rashes, or
  scars.

Forgotten doses: If you are scheduled to take the next dose within a few
  hours, do not take the forgotten dose. Otherwise take the forgotten dose
  as soon as you remember.

ALCOHOL, DRUG, HERB, AND SUPPLEMENT INTERACTIONS

Alcohol should not be used while taking this drug.

Capsaicin and other foods or supplements derived from the capsicum fam-
  ily of plants, including hot peppers, sweet peppers, paprika, and chili
  powder, may interfere with the effects of this drug and should not be
  consumed.

Several OTC drugs used for appetite control, asthma, colds, cough, hay
  fever, or sinus problems may cause an increase in blood pressure when
  taken with this drug. Check with your pharmacist when selecting OTC
  products.

**Taking this drug with any of the ones listed below may change the effect of
either drug with the possibility of causing toxicity or decreasing effectiveness:**
beta blockers†, monoamine oxidase inhibitors†, tolazoline, tricyclic antide-
  pressants†

Severe reactions are possible when this drug is taken with those listed below:
barbiturates†

ALLERGIC REACTIONS AND SIDE EFFECTS

You should tell your doctor about all your allergies and any unexplained symptoms you may have while taking this drug.

MORE COMMON SIDE EFFECTS: Constipation, dizziness, drowsiness, dry mouth, rash*, tiredness*, weakness*

LESS COMMON SIDE EFFECTS: Depression*, eye irritation, fainting, light-headedness, loss of appetite, nausea, nervousness, sexual dysfunction, swelling*, vomiting

RARE SIDE EFFECTS: Breathing difficulty*, cold fingers*, cold toes*, difficulty breathing*, faintness*, nightmares*, small pupils*, slow heartbeat*

PRECAUTIONS

This drug may cause severe withdrawal symptoms, including chest pain and irregular heartbeat, if stopped suddenly. If you wish to stop taking this drug, ask your doctor for specific instructions.

Patches containing this drug may cause discoloration and irritation of the skin.

Be careful driving or handling equipment while taking this drug because the drug may cause drowsiness.

If you have psoriasis or myasthenia gravis, this drug may make those conditions worse.

Do not cut the patches since it may damage the extended-release properties.

If you have a history of depression or Raynaud's syndrome, this drug may make those conditions worse.

This drug may cause dry mouth, which is associated with a greater risk of cavities. Your dentist may recommend that you clean your teeth and mouth differently to avoid infection.

PREGNANCY AND BREAST-FEEDING

Safety during pregnancy has not been established although the drug is known to harm animal fetuses.

Breast-feeding while taking this drug is not recommended.

HELPFUL COMMENTS

Avoid quick movements to minimize dizziness. Dangling your legs over the side of the bed for a few minutes may help reduce dizziness when first waking up.

Sucking on hard sugarless candy or chewing sugarless gum may help relieve dry mouth caused by this drug.

---

†See page 52.   *See page 53.

Try moving the patch to a new location each time it is changed to avoid skin irritation.

If a patch becomes loose, you may hold it in place with adhesive tape or occlusive dressing until it is time to change.

Fold the patches in half when you throw them out to make sure that any remaining drug does not present a risk to children or pets.

If you do not treat high blood pressure, you may develop more serious problems such as heart failure, blood vessel disease, stroke, or kidney disease. Losing weight, exercising, eating more fruits and vegetables, and avoiding salty foods, such as lunchmeat and pickles, may help make drug treatment more successful.

CLOPIDOGREL BISULFATE

Available since November 1997

COMMONLY USED TO TREAT

Circulation problems that could result in a blood clot

DRUG CATEGORY

antiplatelet
Class: ADP blocker

PRODUCTS

Brand-Name Products with No Generic Alternative
Plavix 75 mg tablet ($$$)
No generics available.
Multiple patents that begin to expire in 2003.

DOSING AND FOOD

Doses are taken once a day.
This drug may be taken with or without food.
Adults: Up to 75 mg per day.
Forgotten doses: If you are scheduled to take the next dose within a few hours, do not take the forgotten dose. Otherwise take the forgotten dose as soon as you remember.

ALCOHOL, DRUG, HERB, AND SUPPLEMENT INTERACTIONS

Alcohol may increase some of the side effects from this drug, depending

on the amount consumed. Ask your doctor about the risks caused by drinking alcohol with your condition.

Do not use red clover while taking this drug since it may increase the risk of serious bleeding.

Severe reactions are possible when this drug is taken with those listed below: aspirin, heparin, nonsteroidal antiinflammatories†, warfarin

ALLERGIC REACTIONS AND SIDE EFFECTS

You should tell your doctor about all your allergies and any unexplained symptoms you may have while taking this drug.

MORE COMMON SIDE EFFECTS: Abdominal pain, back pain, bleeding*, bruises*, chest pain*, cough*, dizziness, headache*, heartburn, muscle aches, runny nose*, sneezing*, spots on skin*

LESS COMMON SIDE EFFECTS: Anxiety, bloody vomit*, constipation, depression, diarrhea, fainting*, irregular heartbeat*, itching, joint pain*, leg cramps, nausea, nosebleeds*, numbness, shortness of breath*, skin irritation*, sleep disorders, swelling*, tingling, tiredness, urinary difficulty*, vomiting, weakness

RARE SIDE EFFECTS: Black stools*, bloody urine*, chills*, fever*, mouth sores*, sore throat*, stomach pain*, weakness*

PRECAUTIONS

If you have a history of bleeding problems including ulcers and liver disease, this drug may increase the risk of serious bleeding.

This drug should be stopped 7 days before surgery.

PREGNANCY AND BREAST-FEEDING

Safety during pregnancy has not been established although there was no evidence of harm during studies in animals.

Breast-feeding while taking this drug is not recommended.

HELPFUL COMMENTS

If you cut yourself, it may take longer than usual to stop bleeding.

---

† See page 52.   * See page 53.

CLORAZEPATE DIPOTASSIUM

Available since October 1987

COMMONLY USED TO TREAT

Alcohol withdrawal
Anxiety
Seizures

DRUG CATEGORY

antitremor agent
anxiolytic
sedative-hypnotic
Class: benzodiazepine

PRODUCTS

Brand-Name Products with No Generic Alternative
Tranxene-SD 11.25 mg extended-release tablet ($$$)
Tranxene-SD 22.5 mg extended-release tablet ($$$$)
Brand-Name Products with Generic Alternatives
Tranxene 3.75 mg tablet ($$)
  Generic: clorazepate dipotassium 3.75 mg tablet (¢¢¢)
Tranxene 7.5 mg tablet ($$)
  Generic: clorazepate dipotassium 7.5 mg tablet (¢¢¢¢)
Tranxene 15 mg tablet ($$$)
  Generic: clorazepate dipotassium 15 mg tablet ($$)
Other Generic Product Names
Gen-Xene

DOSING AND FOOD

Doses are taken 2 to 4 times a day. Extended-release products are taken
once a day.
It is best to take this drug on an empty stomach, but taking this drug with
a little food may avoid the stomach upset that some people suffer.
Adults: Up to 90 mg per day in divided doses.
Children age 9 to 12: Up to 60 mg per day in divided doses.
Doses are started low and gradually increased no faster than 7.5 mg
per week.
Forgotten doses: If you are scheduled to take the next dose within a few

hours, do not take the forgotten dose. Otherwise take the forgotten dose as soon as you remember.

ALCOHOL, DRUG, HERB, AND SUPPLEMENT INTERACTIONS

Alcohol should not be used while taking this drug.

Catnip, kava, lady's slipper, lemon balm, passion flower, sassafras, skullcap, and valerian should not be used while taking this drug due to an increased sedative effect.

Taking this drug with any of the ones listed below may change the effect of either drug with the possibility of causing toxicity or decreasing effectiveness: antacids, cimetidine, digoxin, disulfiram, fluvoxamine, haloperidol, itraconazole, ketoconazole, levodopa, nefazodone, oral contraceptives, rifampin

Severe reactions are possible when this drug is taken with those listed below: anesthetics†, antidepressants†, antihistamines†, barbiturates†, monoamine oxidase inhibitors†, narcotics†, phenothiazines†

Increased side effects are possible when this drug is taken with those listed below: aminophylline, theophylline

ALLERGIC REACTIONS AND SIDE EFFECTS

If you are allergic to any benzodiazepines†, you may also be allergic to this drug. You should tell your doctor about all your allergies and any unexplained symptoms you may have while taking this drug.

MORE COMMON SIDE EFFECTS: Drowsiness, lightheadedness

LESS COMMON SIDE EFFECTS: Anxiety*, clumsiness, confusion*, constipation, depression*, diarrhea, difficulty urinating, dizziness, dry mouth, headache, irregular heartbeat*, memory loss*, muscle spasm, nausea, sexual dysfunction, slurry speech, stomach cramps, thirst, trembling, vision changes, vomiting, watery mouth

RARE SIDE EFFECTS: Agitation*, behavior changes*, bleeding*, bruising*, chills*, delusions*, disorientation*, excitement*, eye movement*, fever*, hallucinations*, irritability*, low blood pressure*, mouth sores*, nervousness*, skin irritation*, sleeping difficulty*, sore throat*, spastic movements*, tiredness*, weakness*, yellow eyes or skin*

PRECAUTIONS

This drug may be habit forming and will cause severe withdrawal symptoms if stopped abruptly. If you wish to stop taking this drug, ask your doctor for specific instructions.

---

† See page 52.   * See page 53.

You need to wait 2 weeks after stopping a monoamine oxidase inhibitor†
   before starting this drug.
If you have swallowing difficulty, emphysema, asthma, bronchitis, glaucoma, hyperactivity, mental depression, mental illness, myasthenia gravis,
   porphyria, or sleep apnea, this drug may make those conditions worse.
Heavy smoking may cause this drug to be less effective.
Be careful driving or handling equipment while taking this drug because
   the drug may cause dizziness and drowsiness.

PREGNANCY AND BREAST-FEEDING

There is evidence that this drug may harm the fetus, but the drug may be
   necessary to the health of the mother.
Breast-feeding while taking this drug is not recommended.

HELPFUL COMMENTS

Dangling your legs over the side of the bed for a few minutes may help reduce dizziness when first waking up.
If you need to take an antacid, take it either 2 hours before or after taking
   this drug.

CLOXACILLIN SODIUM

Available for over 20 years

COMMONLY USED TO TREAT

Infection

DRUG CATEGORY

antibiotic
Class: penicillinase-resistant penicillin

PRODUCTS

Brand-Name Products with No Generic Alternative
Cloxacillin sodium 125 mg/5 ml oral solution (n/a)
Brand-Name Products with Generic Alternatives
Cloxapen 250 mg capsule (n/a)
   Generic: cloxacillin sodium 250 mg capsule (¢¢¢)
Cloxapen 500 mg capsule (n/a)
   Generic: cloxacillin sodium 500 mg capsule (¢¢¢¢)

DOSING AND FOOD

Doses are taken 4 times a day.

This drug works best if taken on an empty stomach with a full glass of water, but taking it with food may avoid the stomach upset that some people suffer.

Adults: Up to 2,000 mg per day in divided doses.

Children over 20 kg: Up to 50 mg/kg per day in divided doses.

Forgotten doses: If you are scheduled to take the next dose within a few hours, do not take the forgotten dose. Otherwise take the forgotten dose as soon as you remember.

ALCOHOL, DRUG, HERB, AND SUPPLEMENT INTERACTIONS

Alcohol may increase some of the side effects from this drug, depending on the amount consumed. Ask your doctor about the risks caused by drinking alcohol with your condition.

Taking this drug with any of the ones listed below may change the effect of either drug with the possibility of causing toxicity or decreasing effectiveness: chloramphenicol, erythromycins†, methotrexate, probenecid, sulfonamides†, tetracyclines†

Increased side effects are possible when this drug is taken with those listed below: acetaminophen, amiodarone, androgens†, antithyroid drugs†, carmustine, chloroquine, dantrolene, daunorubicin, disulfiram, divalproex, estrogens†, etretinate, gold salts†, hydroxychloroquine, mercaptopurine, methotrexate, methyldopa, naltrexone, nandrolone, oral contraceptives†, oxandrolone, oxymetholone, phenothiazines†, plicamycin, stanozolol, valproic acid

ALLERGIC REACTIONS AND SIDE EFFECTS

If you are allergic to any penicillins† or cephalosporins†, you may also be allergic to this drug. You should tell your doctor about all your allergies and any unexplained symptoms you may have while taking this drug.

MORE COMMON SIDE EFFECTS: Diarrhea*, headache, mouth sores, vaginal discharge, vaginal itching

LESS COMMON SIDE EFFECTS: Fainting*, fever*, hives*, irregular breathing*, itching*, joint pain*, lightheadedness*, scaly skin*, shortness of breath*, skin rash*, swelling*

RARE SIDE EFFECTS: Abdominal pain*, bleeding*, bruising*, decreased urine output, depression*, nausea*, seizures*, sore throat*, stomach cramps*, vomiting*, yellow eyes or skin*

---

†See page 52.   *See page 53.

PRECAUTIONS

If you have a history of stomach or intestinal disease, you may be at greater risk of developing colitis while taking this drug. Tell your doctor if you get severe or watery diarrhea.

PREGNANCY AND BREAST-FEEDING

Safety during pregnancy has not been established although there was no evidence of harm during studies in animals.

This drug passes into breast milk. Allergic reactions, diarrhea, fungal infections, and skin rash have been reported in babies.

HELPFUL COMMENTS

Contact your doctor if your symptoms do not improve after a couple of days. Do not stop treatment early if you start to feel better. It takes the full prescription for this drug to work completely.

CLOZAPINE

Available since September 1989

COMMONLY USED TO TREAT

Mental disturbances, also known as psychosis

DRUG CATEGORY

antipsychotic
Class: dibenzodiazepine

PRODUCTS

Brand-Name Products with Generic Alternatives
Clozaril 25 mg tablet ($)
　Generic: clozapine 25 mg tablet ($)
Clozaril 100 mg tablet ($$$)
　Generic: clozapine 100 mg tablet ($$$)

DOSING AND FOOD

Doses are taken 1 to 2 times a day.
This drug may be taken with or without food.
Adults: Up to 900 mg per day in divided doses.
Forgotten doses: If you are scheduled to take the next dose within a few

hours, do not take the forgotten dose. Otherwise take the forgotten dose as soon as you remember.

ALCOHOL, DRUG, HERB, AND SUPPLEMENT INTERACTIONS

Alcohol should not be used while taking this drug.

Catnip, kava, lady's slipper, lemon balm, passion flower, sassafras, skullcap, and valerian should not be used due to an increased sedative effect.

Caffeine and nutmeg may reduce the effectiveness of this drug.

Several OTC drugs used for asthma, colds, cough, hay fever, sleep aid, or sinus problems may seriously change the effects and side effects of this drug. Check with your pharmacist when selecting OTC products.

Taking this drug with any of the ones listed below may change the effect of either drug with the possibility of causing toxicity or decreasing effectiveness: antiarrhythmics†, anticholinergics†, anticonvulsants†, antihypertensives†, carbamazepine, cimetidine, digoxin, erythromycin, fluoxetine, fluvoxamine, lithium, paroxetine, phenothiazines†, phenytoin, quinidine, sertraline, warfarin

Severe reactions are possible when this drug is taken with those listed below: antineoplastics†, antithyroid drugs†, azathioprine, benzodiazepines†, chlorambucil, chloramphenicol, colchicine, cyclophosphamide, flucytosine, ganciclovir, interferon, mercaptopurine, methotrexate, plicamycin, zidovudine

Increased side effects are possible when this drug is taken with those listed below: alcohol, anesthetics, antihistamines†, anxiolytics†, barbiturates†, narcotics†, tricyclic antidepressants†

ALLERGIC REACTIONS AND SIDE EFFECTS

You should tell your doctor about all your allergies and any unexplained symptoms you may have while taking this drug.

MORE COMMON SIDE EFFECTS: Constipation, dizziness*, drowsiness*, fever*, headache, irregular heartbeat*, lightheadedness, low blood pressure*, nausea*, salivation*, vomiting*, weight gain

LESS COMMON SIDE EFFECTS: Abdominal pain, anxiety*, blurry vision*, confusion*, dry mouth, heartburn, high blood pressure*, irritability*, nervousness*, restlessness*

RARE SIDE EFFECTS: Appetite changes*, bleeding*, breathing difficulty*, bruising*, chest pain*, chills*, coma*, cough*, dark urine*, depression*, difficulty breathing*, fainting*, hallucinations*, high blood sugar*, lip smacking*, mouth sores*, muscle stiffness*, pale skin*, puffy cheeks*,

---

† See page 52.   * See page 53.

seizures*, sexual dysfunction*, shaking*, shortness of breath*, sleep disturbances*, sore throat*, spastic movements*, sweating*, swelling*, thirst*, tiredness*, tongue movement*, trembling*, urinary changes*, weakness*, yellow eyes or skin*

PRECAUTIONS

It is very important to have weekly blood tests for the first 6 months of taking this drug. Not more than 1 week of drug may be dispensed in a prescription during that time. After 6 months, blood tests are often done every other week.

Be careful driving or handling equipment while taking this drug because the drug may cause drowsiness.

If you have an enlarged prostate, glaucoma, intestinal disorders, blood disease, or blood vessel disease, this drug may make those conditions worse.

People with a history of seizure disorders have an increased risk of having a seizure while taking this drug.

If stopped suddenly, this drug may cause withdrawal symptoms that include a rapid return of psychosis. If you wish to stop taking this drug, ask your doctor for specific instructions.

PREGNANCY AND BREAST-FEEDING

Safety during pregnancy has not been established although there was no evidence of harm during studies in animals.

Breast-feeding while taking this drug is not recommended.

HELPFUL COMMENTS

Sucking on hard sugarless candy or chewing sugarless gum may help relieve dry mouth caused by this drug.

Avoid quick movements to minimize dizziness. Dangling your legs over the side of the bed for a few minutes may help reduce dizziness when first waking up.

Side effects may continue to develop for 4 weeks after this drug is stopped.

CODEINE SULFATE

Available for over 20 years

COMMONLY USED TO TREAT

Cough
Pain

DRUG CATEGORY

analgesic
antidiarrheal
antitussive
Class: narcotic analgesic/opioid

PRODUCTS

Products Only Available as Generics
codeine sulfate 15 mg tablet (¢¢¢)
codeine sulfate 30 mg tablet (¢¢¢)
codeine sulfate 60 mg tablet (¢¢¢¢)

Combination Products That Contain This Drug
Acetaminophen, Aspirin, and Codeine phosphate capsule (n/a)
Ambenyl oral syrup (n/a)
Capital and Codeine oral suspension (¢¢¢)
Fiorinal with Codeine No. 3 capsule ($$)
Mybanil oral syrup (n/a)
Myphetane DC oral syrup (n/a)
Phenaphen with Codeine No. 3 capsule (n/a)
Phenaphen with Codeine No. 4 capsule (n/a)
Phenergan VC with Codeine oral syrup (n/a)
Phenergan with Codeine oral syrup (¢¢¢¢)
Phrenilin with Caffeine and Codeine capsule ($)
Prometh VC with Codeine oral syrup (n/a)
Prometh with Codeine oral syrup (n/a)
Promethazine VC with Codeine oral syrup (¢¢¢¢)
Soma Compound with Codeine tablet ($$$)
Triacin-C oral syrup (¢¢¢)
Tylenol #1 tablet (n/a)
Tylenol #2 tablet (n/a)
Tylenol #3 tablet (¢¢¢)
Tylenol #4 tablet (¢¢¢¢)
Tylenol with Codeine oral elixir (¢¢¢¢)

DOSING AND FOOD

Doses are taken 4 to 6 times a day.
It is best to take this drug on an empty stomach, but taking this drug with
a little food may avoid the stomach upset that some people suffer.
Adults: Up to 120 mg per day in divided doses.

† See page 52.   * See page 53.

Children age 6 to 11: Up to 60 mg per day in divided doses.

Children age 2 to 6: Up to 30 mg per day in divided doses.

Forgotten doses: If you are scheduled to take the next dose within a few hours, do not take the forgotten dose. Otherwise take the forgotten dose as soon as you remember.

ALCOHOL, DRUG, HERB, AND SUPPLEMENT INTERACTIONS

Alcohol should not be used while taking this drug.

Several OTC drugs used for asthma, colds, cough, hay fever, sleep aid, or sinus problems may seriously change the effects and side effects of this drug. Check with your pharmacist when selecting OTC products.

Many combination products that contain this drug also contain aspirin, which may interfere with anticoagulants†.

Taking this drug with any of the ones listed below may change the effect of either drug with the possibility of causing toxicity or decreasing effectiveness: natrexone, rifampin

Severe reactions are possible when this drug is taken with those listed below: anesthetics, anticholinergics†, antihistamines†, barbiturates†, benzodiazepines†, cimetidine, monoamine oxidase inhibitors†, naloxone, narcotics†, phenothiazines†, sedative-hypnotics†, skeletal muscle relaxants†, tricyclic antidepressants†

ALLERGIC REACTIONS AND SIDE EFFECTS

If you are allergic to any narcotics†, you may also be allergic to this drug. You should tell your doctor about all your allergies and any unexplained symptoms you may have while taking this drug.

MORE COMMON SIDE EFFECTS: Constipation, dizziness*, drowsiness*, dry mouth, excitement*, fainting, lightheadedness, nausea, slow breathing*, slow heartbeat*, sweating*, urinary changes*, vomiting

LESS COMMON SIDE EFFECTS: Blurry vision, breathing difficulty*, depression*, flushing*, hallucinations*, headache, hives*, irregular breathing*, irregular heartbeat*, itching*, loss of appetite, mood swings*, nervousness*, restlessness*, ringing in ears*, shortness of breath*, skin rash*, sleep disorders, spastic movements*, stomach cramps, swelling*, tiredness, trembling*, vision changes, weakness*, wheezing*

RARE SIDE EFFECTS: Body aches, clammy skin*, confusion*, diarrhea, fever, goosebumps, irritability, low blood pressure*, runny nose, seizures*, shivering, small pupils*, sneezing, yawning

PRECAUTIONS

Be careful driving or handling equipment while taking this drug because it may cause dizziness and drowsiness.

If you have a history of head injury, brain disease, emphysema, asthma, lung disease, enlarged prostate, urinary disorders, gallbladder disease, or gallstones, you may not be able to take this drug.

People with colitis, heart disease, kidney disease, liver disease, and thyroid disease are at increased risk of developing side effects.

If you have a history of seizures, this drug may make that condition worse.

This drug may cause withdrawal symptoms if stopped suddenly. If you wish to stop taking this drug, ask your doctor for specific instructions.

Side effects may continue to develop even after the drug is stopped.

Because this drug has a high abuse potential, your prescription quantity may be limited.

This drug may cause dry mouth, which is associated with a greater risk of cavities. Your dentist may recommend that you clean your teeth and mouth differently to avoid infection.

PREGNANCY AND BREAST-FEEDING

Safety during pregnancy has not been established although the drug is known to harm animal fetuses.

Breast-feeding while taking this drug is not recommended.

HELPFUL COMMENTS

This drug is more effective in relieving pain when taken in combination with aspirin. If taking a combination product that contains this drug, make sure not to double dose on the aspirin.

If the drug does not seem to be working properly, an increase in dosage may not help. Talk to your doctor about other drugs and treatment options.

Sucking on hard sugarless candy or chewing sugarless gum may help relieve dry mouth caused by this drug.

Lie down for a while after taking a dose of this drug to help reduce the nausea.

Avoid quick movements to minimize dizziness. Dangling your legs over the side of the bed for a few minutes may help reduce dizziness when first waking up.

If being used for pain, this drug works best when taken before the pain gets too severe.

Add more fiber to your diet to help minimize the constipation that occurs

---

† See page 52.   * See page 53.

with this drug. If severe, constipation may need to be treated with a stool softener. Ask your doctor or pharmacist for recommendations.

COLESEVELAM HYDROCHLORIDE

Available since May 2000

COMMONLY USED TO TREAT

High blood lipids including cholesterol, also known as hyperlipidemia

DRUG CATEGORY

antilipemic
Class: bile acid sequestrant

PRODUCTS

Brand-Name Products with No Generic Alternative
Welchol 625 mg tablet (¢¢¢¢¢)
No generics available.
Multiple patents that begin to expire in 2014.

DOSING AND FOOD

Doses are taken 1 to 2 times a day.
This drug should be taken with food and a beverage.
Adults: Up to 4,375 mg per day in divided doses.
Forgotten doses: Do not take a forgotten dose. Just go back to your usual schedule with the next dose.

ALCOHOL, DRUG, HERB, AND SUPPLEMENT INTERACTIONS

This drug may reduce the absorption of fat-soluble drugs including vitamins A, D, E, and K. Make sure your doctor has a complete list of all the drugs and supplements you are taking.

ALLERGIC REACTIONS AND SIDE EFFECTS

You should tell your doctor about all your allergies and any unexplained symptoms you may have while taking this drug.
MORE COMMON SIDE EFFECTS: Belching, constipation*, gas, indigestion, stomachache
LESS COMMON SIDE EFFECTS: Back pain, congestion*, cough*, dry throat*, fever*, hoarseness*, muscle soreness*, nausea, runny nose, swallowing difficulty*

PRECAUTIONS

If you have a history of swallowing disorders, bowel obstruction, or intestinal motility disorders, this drug may make those conditions worse.

PREGNANCY AND BREAST-FEEDING

Safety during pregnancy has not been established although there was no evidence of harm during studies in animals.

It is not known if this drug passes into breast milk. Talk to your doctor about the risks associated with breast-feeding while taking this drug.

HELPFUL COMMENTS

This drug works in the stomach and intestines with relatively no absorption into the body.

COLESTIPOL HYDROCHLORIDE

Available for over 20 years

COMMONLY USED TO TREAT

High blood lipids including cholesterol, also known as hyperlipidemia

DRUG CATEGORY

antilipemic
Class: bile acid sequestrant

PRODUCTS

Brand-Name Products with No Generic Alternative
Colestid 5 g oral granule packet ($$)
Colestid 1 g tablet (¢¢¢¢)
No generics available.
No patents, no exclusivity.

DOSING AND FOOD

Doses are taken 2 to 4 times a day.
This drug should be taken with food.
Adults: Up to 30 g per day in divided doses.
Forgotten doses: If you are scheduled to take the next dose within a few hours, do not take the forgotten dose. Otherwise take the forgotten dose as soon as you remember.

---

† See page 52.   * See page 53.

ALCOHOL, DRUG, HERB, AND SUPPLEMENT INTERACTIONS

This drug may reduce the absorption of fat-soluble drugs including vitamins A, D, E, and K. Make sure your doctor has a complete list of all the drugs and supplements you are taking.

Taking this drug with any of the ones listed below may change the effect of either drug with the possibility of causing toxicity or decreasing effectiveness: anticoagulants†, digoxin, diuretics†, penicillin, propranolol, tetracycline, thyroid hormones†, vancomycin

ALLERGIC REACTIONS AND SIDE EFFECTS

You should tell your doctor about all your allergies and any unexplained symptoms you may have while taking this drug.

MORE COMMON SIDE EFFECTS: Constipation*

LESS COMMON SIDE EFFECTS: Belching, bloating, diarrhea, dizziness, headache, nausea*, stomach pain*, vomiting*

RARE SIDE EFFECTS: Black stools*, joint pain, muscle aches, skin rash, weight loss*

PRECAUTIONS

If you have a history of bleeding disorders, constipation, gallstones, heart disease, hemorrhoids, stomach problems, or thyroid disorders, this drug may make those conditions worse.

PREGNANCY AND BREAST-FEEDING

Safety during pregnancy has not been established although there was no evidence of harm during studies in animals.

It is not known if this drug passes into breast milk. Talk to your doctor about the risks associated with breast-feeding while taking this drug.

HELPFUL COMMENTS

This drug works in the stomach and intestines with relatively no absorption into the body.

Granules should be mixed in about 1/3 cup of carbonated drink, chicken soup, crushed pineapples, fruit cocktail, juice, milk, peaches, pears, tomato soup, or water. After taking the dose, rinse the container with a little bit of water and drink to make sure the entire dose is taken.

CORTISONE ACETATE

Available for over 20 years

COMMONLY USED TO TREAT

Allergic reactions
Severe inflammation

DRUG CATEGORY

antiinflammatory
immunosuppressant
Class: corticosteroid

PRODUCTS

Brand-Name Products with Generic Alternatives
Cortone 25 mg tablet (n/a)
  Generic: cortisone acetate 25 mg tablet (¢)
Products Only Available as Generics
cortisone acetate 5 mg tablet (n/a)
cortisone acetate 10 mg tablet (n/a)

DOSING AND FOOD

Doses are taken 1 to 4 times a day.
It is best to take this drug with food or milk.
Adults: Up to 300 mg per day in divided doses.
Lower doses are used in children.
Forgotten doses: Determining when to take a forgotten dose will depend
on your prescription schedule. If you remember the forgotten dose within a few hours of when it was due, you may take the dose immediately
and continue with your regular schedule. If you are tapering the drug to
avoid withdrawal symptoms, you may need to evaluate the time since the
last dose and the interval between the next doses. A complete change
in schedule may be needed. Talk to your doctor or pharmacist for more
help.

ALCOHOL, DRUG, HERB, AND SUPPLEMENT INTERACTIONS

Alcohol may increase the risk of side effects from this drug, especially
stomach problems. Ask your doctor about the risks caused by drinking
alcohol with your condition.

---

† See page 52.   * See page 53.

Taking this drug with any of the ones listed below may change the effect of either drug with the possibility of causing toxicity or decreasing effectiveness: aminoglutethimide, antacids, anticoagulants†, antidiabetics†, barbiturates†, carbamazepine, cholestyramine, colestipol, diuretics†, estrogens†, griseofulvin, insulin, isoniazid, mitotane, phenylbutazone, phenytoin, primidone, rifampin, salicylates†, somatrem, somatropin

Severe reactions are possible when this drug is taken with those listed below: aspirin, amphotericin B, cardiac glycosides†, immunizations, nonsteroidal antiinflammatories†, ritodrine

ALLERGIC REACTIONS AND SIDE EFFECTS

If you are allergic to any corticosteroids†, you may also be allergic to this drug. You should tell your doctor about all your allergies and any unexplained symptoms you may have while taking this drug.

This drug may cause your eyes to be more sensitive to sunlight, but there are no special risks associated with sunburn while taking this drug.

MORE COMMON SIDE EFFECTS: Indigestion, irregular heartbeat*, leg pain*, nervousness, restlessness*, seizures*, stomach pain*, swelling

LESS COMMON SIDE EFFECTS: Acne*, bloody stools*, bruising*, dizziness, eye pain*, flushing, frequent urination*, hair growth*, headache*, hiccups, increased appetite, lightheadedness, menstrual problems*, muscle cramps*, nausea*, pain*, red eyes*, round face*, skin discoloration, skin irritation*, sleeping difficulty*, spinning sensation, stunted growth*, sweating, tearing of eyes*, thirst*, tiredness*, vision changes*, vomiting*, weakness*, weight gain*, wounds that will not heal*

RARE SIDE EFFECTS: Confusion*, depression*, excitement*, hallucinations*, hives*, mood swings*, skin rash*

PRECAUTIONS

This drug may cause severe and possibly fatal withdrawal symptoms if stopped abruptly. If you wish to stop taking this drug, ask your doctor for specific instructions.

This drug may cause an increase in blood sugar or cholesterol level, calcium loss, and/or retention of fluid.

Avoid contact with anyone who has the chickenpox, measles, or other communicable disease since it may be easier to catch the infection while taking this drug.

Exposure to skin tests, immunizations, and people who have received immunizations may put you at a greater risk of developing the disease when you are taking this drug.

PREGNANCY AND BREAST-FEEDING

Safety during pregnancy has not been established although the drug is known to harm animal fetuses.

Breast-feeding while taking this drug is not recommended.

HELPFUL COMMENTS

If you need to take an antacid, take it either 2 hours before or after taking this drug.

CO-TRIMOXAZOLE
(Sulfamethoxazole/Trimethoprim)

Available for over 20 years

COMMONLY USED TO TREAT

Bronchitis
Cholera infections
Ear infection, specifically known as otitis media
Infections
Lung infections, specifically *Pneumocystis carinii* pneumonitis
Traveler's diarrhea
Urinary tract infections

DRUG CATEGORY

antibiotic
Class: sulfonamides

PRODUCTS

Brand-Name Products with Generic Alternatives
Bactrim tablet (¢¢¢¢¢)
Septra tablet ($)
  Generic: sulfamethoxazole 400 mg, trimethoprim 80 mg tablet (¢¢¢)
Bactrim DS tablet ($$)
Septra DS tablet ($$)
  Generic: sulfamethoxazole 800 mg, trimethoprim 160 mg tablet (¢¢¢¢)
Septra oral suspension (¢¢¢¢)
  Generic: sulfamethoxazole 200 mg/5 ml, trimethoprim 40 mg/5 ml oral suspension (¢¢)

---

† See page 52.   * See page 53.

Other Generic Product Names
Cotrim, Cotrim DS, Sefatrim, SMX-TMP

DOSING AND FOOD

Doses are taken 1 to 4 times a day.

It is best to take this drug on an empty stomach with a full glass of water. Do not eat raw oysters or other raw shellfish at any time while taking this drug.

Adults: Up to 4 regular tablets or 2 DS (double strength) tablets per day in divided doses.

Lower doses are used in children over 2 months old.

Forgotten doses: If you are scheduled to take the next dose within a few hours, do not take the forgotten dose. Otherwise take the forgotten dose as soon as you remember.

ALCOHOL, DRUG, HERB, AND SUPPLEMENT INTERACTIONS

Alcohol may increase some of the side effects from this drug, depending on the amount consumed. Ask your doctor about the risks caused by drinking alcohol with your condition.

Taking this drug with any of the ones listed below may change the effect of either drug with the possibility of causing toxicity or decreasing effectiveness: anticoagulants†, antidiabetics†, cyclosporine, digoxin, sulfonylureas†, tricyclic antidepressants†, zidovudine

Severe reactions are possible when this drug is taken with those listed below: para-aminobenzoic acid, pyrimethamine

Increased side effects are possible when this drug is taken with those listed below: acetaminophen, acetohydroxamic acid, amiodarone, anabolic steroids†, androgens†, antibiotics†, antithyroid drugs†, carbamazepine, carmustine, chloroquine, dantrolene, dapsone, daunorubicin, disulfiram, divalproex, estrogens†, ethotoin, etretinate, furazolidone, gold salts†, hydroxychloroquine, mephenytoin, mercaptopurine, methenamine, methotrexate, methyldopa, naltrexone, nitrofurantoin, oral contraceptives, phenothiazines†, phenytoin, plicamycin, primaquine, procainamide, quinidine, quinine, sulfoxone, valproic acid, vitamin K

ALLERGIC REACTIONS AND SIDE EFFECTS

If you are allergic to furosemide, dichlorphenamide, methazolamide, thiazide diuretics†, antidiabetics†, antiglaucoma drugs†, or any sulfa drugs, you may also be allergic to this drug. You should tell your doctor about all your allergies and any unexplained symptoms you may have while taking this drug.

This drug promotes the effect of sunlight on the body and may cause severe sunburn and increased sensitivity of the eyes.

MORE COMMON SIDE EFFECTS: Diarrhea*, dizziness, fever*, headache, itching*, loss of appetite, nausea, skin rash*, tiredness*, urinary changes*, vomiting

LESS COMMON SIDE EFFECTS: Bleeding*, bruising*, joint pain*, muscle pain*, pale skin*, seizures*, skin irritation*, sore throat*, swallowing difficulty*, weakness*, yellow eyes or skin*

RARE SIDE EFFECTS: Abdominal pain*, back pain*, bloody urine*, mood swings*, swelling*, thirst*

PRECAUTIONS

People with anemia, glucose-6-phosphate dehydrogenase deficiency (G6PD) are at greater risk of developing side effects.

If you have porphyria, this drug may make that condition worse.

This drug may interfere with several diagnostic tests including some urine glucose tests. Diabetics should use glucose oxidase tests or glucose enzyme test strips.

Drink 8 to 10 glasses of water each day while taking this drug to prevent crystals from forming in the kidneys.

This drug causes changes in your blood that put you at greater risk of getting an infection. Be careful not to cut yourself or get bruised. Tell your doctor if you develop signs of infection, such as fever or sore throat. Your dentist may recommend that you clean your teeth and mouth differently to avoid infection.

Be careful driving or handling equipment while taking this drug because it may cause dizziness.

PREGNANCY AND BREAST-FEEDING

Safety during pregnancy has not been established although the drug is known to harm animal fetuses.

Breast-feeding while taking this drug is not recommended.

HELPFUL COMMENTS

Contact your doctor if your symptoms do not improve after a couple of days.

Do not stop treatment early if you start to feel better. It takes the full prescription for this drug to work completely.

---

† See page 52.   * See page 53.

Eye irritation caused by the sun may be reduced by wearing sunglasses when outside.

Do not measure doses of the oral suspension with anything but a measuring cup intended for use with prescription drugs. Slight inaccuracy from other measuring spoons may result in over- or under-dosing.

CYCLOBENZAPRINE HYDROCHLORIDE

Available for over 20 years

COMMONLY USED TO TREAT

Muscle pain and stiffness caused by injury

DRUG CATEGORY

skeletal muscle relaxant
Class: tricyclic antidepressant

PRODUCTS

Brand-Name Products with Generic Alternatives
Flexeril 10 mg tablet ($)
  Generic: cyclobenzaprine hydrochloride 10 mg tablet (¢)

DOSING AND FOOD

Doses are taken 1 to 4 times a day.
This drug may be taken with or without food.
Adults: Up to 60 mg per day in divided doses.
This drug is not used in children under age 15.
Forgotten doses: If more than 1 hour has passed since the forgotten dose, do not take the dose. Just go back to your usual schedule with the next dose.

ALCOHOL, DRUG, HERB, AND SUPPLEMENT INTERACTIONS

Alcohol should not be used while taking this drug.
Several OTC drugs used for asthma, colds, cough, hay fever, sleep aid, or sinus problems may seriously change the effects and side effects of this drug. Check with your pharmacist when selecting OTC products.

Taking this drug with any of the ones listed below may change the effect of either drug with the possibility of causing toxicity or decreasing effectiveness:
guanadrel, guanethidine

Severe reactions are possible when this drug is taken with those listed below: monoamine oxidase inhibitors†

Increased side effects are possible when this drug is taken with those listed below: alcohol, anesthetics, antidyskinetics†, antihistamines†, antimuscarinics†, anxiolytics†, barbiturates†, narcotics†, tricyclic antidepressants†

ALLERGIC REACTIONS AND SIDE EFFECTS

You should tell your doctor about all your allergies and any unexplained symptoms you may have while taking this drug.

MORE COMMON SIDE EFFECTS: Blurry vision, dizziness, drowsiness*, dry mouth, lightheadedness, irregular heartbeat*, seizures*

LESS COMMON SIDE EFFECTS: Bloating, constipation, diarrhea, excitement, gas, headache, indigestion, muscle twitching, nausea, nervousness*, numbness, pain, sleep disorders, speaking difficulty, stomach pain, taste changes, tingling, tiredness, trembling, urinary changes*, vomiting*, weakness*

RARE SIDE EFFECTS: Breathing difficulty*, chest tightness*, clumsiness*, confusion*, depression*, fainting*, fever*, flushed skin*, hallucinations*, hives*, itching*, mood swings*, muscle stiffness*, puffy eyes*, restlessness*, ringing in ears*, shortness of breath*, skin rash*, swelling*, unsteadiness*, urinary difficulty*, vivid dreams*, wheezing*, yellow eyes or skin*

PRECAUTIONS

This drug should not be used for longer than 3 weeks.

You need to wait 2 weeks after stopping a monoamine oxidase inhibitor† before starting this drug.

Be careful driving or handling equipment while taking this drug because the drug may cause drowsiness.

If you have glaucoma or urinary problems, this drug may make those conditions worse.

People with blood vessel disease or hyperthyroidism are at greater risk of developing side effects.

This drug may put you at greater risk of developing problems in the mouth such as cavities, oral thrush, and inflamed gums. Your dentist may recommend that you clean your teeth and mouth differently to avoid infection.

PREGNANCY AND BREAST-FEEDING

Safety during pregnancy has not been established although there was no evidence of harm during studies in animals.

Breast-feeding while taking this drug is not recommended.

† See page 52.   * See page 53.

HELPFUL COMMENTS

Sucking on hard sugarless candy or chewing sugarless gum may help relieve dry mouth caused by this drug. Also consider rinsing your mouth with water and drinking more water.

Avoid quick movements to minimize dizziness. Dangling your legs over the side of the bed for a few minutes may help reduce dizziness when first waking up.

You should tell your dentist if you are taking this drug for more than 2 weeks.

CYCLOPHOSPHAMIDE

Available for over 20 years

COMMONLY USED TO TREAT

Cancer of the breast, eye, bone marrow, lymph system, head, neck, lungs, or ovaries
Hodgkin's disease
Leukemia
Lymphomas
Severe rheumatoid arthritis

DRUG CATEGORY

antineoplastic
immunosuppressant
Class: alkylating agent: nitrogen mustard

PRODUCTS

Brand-Name Products with Generic Alternatives
Cytoxan 25 mg tablet ($$)
  Generic: cyclophosphamide 25 mg tablet ($$)
Cytoxan 50 mg tablet ($$$)
  Generic: cyclophosphamide 50 mg tablet ($$$)

DOSING AND FOOD

Doses are taken 1 to 2 times a day, usually in the morning.
It is best to take this drug with food or milk. Cold foods, such as ice cream, may help to avoid the nausea after taking a dose. Do not eat raw oysters or other raw shellfish at any time while taking this drug.
Adults: Up to 5 mg/kg per day.

Children: Up to 3 mg/kg per day.

Forgotten doses: Do not take a forgotten dose. Just go back to your usual schedule with the next dose.

ALCOHOL, DRUG, HERB, AND SUPPLEMENT INTERACTIONS

Alcohol may increase some of the side effects from this drug, depending on the amount consumed. Ask your doctor about the risks caused by drinking alcohol with your condition.

Taking this drug with any of the ones listed below may change the effect of either drug with the possibility of causing toxicity or decreasing effectiveness: allopurinol, amphotericin B, antithyroid drugs†, azathioprine, barbiturates†, chloramphenicol, chloral hydrate, chloroquine, cocaine, colchicine, corticosteroids†, cyclosporine, cytarabine, flucytosine, ganciclovir, imipramine, interferon, methotrexate, mercaptopurine, muromonab-CD3, plicamycin, phenothiazines†, phenytoin, potassium iodide, probenecid, sulfinpyrazone, tacrolimus, vitamin A, zidovudine

Severe reactions are possible when this drug is taken with those listed below: doxorubicin, succinylcholine

ALLERGIC REACTIONS AND SIDE EFFECTS

You should tell your doctor about all your allergies and any unexplained symptoms you may have while taking this drug.

MORE COMMON SIDE EFFECTS: Back pain*, chills*, cough*, fever*, hoarseness*, loss of appetite, menstrual dysfunction*, nausea, painful urination*, skin color change, vomiting

LESS COMMON SIDE EFFECTS: Agitation*, black stools*, bleeding*, bloody urine*, bruising*, confusion*, diarrhea, dizziness*, fast heartbeat*, flushing, hair loss, headache, hives, itching, joint pain*, shortness of breath*, skin rash, stomach pain, sweating, swelling*, swollen lips, tiredness*, weakness*

RARE SIDE EFFECTS: Mouth sores*, thirst*, urinary changes*, yellow eyes or skin*

PRECAUTIONS

Avoid contact with anyone who has the chickenpox, measles, or other communicable disease since it may be easier to catch the infection while taking this drug.

Exposure to skin tests, immunizations, and people who have received immunizations may put you at a greater risk of developing the disease when you are taking this drug.

†See page 52.   *See page 53.

This drug may increase the level of uric acid in the body, which may lead to gout or kidney stones.

It is very important to drink at least 12 glasses of water each day to ensure that the drug does not irritate the bladder or kidneys.

This drug may cause changes to the blood resulting in an increased risk of blood-clotting problems.

Touching these tablets may cause skin irritation. You should wash your hands immediately after taking the dose.

This drug causes changes in your blood that put you at greater risk of getting an infection. Be careful not to cut yourself or get bruised. Tell your doctor if you develop signs of infection, such as fever or sore throat. Your dentist may recommend that you clean your teeth and mouth differently to avoid infection.

PREGNANCY AND BREAST-FEEDING

There is evidence that this drug may harm the fetus, but the drug may be necessary to the health of the mother.

Breast-feeding while taking this drug is not recommended.

HELPFUL COMMENTS

Some side effects continue even after the drug is stopped.

It is very important to continue taking this drug as ordered by the doctor even if the side effects make you feel ill.

If you vomit shortly after taking this drug, call your doctor to find out if you should repeat the dose.

If you lose your hair while taking this drug it should grow back to normal once the drug is stopped.

CYCLOSERINE

Available for over 20 years

COMMONLY USED TO TREAT

Tuberculosis

DRUG CATEGORY

antibiotic
Class: antimycobacterial

PRODUCTS

Brand-Name Products with No Generic Alternative
Seromycin 250 mg capsule ($$$)
No generics available.
No patents, no exclusivity.

DOSING AND FOOD

Doses are taken 2 to 4 times a day.
Taking this drug with a little food may avoid the stomach upset that some
  people suffer.

Adults: Up to 1,000 mg per day in divided doses.

Children: Up to 20 mg/kg (maximum 750 mg) per day in divided doses.

Forgotten doses: If you are scheduled to take the next dose within a few
  hours, do not take the forgotten dose. Otherwise take the forgotten dose
  as soon as you remember.

ALCOHOL, DRUG, HERB, AND SUPPLEMENT INTERACTIONS

Alcohol should not be used while taking this drug.
Several OTC drugs used for asthma, colds, cough, hay fever, sleep aid, or
  sinus problems may seriously change the effects and side effects of this
  drug. Check with your pharmacist when selecting OTC products.

**Taking this drug with any of the ones listed below may change the effect of
either drug with the possibility of causing toxicity or decreasing effectiveness:**
phenytoin

Severe reactions are possible when this drug is taken with those listed below:
alcohol, ethionamide, isoniazid

ALLERGIC REACTIONS AND SIDE EFFECTS

You should tell your doctor about all your allergies and any unexplained
  symptoms you may have while taking this drug.

MORE COMMON SIDE EFFECTS: Anxiety*, coma*, confusion*, depression*,
dizziness*, drowsiness*, headache, irritability*, mood swings*, nervous-
ness*, nightmares*, restlessness*, seizures*, speaking difficulty*, suicidal
thoughts*, trembling*, twitching*

LESS COMMON SIDE EFFECTS: Numbness*, muscle pain*, skin rash*, tin-
gling*, weakness*

---

†See page 52.   * See page 53.

PRECAUTIONS

Be careful driving or handling equipment while taking this drug because the drug may cause drowsiness.

If you have a history of depression, psychosis, or anxiety, this drug may make those conditions worse.

People with a history of seizures or alcohol abuse are at greater risk of developing a seizure while taking this drug.

PREGNANCY AND BREAST-FEEDING

Safety during pregnancy has not been established although the drug is known to harm animal fetuses.

This drug passes into breast milk, but does not appear to harm the baby. Talk to your doctor about the risks associated with breast-feeding while taking this drug.

HELPFUL COMMENTS

Contact your doctor if your symptoms get worse or do not improve after 2 to 3 weeks.

Do not stop treatment early if you start to feel better. You may have to take this drug for years before your condition is resolved.

Taking vitamin B_6 may be helpful in reducing some of the side effects of this drug.

CYCLOSPORINE

Available since November 1983

COMMONLY USED TO TREAT

Severe rheumatoid arthritis
Severe skin disease, specifically psoriasis
Transplant recipients at risk of organ rejection

DRUG CATEGORY

immunosuppressant
Class: polypeptide antibiotic

PRODUCTS

Brand-Name Products with No Generic Alternative
Restasis 0.05% ophthalmic emulsion (n/a)

Brand-Name Products with Generic Alternatives

Neoral 25 mg capsule§ ($$)
  Generic: Gengraf 25 mg capsule§ ($)
Neoral 50 mg capsule§ (n/a)
  Generic: Gengraf 50 mg capsule§ (n/a)
Neoral 100 mg capsule§ ($$$$)
  Generic: Gengraf 100 mg capsule§ ($$$$)
Neoral 100 mg/ml oral solution§ ($$$$$)
  Generic: Gengraf 100 mg/ml oral solution§ ($$$$$)
Sandimmune 25 mg capsule ($$)
  Generic: cyclosporine 25 mg capsule ($)
Sandimmune 50 mg capsule (n/a)
  Generic: cyclosporine 50 mg capsule (n/a)
Sandimmune 100 mg capsule ($$$$)
  Generic: cyclosporine 100 mg capsule ($$$$)
Sandimmune 100 mg/ml oral solution ($$$$$)
  Generic: cyclosporine 100 mg/ml oral solution ($$$$$)

DOSING AND FOOD

Doses are taken once a day.

It is best to take this drug on an empty stomach. Food interferes with the absorption of this drug but your doctor may suggest you take the drug with a meal to avoid nausea. The type of food you eat will affect the absorption. Do not eat grapefruit or drink grapefruit juice. Do not change your diet while taking this drug.

Adults and children: Up to 15 mg/kg per day.

Forgotten doses: If it is within 12 hours since the forgotten dose, take the dose right away. Otherwise go back to your usual schedule with the next dose.

ALCOHOL, DRUG, HERB, AND SUPPLEMENT INTERACTIONS

Alcohol may increase some of the side effects from this drug, depending on the amount consumed. Ask your doctor about the risks caused by drinking alcohol with your condition.

alfalfa sprouts, astragulus, echinacea, licorice, and St. John's wort may interfere with the effect of this drug and should not be used.

Taking this drug with any of the ones listed below may change the effect of either drug with the possibility of causing toxicity or decreasing effectiveness:
allopurinol, amphotericin B, bromocriptine, cimetidine, clarithromycin, corticosteroids†, co-trimoxazole, danazol, diltiazem, erythromycin, estro-

---

†See page 52.   *See page 53.   § See "Precautions" in this entry.

genst, fluconazole, itraconazole, ketoconazole, nefazodone, nicardipine, phenobarbital, phenytoin, rifampin, verapamil

Severe reactions are possible when this drug is taken with those listed below: amiloride, aminoglycosidest, coal tar, immunosuppressantst, methoxsalen, spironolactone, trioxsalen

Increased side effects are possible when this drug is taken with those listed below: azathioprine, chlorambucil, cyclophosphamide, lovastatin, mercaptopurine, muromonab-CD3, simvastatin

ALLERGIC REACTIONS AND SIDE EFFECTS

You should tell your doctor about all your allergies and any unexplained symptoms you may have while taking this drug.

This drug promotes the effect of sunlight on the body and may cause severe sunburn and increased sensitivity of the eyes.

MORE COMMON SIDE EFFECTS: Hair growth, headache, high blood pressure, nausea*, shaky hands, tender gums*, trembling, vomiting*

LESS COMMON SIDE EFFECTS: Acne, chills*, fever*, frequent urination*, leg cramps, nausea, oily skin, seizures*

RARE SIDE EFFECTS: Bleeding*, bloody urine*, breathing difficulty*, bruising*, confusion*, dark urine*, irregular heartbeat*, mouth sores*, nervousness*, numbness*, pale stools*, shortness of breath*, sore throat*, stomach pain*, tingling*, tiredness*, weakness*, weight loss*, wheezing*

PRECAUTIONS

§Caution: The body absorbs more Neoral and Gengraf than Sandimmune and other generic cyclosporine. These products should not be substituted without a change in prescription.

This drug is not used in people with decreased kidney function.

Your body may retain potassium while taking this drug, which may cause severe side effects if the level gets too high. Potassium levels should be monitored periodically and may need to be treated while taking this drug. Avoid food rich in potassium, such as apricots, bananas, citrus fruit, dates, and tomatoes.

Avoid contact with anyone who has the chickenpox, measles, or other communicable disease since it may be easier to catch the infection while taking this drug.

Exposure to skin tests, immunizations, and people who have received immunizations may put you at a greater risk of developing the disease when you are taking this drug.

If you have cancer or precancerous skin changes, this drug may make those conditions worse.

PREGNANCY AND BREAST-FEEDING

Safety during pregnancy has not been established although the drug is known to harm animal fetuses.

Breast-feeding while taking this drug is not recommended.

HELPFUL COMMENTS

The liquid product should be mixed with a glass of milk (white or chocolate) or fruit juice (not grapefruit) to make it taste better. Rinse the glass with a little water and drink to make sure you take the entire dose.

Dry the dropper used to measure cyclosporine liquid, but do not rinse it with water.

Because this drug may cause tenderness and bleeding of the gums, you may need to talk to your dentist about alternative cleaning methods.

CYPROHEPTADINE HYDROCHLORIDE

Available for over 20 years

COMMONLY USED TO TREAT

Allergies
Headache
Loss of appetite
Rash or hives

DRUG CATEGORY

antihistamine
appetite stimulant
Class: H1 receptor blocker: piperidine

PRODUCTS

Brand-Name Products with Generic Alternatives
Periactin 2 mg/5 ml oral syrup (n/a)
 Generic: cyproheptadine hydrochloride 2 mg/5 ml oral syrup (¢)

Products Only Available as Generics
cyproheptadine hydrochloride 4 mg tablet (¢)

DOSING AND FOOD

Doses are taken 2 to 4 times a day.

It is best to take this drug on an empty stomach, but taking this drug with a little food may avoid the stomach upset that some people suffer.

Adults: Up to 0.5 mg/kg per day in divided doses.

Children age 7 to 14: Up to 16 mg per day in divided doses.

Children age 2 to 6: Up to 12 mg per day in divided doses.

Forgotten doses: If you are scheduled to take the next dose within a few hours, do not take the forgotten dose. Otherwise take the forgotten dose as soon as you remember.

ALCOHOL, DRUG, HERB, AND SUPPLEMENT INTERACTIONS

Alcohol may increase some of the side effects from this drug, depending on the amount consumed. Ask your doctor about the risks caused by drinking alcohol with your condition.

Several OTC drugs used for appetite control, asthma, colds, cough, hay fever, pain, or sinus problems may seriously increase the effects of this drug. Check with your pharmacist when selecting OTC products.

Taking this drug with any of the ones listed below may change the effect of either drug with the possibility of causing toxicity or decreasing effectiveness: anesthetics, anticholinergics†, antihistamines†, anxiolytics†, barbiturates†, narcotics†, tricyclic antidepressants†

Severe reactions are possible when this drug is taken with those listed below: monoamine oxidase inhibitors†, thyrotropin-releasing hormone

Increased side effects are possible when this drug is taken with those listed below: alcohol, antihistamines†

ALLERGIC REACTIONS AND SIDE EFFECTS

If you are allergic to other antihistamines†, you may also be allergic to this drug. You should tell your doctor about all your allergies and any unexplained symptoms you may have while taking this drug.

This drug promotes the effect of sunlight on the body and may cause severe sunburn and increased sensitivity of the eyes.

MORE COMMON SIDE EFFECTS: Drowsiness, dry mouth, fever*, nausea, seizures*, shortness of breath*, skin irritation*, tightness in chest*, weight gain

LESS COMMON SIDE EFFECTS: Belching, bleeding*, body aches, bruising*, clumsiness, confusion, congestion, constipation, cough, diarrhea*, difficult urination, early menstruation, excitement, fast heartbeat, fatigue, fever, headache*, heartburn, hoarseness, indigestion, irritability, joint pain, muscle cramps, nervousness, painful menstruation, restlessness, ringing in ears, runny nose, skin rash, sore throat*, stiffness, stomachache, sweating, swollen glands, swollen joints, tremor, vision changes, vomiting

RARE SIDE EFFECTS: Abdominal pain*, chills*, cough*, dark urine*, dizziness*, facial swelling*, hives*, irregular heartbeat*, itching*, pale stools*, swallowing difficulty*, tingling*, tiredness*, weakness*, wheezing*

PRECAUTIONS

If you have a history of stomach ulcers, glaucoma, enlarged prostate, or difficulty urinating, this drug may make those conditions worse.

This drug may interfere with skin tests used to diagnose allergies and should be stopped for at least 4 days before the test.

Be careful driving or handling equipment while taking this drug because the drug may cause drowsiness.

This drug may cause dry mouth, which is associated with a greater risk of cavities. Your dentist may recommend that you clean your teeth and mouth differently to avoid infection.

PREGNANCY AND BREAST-FEEDING

Safety during pregnancy has not been established although there was no evidence of harm during studies in animals.

Breast-feeding while taking this drug is not recommended.

HELPFUL COMMENTS

Sucking on hard sugarless candy or chewing sugarless gum may help relieve dry mouth caused by this drug.

Several antihistamines are sold without a prescription by the following generic names: brompheniramine, chlorpheniramine, clemastine, diphenhydramine, doxylamine, loratadine. Ask your pharmacist about specific products that contain these drugs.

DANAZOL

Available for over 20 years

COMMONLY USED TO TREAT

Endometriosis

Noncancerous breast cysts, also known as fibrocystic breast disease

Skin disease, specifically herditary angioedema

---

† See page 52.   * See page 53.

DRUG CATEGORY

gonadatropin inhibitor
Class: androgen

PRODUCTS

Brand-Name Products with Generic Alternatives
Danocrine 50 mg capsule ($$)
  Generic: danazol 50 mg capsule ($)
Danocrine 100 mg capsule ($$)
  Generic: danazol 100 mg capsule ($$)
Danocrine 200 mg capsule ($$$)
  Generic: danazol 200 mg capsule ($$$)

DOSING AND FOOD

Doses are taken twice a day.
It is best to take this drug at mealtime.
Adults: Up to 800 mg per day in divided doses.
This drug is rarely used in children.
Forgotten doses: If you are scheduled to take the next dose within a few
  hours, do not take the forgotten dose. Otherwise take the forgotten dose
  as soon as you remember.

ALCOHOL, DRUG, HERB, AND SUPPLEMENT INTERACTIONS

Alcohol may increase some of the side effects from this drug, depending
  on the amount consumed. Ask your doctor about the risks caused by
  drinking alcohol with your condition.

Taking this drug with any of the ones listed below may change the effect of
either drug with the possibility of causing toxicity or decreasing effectiveness:
anticoagulants†, carbamazepine, tacrolimus

ALLERGIC REACTIONS AND SIDE EFFECTS

If you are allergic to any androgens† or anabolic steroids†, you may also be
  allergic to this drug. You should tell your doctor about all your allergies
  and any unexplained symptoms you may have while taking this drug.
This drug promotes the effect of sunlight on the body and may cause
  severe sunburn and increased sensitivity of the eyes.
MORE COMMON SIDE EFFECTS: Menstrual changes*, reduced breast size*,
  weight gain*
LESS COMMON SIDE EFFECTS: Acne*, dark urine*, flushing, mood swings,

nervousness, oily hair*, oily skin*, skin redness, swelling*, tiredness*, vaginal bleeding, vaginal irritation, weakness*, weight gain*

RARE SIDE EFFECTS: Abdominal pain*, bleeding gums*, bleeding*, bloating*, bloody sputum*, bloody urine*, bruising*, chest pain*, chills*, cough*, deep voice in women*, diarrhea*, enlarged clitoris*, eye pain*, fast heartbeat*, fever*, finger pain*, hair growth*, headache*, hives*, hoarseness*, joint pain*, loss of appetite*, muscle aches*, nausea*, nipple discharge*, nosebleeds*, numbness*, pale stools*, reduced testicle size*, restlessness*, semen changes*, shortness of breath*, skin rash*, sore throat*, speech impairment*, swallowing difficulty*, sweating*, tingling*, tiredness*, vision changes*, vomiting*, yellow eyes or skin*

PRECAUTIONS

This drug may cause the body to retain water. If you have a history of headaches, seizures, heart disease, liver disease, or kidney disease, make sure your doctor knows about these conditions before this drug is prescribed.

If you have porphyria, this drug may make that condition worse.

People with blood-clotting disorders, irregular vaginal bleeding, tumors associated with too much male hormone, or severe liver disease may not be able to take this drug.

If you are a diabetic, you may need a change in the dose of your antidiabetic drug† or insulin, since this drug may cause changes in blood sugar.

PREGNANCY AND BREAST-FEEDING

This drug may cause birth defects and should not be used during pregnancy. Breast-feeding while taking this drug is not recommended.

HELPFUL COMMENTS

You may need to stay on this drug for 6 to 9 months before the symptoms of your disease get better.

DANTROLENE SODIUM

Available for over 20 years

COMMONLY USED TO TREAT

Muscle spasms
Surgical patients at risk of developing high fevers, also known as malignant hyperthermia

---

† See page 52.   * See page 53.

DRUG CATEGORY

skeletal muscle relaxant
Class: hydantoin derivative

PRODUCTS

Brand-Name Products with No Generic Alternative
Dantrium 25 mg capsule ($)
Dantrium 50 mg capsule ($$)
Dantrium 100 mg capsule ($$)
No generics available.
No patents, no exclusivity.

DOSING AND FOOD

Doses are taken 1 to 4 times a day.
This drug may be taken with or without food.

Adults: Up to 400 mg per day in divided doses.

Children over age 5: Up to 12 mg/kg (maximum 400 mg) per day in divided doses.

Forgotten doses: If more than 1 hour has passed since the forgotten dose, do not take the dose. Just go back to your usual schedule with the next dose.

ALCOHOL, DRUG, HERB, AND SUPPLEMENT INTERACTIONS

Alcohol should not be used while taking this drug.
Several OTC drugs used for asthma, colds, cough, hay fever, sleep aid, or sinus problems may seriously change the effects or side effects of this drug. Check with your pharmacist when selecting OTC products.

Severe reactions are possible when this drug is taken with those listed below:
anesthetics, antihistamines†, anxiolytics†, barbiturates†, narcotics†, tricyclic antidepressants†, verapamil

Increased side effects are possible when this drug is taken with those listed below:
acetaminophen, amiodarone, anabolic steroids†, androgens†, antibiotics†, antithyroid drugs†, carbamazepine, carmustine, chloroquine, daunorubicin, disulfiram, divelproex, estrogens†, etretinate, gold salts†, hydroxychloroquine, mercaptopurine, methotrexate, methyldopa, naltrexone, oral contraceptives, phenothiazines†, phenytoin, plicamycin, tricyclic antidepressants†, valproic acid

ALLERGIC REACTIONS AND SIDE EFFECTS

You should tell your doctor about all your allergies and any unexplained symptoms you may have while taking this drug.

This drug promotes the effect of sunlight on the body and may cause severe sunburn and increased sensitivity of the eyes.

MORE COMMON SIDE EFFECTS: Confusion*, diarrhea*, dizziness, drowsiness, headache, lightheadedness, muscle weakness, nausea, nervousness, seizures*, sleep disorders, stomachache*, tiredness, vomiting, yellow eyes or skin*

LESS COMMON SIDE EFFECTS: Abdominal pain, bloody urine*, breathing difficulty*, chest pain*, chills, constipation*, dark urine*, depression*, fever, hives*, itching*, loss of appetite, pain*, shortness of breath*, skin discoloration*, skin rash*, speech difficulty, swallowing difficulty*, swelling*, tenderness*, urinary changes*, vision changes

PRECAUTIONS

Be careful driving or handling equipment while taking this drug because the drug may cause drowsiness.

This drug may make it difficult for some people to walk without assistance.

People with emphysema, asthma, bronchitis, lung disease, heart disease, or liver disease may have an increased risk of developing side effects.

This drug is not used for more than 45 days because of the risk of liver damage.

PREGNANCY AND BREAST-FEEDING

Safety during pregnancy has not been established although the drug is known to harm animal fetuses.

Breast-feeding while taking this drug is not recommended.

HELPFUL COMMENTS

Capsules may be opened and the contents mixed with fruit juice or water for easier swallowing.

---

† See page 52.   * See page 53.

DAPSONE

Available for over 20 years

COMMONLY USED TO TREAT

Leprosy, also known as Hansen's disease
Malaria
Pneumonia, specifically *Pneumocystis carinii* pneumonia (PCP)
Protozoa infection, specifically toxoplasmosis

DRUG CATEGORY

antileprotic
antimalarial
antiprotozoal
Class: synthetic sulfone

PRODUCTS

Products Only Available as Generics
dapsone 25 mg tablet (¢¢)
dapsone 100 mg tablet (¢¢)

DOSING AND FOOD

Doses are taken 1 to 2 times a day or 1 to 3 times a week depending on
  the disease.
Taking this drug with a little food may avoid the stomach upset that some
  people suffer.
Adults: Up to 100 mg per day.
Lower doses are used in children.
Forgotten doses: Take the forgotten dose as soon as you remember, then
  continue with the normal schedule.

ALCOHOL, DRUG, HERB, AND SUPPLEMENT INTERACTIONS

Alcohol may increase some of the side effects from this drug, depending
  on the amount consumed. Ask your doctor about the risks caused by
  drinking alcohol with your condition.

**Taking this drug with any of the ones listed below may change the effect of
either drug with the possibility of causing toxicity or decreasing effectiveness:**
activated charcoal, didanosine, paraminobenzoic acid, probenecid, trimethoprim

Severe reactions are possible when this drug is taken with those listed below: methotrexate, pyrithramine

Increased side effects are possible when this drug is taken with those listed below: acetohydroxamic acid, antidiabetics†, furazolidone, methyldopa, nitrofurantoin, primaquine, procainamide, quinidine, quinine, sulfonamides†, vitamin K

ALLERGIC REACTIONS AND SIDE EFFECTS

If you are allergic to any sulfonamide†, you may also be allergic to this drug. You should tell your doctor about all your allergies and any unexplained symptoms you may have while taking this drug.

This drug promotes the effect of sunlight on the body and may cause severe sunburn and increased sensitivity of the eyes.

MORE COMMON SIDE EFFECTS: Blue fingernails*, blue lips*, breathing difficulty*, fever*, loss of appetite*, pains*, pale skin*, skin irritation*, tiredness*, weakness*

RARE SIDE EFFECTS: Bleeding*, bruising*, hair loss*, headache, itching*, mood swings*, nausea, nervousness, numbness*, sleep disorders, sore throat*, tingling*, vomiting, yellow eyes or skin*

PRECAUTIONS

If you have glucose-6-phosphate dehydrogenase deficiency (G6PD), methemoglobin reductase deficiency, or severe anemia, this drug may increase the risk of severe blood disorders.

PREGNANCY AND BREAST-FEEDING

Safety during pregnancy has not been established although the drug is known to harm animal fetuses.

Breast-feeding while taking this drug is not recommended.

HELPFUL COMMENTS

If you have leprosy, it may take 3 to 6 months before the effects of this drug are noticed. Treatment may need to continue for 1 to 2 years.

Do not stop treatment early if you start to feel better. It takes the full prescription for this drug to work completely.

Contact your doctor if you are taking this drug for pneumonia, specifically *Pneumocystis carinii* pneumonia (PCP) and your symptoms do not improve after a week.

---

† See page 52.   * See page 53.

DELAVIRDINE MESYLATE

Available since April 1997

COMMONLY USED TO TREAT

HIV infection

DRUG CATEGORY

antiretroviral
Class: nonnucleodise reverse transcriptase inhibitor (NNRTI)

PRODUCTS

Brand-Name Products with No Generic Alternative
Rescriptor 100 mg tablet (¢¢¢¢¢)
Rescriptor 200 mg tablet ($$)
No generics available.
Multiple patents that begin to expire in 2013.

DOSING AND FOOD

Doses are taken 3 times a day.
This drug may be taken with or without food.
Adults: Up to 1,200 mg per day in divided doses.
Forgotten doses: If you are scheduled to take the next dose within a few
hours, do not take the forgotten dose. Otherwise take the forgotten dose
as soon as you remember.

ALCOHOL, DRUG, HERB, AND SUPPLEMENT INTERACTIONS

Alcohol may increase some of the side effects from this drug, depending
on the amount consumed. Ask your doctor about the risks caused by
drinking alcohol with your condition.
St. John's wort may decrease the effectiveness of this drug and should not
be used during treatment.

**Taking this drug with any of the ones listed below may change the effect of
either drug with the possibility of causing toxicity or decreasing effectiveness:**
amphetamines, antacids, antihistamines†, astemizole, benzodiazepines†,
calcium channel blockers†, carbamazepine, clarithromycin, dapsone,
didanosine, ergot alkaloids†, fluoxetine, H2 receptor antagonists†, in-
dinavir, ketoconazole, phenobarbital, phenytoin, quinidine, refabutin,
rifampin, saquinavir, sedative-hypnotics†, warfarin

ALLERGIC REACTIONS AND SIDE EFFECTS

You should tell your doctor about all your allergies and any unexplained symptoms you may have while taking this drug.

MORE COMMON SIDE EFFECTS: Diarrhea, headache, itching*, nausea, skin rash*, slow heartbeat*, stomachache*, tiredness, weakness, yellow eyes or skin*

LESS COMMON SIDE EFFECTS: Blisters*, fever*, joint aches*, muscle aches*, mouth sores*, swelling*, swollen eyes*, vomiting

RARE SIDE EFFECTS: Bleeding gums, breathing difficulty*, increased appetite, thirst

PRECAUTIONS

This drug is not a cure for HIV infection but may slow the progression of the disease. The HIV virus can still be transmitted while taking this drug.

Skin rash that develops while taking this drug may become life threatening and should be reported immediately to your doctor.

This drug is usually prescribed in combination with another antiretroviral drug. Ask your pharmacist about the type of drug interaction that may occur between antiretroviral drugs† to coordinate the administration times of multiple drugs.

PREGNANCY AND BREAST-FEEDING

Safety during pregnancy has not been established although the drug is known to harm animal fetuses.

Breast-feeding while taking this drug is not recommended.

HELPFUL COMMENTS

If you need to take an antacid, take it either 2 hours before or after taking this drug.

Tablets may be dissolved in about 1/3 to 1/2 cup of water for easier swallowing.

---

† See page 52.   * See page 53.

DEMECLOCYCLINE HYDROCHLORIDE

Available for over 20 years

COMMONLY USED TO TREAT

Infection

DRUG CATEGORY

antibiotic
Class: tetracycline

PRODUCTS

Brand-Name Products with No Generic Alternative
Declomycin 150 mg tablet ($$$$)
Declomycin 300 mg tablet ($$$$)
No generics available.
No patents, no exclusivity.

DOSING AND FOOD

Doses are taken 2 to 4 times a day.
It is best to take this drug on an empty stomach, but taking this drug with
a little food may avoid the stomach upset that some people suffer. Do
not drink milk or eat dairy products within 2 hours of taking this drug.
Adults: Up to 600 mg per day in divided doses.
Children over age 8: Up to 13.2 mg/kg per day in divided doses.
This drug is not used in children under age 8 because of potential damage
to developing teeth and bones.
Forgotten doses: If you are scheduled to take the next dose within a few
hours, do not take the forgotten dose. Otherwise take the forgotten dose
as soon as you remember.

ALCOHOL, DRUG, HERB, AND SUPPLEMENT INTERACTIONS

Alcohol may increase some of the side effects from this drug, depending
on the amount consumed. Ask your doctor about the risks caused by
drinking alcohol with your condition.
Many OTC drugs including antacids, laxatives, and mineral supplements
such as calcium, magnesium, or iron, may decrease the effects of this
drug when taken at the same time as this drug. If you need to take an
OTC drug, take it either 2 hours before or after taking this drug.

Taking this drug with any of the ones listed below may change the effect of either drug with the possibility of causing toxicity or decreasing effectiveness: antacids, calcium supplements, cholestyramine, colestipol, iron supplements, mineral supplements, oral contraceptives, penicillins†

ALLERGIC REACTIONS AND SIDE EFFECTS

If you are allergic to any tetracyclines†, you may also be allergic to this drug. You should tell your doctor about all your allergies and any unexplained symptoms you may have while taking this drug.

This drug promotes the effect of sunlight on the body and may cause severe sunburn and increased sensitivity of the eyes. This effect may last as long as 2 to 4 weeks after the drug is stopped.

MORE COMMON SIDE EFFECTS: Diarrhea, stomach cramps, sun sensitivity*

LESS COMMON SIDE EFFECTS: Itching, mouth sores, thirst*, tiredness*, urinary changes*, weakness*

RARE SIDE EFFECTS: Abdominal pain*, headache*, loss of appetite*, nausea*, vomiting*, vision changes*, yellow eyes or skin*

PRECAUTIONS

If you have diabetes insipidus, this drug may make that condition worse.

People with kidney disease may be at greater risk of developing side effects while taking this drug.

This drug decomposes after the expiration date and may be harmful if taken. Make sure you destroy any leftover tablets as soon as you are done with the prescription.

Some people get a discolored tongue when taking this drug, but the coloring will return to normal when the drug is stopped.

PREGNANCY AND BREAST-FEEDING

This drug may cause toxic effects to the fetus and should not be used during pregnancy.

Breast-feeding while taking this drug is not recommended.

HELPFUL COMMENTS

Oral contraceptives may not work properly when taken with this drug. You need to use a barrier contraceptive, such as a condom, or other nonhormonal contraceptive to prevent pregnancy.

Contact your doctor if your symptoms do not improve after a couple of days.

Do not stop treatment early if you start to feel better. It takes the full prescription for this drug to work completely.

† See page 52.   * See page 53.

DESIPRAMINE HYDROCHLORIDE

Available for over 20 years

COMMONLY USED TO TREAT

Depression

DRUG CATEGORY

antibulemic
anticataplectic
antidepressant
antineuralgic
antipanic
Class: tricyclic antidepressant

PRODUCTS

Brand-Name Products with Generic Alternatives
Norpramin 10 mg tablet (¢¢¢¢)
  Generic: desipramine hydrochloride 10 mg tablet (¢¢¢)
Norpramin 25 mg tablet (¢¢¢¢¢)
  Generic: desipramine hydrochloride 25 mg tablet (¢¢)
Norpramin 50 mg tablet ($)
  Generic: desipramine hydrochloride 50 mg tablet (¢¢¢¢)
Norpramin 75 mg tablet ($$)
  Generic: desipramine hydrochloride 75 mg tablet (¢¢¢¢¢)
Norpramin 100 mg tablet ($$$)
  Generic: desipramine hydrochloride 100 mg tablet ($)
Norpramin 150 mg tablet ($$$)
  Generic: desipramine hydrochloride 150 mg tablet ($$)

DOSING AND FOOD

Doses are taken once a day at bedtime.
Taking this drug with food or milk may avoid the stomach upset that some
  people suffer.
Adults: Up to 300 mg per day.
Lower doses are used in teens and adults over age 65.
This drug is not used in children under age 12.
Forgotten doses: Do not take a forgotten dose. Just go back to your usual
  schedule with the next dose.

ALCOHOL, DRUG, HERB, AND SUPPLEMENT INTERACTIONS

Alcohol should not be used while taking this drug.

Evening primrose oil, yohimbe, SAMe, and St. John's wort may cause serious reactions when taken with this drug. Tell your doctor if you are taking any of these supplements.

Several OTC drugs used for asthma, colds, cough, hay fever, sleep aid, or sinus problems may seriously change the effects and side effects of this drug. Check with your pharmacist when selecting OTC products.

Taking this drug with any of the ones listed below may change the effect of either drug with the possibility of causing toxicity or decreasing effectiveness:
antipsychotics†, anxiolytics†, beta blockers†, cimetidine, clonidine, fluoxetine, fluvoxamine, guanabenz, guanadrel, guanethidine, haloperidol, methyldopa, methylphenidate, oral contraceptives, phenothiazines†, propoxyphene, reserpine

Severe reactions are possible when this drug is taken with those listed below:
amphetamines†, anesthetics, antiarrhythmics†, anticholinergics†, antidyskinetics†, antihistamines†, antithyroid drugs†, anxiolytics†, appetite suppressants, barbiturates†, disopyramide, disulfiram, ephedrine, epinephrine, ethchlorvynol, isoproterenol, meperidine, metrizamide, monoamine oxidase inhibitors†, narcotics†, phenylephrine, pimozide, procainamide, quinidine, SSRI†, tricyclic antidepressants†, warfarin

Increased side effects are possible when this drug is taken with those listed below:
alseroxylon, deserpidine, metoclopramide, metyrosine, pemoline, pimozide, promethazine, rauwolfia serpentine, reserpine, trimeprazine

ALLERGIC REACTIONS AND SIDE EFFECTS

If you are allergic to carbamazepine, maprotiline, trazodone, or any tricyclic antidepressants†, you may also be allergic to this drug. You should tell your doctor about all your allergies and any unexplained symptoms you may have while taking this drug.

This drug promotes the effect of sunlight on the body and may cause severe sunburn and increased sensitivity of the eyes.

MORE COMMON SIDE EFFECTS: Blurry vision*, constipation*, dizziness, drowsiness, dry mouth, irregular heartbeat*, nausea, seizures*, sweating, tiredness, urinary changes*

LESS COMMON SIDE EFFECTS: Confusion*, diarrhea, expressionless face*, eye pain*, fainting*, hallucinations*, headache, heartburn, increased appetite, loss of balance*, nervousness*, restlessness*, shakiness*, shuf-

† See page 52.   * See page 53.

- fling walk*, sleeping difficulty*, slowed movements*, stiffness*, swallowing difficulty*, taste changes, trembling*, vomiting, weakness*, weight gain
- **RARE SIDE EFFECTS:** Anxiety*, breast enlargement*, fever*, hair loss, irritability*, muscle twitching*, ringing in ears*, skin rash*, sore throat*, swelling*, teeth or gum problems*, yellow eyes or skin*

PRECAUTIONS

You need to wait 2 weeks after stopping a monoamine oxidase inhibitor† or SSRI† before starting this drug.

Be careful driving or handling equipment while taking this drug because it may cause drowsiness and dizziness.

Stopping this drug abruptly may result in withdrawal symptoms that include nausea, headache, and general discomfort.

If you have a history of asthma, blood disorders, seizures, enlarged prostate, glaucoma, heart disease, high blood pressure, urinary difficulty, schizophrenia, or manic depression, this drug may make those conditions worse.

This drug may cause dry mouth, which is associated with a greater risk of cavities. Your dentist may recommend that you clean your teeth and mouth differently to avoid infection.

PREGNANCY AND BREAST-FEEDING

Safety during pregnancy has not been established although the drug is known to harm animal fetuses. There have been reports of babies suffering from muscle spasms, heart problems, breathing difficulty, and urinary problems when the mother was taking this drug.

Breast-feeding while taking this drug is not recommended.

HELPFUL COMMENTS

Heavy smoking may decrease the effectiveness of this drug.

You may need to take this drug for 4 weeks or longer before you notice the effects.

Sucking on hard sugarless candy or chewing sugarless gum may help relieve dry mouth caused by this drug.

DESLORATADINE

Available since December 2001

COMMONLY USED TO TREAT

Allergies

DRUG CATEGORY

antihistamine
Class: H1 receptor blocker: piperidine

PRODUCTS

Brand-Name Products with No Generic Alternative
Clarinex 5 mg tablet ($$)
No generics available.
Exclusivity until 2006.

DOSING AND FOOD

Doses are taken once a day.
Taking this drug with a little food may avoid the stomach upset that some
people suffer.
Adults: Up to 5 mg per day.
Lower doses are used in children under age 12.
Lower doses may be needed in people with kidney disease.
Forgotten doses: This drug should be taken no more often than once
every 24 hours. If you have forgotten a dose and are having symptoms,
take the dose right away and reschedule the next dose for 24 hours later.

ALCOHOL, DRUG, HERB, AND SUPPLEMENT INTERACTIONS

Alcohol may increase some of the side effects from this drug, depending
on the amount consumed. Ask your doctor about the risks caused by
drinking alcohol with your condition.
Several OTC drugs used for appetite control, asthma, colds, cough, hay
fever, pain, or sinus problems may seriously increase the effects of this
drug. Check with your pharmacist when selecting OTC products.

**Taking this drug with any of the ones listed below may change the effect of
either drug with the possibility of causing toxicity or decreasing effectiveness:**
anticholinergics†

Severe reactions are possible when this drug is taken with those listed below:
monoamine oxidase inhibitors†

---

†*See page 52.*   **See page 53.*

Increased side effects are possible when this drug is taken with those listed below: alcohol, anesthetics, antihistamines†, anxiolytics†, barbiturates†, narcotics†, tricyclic antidepressants†

ALLERGIC REACTIONS AND SIDE EFFECTS

If you are allergic to other antihistamines†, you may also be allergic to this drug. You should tell your doctor about all your allergies and any unexplained symptoms you may have while taking this drug.

This drug promotes the effect of sunlight on the body and may cause severe sunburn and increased sensitivity of the eyes.

MORE COMMON SIDE EFFECTS: Drowsiness, dry mouth, headache*, increased appetite, nausea, stomachache, thick mucus, weight gain

LESS COMMON SIDE EFFECTS: Appetite changes, belching, bleeding*, body aches, bruising*, clumsiness, confusion, congestion, constipation, cough, diarrhea, difficulty urinating, early menstruation, excitement, fatigue, fever*, heartburn, hoarseness, indigestion, irregular heartbeat*, irritability, joint pain, muscle cramps, nervousness, painful menstruation, restlessness, ringing in ears, runny nose, skin rash, sore throat*, stiffness, sweating, swollen glands, swollen joints, tremor, vision changes, vomiting

RARE SIDE EFFECTS: Abdominal pain*, chills*, cough*, dark urine*, diarrhea*, dizziness*, facial swelling*, hives*, itching*, pale stools*, seizures*, shortness of breath*, skin irritation*, swallowing difficulty*, tightness of chest*, tingling*, tiredness*, weakness*, wheezing*

PRECAUTIONS

If you have glaucoma, an enlarged prostate, or urinary difficulty, this drug may make those conditions worse.

This drug may interfere with skin tests used to diagnose allergies and should be stopped for at least 4 days before the test.

You need to wait 2 weeks after stopping a monoamine oxidase inhibitor† before starting this drug.

Be careful driving or handling equipment while taking this drug because the drug may cause drowsiness.

This drug may cause dry mouth, which is associated with a greater risk of cavities. Your dentist may recommend that you clean your teeth and mouth differently to avoid infection.

PREGNANCY AND BREAST-FEEDING

Safety during pregnancy has not been established although there was no evidence of harm during studies in animals.

Breast-feeding while taking this drug is not recommended.

HELPFUL COMMENTS

Sucking on hard sugarless candy or chewing sugarless gum may help relieve dry mouth caused by this drug.

Several antihistamines are sold without a prescription by the following generic names: brompheniramine, chlorpheniramine, clemastine, diphenhydramine, doxylamine, loratadine. Ask your pharmacist about specific products that contain these drugs.

DESMOPRESSIN ACETATE

Available for over 20 years

COMMONLY USED TO TREAT

Bed-wetting in people with brain injury
Hemophilia A (mild to moderate disease)
Von Willebrand's disease (mild to moderate disease)
Water loss and thirst in people with diabetes insipidus

DRUG CATEGORY

antidiuretic
hemostatic
Class: posterior pituitary hormone

PRODUCTS

Brand-Name Products with No Generic Alternative
DDAVP 0.1 mg tablet ($$)
DDAVP 0.2 mg tablet ($$$)
DDAVP 0.01% nasal solution ($$$$$)
Stimate 0.15 mg nasal spray ($$$$$)
Multiple patents that begin to expire in 2008.

Brand-Name Products with Generic Alternatives
DDAVP 0.01 mg nasal spray ($$$$$)
  Generic: desmopressin acetate 0.01 mg nasal spray ($$$$$)

DOSING AND FOOD

Doses are taken 1 to 3 times a day.
This drug may be taken with or without food.

---

† *See page 52.*   * *See page 53.*

Adults: Up to 1.2 mg by mouth per day in divided doses. Up to 4 nasal sprays per day in divided doses.

Higher doses are used in people with bleeding disorders but are not used on a regular schedule.

Lower doses are used in children.

Forgotten doses: If you are scheduled to take the next dose within a few hours, do not take the forgotten dose. Otherwise take the forgotten dose as soon as you remember.

ALCOHOL, DRUG, HERB, AND SUPPLEMENT INTERACTIONS

Alcohol may increase some of the side effects from this drug, depending on the amount consumed. Ask your doctor about the risks caused by drinking alcohol with your condition.

Several OTC drugs used for asthma, colds, cough, hay fever, pain, or sinus problems may seriously decrease the effects of this drug. Check with your pharmacist when selecting OTC products.

Taking this drug with any of the ones listed below may change the effect of either drug with the possibility of causing toxicity or decreasing effectiveness: demeclocycline, epinephrine, heparin, lithium, norepinephrine

Severe reactions are possible when this drug is taken with those listed below: carbamazepine, chlorpropamide, clofibrate

ALLERGIC REACTIONS AND SIDE EFFECTS

You should tell your doctor about all your allergies and any unexplained symptoms you may have while taking this drug.

RARE SIDE EFFECTS: Breathing difficulty*, chest tightness*, chills*, confusion*, decreased urination*, drowsiness*, fast heartbeat, fever*, headache*, hives*, itching*, seizures*, shortness of breath*, skin rash*, weight gain*, wheezing*

PRECAUTIONS

Teens and adults over age 65 may need to reduce the amount of fluid they drink to avoid water intoxication while taking this drug. Talk to your doctor about this concern.

Large doses of this drug may cause changes in blood pressure.

This drug is very poorly absorbed after an oral dose. Since the drug is absorbed into the body from the nose, nasal sprays may provide more reliable dosing. A stuffy nose may interfere with drug absorption when using a nasal spray.

Nasal spray products must be squeezed about 4 times when first used to make sure the spray will contain the full dose.

PREGNANCY AND BREAST-FEEDING

Safety during pregnancy has not been established although there was no evidence of harm during studies in animals.

This drug passes into breast milk, but does not appear to harm the baby. Talk to your doctor about the risks associated with breast-feeding while taking this drug.

HELPFUL COMMENTS

Clear your nasal passageways by blowing your nose before using the nasal spray to make sure there is a clear path for more drug to be absorbed.

Make sure you keep your head upright, block the other nostril, and sniff at the same time as squeezing the nasal spray.

DEXAMETHASONE

Available for over 20 years

COMMONLY USED TO TREAT

Allergic reactions
Severe inflammation

DRUG CATEGORY

antiinflammatory
immunosuppressant
Class: corticosteroid

PRODUCTS

Brand-Name Products with No Generic Alternative
Dexamethasone Intensol 1 mg/ml oral concentrate ($$$)
Maxidex 0.1% ophthalmic suspension ($$$$$)

Brand-Name Products with Generic Alternatives
Decadron 0.25 mg tablet (n/a)
   Generic: dexamethasone 0.25 mg tablet (¢¢)
Decadron 0.5 mg tablet (¢¢¢¢)
   Generic: dexamethasone 0.5 mg tablet (¢¢)
Decadron 0.75 mg tablet (¢¢¢¢¢)
   Generic: dexamethasone 0.75 mg tablet (¢¢¢)

† See page 52.   * See page 53.

Decadron 1.5 mg tablet (n/a)
  Generic: dexamethasone 1.5 mg tablet (¢¢¢¢¢)
Decadron 4 mg tablet ($$)
  Generic: dexamethasone 4 mg tablet ($$)
Decadron 6 mg tablet (n/a)
  Generic: dexamethasone 6 mg tablet ($$)
Decadron 0.5 mg/5 ml oral elixir (n/a)
  Generic: dexamethasone 0.5 mg/5 ml oral elixir (¢¢)
Decadron 0.1% ophthalmic solution ($$$$$)
  Generic: dexamethasone sodium phosphate 0.1% ophthalmic solution ($$$$$)

Other Generic Product Names
Hexadrol, Mymethasone

Combination Products That Contain This Drug
Dexacidin ophthalmic suspension ($$$$)
Dexasporin ophthalmic suspension (¢¢¢¢)
Maxitrol ophthalmic ointment ($$$$$)
Maxitrol ophthalmic suspension ($$$$$)
Tobradex ophthalmic ointment ($$$$$)
Tobradex ophthalmic suspension ($$$$$)

DOSING AND FOOD

Doses are taken 1 to 4 times a day.
The oral form of this drug should be taken with food.
Adults: Up to 9 mg per day in divided doses.
Children: Up to 0.34 mg/kg per day in divided doses.
Eyedrops: 1 to 2 drops per dose.
Forgotten doses: Determining when to take a forgotten dose will depend on your prescription schedule. If you remember the forgotten dose within a few hours of when it was due, you may take the dose immediately and continue with your regular schedule. If you are tapering the drug to avoid withdrawal symptoms, you may need to evaluate the time since the last dose and the interval between the next doses. A complete change in schedule may be needed. Talk to your doctor or pharmacist for more help.

ALCOHOL, DRUG, HERB, AND SUPPLEMENT INTERACTIONS

Alcohol may increase the risk of side effects from this drug, especially stomach problems. Ask your doctor about the risks caused by drinking alcohol with your condition.

Taking this drug with any of the ones listed below may change the effect of either drug with the possibility of causing toxicity or decreasing effectiveness: aminoglutethimide, antacids, anticoagulants†, antidiabetics†, barbiturates†, carbamazepine, cholestyramine, colestipol, diuretics†, estrogens†, griseofulvin, insulin, isoniazid, mitotane, phenylbutazone, phenytoin, primidone, rifampin, salicylates†, somatrem, somatropin

Severe reactions are possible when this drug is taken with those listed below: aspirin, amphotericin B, cardiac glycosides†, immunizations, nonsteroidal antiinflammatories†, ritodrine

ALLERGIC REACTIONS AND SIDE EFFECTS

If you are allergic to any corticosteroids†, you may also be allergic to this drug. You should tell your doctor about all your allergies and any unexplained symptoms you may have while taking this drug.

This drug may cause your eyes to be more sensitive to sunlight, but there are no special risks associated with sunburn while taking this drug.

MORE COMMON SIDE EFFECTS: Excitement*, indigestion, irregular heartbeat*, leg pain*, nervousness, restlessness*, seizures*, sleep disorders, stomach pain*, swelling*

LESS COMMON SIDE EFFECTS: Acne*, bloody stools*, bruising*, dizziness, eye pain*, flushing, frequent urination*, hair growth*, headache*, hiccups, increased appetite, lightheadedness, menstrual problems*, muscle cramps*, nausea*, pain*, red eyes*, rounding of the face*, skin discoloration, skin irritation*, sleeping difficulty*, spinning sensation, stunted growth*, sweating, tearing of eyes*, thirst*, tiredness*, vision changes*, vomiting*, weakness*, weight gain*

RARE SIDE EFFECTS: Confusion*, depression*, hallucinations*, hives*, mood swings*, skin rash*

PRECAUTIONS

This drug may cause severe and possibly fatal withdrawal symptoms if stopped abruptly. If you wish to stop taking this drug, ask your doctor for specific instructions.

The eyedrops work only on the eye and are not absorbed very well into the body. Most of the interactions and warnings in this summary do not apply to the eyedrops.

This drug may cause an increase in blood sugar or cholesterol level, calcium loss, and/or retention of fluid.

Avoid contact with anyone who has the chickenpox, measles, or other com-

---

† See page 52.   * See page 53.

municable disease since it may be easier to catch the infection while taking this drug.

Exposure to skin tests, immunizations, and people who have received immunizations may put you at a greater risk of developing the disease when you are taking this drug.

PREGNANCY AND BREAST-FEEDING

Safety during pregnancy has not been established although the drug is known to harm animal fetuses.

Breast-feeding while taking this drug is not recommended.

HELPFUL COMMENTS

If you need to take an antacid, take it either 2 hours before or after taking this drug.

DEXCHLORPHENIRAMINE MALEATE

Available for over 20 years

COMMONLY USED TO TREAT

Allergies

DRUG CATEGORY

antihistamine
Class: H1 receptor antagonist

PRODUCTS

Brand-Name Products with Generic Alternatives
Polaramine 2 mg tablet (¢¢¢¢)
  Generic: dexchlorpheniramine maleate 2 mg tablet (n/a)
Polaramine 2 mg/5 ml oral syrup (n/a)
  Generic: mylaramine 2 mg/5 ml oral syrup (n/a)

DOSING AND FOOD

Doses are taken 4 to 6 times a day.
Taking this drug with a little food may avoid the stomach upset that some people suffer.
Adults and children over age 12: Up to 12 mg per day in divided doses.
Children age 5 to 12: Up to 6 mg per day in divided doses.
Children age 2 to 5: Up to 3 mg per day in divided doses.

Forgotten doses: If you are scheduled to take the next dose within a few hours, do not take the forgotten dose. Otherwise take the forgotten dose as soon as you remember.

ALCOHOL, DRUG, HERB, AND SUPPLEMENT INTERACTIONS

Alcohol may increase some of the side effects from this drug, depending on the amount consumed. Ask your doctor about the risks caused by drinking alcohol with your condition.

Several OTC drugs used for appetite control, asthma, colds, cough, hay fever, pain, or sinus problems may seriously increase the effects of this drug. Check with your pharmacist when selecting OTC products.

Taking this drug with any of the ones listed below may change the effect of either drug with the possibility of causing toxicity or decreasing effectiveness: anticholinergics†

Severe reactions are possible when this drug is taken with those listed below: monoamine oxidase inhibitors†

Increased side effects are possible when this drug is taken with those listed below: alcohol, anesthetics, antihistamines†, anxiolytics†, barbiturates†, narcotics†, tricyclic antidepressants†

ALLERGIC REACTIONS AND SIDE EFFECTS

If you are allergic to other antihistamines†, you may also be allergic to this drug. You should tell your doctor about all your allergies and any unexplained symptoms you may have while taking this drug.

This drug promotes the effect of sunlight on the body and may cause severe sunburn and increased sensitivity of the eyes.

MORE COMMON SIDE EFFECTS: Drowsiness, dry mouth, headache*, increased appetite, nausea, stomachache, thick mucus, weight gain

LESS COMMON SIDE EFFECTS: Appetite changes, belching, bleeding*, body aches, bruising*, clumsiness, confusion, congestion, constipation, cough, diarrhea, early menstruation, excitement, fast heartbeat, fatigue, fever, heartburn, hoarseness, indigestion, irritability, joint pain, muscle cramps, nervousness, nightmares, painful menstruation, restlessness, ringing in ears, runny nose, skin rash, sore throat*, stiffness, sweating, swollen glands, swollen joints, tremor, urinary difficulty, vision changes, vomiting

RARE SIDE EFFECTS: Abdominal pain*, chest tightness*, chills*, cough*, dark urine*, diarrhea*, dizziness*, facial swelling*, fever*, hives*, irregular heartbeat*, itching*, pale stools*, seizures*, shortness of breath*, skin irritation*, swallowing difficulty*, tingling*, tiredness*, weakness*, wheezing*

---

† See page 52.   * See page 53.

PRECAUTIONS

If you have glaucoma, an enlarged prostate, or difficulty urinating, this drug may make those conditions worse.

This drug may interfere with skin tests used to diagnose allergies and should be stopped for at least 4 days before the test.

You need to wait 2 weeks after stopping a monoamine oxidase inhibitor† before starting this drug.

Be careful driving or handling equipment while taking this drug because the drug may cause drowsiness.

This drug may cause dry mouth, which is associated with a greater risk of cavities. Your dentist may recommend that you clean your teeth and mouth differently to avoid infection.

PREGNANCY AND BREAST-FEEDING

Safety during pregnancy has not been established although there was no evidence of harm during studies in animals.

Breast-feeding while taking this drug is not recommended.

HELPFUL COMMENTS

Sucking on hard sugarless candy or chewing sugarless gum may help relieve dry mouth caused by this drug.

Several antihistamines are sold without a prescription by the following generic names: brompheniramine, chlorpheniramine, clemastine, diphenhydramine, doxylamine, loratadine. Ask your pharmacist about specific products that contain these drugs.

DIAZEPAM

Available for over 20 years

COMMONLY USED TO TREAT

Alcohol withdrawal
Anxiety
Muscle twitches
Seizures

DRUG CATEGORY

anticonvulsant
antipanic
antitremor

anxiolytic
sedative-hypnotic
skeletal muscle relaxant
Class: benzodiazepine

PRODUCTS

Brand-Name Products with No Generic Alternative
Diastat 2.5 mg/0.5 ml rectal gel ($$$$$)
Diastat 5 mg/1 ml rectal gel ($$$$$)
Diastat 10 mg/2 ml rectal gel ($$$$$)
Diastat 15 mg/3 ml rectal gel ($$$$$)
Diastat 20 mg/4 ml rectal gel ($$$$$)
Brand-Name Products with Generic Alternatives
Valium 2 mg tablet (¢¢¢¢)
  Generic: diazepam 2 mg tablet (¢)
Valium 5 mg tablet (¢¢¢¢¢)
  Generic: diazepam 5 mg tablet (¢)
Valium 10 mg tablet ($$)
  Generic: diazepam 10 mg tablet (¢)
Products Only Available as Generics
diazepam intensol 5 mg/ml oral concentrate ($$$)

DOSING AND FOOD

Doses are taken 2 to 4 times a day.
Taking this drug with food may avoid the stomach upset some people suffer.
Adults: Up to 40 mg per day in divided doses.
Children over age 6 months: Up to 10 mg per day in divided doses.
Forgotten doses: If you are scheduled to take the next dose within a few
  hours, do not take the forgotten dose. Otherwise take the forgotten dose
  as soon as you remember.

ALCOHOL, DRUG, HERB, AND SUPPLEMENT INTERACTIONS

Alcohol should not be used while taking this drug.
Catnip, kava, lady's slipper, lemon balm, passion flower, sassafras, skullcap,
  and valerian should not be used while taking this drug due to an increased sedative effect.

**Taking this drug with any of the ones listed below may change the effect of
either drug with the possibility of causing toxicity or decreasing effectiveness:**
antacids, cimetidine, digoxin, disulfiram, fluvoxamine, haloperidol, itraconazole, ketoconazole, levodopa, nefazodone, oral contraceptives, rifampin

†See page 52.   *See page 53.

Severe reactions are possible when this drug is taken with those listed below:
anesthetics, antidepressants†, antihistamines†, barbiturates†, monoamine
oxidase inhibitors†, narcotics†, neuromuscular blockers†, phenothiazines†

Increased side effects are possible when this drug is taken with those listed below:
aminophylline, theophylline

ALLERGIC REACTIONS AND SIDE EFFECTS

If you are allergic to any benzodiazepines†, you may also be allergic to this
drug. You should tell your doctor about all your allergies and any unexplained symptoms you may have while taking this drug.

MORE COMMON SIDE EFFECTS: Clumsiness, dizziness, drowsiness, joint pain,
lightheadedness, slow heartrate*, shallow breathing*, yellow eyes or skin*

LESS COMMON SIDE EFFECTS: Anxiety*, confusion*, constipation, depression*, diarrhea, difficulty urinating, dry mouth, headache, irregular heartbeat*, memory loss*, muscle spasm, nausea, sexual dysfunction, slurry
speech, stomach cramps, thirst, trembling, vision changes, vomiting,
watery mouth

RARE SIDE EFFECTS: Agitation*, behavior changes*, bleeding*, bruising*,
chills*, delusions*, disorientation*, excitement*, eye movement*, fever*,
hallucinations*, irritability*, low blood pressure*, mouth sores*, nervousness*, skin irritation*, sleeping difficulty*, sore throat*, tiredness*,
weakness*

PRECAUTIONS

This drug may be habit forming and will cause severe withdrawal symptoms if stopped abruptly. If you wish to stop taking this drug, ask your
doctor for specific instructions.

You need to wait 2 weeks after stopping a monoamine oxidase inhibitor†
before starting this drug.

If you have difficulty swallowing, emphysema, asthma, bronchitis, glaucoma, hyperactivity, mental depression, mental illness, myasthenia gravis,
porphyria, or sleep apnea, this drug may make those conditions worse.

Heavy smoking may cause this drug to be less effective.

Be careful driving or handling equipment while taking this drug because
the drug may cause dizziness and drowsiness.

PREGNANCY AND BREAST-FEEDING

There is evidence that this drug may harm the fetus, but the drug may be
necessary to the health of the mother.

Breast-feeding while taking this drug is not recommended.

HELPFUL COMMENTS

Dangling your legs over the side of the bed for a few minutes may help reduce dizziness when first waking up.

If you need to take an antacid, take it either 2 hours before or after taking this drug.

DIAZOXIDE

Available for over 20 years

COMMONLY USED TO TREAT

Low blood sugar, also known as hypoglycemia

DRUG CATEGORY

antihypertensive
antihypoglycemic
Class: peripheral vasodilator

PRODUCTS

Brand-Name Products with No Generic Alternative
Proglycem 50 mg/ml oral suspension ($$$$$)
No generics available.
No patents, no exclusivity.

DOSING AND FOOD

Doses are taken 2 to 3 times a day.
This drug may be taken with or without food.
Children and Adults: Up to 8 mg/kg per day in divided doses.
Higher doses may be used in infants.
Forgotten doses: If you are scheduled to take the next dose within a few hours, do not take the forgotten dose. Otherwise take the forgotten dose as soon as you remember.

ALCOHOL, DRUG, HERB, AND SUPPLEMENT INTERACTIONS

Alcohol may increase some of the side effects from this drug, depending on the amount consumed. Ask your doctor about the risks caused by drinking alcohol with your condition.

aloe, bilberry leaf, bitter melon, burdock, dandelion, fenugreek, garlic,

---

† See page 52.   * See page 53.

ginkgo biloba, and ginseng may lower blood sugar and should not be used when taking this drug. Tell your doctor if you are taking any of these supplements.

Taking this drug with any of the ones listed below may change the effect of either drug with the possibility of causing toxicity or decreasing effectiveness: antidiabetics†, ethotoin, mephenytoin, phenytoin, warfarin

Increased side effects are possible when this drug is taken with those listed below: amantadine, antidepressants†, antihypertensives†, antipsychotics†, bromocriptine, cyclandelate, deferoxamine, diuretics†, hydralazine, isoxsuprine, levobunolol, levodopa, metapranolol, nabilone, narcotics†, nimodipine, nylidrin, papaverine, pentamidine, pimozide, promethazine, timolol, trimeprazine

ALLERGIC REACTIONS AND SIDE EFFECTS

If you are allergic to any sulfonamides† or thiazide diuretics†, you may also be allergic to this drug. You should tell your doctor about all your allergies and any unexplained symptoms you may have while taking this drug.

MORE COMMON SIDE EFFECTS: Hair growth, irregular heartbeat*, seizures*, stiffness*, swelling*, urinary changes*, weight gain*

LESS COMMON SIDE EFFECTS: Constipation, dizziness*, fast heartbeat*, loss of appetite, nausea, stomach pain, taste changes, vomiting

RARE SIDE EFFECTS: Bleeding*, breath odor*, bruising*, chest pain*, confusion*, drowsiness*, fever*, flushing*, numbness*, shaky hands*, shortness of breath*, skin rash*, thirst*, trembling*

PRECAUTIONS

If you have gout, this drug may make that condition worse.

This drug may cause sodium and water retention. If your weight changes more than 5 pounds in a week, call your doctor.

This drug may interfere with glucagon diagnostic tests.

PREGNANCY AND BREAST-FEEDING

Safety during pregnancy has not been established although the drug is known to harm animal fetuses.

Breast-feeding while taking this drug is not recommended.

HELPFUL COMMENTS

It takes about 1 hour for this drug to begin working.

Avoid quick movements to minimize dizziness. Dangling your legs over the side of the bed for a few minutes may help reduce dizziness when first waking up.

Hair growth will return to normal once the drug is stopped.

DICLOFENAC POTASSIUM

Available since June 1988

COMMONLY USED TO TREAT

Arthritis
Menstrual pain
Pain

DRUG CATEGORY

analgesic
antiarthritic
antidysmenorrheal
antigout
Class: nonsteroidal antiinflammatory

PRODUCTS

Brand-Name Products with No Generic Alternative

Solaraze 3% topical gel (¢¢¢¢)
Voltaren 0.1% ophthalmic solution ($$$$$)

Brand-Name Products with Generic Alternatives

Cataflam 50 mg tablet ($$)
  Generic: diclofenac potassium 50 mg tablet ($$)
Voltaren 25 mg delayed-release tablet (¢¢¢¢¢)
  Generic: diclofenac sodium 25 mg delayed-release tablet (¢¢¢)
Voltaren 50 mg delayed-release tablet ($)
  Generic: diclofenac sodium 50 mg delayed-release tablet (¢¢)
Voltaren 75 mg delayed-release tablet ($$)
  Generic: diclofenac sodium 75 mg delayed-release tablet (¢¢)
Voltaren XR 100 mg extended-release tablet ($$$)
  Generic: diclofenac sodium 100 mg extended-release tablet ($$$)

Combination Products That Contain This Drug

Arthrotec extended-release tablet ($$)

---

† See page 52.   * See page 53.

DOSING AND FOOD

Doses are taken 2 to 5 times a day. Extended-release products are taken 1 to 4 times a day.

It is best to take this drug with food.

Adults: Up to 225 mg per day in divided doses.

Forgotten doses: If you are scheduled to take the next dose within a few hours, do not take the forgotten dose. Otherwise take the forgotten dose as soon as you remember.

ALCOHOL, DRUG, HERB, AND SUPPLEMENT INTERACTIONS

Alcohol may increase the risk of serious side effects from this drug. Ask your doctor about the risks caused by drinking alcohol with your condition.

Do not use dong quai, feverfew, garlic, ginger, horse chestnut, red clover, or St. John's wort while taking this drug since they may increase the risk of serious side effects.

Taking this drug with any of the ones listed below may change the effect of either drug with the possibility of causing toxicity or decreasing effectiveness: ACE inhibitors†, acetaminophen, antihypertensives†, digoxin, diuretics†, furosemide, hydrochlorothiazide, nifedipine, lithium, methotrexate, phenytoin, probenecid, sulfonylureas†, sulindac, verapamil

Severe reactions are possible when this drug is taken with those listed below: antibiotics†, anticoagulants†, aspirin, cefamandole, cefoperazone, cefotetan, corticosteroids†, cyclosporine, dipyridamole, gold salts, heparin, mezlocillin, nonsteroidal antiinflammatories†, penicillamine, piperacillin, plicamycin, salicylates†, sulfinpyrazone, ticarcillin, valproic acid, warfarin

ALLERGIC REACTIONS AND SIDE EFFECTS

If you are allergic to aspirin, zomepirac, salicylates†, or other nonsteroidal antiinflammatories†, you may also be allergic to this drug. You should tell your doctor about all your allergies and any unexplained symptoms you may have while taking this drug.

This drug promotes the effect of sunlight on the body and may cause severe sunburn and increased sensitivity of the eyes.

MORE COMMON SIDE EFFECTS: Abdominal pain, diarrhea, dizziness, drowsiness, headache, heartburn*, indigestion*, itching*, mouth sores*, nausea*, skin rash*, swelling*, weight gain*

LESS COMMON SIDE EFFECTS: Bruising*, constipation, gas, high blood pressure*, sweating, vomiting

RARE SIDE EFFECTS: Back pain*, black stools*, bloody urine*, bloody vomit, blue fingernails*, blue lips*, breathing difficulty*, chest pain*, chest tightness*, chills*, confusion*, cough*, dark urine*, fainting*, fever*, hallucinations*, hearing loss*, hives*, hoarseness*, lip sores*, loss of appetite*, low blood pressure*, mood swings*, muscle cramps*, nosebleeds*, pain*, pale skin*, pale stools*, puffy eyes*, rectal bleeding*, restlessness*, ringing in ears*, runny nose*, seizures*, shortness of breath*, sore throat*, stiff neck*, thirst*, tiredness*, urinary changes*, vision changes*, weakness*, wheezing*, yellow eyes or skin*

PRECAUTIONS

This drug may cause serious stomach problems and possibly ulcers. Be careful to take this drug as directed with food and let your doctor know if you develop any stomach-related symptoms.

Do not crush, break, or chew the extended-release products.

Be careful driving or handling equipment while taking this drug because the drug may cause drowsiness.

Do not lie down for about 30 minutes after taking this drug, to help reduce the risk of heartburn and throat irritation.

If you use tobacco or have a history of alcohol abuse, stomach problems, intestinal problems, hemorrhoids, diabetes mellitus, severe fluid retention, or systemic lupus erythematosus, there may be an increased risk of developing side effects while taking this drug.

PREGNANCY AND BREAST-FEEDING

Safety during pregnancy has not been established although the drug is known to harm animal fetuses.

Breast-feeding while taking this drug is not recommended.

HELPFUL COMMENTS

Avoid quick movements to minimize dizziness. Dangling your legs over the side of the bed for a few minutes may help reduce dizziness when first waking up.

Several nonsteroidal antiinflammatories are available without a prescription in lower, nonprescription strengths including ibuprofen, ketoprofen, and naproxen.

---

† See page 52.   * See page 53.

DICLOXACILLIN SODIUM

Available for over 20 years

COMMONLY USED TO TREAT

Infection

DRUG CATEGORY

antibiotic
Class: penicillinase-resistant penicillin

PRODUCTS

Brand-Name Products with Generic Alternatives
Pathocil 250 mg capsule (n/a)
  Generic: dicloxacillin 250 mg capsule (¢¢¢)
Pathocil 500 mg capsule (n/a)
  Generic: dicloxacillin 500 mg capsule (¢¢¢)
Pathocil 62.5 mg/5 ml oral suspension (n/a)
  Generic: dicloxacillin 62.5 mg/5 ml oral suspension (n/a)

DOSING AND FOOD

Doses are taken 4 times a day.
This drug works best if taken on an empty stomach with a full glass of
water, but taking it with food may avoid the stomach upset that some
people suffer.
Adults: Up to 2 g per day in divided doses.
Children more than 40 kg: Up to 25 mg/kg per day in divided doses.
Forgotten doses: If you are scheduled to take the next dose within a few
hours, do not take the forgotten dose. Otherwise take the forgotten dose
as soon as you remember.

ALCOHOL, DRUG, HERB, AND SUPPLEMENT INTERACTIONS

Alcohol may increase some of the side effects from this drug, depending
on the amount consumed. Ask your doctor about the risks caused by
drinking alcohol with your condition.

**Taking this drug with any of the ones listed below may change the effect of
either drug with the possibility of causing toxicity or decreasing effectiveness:**
chloramphenicol, erythromycins†, methotrexate, probenecid, sulfona-
mides†, tetracyclines†

Increased side effects are possible when this drug is taken with those listed below:
acetaminophen, amiodarone, androgens†, antithyroid drugs†, carmustine, chloroquine, dantrolene, daunorubicin, disulfiram, divalproex, estrogens†, etretinate, gold salts†, hydroxychloroquine, mercaptopurine, methotrexate, methyldopa, naltrexone, nandrolone, oral contraceptives, oxandrolone, oxymetholone, phenothiazines†, plicamycin, stanozolol, valproic acid

ALLERGIC REACTIONS AND SIDE EFFECTS

If you are allergic to any penicillins† or cephalosporins†, you may also be allergic to this drug. You should tell your doctor about all your allergies and any unexplained symptoms you may have while taking this drug.

MORE COMMON SIDE EFFECTS: Headache, diarrhea*, mouth sores, vaginal discharge, vaginal itching

LESS COMMON SIDE EFFECTS: Fainting*, fever*, hives*, irregular breathing*, itching*, joint pain*, lightheadedness*, scaly skin*, shortness of breath*, skin rash*, swelling*

RARE SIDE EFFECTS: Abdominal pain*, bleeding*, bruising*, decreased urine output, depression*, nausea*, seizures*, sore throat*, stomach cramps*, vomiting*, yellow eyes or skin*

PRECAUTIONS

If you have a history of stomach or intestinal disease, you may be at greater risk of developing colitis while taking this drug. Tell your doctor if you get severe or watery diarrhea.

PREGNANCY AND BREAST-FEEDING

Safety during pregnancy has not been established although there was no evidence of harm during studies in animals.

This drug passes into breast milk. Allergic reactions, diarrhea, fungal infections, and skin rash have been reported in babies.

HELPFUL COMMENTS

Contact your doctor if your symptoms do not improve after a couple of days.

Do not stop treatment early if you start to feel better. It takes the full prescription for this drug to work completely.

---

† See page 52.   * See page 53.

DICYCLOMINE HYDROCHLORIDE

Available since October 1984

COMMONLY USED TO TREAT

Infant colic
Intestinal disorders
Irritable bowel syndrome (IBS)

DRUG CATEGORY

antispasmodic
Class: anticholinergic

PRODUCTS

Brand-Name Products with No Generic Alternative
Bentyl 10 mg/5 ml oral syrup (¢¢¢)
Brand-Name Products with Generic Alternatives
Bentyl 10 mg capsule (¢¢¢)
   Generic: dicyclomine hydrochloride 10 mg capsule (¢¢)
Bentyl 20 mg tablet (¢¢¢)
   Generic: dicyclomine hydrochloride 20 mg tablet (¢)
Other Generic Product Names
Dicyclocot

DOSING AND FOOD

Doses are taken 3 to 4 times a day.
It is best to take this drug on an empty stomach at least 30 minutes before
   meals.
Adults: Up to 160 mg per day in divided doses.
Children: Up to 40 mg per day in divided doses.
Forgotten doses: If you are scheduled to take the next dose within a few
   hours, do not take the forgotten dose. Otherwise take the forgotten dose
   as soon as you remember.

ALCOHOL, DRUG, HERB, AND SUPPLEMENT INTERACTIONS

Alcohol may increase some of the side effects from this drug, depending
   on the amount consumed. Ask your doctor about the risks caused by
   drinking alcohol with your condition.
OTC drugs used to treat diarrhea may contain an ingredient that can inter-

fere with the effects of this drug. Ask your pharmacist for help when selecting an OTC product.

Taking this drug with any of the ones listed below may change the effect of either drug with the possibility of causing toxicity or decreasing effectiveness: antacids, anticholinergics†, attapulgite, digoxin, kaolin, ketoconazole, levodopa, tricyclic antidepressants†

Increased side effects are possible when this drug is taken with those listed below: amantadine, antihistamines†, antidyskinetics†, disopyramide, glutethimide, meperidine, methotrimeprazine, phenothiazines, potassium supplements, procainamide, quinidine

ALLERGIC REACTIONS AND SIDE EFFECTS

If you are allergic to any belladonna alkaloids†, you may also be allergic to this drug. You should tell your doctor about all your allergies and any unexplained symptoms you may have while taking this drug.

This drug may cause your eyes to be more sensitive to sunlight, but there are no special risks associated with sunburn while taking this drug.

MORE COMMON SIDE EFFECTS: Constipation, decreased sweating, dizziness*, dry mouth*, headache, irregular heartbeat*, urinary difficulty

LESS COMMON SIDE EFFECTS: Bloated feeling, blurry vision, decreased breast milk, drowsiness*, dry skin*, memory loss, nausea, swallowing difficulty*, tiredness*, vomiting, weakness*

RARE SIDE EFFECTS: Breathing difficulty*, clumsiness*, confusion*, excitement*, eye pain*, fainting*, fever*, flushing*, hallucinations, hives*, irritability*, lightheadedness*, nervousness*, restlessness*, seizures*, skin rash*, slurry speech*, unsteadiness*, vision changes*

PRECAUTIONS

Be careful driving or handling equipment while taking this drug because it may cause dizziness and sensitivity of the eyes to light.

If you have colitis, enlarged prostate, fever, glaucoma, heart disease, hernia, high blood pressure, intestinal blockage, lung disease, myasthenia gravis, or urinary difficulty, this drug may make those conditions worse.

People with hyperthyroidism or Down's syndrome may experience an increase in heart rate from this drug.

You are more likely to overheat when taking this drug and should avoid exercising in hot weather and using a sauna or hot tub.

This drug may cause dry mouth, which is associated with a greater risk of cavities. Your dentist may recommend that you clean your teeth and mouth differently to avoid infection.

† See page 52.   * See page 53.

PREGNANCY AND BREAST-FEEDING

Safety during pregnancy has not been established although there was no evidence of harm during studies in animals.

Breast-feeding while taking this drug is not recommended.

HELPFUL COMMENTS

If you need to take an antacid, take it either 2 hours before or after taking this drug.

Eye irritation caused by the sun may be reduced by wearing sunglasses when outside.

Sucking on hard sugarless candy or chewing sugarless gum may help relieve dry mouth caused by this drug.

You may need to drink more water to reduce the constipation that many people suffer when taking this drug.

DIDANOSINE

Available since October 1991

COMMONLY USED TO TREAT

HIV infection

DRUG CATEGORY

antiretroviral
Class: nucleoside reverse transcriptase inhibitor (NsRTI)

PRODUCTS

Brand-Name Products with No Generic Alternative
Videx 25 mg chewable tablet (¢¢¢¢)
Videx 50 mg chewable tablet ($)
Videx 100 mg chewable tablet ($$)
Videx 150 mg chewable tablet ($$$)
Videx 200 mg chewable tablet ($$$)
Videx 100 mg packet for oral solution ($$)
Videx 167 mg packet for oral solution ($$$)
Videx 250 mg packet for oral solution ($$$$)
Videx 10 mg/ml oral solution ($$)
Videx EC 125 mg delayed-release capsule ($$$)
Videx EC 200 mg delayed-release capsule ($$$)

Videx EC 250 mg delayed-release capsule ($$$$)
Videx EC 400 mg delayed-release capsule ($$$$)
No generics available.
Multiple patents that begin to expire in 2006.

DOSING AND FOOD

Doses are taken 1 to 2 times a day. Extended-release products are taken
once daily.

Take this drug on an empty stomach at least 30 minutes before eating for
best absorption. Do not mix oral solution with fruit juice or other acidic
beverage.

Adults: Up to 400 mg per day in divided doses.

Lower doses are used in children and adults less than 132 pounds.

Forgotten doses: If you are scheduled to take the next dose within a few
hours, do not take the forgotten dose. Otherwise take the forgotten dose
as soon as you remember.

ALCOHOL, DRUG, HERB, AND SUPPLEMENT INTERACTIONS

Alcohol may increase the risk of serious side effects from this drug. Ask your
doctor about the risks caused by drinking alcohol with your condition.

**Taking this drug with any of the ones listed below may change the effect of
either drug with the possibility of causing toxicity or decreasing effectiveness:**
allopurinol, ciprofloxacin, dapsone, delavirdine, enoxacin, fluoroquino-
lones†, ganciclovir, indinavir, itraconazole, ketoconazole, lomefloxacin,
norfloxacin, ofloxacin, tetracycline

Severe reactions are possible when this drug is taken with those listed below:
alcohol, aspraginase, azathioprine, chloramphenicol, cisplatin, co-trimoxazole, estrogens†, ethambutol, ethionamide, furosemide, hydralazine,
isoniazid, lithium, methyldopa, metronidazole, nitrofurantoin, nitrous
oxide, pentamidine, phenytoin, stavudine, sulfonamides†, sulindac,
thiazide diuretics†, valproic acid, vincristine, zalcitabine

Increased side effects are possible when this drug is taken with those listed below:
antacids

ALLERGIC REACTIONS AND SIDE EFFECTS

You should tell your doctor about all your allergies and any unexplained
symptoms you may have while taking this drug.

---

†*See page 52.*   **See page 53.*

MORE COMMON SIDE EFFECTS: Abdominal pain*, anxiety, diarrhea, dry mouth, headache, irritability, numbness*, restlessness, seizures*, sleep disorders, tingling*

LESS COMMON SIDE EFFECTS: Chills*, fever*, nausea*, stomach pain*, vomiting*, yellow eyes or skin*

RARE SIDE EFFECTS: Bleeding*, bruising*, itching*, shortness of breath*, skin rash*, sore throat*, swelling*, tiredness*, weakness*

PRECAUTIONS

This drug is usually prescribed in combination with another antiretroviral drug. Ask your pharmacist about the type of drug interaction that may occur between antiretroviral drugs† to coordinate the administration times of multiple drugs.

Do not open, crush, break, or chew the extended-release products.

Tablets should be chewed completely before swallowing.

Chewable tablets contain phenylalanine, which should not be used in people with phenylketonuria.

People with a history of alcoholism, pancreatitis, or elevated triglycerides may be at greater risk of developing serious and possibly fatal pancreatitis (inflammation of the pancreas).

If you have peripheral neuropathy or gout, this drug may make those conditions worse.

This drug may cause dry mouth, which is associated with a greater risk of cavities. Your dentist may recommend that you clean your teeth and mouth differently to avoid infection.

PREGNANCY AND BREAST-FEEDING

Safety during pregnancy has not been established although there was no evidence of harm during studies in animals.

Breast-feeding while taking this drug is not recommended.

HELPFUL COMMENTS

This drug is also called by the generic name ddI.

Several drug interactions, including antacids, may be avoided by taking the dose of this drug 2 hours before or after taking anything else.

The packets for oral solution should be mixed with about $1/2$ cup of water for 2 to 3 minutes for the drug to completely dissolve. Do not mix doses in advance. Do not take the powder without mixing.

DIFLUNISAL

Available for over 20 years

COMMONLY USED TO TREAT

Arthritis
Pain

DRUG CATEGORY

analgesic
antiarthritic
antigout
Class: salicylate

PRODUCTS

Brand-Name Products with Generic Alternatives
Dolobid 250 mg tablet ($)
  Generic: diflunisal 250 mg tablet (¢¢¢¢¢)
Dolobid 500 mg tablet ($)
  Generic: diflunisal 500 mg tablet (¢¢¢¢¢)

DOSING AND FOOD

Doses are taken 2 to 3 times a day.
It is best to take this drug with food.
Adults: Up to 1,500 mg per day in divided doses.
Forgotten doses: If you are scheduled to take the next dose within a few hours, do not take the forgotten dose. Otherwise take the forgotten dose as soon as you remember.

ALCOHOL, DRUG, HERB, AND SUPPLEMENT INTERACTIONS

Alcohol may increase the risk of serious side effects from this drug. Ask your doctor about the risks caused by drinking alcohol with your condition.

Do not use dong quai, feverfew, garlic, ginger, horse chestnut, red clover, or St. John's wort while taking this drug since they may increase the risk of serious side effects.

Taking this drug with any of the ones listed below may change the effect of either drug with the possibility of causing toxicity or decreasing effectiveness: acetaminophen, antihypertensives†, digoxin, diuretics†, furosemide, hydrochlorothiazide, nifedipine, lithium, methotrexate, probenecid, sulfonylureas†, sulindac, verapamil

†See page 52.   *See page 53.

Severe reactions are possible when this drug is taken with those listed below
antibiotics†, anticoagulants†, aspirin, cefamandole, cefoperazone, cefote
tan, corticosteroids†, cyclosporine, gold salts†, heparin, nonsteroidal an
tiinflammatories†, penicillamine, plicamycin, salicylates†, valproic acid
warfarin

ALLERGIC REACTIONS AND SIDE EFFECTS

If you are allergic to aspirin, zomepirac, salicylates†, or other nonsteroida
antiinflammatories†, you may also be allergic to this drug. You should
tell your doctor about all your allergies and any unexplained symptoms
you may have while taking this drug.

This drug promotes the effect of sunlight on the body and may cause
severe sunburn and increased sensitivity of the eyes.

MORE COMMON SIDE EFFECTS: Abdominal pain, diarrhea, dizziness, drowsiness, headache, heartburn*, indigestion*, itching*, mouth sores*, nausea*, skin rash*, swelling*, weight gain*

LESS COMMON SIDE EFFECTS: Bruising*, constipation, gas, high blood pressure*, sweating, vomiting

RARE SIDE EFFECTS: Back pain*, black stools*, bloody urine*, bloody vomit, blue fingernails*, blue lips*, breathing difficulty*, chest pain*, chest
tightness*, chills*, confusion*, cough*, dark urine*, fainting*, fever*, hallucinations*, hearing loss*, hives*, hoarseness*, lip sores*, loss of appetite*, low blood pressure*, mood swings*, muscle cramps*, nosebleeds*,
pain*, pale skin*, pale stools*, puffy eyes*, rectal bleeding*, restlessness*,
ringing in ears*, runny nose*, seizures*, shortness of breath*, sore
throat*, stiff neck*, swollen glands*, swollen tongue*, thirst*, tiredness*,
urinary changes*, vision changes*, weakness*, wheezing*, yellow eyes or
skin*

PRECAUTIONS

This drug may cause serious stomach problems and possibly ulcers. Be
careful to take this drug as directed with food, and let your doctor know
if you develop any stomach-related symptoms.

Do not crush, break, or chew the tablets.

Be careful driving or handling equipment while taking this drug because
the drug may cause drowsiness.

Do not lie down for about 30 minutes after taking this drug to help reduce
the risk of heartburn and throat irritation.

If you use tobacco or have a history of alcohol abuse, stomach problems,
intestinal problems, hemorrhoids, diabetes mellitus, severe fluid reten-

tion, or systemic lupus erythematosus, there may be an increased risk of developing side effects while taking this drug.

PREGNANCY AND BREAST-FEEDING

Safety during pregnancy has not been established although the drug is known to harm animal fetuses.

Breast-feeding while taking this drug is not recommended.

HELPFUL COMMENTS

Avoid quick movements to minimize dizziness.

Several nonsteroidal antiinflammatories† are available without a prescription in lower, nonprescription strengths, including ibuprofen, ketoprofen, and naproxen.

DIGOXIN

Available for over 20 years

COMMONLY USED TO TREAT

Irregular heartbeat
Heart failure

DRUG CATEGORY

antiarrhythmic
inotrope
Class: cardiac glycoside

PRODUCTS

Brand-Name Products with No Generic Alternative
Lanoxicap 0.05 mg capsule (¢¢¢)
Lanoxicap 0.1 mg capsule (¢¢¢)
Lanoxicap 0.2 mg capsule (¢¢¢)

Brand-Name Products with Generic Alternatives
Lanoxin 0.125 mg tablet (¢¢)
  Generic: digoxin 0.125 mg tablet (¢)
Lanoxin 0.25 mg tablet (¢¢)
  Generic: digoxin 0.25 mg tablet (¢)
Lanoxin 0.05 mg/ml oral elixir ($$)
  Generic: digoxin 0.05 mg/ml oral elixir ($$)

---

†See page 52.   *See page 53.

Other Generic Product Names
Digitek

DOSING AND FOOD

Doses are taken 3 to 4 times a day for the first 24 hours, then 1 to 2 times a day.

Taking this drug with food may avoid the stomach upset some people suffer.

Adults (tablets and elixir): Up to 0.5 mg per day.

Adults (capsules): Up to 0.35 mg per day.

Lower doses are used in children based on age and weight.

Forgotten doses: If more than 12 hours have passed since the forgotten dose, do not take the dose. Otherwise take the forgotten dose as soon as you remember.

ALCOHOL, DRUG, HERB, AND SUPPLEMENT INTERACTIONS

Alcohol may increase some of the side effects from this drug, depending on the amount consumed. Ask your doctor about the risks caused by drinking alcohol with your condition.

Betel palm, fumitory, goldenseal, gossypol, hawthorn, licorice, lily of the valley, motherwort, oleander, plantain, rue, shepherd's purse, siberian ginseng, squill, and St. John's wort may change the effects or side effects of this drug and should not be used.

Several OTC drugs used for asthma, colds, cough, hay fever, sleep aid, or sinus problems may seriously change the effects of this drug. Check with your pharmacist when selecting OTC products.

OTC drugs used to treat diarrhea may contain an ingredient that can interfere with the effects of this drug. Ask your pharmacist for help when selecting an OTC product.

Taking this drug with any of the ones listed below may change the effect of either drug with the possibility of causing toxicity or decreasing effectiveness: amiloride, aminosalicylic acids, amphotericin B, antacids, antiarrhythmics†, antibiotics†, anticholinergics†, calcium channel blockers†, carbenicillin, cholestyramine, colestipol, corticosteroids†, corticotropin, edentate disodium, glucagon, kaolin, laxatives, metoclopramide, pectin, propafenone, quinidine, sodium polystyrene sulfonate, sulfasalazine, ticarcillin

Severe reactions are possible when this drug is taken with those listed below: amphetamines, appetite suppressants, procainamide, sympathomimetics†

Increased side effects are possible when this drug is taken with those listed below: beta blockers†, diuretics†

ALLERGIC REACTIONS AND SIDE EFFECTS

You should tell your doctor about all your allergies and any unexplained symptoms you may have while taking this drug.

This drug may cause your eyes to be more sensitive to sunlight, but there are no special risks associated with sunburn while taking this drug.

MORE COMMON SIDE EFFECTS: Agitation, blurry vision*, hallucinations, loss of appetite*, nausea*, tiredness, vision changes*, weakness

LESS COMMON SIDE EFFECTS: Diarrhea*, dizziness*, eye sensitivity, headache*, vomiting*

RARE SIDE EFFECTS: Anxiety*, bleeding gums*, breast enlargement in men*, confusion*, depression*, fainting*, irregular heartbeat*, nosebleeds*, skin rash*, stomach upset*

PRECAUTIONS

The absorption of drug from the capsule products is greater than from the tablets or elixir. The tablet and capsule products should not be substituted for each other without a change in prescription.

Learn how to measure your heart rate and call your doctor if it falls below 60 beats per minute.

This drug may easily reach toxic levels in the body. Dosing must be very exact and regular blood tests are needed to assure safety.

People with a history of thyroid disease may require an adjustment in the dose of this drug.

PREGNANCY AND BREAST-FEEDING

Safety during pregnancy has not been established although the drug is known to harm animal fetuses.

This drug passes into breast milk, but it has been used while breast-feeding. Safety has not been fully established. Talk to your doctor about the risks associated with breast-feeding while taking this drug.

HELPFUL COMMENTS

If you need to take an antacid, take it either 2 hours before or after taking this drug.

Do not measure doses of the oral elixir with anything but the dropper that comes with the prescription. Slight inaccuracy from other measuring spoons may result in over- or under-dosing.

---

† See page 52.   * See page 53.

DILTIAZEM

Available for over 20 years

COMMONLY USED TO TREAT

Chest pain, also known as angina
High blood pressure, also known as hypertension
Irregular heartbeat, also known as arrhythmias

DRUG CATEGORY

antianginal
antiarrhythmic
antihypertensive
Class: calcium channel blocker

PRODUCTS

Brand-Name Products with No Generic Alternative
Cardizem LA 120 mg extended-release tablet (n/a)
Cardizem LA 180 mg extended-release tablet (n/a)
Cardizem LA 240 mg extended-release tablet (n/a)
Cardizem LA 300 mg extended-release tablet (n/a)
Cardizem LA 360 mg extended-release tablet (n/a)
Cardizem LA 420 mg extended-release tablet (n/a)
Tiamate 120 mg extended-release tablet (n/a)
Tiamate 180 mg extended-release tablet (n/a)
Tiamate 240 mg extended-release tablet (n/a)
Tiazac 360 mg extended-release 24-hour capsule ($$)
Tiazac 420 mg extended-release 24-hour capsule ($$$)

Brand-Name Products with Generic Alternatives
Cardizem 30 mg tablet (¢¢¢¢)
  Generic: diltiazem hydrochloride 30 mg tablet (¢)
Cardizem 60 mg tablet (¢¢¢¢¢)
  Generic: diltiazem hydrochloride 60 mg tablet (¢¢)
Cardizem 90 mg tablet ($)
  Generic: diltiazem hydrochloride 90 mg tablet (¢¢¢)
Cardizem 120 mg tablet ($$)
  Generic: diltiazem hydrochloride 120 mg tablet ($)
Cardizem SR 60 mg extended-release 12-hour capsule ($)
  Generic: diltiazem hydrochloride 60 mg extended-release
  12-hour capsule (¢¢¢¢)

Cardizem SR 90 mg extended-release 12-hour capsule ($)
  Generic: diltiazem hydrochloride 90 mg extended-release
  12-hour capsule (¢¢¢¢¢)
Cardizem SR 120 mg extended-release 12-hour capsule ($$)
  Generic: diltiazem hydrochloride 120 mg extended-release
  12-hour capsule ($)
Cardizem CD 120 mg extended-release 24-hour capsule ($)
  Generic: diltiazem hydrochloride 120 mg extended-release
  24-hour capsule (¢¢¢¢¢)
Cardizem CD 180 mg extended-release 24-hour capsule ($$)
  Generic: diltiazem hydrochloride 180 mg extended-release
  24-hour capsule ($)
Cardizem CD 240 mg extended-release 24-hour capsule ($$)
  Generic: diltiazem hydrochloride 240 mg extended-release
  24-hour capsule ($)
Cardizem CD 300 mg extended-release 24-hour capsule ($$$)
  Generic: diltiazem hydrochloride 300 mg extended-release
  24-hour capsule ($$$)

Other Generic Product Names
Cartia XT, Dilacor XR, Diltia XT, Tiazac

Combination Products That Contain This Drug
Teczem extended-release tablet (n/a)

DOSING AND FOOD

Doses are taken 3 to 4 times a day. Extended-release products are taken
1 to 2 times a day.
It is best to take this drug on an empty stomach, but taking this drug with
a little food may avoid the stomach upset that some people suffer.
Adults: Up to 480 mg per day in divided doses.
Forgotten doses: If you are scheduled to take the next dose within a few
hours, do not take the forgotten dose. Otherwise take the forgotten dose
as soon as you remember.

ALCOHOL, DRUG, HERB, AND SUPPLEMENT INTERACTIONS

Alcohol may increase some of the side effects from this drug, depending
on the amount consumed. Ask your doctor about the risks caused by
drinking alcohol with your condition.
Several OTC drugs used for appetite control, asthma, colds, cough, hay
fever, or sinus problems may cause an increase in blood pressure when

---

†See page 52.   *See page 53.

taken with this drug. Check with your pharmacist when selecting OTC products.

Taking this drug with any of the ones listed below may change the effect of either drug with the possibility of causing toxicity or decreasing effectiveness: anesthetics, benzodiazepines†, carbamazepine, cimetidine, cyclosporine, digoxin, lovastatin, procainamide, quinidine, rifampin

Severe reactions are possible when this drug is taken with those listed below: beta blockers†

ALLERGIC REACTIONS AND SIDE EFFECTS

If you are allergic to any other calcium channel blocker†, you may also be allergic to this drug. You should tell your doctor about all your allergies and any unexplained symptoms you may have while taking this drug.

MORE COMMON SIDE EFFECTS: Constipation, headache, fluid retention, irregular heartbeat*, nausea, skin rash*, swelling*

LESS COMMON SIDE EFFECTS: Breathing difficulty*, cough*, diarrhea, dizziness, flushing, shortness of breath*, tiredness, weakness, wheezing*

RARE SIDE EFFECTS: Chest pain*, fainting*, tender gums*

PRECAUTIONS

Do not open, crush, break, or chew the extended-release products.

This drug may cause changes to your gums and mouth. Your dentist may recommend that you clean your teeth and mouth differently to avoid infection.

Learn how to measure your heart rate and call your doctor if it falls below 60 beats per minute.

People with heart failure or liver disease may not be able to use this drug.

PREGNANCY AND BREAST-FEEDING

Safety during pregnancy has not been established although the drug is known to harm animal fetuses.

Breast-feeding while taking this drug is not recommended.

HELPFUL COMMENTS

Avoid quick movements to minimize dizziness. Dangling your legs over the side of the bed for a few minutes may help reduce dizziness when first waking up.

If you do not treat high blood pressure, you may develop more serious problems such as heart failure, blood vessel disease, stroke, or kidney disease. Losing weight, exercising, eating more fruits and vegetables, and avoiding salty foods, such as lunchmeat and pickles, may help make drug treatment more successful.

DIPYRIDAMOLE

Available since December 1986

COMMONLY USED TO TREAT

People at risk of developing blood clots

DRUG CATEGORY

antiplatelet
Class: pyrimidine analogue

PRODUCTS

Brand-Name Products with Generic Alternatives
Persantine 25 mg tablet
  Generic: dipyridamole 25 mg tablet
Persantine 50 mg tablet
  Generic: dipyridamole 50 mg tablet
Persantine 75 mg tablet
  Generic: dipyridamole 75 mg tablet
Combination Products That Contain This Drug
Aggrenox extended-release capsule ($$)

DOSING AND FOOD

Doses are taken 3 to 4 times a day.
It is best to take this drug on an empty stomach with a full glass of water at
  least 1 hour before meals.
Adults: Up to 400 mg per day in divided doses.
Forgotten doses: If you are scheduled to take the next dose within 4
  hours, do not take the forgotten dose. Otherwise take the forgotten dose
  as soon as you remember.

ALCOHOL, DRUG, HERB, AND SUPPLEMENT INTERACTIONS

Alcohol may increase some of the side effects from this drug, depending
on the amount consumed. Ask your doctor about the risks caused by
drinking alcohol with your condition.

† See page 52.   * See page 53.

Taking this drug with any of the ones listed below may change the effect of either drug with the possibility of causing toxicity or decreasing effectiveness: aminophylline

Increased side effects are possible when this drug is taken with those listed below: aspirin, cefamandole, cefoperazone, cefotetan, divalproex, heparin, non-steroidal antiinflammatories†, pentoxifylline, plicamycin, sulfinpyrazone, ticarcillin, ticlopidine, valproic acid

ALLERGIC REACTIONS AND SIDE EFFECTS

You should tell your doctor about all your allergies and any unexplained symptoms you may have while taking this drug.

MORE COMMON SIDE EFFECTS: Diarrhea, dizziness, headache, lightheadedness, nausea, stomach cramps

LESS COMMON SIDE EFFECTS: Flushing, vomiting, weakness*

RARE SIDE EFFECTS: Bleeding*, chest pain*, gallstones*, hair loss, joint pain, muscle pain, neck swelling*, runny nose, sneezing, tiredness*, yellow eyes or skin*

PRECAUTIONS

Although your doctor may prescribe aspirin or an anticoagulant† while taking this drug, there may be a greater risk of bleeding when these drugs are combined.

Be careful driving or handling equipment while taking this drug because it may cause dizziness.

PREGNANCY AND BREAST-FEEDING

Safety during pregnancy has not been established although there was no evidence of harm during studies in animals.

This drug passes into breast milk, but does not appear to harm the baby. Talk to your doctor about the risks associated with breast-feeding while taking this drug.

HELPFUL COMMENTS

It may take 2 to 3 months before the full effects of this drug are noticed.

DIRITHROMYCIN

Available since June 1995

COMMONLY USED TO TREAT

Infection

DRUG CATEGORY

Antibiotic
Class: macrolide

PRODUCTS

Brand-Name Products with No Generic Alternative
Dynabac 250 mg extended-release tablet ($$$)
No generics available.
No patents, no exclusivity.

DOSING AND FOOD

Doses are taken once a day.
It is best to take this drug with food or milk.
Adults and children over age 12: Up to 500 mg per day.
Forgotten doses: If you are scheduled to take the next dose within a few hours, do not take the forgotten dose. Otherwise take the forgotten dose as soon as you remember.

ALCOHOL, DRUG, HERB, AND SUPPLEMENT INTERACTIONS

Alcohol may increase some of the side effects from this drug, depending on the amount consumed. Ask your doctor about the risks caused by drinking alcohol with your condition.

Taking this drug with any of the ones listed below may change the effect of either drug with the possibility of causing toxicity or decreasing effectiveness:
alfentanil, anticoagulants†, bromocriptine, carbamazepine, cyclosporine, digoxin, disopyramide, ergotamine, H2 antagonists†, hexobarbital, lovastatin, phenytoin, theophylline, triazolam, valproate

ALLERGIC REACTIONS AND SIDE EFFECTS

If you are allergic to any macrolides†, or erythromycin, you may also be allergic to this drug. You should tell your doctor about all your allergies and any unexplained symptoms you may have while taking this drug.

---

† See page 52.   * See page 53.

LESS COMMON SIDE EFFECTS: Diarrhea*, dizziness, headache, nausea, vomiting, weakness

RARE SIDE EFFECTS: Abdominal pain*, fever*

PRECAUTIONS

Do not crush, break, or chew the extended-release products.

PREGNANCY AND BREAST-FEEDING

Safety during pregnancy has not been established although the drug is known to harm animal fetuses.

Breast-feeding while taking this drug is not recommended.

HELPFUL COMMENTS

Contact your doctor if your symptoms do not improve after a couple of days. Do not stop treatment early if you start to feel better. It takes the full prescription for this drug to work completely.

DISOPYRAMIDE PHOSPHATE

Available for over 20 years

COMMONLY USED TO TREAT

Irregular heartbeat, also known as arrhythmias

DRUG CATEGORY

antiarrhythmic
Class: pyridine derivative

PRODUCTS

Brand-Name Products with No Generic Alternative
Norpace CR 100 mg extended-release capsule (¢¢¢¢¢)

Brand-Name Products with Generic Alternatives
Norpace CR 150 mg extended-release capsule ($)
  Generic: disopyramide phosphate 150 mg extended-release capsule ($)
Norpace 100 mg capsule (¢¢¢¢¢)
  Generic: disopyramide phosphate 100 mg capsule (¢¢)
Norpace 150 mg capsule (¢¢¢¢¢)
  Generic: disopyramide phosphate 150 mg capsule (¢¢)

DOSING AND FOOD

Doses are taken 4 times a day. Extended-release products are taken twice a day.

This drug may be taken with or without food.

Adults: Up to 600 mg per day in divided doses.

Children age 4 to 18: Up to 15 mg/kg per day in divided doses.

Children age 1 to 4: Up to 20 mg/kg per day in divided doses.

Children under age 1: Up to 30 mg/kg per day in divided doses.

Lower doses are used in people with kidney disease, liver disease, and
. adults over age 65.

Forgotten doses: If more than 2 hours have passed since the forgotten dose, do not take the dose. Otherwise take the forgotten dose as soon as you remember.

ALCOHOL, DRUG, HERB, AND SUPPLEMENT INTERACTIONS

Alcohol may increase some of the side effects from this drug, depending on the amount consumed. Ask your doctor about the risks caused by drinking alcohol with your condition.

Do not use jimsonweed while taking this drug.

Taking this drug with any of the ones listed below may change the effect of either drug with the possibility of causing toxicity or decreasing effectiveness: antiarrhythmics†, anticholinergics†, astemizole, chloroquine, cisapride, clarithromycin, diphenhydramine, erythromycin, fludrocortisone, halofantrine, haloperidole, indapamide, maprotiline, pentamidine, phenothiazines†, pimozide, rifampin, risperidone, sparfloxacin, sulfamethoxazole, tamoxifen, thiothixene, tricyclic antidepressants†, trimethoprim, warfarin

Severe reactions are possible when this drug is taken with those listed below: antidiabetics†, insulin

ALLERGIC REACTIONS AND SIDE EFFECTS

You should tell your doctor about all your allergies and any unexplained symptoms you may have while taking this drug.

MORE COMMON SIDE EFFECTS: Blurry vision, constipation, dizziness*, dry eyes, dry mouth, fainting*, irregular heartbeat*, shortness of breath*, tiredness, urinary changes

LESS COMMON SIDE EFFECTS: Bloating, chest pain*, diarrhea, headache*, impotence, itching*, lightheadedness*, loss of appetite, nausea*, nerv-

---

†See page 52.   *See page 53.

ousness*, rash*, sleep disorders, stomach pain, swelling*, weakness*, weight gain*

RARE SIDE EFFECTS: Anxiety*, bleeding gums*, breast enlargement*, chills*, cold sweats*, confusion*, depression*, drowsiness*, fever*, hunger*, nosebleeds*, pale skin*, shakiness*, sore throat*, yellow eyes or skin*

PRECAUTIONS

Do not open, crush, break, or chew the extended-release products.

Be careful driving or handling equipment while taking this drug because it may cause dizziness and blurry vision.

This drug may lower your blood sugar, which may require adjusting doses of antidiabetic† drugs or insulin.

If you have glaucoma or myasthenia gravis, this drug may make those conditions worse.

This drug may cause changes to your gums and mouth. Your dentist may recommend that you clean your teeth and mouth differently to avoid infection.

People with an enlarged prostate or a history of urinary disorders may be at greater risk of developing urinary difficulty.

You are more likely to overheat when taking this drug and should avoid exercising in hot weather and using a sauna or hot tub.

PREGNANCY AND BREAST-FEEDING

Safety during pregnancy has not been established although the drug is known to harm animal fetuses.

Breast-feeding while taking this drug is not recommended.

HELPFUL COMMENTS

Sucking on hard sugarless candy or chewing sugarless gum may help relieve dry mouth caused by this drug.

Avoid quick movements to minimize dizziness. Dangling your legs over the side of the bed for a few minutes may help reduce dizziness when first waking up.

If this drug causes constipation, you may need to add more fiber to your diet.

DISULFIRAM

Available since December 1983

COMMONLY USED TO TREAT

Alcoholism

DRUG CATEGORY

alcohol deterrent
Class: aldehyde dehydrogenase inhibitor

PRODUCTS

Brand-Name Products with No Generic Alternative
Antabuse 250 mg tablet ($)
Antabuse 500 mg tablet (n/a)
No generics available.
No patents, no exclusivity.

DOSING AND FOOD

Doses are taken once a day in the morning.
This drug may be taken with or without food.
Adults: Up to 500 mg per day.
Forgotten doses: If more than 3 hours have passed since the forgotten dose, do not take the dose. Otherwise take the forgotten dose as soon as you remember.

ALCOHOL, DRUG, HERB, AND SUPPLEMENT INTERACTIONS

Consuming any alcohol while on this drug will cause a severe reaction that includes anxiety, blurry vision, breathing difficulty*, chest pain, confusion, dizziness, fainting, flushing, headache, irregular heartbeat, muscle weakness, nausea, sweating, thirst, and vomiting. This reaction can also be triggered by the alcohol found in food, herbs, supplements, and OTC drugs.

Passion flower, pill-bearing spurge, pokeweek, squaw vine, sundew, sweet flag, tormentil, valerian, and yarrow should not be used while taking this drug.

Caffeine and marijuana should not be used while taking this drug since the effects may be increased.

Taking this drug with any of the ones listed below may change the effect of either drug with the possibility of causing toxicity or decreasing effectiveness: alfentanil, anesthetics, anticoagulants†, antihistamines†, anxiolytics†, bar-

† See page 52.   * See page 53.

biturates, chlordiazepoxide, diazepam, ethotoin, mephenytoin, midazolam, narcotics†, phenytoin, tricyclic antidepressants†, warfarin

Severe reactions are possible when this drug is taken with those listed below: bacampicillin, isoniazid, metronidazole, paraldehyde, tricyclic antidepressants†

ALLERGIC REACTIONS AND SIDE EFFECTS

You should tell your doctor about all your allergies and any unexplained symptoms you may have while taking this drug.

MORE COMMON SIDE EFFECTS: Drowsiness

LESS COMMON SIDE EFFECTS: Eye pain*, headache, mood swings*, muscle pain*, numbness*, sexual dysfunction, skin rash, taste changes, tingling*, tiredness, vision changes*

RARE SIDE EFFECTS: Dark urine*, pale stools*, stomach pain*, yellow eyes or skin*

PRECAUTIONS

Make sure your food does not contain any type of cooking alcohol, such as wine, vinegar, or sherry. Topical products that contain alcohol, such as aftershave, perfume, and rubbing alcohol, may also cause a reaction. Fumes from paint thinner, varnish, shellac, and other chemical solvents may also cause a severe alcohol-type reaction.

If you have asthma, diabetes mellitus, seizure disorders, hypothyroidism, heart disease, kidney disease, or liver disease, an alcohol-induced reaction to this drug may make those conditions worse.

Make sure you have not had any alcohol in the 12 hours before your first dose.

If you have depression or mental illness, this drug may make those conditions worse.

The effects of this drug will continue for about 2 weeks after this drug is stopped.

Be careful driving or handling equipment while taking this drug because the drug may cause drowsiness.

Never give this drug to a patient without their knowledge.

PREGNANCY AND BREAST-FEEDING

Safety during pregnancy has not been established although the drug is known to harm animal fetuses.

This drug passes into breast milk, but does not appear to harm the baby.

Talk to your doctor about the risks associated with breast-feeding while taking this drug.

HELPFUL COMMENTS

Carry a medical-alert card that includes a contact person's name and phone number and your doctor's name and phone number so help may be called in case of a reaction.

DOFETILIDE

Available since October 1999

COMMONLY USED TO TREAT

Irregular heartbeat, also known as arrhythmias

DRUG CATEGORY

antiarrhythmic
Class: unclassified

PRODUCTS

Brand-Name Products with No Generic Alternative
Tikosyn 0.125 mg capsule ($$)
Tikosyn 0.25 mg capsule ($$)
Tikosyn 0.5 mg capsule ($$)
No generics available.
Patent expires in 2018. Exclusivity until 2004.

DOSING AND FOOD

Doses are taken twice a day.
This drug may be taken with or without food. Do not drink grapefruit juice while taking this drug.
Adults: Up to 1 mg per day in divided doses.
Lower doses are used in people with kidney disease.
Forgotten doses: Do not take a forgotten dose. Just go back to your usual schedule with the next dose.

ALCOHOL, DRUG, HERB, AND SUPPLEMENT INTERACTIONS

Alcohol may increase some of the side effects from this drug, depending on the amount consumed. Ask your doctor about the risks caused by drinking alcohol with your condition.

† See page 52.   * See page 53.

Cimetidine (Tagamet), the OTC drug used for treatment of heartburn and stomach upset, may cause a potentially toxic interaction with this drug and should not be used. Check with your pharmacist for another OTC drug that may be used as an alternative.

Taking this drug with any of the ones listed below may change the effect of either drug with the possibility of causing toxicity or decreasing effectiveness: amiloride, amiodarone, cimetidine, diltiazem, ketoconazole, macrolides†, megestrol, metformin, nefazodone, norfloxacin, prochlorperazine, protease inhibitors†, sulfamethoxazole, triamterene, trimethoprim, verapamil, zafirlukast

Severe reactions are possible when this drug is taken with those listed below: antiarrhythmics†, bepridil, diuretics†, phenothiazines†, tricyclic antidepressants†

ALLERGIC REACTIONS AND SIDE EFFECTS

You should tell your doctor about all your allergies and any unexplained symptoms you may have while taking this drug.

MORE COMMON SIDE EFFECTS: Dizziness*, fainting*, headache, irregular heartbeat*, slow heart rate*, swelling*

LESS COMMON SIDE EFFECTS: Back pain, breathing difficulty*, chest pain*, chills, confusion*, cough, diarrhea, fever, flulike symptoms, joint pain, loss of appetite, migraine, muscle aches, nausea, numbness*, paralysis*, rash, runny nose, shivering, shortness of breath*, sleep disorders, slurry speech*, sneezing, sore throat, stomach pain, sweating, tingling*, tiredness*, vomiting, weakness*, weight gain*, yellow eyes or skin*

PRECAUTIONS

Be careful driving or handling equipment while taking this drug because it may cause dizziness.

Recurrent diarrhea, sweating, or vomiting may increase the risk of developing irregular heart rhythm.

PREGNANCY AND BREAST-FEEDING

Safety during pregnancy has not been established although the drug is known to harm animal fetuses.

Breast-feeding while taking this drug is not recommended.

HELPFUL COMMENTS

Avoid quick movements to minimize dizziness. Dangling your legs over the side of the bed for a few minutes may help reduce dizziness when first waking up.

DOLASETRON MESYLATE

Available since September 1997

COMMONLY USED TO TREAT

Nausea and vomiting after surgery or cancer treatment

DRUG CATEGORY

antiemetic
Class: selective 5-HT3 receptor antagonist

PRODUCTS

Brand-Name Products with No Generic Alternative
Anzemet 50 mg tablet ($$$$$)
Anzemet 100 mg tablet ($$$$$)
No generics available.
Patent expires in 2011.

DOSING AND FOOD

A singe dose is taken 1 to 2 hours before the surgery or 1 hour before
  chemotherapy.
This drug may be taken with or without food.
Adults: Up to 100 mg per dose.
Children age 2 to 16: Up to 1.8 mg/kg (maximum 100 mg) per dose.

ALCOHOL, DRUG, HERB, AND SUPPLEMENT INTERACTIONS

Alcohol may increase some of the side effects from this drug, depending
  on the amount consumed. Ask your doctor about the risks caused by
  drinking alcohol with your condition.

Taking this drug with any of the ones listed below may change the effect of
either drug with the possibility of causing toxicity or decreasing effectiveness:
cimetidine, rifampin

Severe reactions are possible when this drug is taken with those listed below:
antiarrhythmics†, diuretics†

ALLERGIC REACTIONS AND SIDE EFFECTS

You should tell your doctor about all your allergies and any unexplained
  symptoms you may have while taking this drug.
MORE COMMON SIDE EFFECTS: Diarrhea, headache, irregular heartbeat*,
  slow heart rate

---

†*See page 52.*   **See page 53.*

LESS COMMON SIDE EFFECTS: Blood pressure changes*, chills, dizziness, fever, lightheadedness, stomach pain*, tiredness

RARE SIDE EFFECTS: Bloody urine*, breathing difficulty*, chest pain*, hives*, itching*, nausea*, pain*, skin rash*, swelling*, urinary difficulty*, vomiting*

PRECAUTIONS

It is very important to take this drug at the specified time in order for it to work properly.

People with a history of arrhythmias may not be able to take this drug.

PREGNANCY AND BREAST-FEEDING

Safety during pregnancy has not been established although there was no evidence of harm during studies in animals.

It is not known if this drug passes into breast milk. Talk to your doctor about possible risks to the baby.

HELPFUL COMMENTS

There is an injectable form of this drug that may be mixed with juice and taken by mouth for people who have difficulty swallowing. These doses should not be mixed more than 2 hours in advance.

Tell your doctor if you have any nausea or vomiting after taking a dose of this drug.

DONEPEZIL HYDROCHLORIDE

Available since November 1996

COMMONLY USED TO TREAT

Alzheimer's disease

DRUG CATEGORY

antidementia
Class: cholinesterase inhibitor

PRODUCTS

Brand-Name Products with No Generic Alternative
Aricept 5 mg tablet ($$$)
Aricept 10 mg tablet ($$$)
No generics available.

Multiple patents that begin to expire in 2010.

DOSING AND FOOD

Doses are taken once a day at bedtime.
This drug may be taken with or without food.

Adults: Up to 10 mg per day.

Forgotten doses: Do not take a forgotten dose. Just go back to your usual schedule with the next dose.

ALCOHOL, DRUG, HERB, AND SUPPLEMENT INTERACTIONS

Alcohol may increase some of the side effects from this drug, depending on the amount consumed. Ask your doctor about the risks caused by drinking alcohol with your condition.

Jaborandi and pill-bearing spurge may increase the risk of toxicity from this drug and should not be taken.

Taking this drug with any of the ones listed below may change the effect of either drug with the possibility of causing toxicity or decreasing effectiveness: acetylcholinesterase inhibitors†, anticholinergics†, bethanechol, carbamazepine, dexamethasone, phenobarbital, phenytoin, rifampin, succinylcholine

ALLERGIC REACTIONS AND SIDE EFFECTS

If you are allergic to biperiden, bupivacaine, methylphenidate, paroxetine, rifabutin, or trihexyphenidyl, you may also be allergic to this drug. You should tell your doctor about all your allergies and any unexplained symptoms you may have while taking this drug.

MORE COMMON SIDE EFFECTS: Black stools*, diarrhea*, headache*, loss of appetite*, muscle cramps*, nausea*, seizures*, sleep disorders*, stomach pain*, tiredness*, weakness*, vomiting*

LESS COMMON SIDE EFFECTS: Abnormal dreams*, bleeding*, bruising*, constipation*, depression*, dizziness*, drowsiness*, fainting*, frequent urination*, stiffness*, swelling*, weight loss*

RARE SIDE EFFECTS: Aggression*, agitation*, bloating*, blood pressure change*, bloody urine*, blurry vision*, cataracts*, chest pain*, chills*, clumsiness*, confusion*, congestion*, cough*, crying*, delusions*, dry mouth*, fever*, flushing*, heart rate changes*, hives*, hot flashes*, irregular heartbeat*, irritability*, itching*, low blood pressure*, mood swings*, nervousness*, poor bowel control*, restlessness*, runny nose*, sexual craving*, shortness of breath*, sneezing*, sore eyes*, sore throat*,

---

† *See page 52.*   * *See page 53.*

speaking difficulty*, sweating*, thirst*, tingling*, tremor*, unsteadiness*, urinary changes*, watery mouth*, wheezing*, wrinkled skin*

PRECAUTIONS

If you have asthma, lung disease, peptic ulcer, seizures, or urinary difficulty, this drug may make those conditions worse.

Be careful driving or handling equipment while taking this drug because the drug may cause drowsiness.

PREGNANCY AND BREAST-FEEDING

Safety during pregnancy has not been established although the drug is known to harm animal fetuses.

Breast-feeding while taking this drug is not recommended.

HELPFUL COMMENTS

It takes 4 to 6 weeks for the full effects of this drug to be noticed.

DOXAZOSIN MESYLATE

Available since November 1990

COMMONLY USED TO TREAT

Enlarged prostate, also known as benign (noncancerous) protatic hyperplasia or BPH

High blood pressure, also known as hypertension

DRUG CATEGORY

antihypertensive
Class: alpha adrenergic blocker

PRODUCTS

Brand-Name Products with Generic Alternatives
Cardura 1 mg tablet ($)
  Generic: doxazosin mesylate 1 mg tablet (¢¢¢¢¢)
Cardura 2 mg tablet ($)
  Generic: doxazosin mesylate 2 mg tablet (¢¢¢¢¢)
Cardura 4 mg tablet ($)
  Generic: doxazosin mesylate 4 mg tablet (¢¢¢¢¢)
Cardura 8 mg tablet ($)
  Generic: doxazosin mesylate 8 mg tablet ($)

DOSING AND FOOD

Doses are taken once a day.

It is best to take this drug on an empty stomach, but taking this drug with a little food may avoid the stomach upset that some people suffer.

Adults: Up to 16 mg per day.

Forgotten doses: If you are scheduled to take the next dose within a few hours, do not take the forgotten dose. Otherwise take the forgotten dose as soon as you remember.

ALCOHOL, DRUG, HERB, AND SUPPLEMENT INTERACTIONS

Alcohol may cause your blood pressure to rise, making this drug less effective, and may increase the risk of side effects caused by this drug. Ask your doctor about the risks caused by drinking alcohol with your condition.

Butcher's broom may reduce the effect of this drug and should not be used.

Several OTC drugs used for appetite control, asthma, colds, cough, hay fever, or sinus problems may cause an increase in blood pressure when taken with this drug. Check with your pharmacist when selecting OTC products.

Taking this drug with any of the ones listed below may change the effect of either drug with the possibility of causing toxicity or decreasing effectiveness: clonidine

ALLERGIC REACTIONS AND SIDE EFFECTS

If you are allergic to prazosin or terazosin, you may also be allergic to this drug. You should tell your doctor about all your allergies and any unexplained symptoms you may have while taking this drug.

MORE COMMON SIDE EFFECTS: Dizziness*, headache, irregular heartbeat*, lightheadedness*, tiredness

LESS COMMON SIDE EFFECTS: Drowsiness, fainting*, irritability, itching, nausea, nervousness, rash, runny nose, shortness of breath*, sleepiness, swelling*

RARE SIDE EFFECTS: Prolonged penile erection*

PRECAUTIONS

Men have a very small risk of developing painful, prolonged erection of the penis, which requires treatment by a doctor. If this happens, go to your doctor or the nearest emergency room immediately.

Be careful driving or handling equipment while taking this drug because it may cause dizziness.

†See page 52.   * See page 53.

People on a dose higher than 4 mg per day have a greater risk of developing side effects.

PREGNANCY AND BREAST-FEEDING

Safety during pregnancy has not been established although the drug is known to harm animal fetuses.

Breast-feeding while taking this drug is not recommended.

HELPFUL COMMENTS

Avoid quick movements to minimize dizziness. Dangling your legs over the side of the bed for a few minutes may help reduce dizziness when first waking up.

It takes about 2 weeks for the effects of this drug to be noticed.

Take your first dose of this drug at bedtime so you do not feel the light-headedness and dizziness that is more severe with the first dose. Be careful when getting up during the night. Dangle your feel over the side of the bed for a few minutes before standing.

If you do not treat high blood pressure, you may develop more serious problems such as heart failure, blood vessel disease, stroke, or kidney disease. Losing weight, exercising, eating more fruits and vegetables, and avoiding salty foods, such as lunchmeat and pickles, may help make drug treatment more successful.

DOXEPIN HYDROCHLORIDE

Available for over 20 years

COMMONLY USED TO TREAT

Anxiety
Depression
Itching caused by eczema (topical products only)

DRUG CATEGORY

antidepressant
antineuralgic
antipruretic
Class: tricyclic antidepressant

PRODUCTS

Brand-Name Products with No Generic Alternative
Zonalon 5% topical cream (¢¢¢¢)

Brand-Name Products with Generic Alternatives

Sinequan 10 mg capsule (¢¢)
  Generic: doxepin hydrochloride 10 mg capsule (¢)
Sinequan 25 mg capsule (¢¢¢¢)
  Generic: doxepin hydrochloride 25 mg capsule (¢)
Sinequan 50 mg capsule (¢¢¢¢¢)
  Generic: doxepin hydrochloride 50 mg capsule (¢¢)
Sinequan 75 mg capsule ($)
  Generic: doxepin hydrochloride 75 mg capsule (¢¢)
Sinequan 100 mg capsule ($)
  Generic: doxepin hydrochloride 100 mg capsule (¢¢¢)
Sinequan 150 mg capsule ($)
  Generic: doxepin hydrochloride 150 mg capsule ($$)
Sinequan 100 mg/ ml oral concentrate ($$)
  Generic: doxepin hydrochloride 100 mg/ml oral concentrate (¢¢¢¢¢)

DOSING AND FOOD

Doses are taken 1 to 3 times a day.

Taking this drug with food or milk may avoid the stomach upset that some people suffer. Do not drink carbonated beverages when taking your dose. Do not eat grapefruit or drink grapefruit juice while taking this drug.

Adults: Up to 300 mg per day.

Lower doses are used in teens and adults over age 65.

Topical cream is used 4 times a day. Apply a thin layer and leave the area uncovered.

Forgotten doses: If you are scheduled to take the next dose within a few hours, do not take the forgotten dose. Otherwise take the forgotten dose as soon as you remember.

ALCOHOL, DRUG, HERB, AND SUPPLEMENT INTERACTIONS

Alcohol should not be used while taking this drug.

Evening primrose oil, SAMe, St. John's wort, and yohimbe may cause serious reactions when taken with this drug. Tell your doctor if you are taking any of these supplements.

Several OTC drugs used for asthma, colds, cough, hay fever, sleep aid, or sinus problems may seriously change the effects and side effects of this drug. Check with your pharmacist when selecting OTC products.

Taking this drug with any of the ones listed below may change the effect of either drug with the possibility of causing toxicity or decreasing effectiveness: anesthetics, antipsychotics†, anxiolytics†, barbiturates†, beta blockers†,

---

† *See page 52.*   * *See page 53.*

cimetidine, clonidine, fluoxetine, guanabenz, guanadrel, guanethidine, haloperidol, methyldopa, methylphenidate, narcotics†, oral contraceptives, phenothiazines†, propoxyphene, reserpine, sertraline

Severe reactions are possible when this drug is taken with those listed below: amphetamines†, anesthetics, antiarrhythmics†, anticholinergics†, antidyskinetics†, antihistamines†, antithyroid drugs†, anxiolytics†, appetite suppressants, barbiturates†, disopyramide, disulfiram, ephedrine, epinephrine, ethchlorvynol, isoproterenol, meperidine, metrizamide, monoamine oxidase inhibitors†, narcotics†, phenylephrine, pimozide, procainamide, quinidine, tricyclic antidepressants†, warfarin

Increased side effects are possible when this drug is taken with those listed below: alseroxylon, deserpidine, metoclopramide, metyrosine, pemoline, pimozide, promethazine, rauwolfia serpentine, reserpine, trimeprazine

ALLERGIC REACTIONS AND SIDE EFFECTS

If you are allergic to carbamazepine, maprotiline, trazodone, or any tricyclic antidepressants†, you may also be allergic to this drug. You should tell your doctor about all your allergies and any unexplained symptoms you may have while taking this drug.

This drug promotes the effect of sunlight on the body and may cause severe sunburn and increased sensitivity of the eyes.

MORE COMMON SIDE EFFECTS: Blurry vision*, constipation*, dizziness, drowsiness, dry mouth, irregular heartbeat*, seizures*, sweating, tiredness

LESS COMMON SIDE EFFECTS: Confusion*, decreased appetite, diarrhea, expressionless face*, eye pain*, fainting*, hallucinations*, headache, heartburn, loss of balance*, nausea, nervousness*, restlessness*, shakiness*, shuffling walk*, sleeping difficulty*, slowed movements*, stiffness*, swallowing difficulty*, taste changes, trembling*, urinary changes*, vomiting, weakness*, weight gain

RARE SIDE EFFECTS: Anxiety*, breast enlargement*, fever*, hair loss, irritability*, muscle twitching*, ringing in ears*, skin rash*, sore throat*, swelling*, teeth or gum problems*, yellow eyes or skin*

PRECAUTIONS

The topical form of this drug is absorbed through the skin and may be associated with the same warnings as the oral products.

You need to wait 2 weeks after stopping a monoamine oxidase inhibitor† or SSRI† before starting this drug.

Be careful driving or handling equipment while taking this drug because it may cause drowsiness and dizziness.

Stopping this drug abruptly may result in withdrawal symptoms that include nausea, headache, and general discomfort.

If you have a history of asthma, blood disorders, seizures, enlarged prostate, glaucoma, heart disease, high blood pressure, urinary difficulty, schizophrenia, or manic depression, this drug may make those conditions worse.

This drug may cause dry mouth, which is associated with a greater risk of cavities. Your dentist may recommend that you clean your teeth and mouth differently to avoid infection.

PREGNANCY AND BREAST-FEEDING

Safety during pregnancy has not been established although the drug is known to harm animal fetuses. There have been reports of babies suffering from muscle spasms, heart problems, breathing difficulty, and urinary problems when the mother was taking this drug.

Breast-feeding while taking this drug is not recommended.

HELPFUL COMMENTS

Oral-concentrate products should be diluted with $1/2$ cup of water, milk, orange juice, pineapple juice, prune juice, or tomato juice. Do not mix with carbonated beverages or grapefruit juice.

Heavy smoking may decrease the effectiveness of this drug.

Sucking on hard sugarless candy or chewing sugarless gum may help relieve dry mouth caused by this drug.

If you are using the topical product and your symptoms do not improve after a couple of days, call your doctor.

DOXYCYCLINE

Available for over 20 years

COMMONLY USED TO TREAT

Infection

DRUG CATEGORY

antibiotic
Class: tetracycline

---

† See page 52.　　* See page 53.

PRODUCTS

Brand-Name Products with No Generic Alternative
Atridox 10% extended-release periodontal liquid ($$$$$)
Doryx 75 mg capsule ($$$)
Doryx 100 mg capsule ($$$)
Periostat 20 mg tablet (¢¢¢¢¢)
Vibramycin 25 mg/5 ml oral suspension ($)
Vibramycin 50 mg/5 ml oral suspension ($$)

Brand-Name Products with Generic Alternatives
Vibramycin 50 mg capsule ($$)
  Generic: doxycycline hyclate 50 mg capsule (¢¢)
Vibramycin 100 mg capsule ($$$)
  Generic: doxycycline hyclate 100 mg capsule (¢¢)
Vibra-Tabs 100 mg tablet ($$$)
  Generic: doxycycline hyclate 100 mg tablet (¢¢)

Products Only Available as Generics
doxycycline monohydrate 50 mg capsule ($)
doxycycline monohydrate 100 mg capsule ($$)

Other Generic Product Names
Monodox

DOSING AND FOOD

Doses are taken 1 to 2 times a day.
This drug may be taken with or without food although dairy products may decrease the drug's absorption.

Adults: Up to 200 mg per day in divided doses.

Children over age 8: Up to 4.4 mg/kg per day in divided doses.
This drug is not used in children under age 8 because of potential damage to developing teeth and bones.

Forgotten doses: If you are scheduled to take the next dose within a few hours, do not take the forgotten dose. Otherwise take the forgotten dose as soon as you remember.

ALCOHOL, DRUG, HERB, AND SUPPLEMENT INTERACTIONS

Alcohol should not be used while taking this drug since it may decrease the effectiveness.
Many OTC drugs including antacids, laxatives, and mineral supplements, such as calcium, magnesium, or iron, may decrease the effects of this

drug when taken at the same time as this drug. If you need to take an OTC drug take it either 2 hours before or after taking this drug.

Taking this drug with any of the ones listed below may change the effect of either drug with the possibility of causing toxicity or decreasing effectiveness: antacids, anticoagulants†, barbiturates†, calcium supplements, carbamazepine, cholestyramine, cimetidine, colestipol, digoxin, iron supplements, mineral supplements, oral contraceptives, penicillins, phenytoin, sodium bicarbonate, zinc

Severe reactions are possible when this drug is taken with those listed below: methoxyflurane, tetracycline

ALLERGIC REACTIONS AND SIDE EFFECTS

If you are allergic to any tetracyclines†, you may also be allergic to this drug. You should tell your doctor about all your allergies and any unexplained symptoms you may have while taking this drug.

This drug promotes the effect of sunlight on the body and may cause severe sunburn and increased sensitivity of the eyes. This effect may last as long as 2 to 4 weeks after the drug is stopped.

MORE COMMON SIDE EFFECTS: Diarrhea, heartburn, loss of appetite*, nausea*, stomach cramps, skin rash*, sun sensitivity*, vomiting*

LESS COMMON SIDE EFFECTS: Dizziness, genital itch, lightheadedness, mouth sores, rectal itch

RARE SIDE EFFECTS: Abdominal pain*, headache*, visual changes*, yellow eyes or skin*

PRECAUTIONS

This drug may interfere with urine glucose tests, providing false negative results.

People with kidney disease or liver disease may be at greater risk of developing side effects.

This drug decomposes after the expiration date and may be harmful if taken. Make sure you destroy any leftover doses as soon as you are done with the prescription.

The last dose of the day should be taken with a full glass of water at least 1 hour before bedtime to avoid heartburn.

Be careful driving or handling equipment while taking this drug because the drug may cause dizziness.

Some people get a discolored tongue while taking this drug, but the coloring will return to normal when the drug is stopped.

---

† See page 52.   * See page 53.

Do not crush of break the capsules.

PREGNANCY AND BREAST-FEEDING

This drug may cause toxic effects to the fetus and should not be used during pregnancy.

Breast-feeding while taking this drug is not recommended.

HELPFUL COMMENTS

Oral contraceptives may not work properly when taken with this drug. You need to use a barrier contraceptive, such as a condom, or other non-hormonal contraceptive to prevent pregnancy.

Contact your doctor if your symptoms do not improve after a couple of days.

Do not stop treatment early if you start to feel better. It takes the full prescription for this drug to work completely.

DRONABINOL

Available since May 1985

COMMONLY USED TO TREAT

Lack of appetite in AIDS patients
Nausea and vomiting caused by cancer treatment

DRUG CATEGORY

antiemetic
Class: cannabinoid

PRODUCTS

Brand-Name Products with No Generic Alternative
Marinol 2.5 mg capsule ($$$)
Marinol 5 mg capsule ($$$$)
Marinol 10 mg capsule ($$$$$)
No generics available.
No patents, no exclusivity.

DOSING AND FOOD

Doses are taken twice a day.
It is best to take this drug on an empty stomach before lunch and dinner.
Adults and teens: Up to 20 mg per day in divided doses.

Lower doses are used in children based on their body size.

Forgotten doses: If you are scheduled to take the next dose within a few hours, do not take the forgotten dose. Otherwise take the forgotten dose as soon as you remember.

ALCOHOL, DRUG, HERB, AND SUPPLEMENT INTERACTIONS

Alcohol should not be used while taking this drug.

Many OTC drugs used for appetite control, asthma, colds, cough, hay fever, pain, or sinus problems affect the central nervous system and may change the effects or side effects of this drug. Check with your pharmacist for products to avoid.

Increased side effects are possible when this drug is taken with those listed below: anesthetics, antihistamines†, anxiolytics†, barbiturates†, narcotics†, tricyclic antidepressants†

ALLERGIC REACTIONS AND SIDE EFFECTS

If you are allergic to sesame oil or marijuana, you may also be allergic to this drug. You should tell your doctor about all your allergies and any unexplained symptoms you may have while taking this drug.

MORE COMMON SIDE EFFECTS: Clumsiness, dizziness, drowsiness*, nausea, poor concentration, unsteadiness, vomiting

LESS COMMON SIDE EFFECTS: Anxiety*, blurry vision, confusion*, delusions*, depression*, dry mouth*, flushing, hallucinations*, irregular heartbeat*, lightheadedness*, memory loss*, mood swings*, nervousness*, restlessness, tiredness, vision changes, weakness

RARE SIDE EFFECTS: Constipation*, forgetfulness*, panic attacks*, poor coordination*, red eyes*, seizures*, sensory changes*, sluggishness*, slurry speech*, urinary changes*

PRECAUTIONS

This drug may be habit forming and will cause severe withdrawal symptoms if stopped abruptly after long-term use. If you wish to stop taking this drug, ask your doctor for specific instructions.

People with a history of alcohol or drug abuse are at greater risk of developing dependence on this drug.

Be careful driving or handling equipment while taking this drug because it may cause drowsiness and dizziness.

If you have heart disease, high blood pressure, manic-depressive disorder, or other mental illness, this drug may make those conditions worse.

---

† See page 52.   * See page 53.

Toxicity may occur if too much of this drug is taken or if it is mixed with other drugs. Signs of toxicity include mood swings, confusion, hallucinations, depression, anxiety, or irregular heartbeat.

This drug is detectable in the urine for months after it is stopped. If you have a pre-employment drug-screening test, make sure the laboratory knows that you are taking this drug.

PREGNANCY AND BREAST-FEEDING

Safety during pregnancy has not been established although the drug is known to harm animal fetuses.

Breast-feeding while taking this drug is not recommended.

HELPFUL COMMENTS

This drug is also called by the generic name delta-9-tetrahydrocannabinol or THC.

Avoid quick movements to minimize dizziness.

It takes about 30 to 60 minutes for the effects of this drug to be noticed. The appetite-stimulation effect usually lasts about 24 hours.

DUTASTERIDE

Available since January 2003

COMMONLY USED TO TREAT

Enlarged prostate, also known as benign (noncancerous) prostatic hyperplasia or BPH

DRUG CATEGORY

androgen synthesis inhibitor
Class: steroid derivative

PRODUCTS

Brand-Name Products with No Generic Alternative
Avodart 0.5 mg capsule (n/a)
No generics available.
Multiple patents that begin to expire in 2013. Exclusivity until 2006.

DOSING AND FOOD

Doses are taken once a day.

This drug may be taken with or without food. Do not drink grapefruit juice while taking this drug.

Men: Up to 0.5 mg per day.

Forgotten doses: If you are scheduled to take the next dose within a few hours, do not take the forgotten dose. Otherwise take the forgotten dose as soon as you remember.

ALCOHOL, DRUG, HERB, AND SUPPLEMENT INTERACTIONS

Alcohol may increase some of the side effects from this drug, depending on the amount consumed. Ask your doctor about the risks caused by drinking alcohol with your condition.

Taking this drug with any of the ones listed below may change the effect of either drug with the possibility of causing toxicity or decreasing effectiveness: cimetidine, ciprofloxacin, diltiazem, ketoconazole, ritonavir, verapamil

ALLERGIC REACTIONS AND SIDE EFFECTS

If you are allergic to finasteride, you may also be allergic to this drug. You should tell your doctor about all your allergies and any unexplained symptoms you may have while taking this drug.

MORE COMMON SIDE EFFECTS: Breast enlargement, sexual dysfunction

LESS COMMON SIDE EFFECTS: Breast tenderness

PRECAUTIONS

Do not donate blood while taking this drug and for 6 months after the drug is stopped.

Pregnant women should not touch this drug.

PREGNANCY AND BREAST-FEEDING

This drug may cause birth defects and should not be used during pregnancy. Any exposure to the drug including touching broken capsules may also be associated with birth defects.

This drug is not indicated for use in women; therefore, breast-feeding while taking this drug is not recommended.

HELPFUL COMMENTS

The effects of this drug should be noticed in 1 to 2 weeks.

---

†See page 52.   *See page 53.

EFAVIRENZ

Available since September 1998

COMMONLY USED TO TREAT

HIV infection

DRUG CATEGORY

antiretroviral
Class: nonnucleodise reverse transcriptase inhibitor (NNRTI)

PRODUCTS

Brand-Name Products with No Generic Alternative
Sustiva 50 mg capsule ($)
Sustiva 100 mg capsule ($$)
Sustiva 200 mg capsule ($$$)
Sustiva 300 mg capsule (n/a)
Sustiva 600 mg tablet ($$$)
No generics available.
Multiple patents that begin to expire in 2013.

DOSING AND FOOD

Doses are taken once a day usually at bedtime.
Taking this drug with fatty foods will help increase absorption of the drug.
  Be careful not to eat too much fatty food.
Adults and children more than 88 pounds: Up to 600 mg per day.
Children over age 3 weighing 71.5 to 88 pounds: Up to 400 mg per day.
Children over age 3 weighing 55 to 71.5 pounds: Up to 350 mg per day.
Children over age 3 weighing 44 to 55 pounds: Up to 300 mg per day.
Children over age 3 weighing 33 to 44 pounds: Up to 250 mg per day.
Children over age 3 weighing 22 to 33 pounds: Up to 200 mg per day.
Forgotten doses: If you are scheduled to take the next dose within a few
  hours, do not take the forgotten dose. Otherwise take the forgotten dose
  as soon as you remember.

ALCOHOL, DRUG, HERB, AND SUPPLEMENT INTERACTIONS

Alcohol should not be used while taking this drug.
St. John's wort may decrease the effectiveness of this drug and should not
  be taken.

Many OTC drugs used for appetite control, asthma, colds, cough, hay fever, pain, or sinus problems affect the central nervous system and may increase the risk of side effects from this drug. Check with your pharmacist for products to avoid.

Taking this drug with any of the ones listed below may change the effect of either drug with the possibility of causing toxicity or decreasing effectiveness: amprenavir, astemizole, cisapride, clarithromycin, ergot alkaloids†, estrogens†, indinavir, midazolam, oral contraceptives, phenobarbital, rifabutin, rifampin, saquinavir, triazolam, warfarin

Severe reactions are possible when this drug is taken with those listed below: CNS stimulants†

Increased side effects are possible when this drug is taken with those listed below: Ritonavir

ALLERGIC REACTIONS AND SIDE EFFECTS

You should tell your doctor about all your allergies and any unexplained symptoms you may have while taking this drug.

MORE COMMON SIDE EFFECTS: Agitation, anxiety, depression*, diarrhea, dizziness, drowsiness, euphoria, fatigue, hallucinations*, headache*, itching*, poor concentration, skin rash*, sleep disorders, sweating, vivid dreams

LESS COMMON SIDE EFFECTS: Back pain*, belching, bloody urine*, dry mouth, flushing, gas, hair loss, heartburn, indigestion, joint pain, loss of sensitivity to touch, memory loss, mood swings, nervousness, ringing in ears, stomachache, taste changes, urinary difficulty*, weakness

RARE SIDE EFFECTS: Abdominal pain*, blisters*, breathing difficulties*, chest tightness*, chills*, clumsiness*, confusion*, cough*, dark urine*, delusions*, fainting*, fever*, hives*, irregular heartbeat*, loss of appetite*, mouth sores*, muscle cramps*, nausea*, nerve pain*, seizures*, speech disorders*, suicidal thoughts*, swelling*, tingling*, tiredness*, tremor*, unsteadiness*, vision changes*, vomiting*, weight changes*, wheezing*, yellow eyes or skin*

PRECAUTIONS

This drug is usually prescribed in combination with another antiretroviral drug. Ask your pharmacist about the type of drug interaction that may occur between antiretroviral drugs† to coordinate the administration times of multiple drugs.

---

†See page 52.   *See page 53.

Be careful driving or handling equipment while taking this drug because it
   may cause dizziness.
This drug may cause a false positive result from urine drug-screening tests.
Oral contraceptives may not work properly when taken with this drug. You
   need to use a barrier contraceptive, such as a condom or other nonhormonal contraceptive, in addition to the oral contraception to prevent
   pregnancy.

PREGNANCY AND BREAST-FEEDING

Safety during pregnancy has not been established although the drug is
   known to harm animal fetuses.
Breast-feeding while taking this drug is not recommended.

HELPFUL COMMENTS

The dizziness, drowsiness, and sleep disorders that some people suffer may
   start to diminish 2 to 4 weeks after starting this drug.

ENALAPRIL MALEATE

Available since December 1985

COMMONLY USED TO TREAT

Heart failure
High blood pressure, also known as hypertension

DRUG CATEGORY

antihypertensive
Class: ACE inhibitor

PRODUCTS

Brand-Name Products with Generic Alternatives
Vasotec 2.5 mg tablet (¢¢¢¢)
   Generic: enalapril 2.5 mg tablet (¢¢¢¢¢)
Vasotec 5 mg tablet (¢¢¢¢¢)
   Generic: enalapril 5 mg tablet (¢¢¢)
Vasotec 10 mg tablet ($)
   Generic: enalapril 10 mg tablet (¢¢)
Vasotec 20 mg tablet ($$)
   Generic: enalapril 20 mg tablet (¢¢)

Combination Products That Contain This Drug
Lexxel extended-release tablet ($)
Teczem extended-release tablet (n/a)
Vasoretic tablet ($)

DOSING AND FOOD

Doses are taken 1 to 2 times a day.

This drug may be taken with or without food.

Adults: Up to 40 mg per day in divided doses.

Lower doses are used in people with kidney disease and heart failure.

This drug is rarely used in children.

Forgotten doses: If you are scheduled to take the next dose within a few hours, do not take the forgotten dose. Otherwise take the forgotten dose as soon as you remember.

ALCOHOL, DRUG, HERB, AND SUPPLEMENT INTERACTIONS

Alcohol may cause your blood pressure to rise making this drug less effective. Ask your doctor about the risks caused by drinking alcohol with your condition.

Licorice may interfere with the effects of this drug.

Capsaicin and other foods or supplements, including hot peppers, sweet peppers, paprika, and chili powder, derived from the capsicum family of plants may increase the risk of developing a cough and should not be taken with this drug.

Several OTC drugs used for appetite control, asthma, colds, cough, hay fever, or sinus problems may cause an increase in blood pressure when taken with this drug. Check with your pharmacist when selecting OTC products.

Taking this drug with any of the ones listed below may change the effect of either drug with the possibility of causing toxicity or decreasing effectiveness: antidiabetics†, antihypertensives†, aspirin, digoxin, diuretics†, insulin, lithium, nonsteroidal antiinflammatories†, phenothiazines†, potassium supplements, rifampin

ALLERGIC REACTIONS AND SIDE EFFECTS

If you are allergic to any ACE inhibitors†, you may also be allergic to this drug. You should tell your doctor about all your allergies and any unexplained symptoms you may have while taking this drug.

---

†See page 52. *See page 53.

MORE COMMON SIDE EFFECTS: Cough, headache

LESS COMMON SIDE EFFECTS: Diarrhea, dizziness*, fainting*, fever*, joint pain*, lightheadedness*, loss of taste, nausea, skin rash*, tiredness*

RARE SIDE EFFECTS: Abdominal pain*, breathing difficulty*, chest pain*, chills*, confusion*, hoarseness*, irregular heartbeat*, itching*, nausea*, nervousness*, numbness*, swallowing difficulty*, swelling*, vomiting*, weakness*, yellow eyes or skin*

PRECAUTIONS

Be careful driving or handling equipment while taking this drug because the drug may cause dizziness.

If you have kidney disease, this drug may make that condition worse.

People with systemic lupus erythematosus may be at greater risk of developing blood problems while taking this drug.

Do not use potassium-containing products, including salt substitutes, while taking this drug.

Diuretics† should be stopped 2 to 3 days prior to starting this drug. If it is not possible to stop the diuretic, the dose of this drug should be lowered.

Drink plenty of fluids to avoid dehydration when sweating, such as in hot weather and during exercise.

PREGNANCY AND BREAST-FEEDING

Safety during pregnancy has not been established although the drug is known to harm animal fetuses.

Breast-feeding while taking this drug is not recommended.

HELPFUL COMMENTS

It may take several weeks before the full effects of this drug are noticed.

A persistent dry cough may appear while taking this drug, but it will go away when the drug is stopped.

Avoid quick movements to minimize dizziness. Dangling your legs over the side of the bed for a few minutes may help reduce dizziness when first waking up.

If you do not treat high blood pressure, you may develop more serious problems such as heart failure, blood vessel disease, stroke, or kidney disease. Losing weight, exercising, eating more fruits and vegetables, and avoiding salty foods, such as lunchmeat and pickles, may help make drug treatment more successful.

ENOXAPARIN SODIUM

Available since May 1993

COMMONLY USED TO TREAT

People at risk of developing blood clots

DRUG CATEGORY

anticoagulant
Class: heparin anticoagulant

PRODUCTS

Brand-Name Products with No Generic Alternative
Lovenox 30 mg/0.3 ml subcutaneous injection ($$$$$)
Lovenox 40 mg/0.4 ml subcutaneous injection ($$$$$)
Lovenox 60 mg/0.6 ml subcutaneous injection ($$$$$)
Lovenox 80 mg/0.8 ml subcutaneous injection ($$$$$)
Lovenox 100 mg/1 ml subcutaneous injection ($$$$$)
Lovenox 120 mg/0.8 ml subcutaneous injection ($$$$$)
Lovenox 150 mg/1 ml subcutaneous injection ($$$$$)
No generics available.
Multiple patents that begin to expire in 2004.

DOSING AND FOOD

Doses are injected 1 to 2 times a day.
Adults: Up to 325 mg per day in divided doses.
Forgotten doses: If you are scheduled to take the next dose in less than 5
hours, do not take the forgotten dose. Otherwise take the forgotten dose
as soon as you remember.

ALCOHOL, DRUG, HERB, AND SUPPLEMENT INTERACTIONS

Alcohol may increase some of the side effects from this drug, depending
on the amount consumed. Ask your doctor about the risks caused by
drinking alcohol with your condition.
Several OTC drugs used for pain, heartburn, and stomach distress may increase the risk of bleeding when taken with this drug. Check with your
pharmacist when selecting OTC products.

Severe reactions are possible when this drug is taken with those listed below:
anticoagulants†, antiplatelet drugs†, aspirin, dipyridamole, divalproex,

---

† See page 52.   * See page 53.

ketorolac, nonsteroidal antiinflammatories†, plicamycin, salicylates†, sulfinpyrazone, ticlopidine, valproic acid

ALLERGIC REACTIONS AND SIDE EFFECTS

If you are allergic to any pork products, you may also be allergic to this drug. You should tell your doctor about all your allergies and any unexplained symptoms you may have while taking this drug.

MORE COMMON SIDE EFFECTS: Black stools*, bleeding gums*, bleeding*, bloody urine*, breathing difficulty*, bruising*, coughing up blood*, dizziness*, headache*, increased menstrual flow*, nosebleeds*, numbness*, pain*, pale skin*, paralysis*, shortness of breath*, skin irritation*, swallowing difficulty*, swelling*, tiredness*, vaginal bleeding*, weakness*

LESS COMMON SIDE EFFECTS: Back pain*, blood blisters*, chest discomfort*, confusion*, convulsions*, diarrhea, fever*, irritability*, irritation at site of injection, lightheadedness*, nausea, urinary pain*, vomiting, wheezing*

RARE SIDE EFFECTS: Chest pain*, chills*, cough*, fainting*, hives*, irregular heartbeat*, sneezing*, sore throat*, thick sputum*, tingling*

PRECAUTIONS

People with a history of blood disease, bleeding disorders, heart disease, high blood pressure, kidney disease, liver disease, ulcers, or high-risk pregnancy, may not be able to use this drug.

Before starting this drug, make sure your doctor knows if you have recently had dental surgery, miscarriage, childbirth, suffered a fall, or been battered in any way that would increase the risk of bleeding.

Do not mix with other injectable drugs.

Make sure you understand the instructions for injecting this drug, especially the difference between a subcutaneous injection and an intramuscular injection.

Used syringes should be put into a puncture-resistant container for disposal, such as an empty liquid-laundry-detergent jug. Ask your pharmacy if they have a syringe-return program for easy disposal.

This drug may cause changes to your gums and mouth. Your dentist may recommend that you clean your teeth and mouth differently to avoid infection.

Air bubbles in the syringe should not be pushed out before injection since some of the drug may be lost in the process.

Do not perform physical activities that could lead to bruising or bleeding while taking this drug.

PREGNANCY AND BREAST-FEEDING

Safety during pregnancy has not been established although there was no evidence of harm during studies in animals.

t is not known if this drug passes into breast milk. Talk to your doctor about the risks associated with breast-feeding while taking this drug.

HELPFUL COMMENTS

This drug is used for only a short period of time, usually less than 2 weeks.
Watch for any signs of bleeding while taking this drug and report them to your doctor immediately.

ENTACAPONE

Available since October 1999

COMMONLY USED TO TREAT

Parkinson's disease

DRUG CATEGORY

antidyskinetic
Class: COMT inhibitor

PRODUCTS

Brand-Name Products with No Generic Alternative
Comtan 200 mg tablet ($$)
No generics available.
Multiple patents that begin to expire in 2007.

DOSING AND FOOD

Doses are taken 1 to 8 times a day with each dose of levodopa and carbidopa.
This drug may be taken with or without food.
Adults: Up to 1,600 mg per day in divided doses.
Forgotten doses: If you are scheduled to take the next dose within a few hours, do not take the forgotten dose. Otherwise take the forgotten dose as soon as you remember.

ALCOHOL, DRUG, HERB, AND SUPPLEMENT INTERACTIONS

Alcohol should not be used while taking this drug.

---

† See page 52.   * See page 53.

Many OTC drugs used for appetite control, asthma, colds, cough, hay fever, pain, or sinus problems affect the central nervous system and may increase the side effects of this drug. Check with your pharmacist for products to avoid.

Taking this drug with any of the ones listed below may change the effect of either drug with the possibility of causing toxicity or decreasing effectiveness: ampicillin, apomorphine, bitolterol, chloramphenicol, cholestyramine, dobutamine, dopamine, epinephrine, erythromycin, isoetharine, isoproterenol, methyldopa, norepinephrine, probenecid

Severe reactions are possible when this drug is taken with those listed below: anesthetics, antihistamines†, anxiolytics†, barbiturates†, monoamine oxidase inhibitors†, narcotics†, tricyclic antidepressants†

ALLERGIC REACTIONS AND SIDE EFFECTS

You should tell your doctor about all your allergies and any unexplained symptoms you may have while taking this drug.

MORE COMMON SIDE EFFECTS: Abdominal pain, diarrhea, dizziness, fatigue, hallucinations*, hyperactivity*, motionlessness*, nausea, twisting*, twitching*, uncontrolled movements*, urine color change*

LESS COMMON SIDE EFFECTS: Anxiety, back pain*, belching, breathing difficulty*, bruising, chest tightness, chills*, constipation, cough*, drowsiness, dry mouth, fever*, gas, heartburn, hoarseness*, indigestion, insomnia, irritability, loss of strength, muscle pain*, nervousness, restlessness, shortness of breath, skin irritation, sleepiness, sour stomach, sweating, taste changes, tenderness, tremor, urinary difficulty*, weakness*, wheezing

RARE SIDE EFFECTS: Confusion*, stiffness*, tiredness*

PRECAUTIONS

This drug must be given with levodopa and carbidopa in order to be effective. Any forms of those drugs are acceptable including the extended-release products.

Be careful driving or handling equipment while taking this drug because the drug may cause drowsiness.

Do not crush, break, or chew tablets.

Drink plenty of fluids to avoid dehydration when sweating, such as in hot weather and during exercise.

Stopping this drug suddenly may cause severe symptoms. If you wish to stop taking this drug, ask your doctor for specific instructions.

ome monoamine oxidase inhibitors† may be taken while on this drug. Talk to your doctor or pharmacist to determine which drugs are acceptable.

PREGNANCY AND BREAST-FEEDING

afety during pregnancy has not been established although the drug is known to harm animal fetuses.

t is not known if this drug passes into breast milk. Talk to your doctor about the risks associated with breast-feeding while taking this drug.

HELPFUL COMMENTS

Expect your urine to turn a brownish orange color.

Sucking on hard sugarless candy or chewing sugarless gum may help relieve dry mouth caused by this drug.

Avoid quick movements to minimize dizziness. Dangling your legs over the side of the bed for a few minutes may help reduce dizziness when first waking up.

EPLERENONE

Available since September 2002

COMMONLY USED TO TREAT

High blood pressure, also known as hypertension

DRUG CATEGORY

antihypertensive
Class: aldosterone blocker

PRODUCTS

Brand-Name Products with No Generic Alternative
Inspra 25 mg tablet (n/a)
Inspra 50 mg tablet (n/a)
Inspra 100 mg tablet (n/a)
No generics available.
Multiple patents that begin to expire in 2004. Exclusivity until 2007.

DOSING AND FOOD

Doses are taken 1 to 2 times a day.
This drug may be taken with or without food. Do not drink grapefruit juice while taking this drug.

† See page 52.   * See page 53.

Adults: Up to 100 mg per day in divided doses.

Forgotten doses: If you are scheduled to take the next dose within a few hours, do not take the forgotten dose. Otherwise take the forgotten dose as soon as you remember.

ALCOHOL, DRUG, HERB, AND SUPPLEMENT INTERACTIONS

Alcohol may increase some of the side effects from this drug, depending on the amount consumed. Ask your doctor about the risks caused by drinking alcohol with your condition.

Several OTC drugs used for appetite control, asthma, colds, cough, hay fever, or sinus problems may cause an increase in blood pressure when taken with this drug. Check with your pharmacist when selecting OTC products.

Taking this drug with any of the ones listed below may change the effect of either drug with the possibility of causing toxicity or decreasing effectiveness: erythromycin, fluconazole, ketoconazole, lithium, nonsteroidal antiinflammatories†, saquinavir, verapamil

Severe reactions are possible when this drug is taken with those listed below: ACE inhibitors†, angiotensin II receptor antagonists†, midamor, potassium supplements, spironolactone, triamterene

ALLERGIC REACTIONS AND SIDE EFFECTS

You should tell your doctor about all your allergies and any unexplained symptoms you may have while taking this drug.

MORE COMMON SIDE EFFECTS: Abdominal pain, chest pain*, cough, diarrhea, dizziness, headache, irregular heartbeat*, pale skin*, tiredness

LESS COMMON SIDE EFFECTS: Breast enlargement, confusion*, loss of energy*, sexual dysfunction, tingling*, vaginal bleeding, weakness*

PRECAUTIONS

If you have diabetes, kidney disease, or high potassium levels, you may not be able to take this drug.

Your body may retain potassium while taking this drug, which may cause severe side effects if the level gets too high. Potassium levels should be monitored periodically and may need to be treated while taking this drug. Avoid food rich in potassium, such as apricots, bananas, citrus fruit, dates, and tomatoes. Do not use potassium supplements such as salt substitutes.

If you have type 2 diabetes or microalbuminurea, you may be at greater risk of developing side effects caused by high potassium levels.

PREGNANCY AND BREAST-FEEDING

Safety during pregnancy has not been established although there was no evidence of harm during studies in animals.

Breast-feeding while taking this drug is not recommended.

HELPFUL COMMENTS

It may take 4 weeks before the full effects of this drug are noticed.

If you do not treat high blood pressure, you may develop more serious problems such as heart failure, blood vessel disease, stroke, or kidney disease. Losing weight, exercising, eating more fruits and vegetables, and avoiding salty foods, such as lunchmeat and pickles, may help make drug treatment more successful.

EPROSARTAN MESYLATE

Available since December 1997

COMMONLY USED TO TREAT

High blood pressure, also known as hypertension

DRUG CATEGORY

antihypertensive
Class: angiotensin II receptor antagonist (AIIRB)

PRODUCTS

Brand-Name Products with No Generic Alternative
Teveten 300 mg tablet (n/a)
Teveten 400 mg tablet ($)
Teveten 600 mg tablet ($)
No generics available.
Multiple patents that begin to expire in 2010.
Combination Products That Contain This Drug
Teveten HCT tablet

DOSING AND FOOD

Doses are taken 1 to 2 times a day.
This drug may be taken with or without food.
Adults: Up to 800 mg per day in divided doses.
Forgotten doses: If you are scheduled to take the next dose within a few

† *See page 52.*   * *See page 53.*

hours, do not take the forgotten dose. Otherwise take the forgotten dose as soon as you remember.

ALCOHOL, DRUG, HERB, AND SUPPLEMENT INTERACTIONS

Alcohol may cause your blood pressure to rise, making this drug less effective. Ask your doctor about the risks caused by drinking alcohol with your condition.

Several OTC drugs used for appetite control, asthma, colds, cough, hay fever, or sinus problems may cause an increase in blood pressure when taken with this drug. Check with your pharmacist when selecting OTC products.

ALLERGIC REACTIONS AND SIDE EFFECTS

You should tell your doctor about all your allergies and any unexplained symptoms you may have while taking this drug.

MORE COMMON SIDE EFFECTS: Fever*, sore throat*, swelling*

LESS COMMON SIDE EFFECTS: Abdominal pain, cough*, joint pain, tiredness, urinary changes*

RARE SIDE EFFECTS: Dizziness*, fainting*, lightheadedness*

PRECAUTIONS

People who are dehydrated or are low on sodium, may experience an increase in the blood-pressure-lowering effect of this drug.

Drink plenty of fluids to avoid dehydration when sweating, such as in hot weather and during exercise.

If you have congestive heart failure, this drug may make that condition worse.

PREGNANCY AND BREAST-FEEDING

There is evidence that this drug may harm the fetus, but the drug may be necessary to the health of the mother.

Breast-feeding while taking this drug is not recommended.

HELPFUL COMMENTS

It may take 2 to 3 weeks before the full effects of this drug are noticed.

If you do not treat high blood pressure, you may develop more serious problems such as heart failure, blood vessel disease, stroke, or kidney disease. Losing weight, exercising, eating more fruits and vegetables, and avoiding salty foods, such as lunchmeat and pickles, may help make drug treatment more successful.

ERGOLOID MESYLATES

Available for over 20 years

COMMONLY USED TO TREAT

Decreased mental ability related to aging, stroke, or Alzheimer's disease

DRUG CATEGORY

antidementia
Class: ergot alkaloid

PRODUCTS

Brand-Name Products with Generic Alternatives
Hydergine 1 mg tablet (n/a)
  Generic: ergoloid mesylates 1 mg tablet (¢¢¢¢¢)
Hydergine 0.5 mg sublingual tablet (n/a)
  Generic: ergoloid mesylates 0.5 mg sublingual tablet (n/a)
Hydergine 1 mg sublingual tablet (n/a)
  Generic: ergoloid mesylates 1 mg sublingual tablet (¢¢¢¢¢)

Other Generic Product Names
Gerimal, Hydrogenated ergot alkaloids

DOSING AND FOOD

Doses are taken 3 times a day.
This drug may be taken with or without food.
Adults: Up to 6 mg per day in divided doses.
Forgotten doses: Do not take a forgotten dose. Just go back to your usual
  schedule with the next dose.

ALCOHOL, DRUG, HERB, AND SUPPLEMENT INTERACTIONS

Alcohol may increase some of the side effects from this drug, depending
  on the amount consumed. Ask your doctor about the risks caused by
  drinking alcohol with your condition.

Severe reactions are possible when this drug is taken with those listed below:
cocaine, epinephrine, ergoloid, ergonovine, methylergonovine, methysergide, sympathomimetics†

ALLERGIC REACTIONS AND SIDE EFFECTS

If you are allergic to any other ergot alkaloid†, you may also be allergic to

---

†See page 52.   *See page 53.

this drug. You should tell your doctor about all your allergies and any un-explained symptoms you may have while taking this drug.

LESS COMMON SIDE EFFECTS: Dizziness*, drowsiness*, lightheadedness*, skin rash*, slow pulse*, sore tongue

RARE SIDE EFFECTS: Blurry vision*, fainting*, flushing*, headache*, loss of appetite*, nausea*, vomiting*, stomach cramps*, stuffy nose*

PRECAUTIONS

This drug comes in sublingual tablets that should be placed under the tongue until they dissolve. The drug is absorbed into the body through the mouth, so the drug should not be chewed or swallowed. Do not put anything else in your mouth while the tablet is under the tongue.

Smoking may increase the side effects of this drug. You should stop smoking while taking this drug, or wait several hours after taking your dose before smoking.

Learn how to measure your heart rate and call your doctor if it falls below 60 beats per minute.

PREGNANCY AND BREAST-FEEDING

Safety during pregnancy has not been established although the drug is known to harm animal fetuses.

Breast-feeding while taking this drug is not recommended.

HELPFUL COMMENTS

It may take over a month for the effects of this drug to be noticed.

ERGONOVINE MALEATE

Available for over 20 years

COMMONLY USED TO TREAT

Uterine bleeding after childbirth

DRUG CATEGORY

oxytocic
Class: ergot alkaloid

PRODUCTS

Products Only Available as Generics
ergonovine maleate 0.2 mg tablet (¢¢¢)

DOSING AND FOOD

Doses are taken 2 to 4 times a day.

This drug may be taken with or without food.

Women: Up to 1.6 mg per day in divided doses.

Forgotten doses: Do not take a forgotten dose. Just go back to your usual schedule with the next dose.

ALCOHOL, DRUG, HERB, AND SUPPLEMENT INTERACTIONS

Alcohol may increase some of the side effects from this drug, depending on the amount consumed. Ask your doctor about the risks caused by drinking alcohol with your condition.

Taking this drug with any of the ones listed below may change the effect of either drug with the possibility of causing toxicity or decreasing effectiveness: digoxin, digitoxin, nitrates

Severe reactions are possible when this drug is taken with those listed below: bromocriptine, epinephrine, ergoloid, ergonovine, ergotamine, methylergonovine, methysergide, sympathomimetics†

ALLERGIC REACTIONS AND SIDE EFFECTS

If you are allergic to any other ergot alkaloid†, you may also be allergic to this drug. You should tell your doctor about all your allergies and any unexplained symptoms you may have while taking this drug.

MORE COMMON SIDE EFFECTS: Nausea*, uterine cramps, vomiting*

LESS COMMON SIDE EFFECTS: Anxiety*, blisters*, chest pain*, coldness*, confusion*, diarrhea*, dizziness*, drowsiness*, dry mouth, excitement*, headache*, increased blood pressure*, irregular heartbeat*, itching*, muscle pain*, nervousness, numbness*, pale skin*, restlessness, seizures*, shortness of breath*, stomach pain*, swelling*, tingling*, thirst*, vision changes*, weakness*

PRECAUTIONS

Smoking may increase the side effects of this drug. You should stop smoking while taking this drug, or wait several hours after taking your dose before smoking.

PREGNANCY AND BREAST-FEEDING

Safety during pregnancy has not been established although the drug is known to harm animal fetuses.

Breast-feeding while taking this drug is not recommended.

---

† See page 52.   * See page 53.

HELPFUL COMMENTS

This drug is used for only 2 to 7 days.

ERGOTAMINE TARTRATE

Available for over 20 years

COMMONLY USED TO TREAT

Headache

DRUG CATEGORY

antihypotensive
antimigraine
Class: ergot alkaloid

PRODUCTS

Brand-Name Products with No Generic Alternative
Ergomar 2 mg sublingual tablet (n/a)
No generics available.
No patents, no exclusivity.
Combination Products That Contain This Drug
Cafergot rectal suppository ($$$$)
Ercatab tablet (n/a)

DOSING AND FOOD

Doses are not taken on a regular schedule.
This drug may be taken with or without food.
Adults: Up to 6 mg per day (maximum 10 mg per week) in divided doses.
Children age 6 and older: Up to 3 mg per day (maximum 6 mg per week)
in divided doses.

ALCOHOL, DRUG, HERB, AND SUPPLEMENT INTERACTIONS

Alcohol may make your headache worse. Ask your doctor about the risks
caused by drinking alcohol with your condition.

Taking this drug with any of the ones listed below may change the effect of
either drug with the possibility of causing toxicity or decreasing effectiveness:
beta blockers†, caffeine, erythromycin, macrolides†

Severe reactions are possible when this drug is taken with those listed below:
cocaine, epinephrine, ergoloid, ergonovine, methylergonovine, methysergide

ALLERGIC REACTIONS AND SIDE EFFECTS

If you are allergic to atropine, barbiturates†, belladonna alkaloids†, pento-barbital, caffeine, cyclizine, dimenhydrinate, diphenhydramine, or any other ergot alkaloid†, you may also be allergic to this drug. You should tell your doctor about all your allergies and any unexplained symptoms you may have while taking this drug.

MORE COMMON SIDE EFFECTS: Coldness*, diarrhea*, dizziness*, drowsiness*, dry mouth, itching*, nausea*, nervousness, numbness*, restlessness, swelling*, tingling*, vomiting*, weakness*

LESS COMMON SIDE EFFECTS: Anxiety*, blisters*, chest pain*, confusion*, excitement*, headache*, increased blood pressure*, irregular heartbeat*, muscle pain*, pale skin*, seizures*, shortness of breath*, stomach pain*, vision changes*

PRECAUTIONS

This drug is not a general pain reliever but is used effectively for all types of headaches.

Be careful driving or handling equipment while taking this drug because it may cause dizziness and drowsiness.

Smoking may increase the side effects of this drug. You should stop smoking while taking this drug, or wait several hours after taking your dose before smoking.

If you have an enlarged prostate, urinary problems, glaucoma, high blood pressure, infection, intestinal problems, depression, or a thyroid condition, you may be at greater risk of developing side effects while taking this drug.

This drug comes in sublingual tablets that should be placed under the tongue until they dissolve. The drug is absorbed into the body through the mouth, so the drug should not be chewed or swallowed. Do not put anything else in your mouth while the tablet is under the tongue.

If a second dose is needed to treat your headache, make sure the doses are taken 30 to 60 minutes apart.

This drug may cause dry mouth, which is associated with a greater risk of cavities. Your dentist may recommend that you clean your teeth and mouth differently to avoid infection.

PREGNANCY AND BREAST-FEEDING

This drug may cause birth defects and should not be used during pregnancy. Breast-feeding while taking this drug is not recommended.

---

† See page 52.   * See page 53.

HELPFUL COMMENTS

This drug does not prevent headaches from returning. Ask your doctor about other drugs, such as beta blockers† or calcium channel blockers†, that may be used to prevent headaches, depending on your condition.

This drug is used most often in combination products, especially with caffeine, which may increase absorption of the drug.

Dress warmly while taking this drug since it may cause you to be more sensitive to cold temperatures.

If using a suppository, remove the foil and run under cold water before inserting.

ERYTHROMYCIN

Available for over 20 years

COMMONLY USED TO TREAT

Acne
Infection

DRUG CATEGORY

antiacne
antibiotic
Class: macrolide

PRODUCTS

Brand-Name Products with No Generic Alternative
Akne-Mycin 2% topical ointment (¢¢¢)
Eryped 400 mg/5 ml oral granules for suspension (¢¢¢¢)
E-Solve 2% topical lotion (n/a)
PCE 333 mg tablet ($$)
PCE 500 mg tablet ($$$)
Saticin 1.5% topical solution (¢¢)

Brand-Name Products with Generic Alternatives
E.E.S. 200 mg chewable tablet (n/a)
  Generic: erythromycin ethylsuccinate 200 mg chewable tablet (n/a)
Erythrocin stearate 250 mg tablet (¢¢)
  Generic: erythromycin stearate 250 mg tablet (¢¢)
EryC 250 mg delayed-release capsule (¢¢¢¢)
  Generic: erythromycin base 250 mg delayed-release capsule (¢¢¢)

Ery-Tab 250 mg delayed-release tablet (¢¢)
  Generic: erythromycin base 250 mg delayed-release tablet (¢¢¢)
Ery-Tab 333 mg delayed-release tablet (¢¢¢)
  Generic: erythromycin base 333 mg delayed-release tablet (¢¢¢)
E.E.S. 400 mg tablet (¢¢)
  Generic: erythromycin ethylsuccinate 400 mg tablet (¢¢¢)
Ery-Tab 500 mg delayed-release tablet (¢¢¢)
  Generic: erythromycin base 500 mg delayed-release tablet (¢¢¢)
Erythrocin stearate 500 mg tablet (¢¢¢)
  Generic: erythromycin stearate 500 mg tablet (¢¢¢)
Ilosone 125 mg/5 ml oral suspension (n/a)
  Generic: erythromycin estolate 125 mg/5 ml oral suspension (¢¢¢)
Eryped 200 mg/5 ml oral granules for suspension (¢¢¢)
  Generic: erythromycin ethylsuccinate 200 mg/5 ml oral granules
  for suspension (¢¢¢)
E.E.S. 200 mg/5 ml oral suspension (¢¢)
  Generic: erythromycin ethylsuccinate 200 mg/5 ml oral suspension (¢¢¢)
Ilosone 250 mg/5 ml oral suspension (n/a)
  Generic: erythromycin estolate 250 mg/5 ml oral suspension (¢¢¢¢)
E.E.S. 400 mg/5 ml oral suspension (¢¢¢)
  Generic: erythromycin ethylsuccinate 400 mg/5 ml oral suspension (¢¢¢)
Erygel 2% topical gel (¢¢¢)
  Generic: erythromycin 2% topical gel (¢¢¢)
Ilotycin 0.5% ophthalmic ointment (n/a)
  Generic: erythromycin 0.5% ophthalmic ointment (¢¢¢)
T-Stat 2% topical solution (¢¢)
  Generic: erythromycin 2% topical solution (¢)
Erycette 2% topical swab (¢¢¢)
  Generic: erythromycin 2% topical swab (¢¢¢)

Products Only Available as Generics
erythromycin base 250 mg tablet (¢¢)
erythromycin base 500 mg tablet (¢¢)
erythromycin estolate 250 mg capsule (n/a)

Other Generic Product Names
A/T/S, E Base, E Glades, E Mycin, Emgel, Erycette, Eryderm, Erymax, Ery-thra Derm, Erythro, Pediamycin, Sansac, Statin

Combination Products That Contain This Drug
Eryzole oral granules (¢¢¢¢)
Pediazole oral granules (¢¢¢¢¢)

DOSING AND FOOD

Doses are taken 4 times a day.

It is best to take this drug 1 hour before or 2 hours after meals with a full glass of water.

This drug is used in adults and children, but the dose varies depending on the product.

Topical products are applied in a thin layer to the entire affected area, not just on pimples.

Forgotten doses: If you are scheduled to take the next dose within a few hours, do not take the forgotten dose. Otherwise take the forgotten dose as soon as you remember.

ALCOHOL, DRUG, HERB, AND SUPPLEMENT INTERACTIONS

Alcohol may increase some of the side effects from this drug, depending on the amount consumed. Ask your doctor about the risks caused by drinking alcohol with your condition.

Pill-bearing spurge should not be used while taking this drug since it may increase the risk of toxicity and side effects.

Taking this drug with any of the ones listed below may change the effect of either drug with the possibility of causing toxicity or decreasing effectiveness: anticoagulants†, carbamazepine, clindamycin, cyclosporine, digoxin, disopyramide, lincomycin, midazolam, theophylline, triazolam

Severe reactions are possible when this drug is taken with those listed below: astemizole, terfenadine

Increased side effects are possible when this drug is taken with those listed below: acetaminophen, aminophylline, amiodarone, anabolic steroids†, androgens†, antibiotics†, antithyroid drugs†, caffeine, carmustine, chloroquine, dantrolene, daunorubicin, disulfiram, divalproex, estrogens†, etretinate, gold salts, hydroxychloroquine, mercaptopurine, methotrexate, methyldopa, naltrexone, oral contraceptives, oxtriphylline, phenothiazines†, phenytoin, plicamycin, valproic acid

ALLERGIC REACTIONS AND SIDE EFFECTS

If you are allergic to other macrolides†, you may also be allergic to this drug. You should tell your doctor about all your allergies and any unexplained symptoms you may have while taking this drug.

MORE COMMON SIDE EFFECTS: Abdominal pain, allergy*, diarrhea, dry skin, irregular heartbeat*, nausea*, stomach cramps, vomiting*

LESS COMMON SIDE EFFECTS: Fever*, itching*, skin rash*, mouth sores, tiredness*, vaginal discharge, vaginal itching, weakness*, yellow eyes or skin*

RARE SIDE EFFECTS: Fainting*, loss of hearing*

PRECAUTIONS

People with kidney or liver disease have a greater risk of losing their hearing while taking this drug. This side effect is temporary and hearing should return to normal after the drug is stopped.

Do not open, crush, break, or chew the delayed-release products.

Chewable tablets must be thoroughly chewed before swallowing.

Very small amounts of this drug are absorbed into the body when using the topical or ophthalmic products. The warning and precautions in the summary do not apply to these products. Instead, watch for irritation where the drug is used, as an indication of possible allergy.

Topical products may be extremely irritating if they get into the eye, nose, or mouth.

Do not smoke while applying topical products since they contain alcohol and are flammable.

PREGNANCY AND BREAST-FEEDING

Safety during pregnancy has not been established although there was no evidence of harm during studies in animals.

This drug passes into breast milk, but does not appear to harm the baby. Talk to your doctor about the risks associated with breast-feeding while taking this drug.

HELPFUL COMMENTS

Contact your doctor if your symptoms do not improve after a couple of days.

Do not stop treatment early if you start to feel better. It takes the full prescription for this drug to work completely.

Make sure to wash your hands before and after using topical or ophthalmic products.

ESOMEPRAZOLE MAGNESIUM

Available since February 2001

COMMONLY USED TO TREAT

Heartburn, specifically gastroesophageal reflux disease (GERD)

---

† *See page 52.*   * *See page 53.*

DRUG CATEGORY

antiulcer
Class: proton pump inhibitor

PRODUCTS

Brand-Name Products with No Generic Alternative
Nexium 20 mg delayed-release capsule ($$$)
Nexium 40 mg delayed-release capsule ($$$)
No generics available.
Multiple patents that begin to expire in 2005.

DOSING AND FOOD

Doses are taken once a day.
It is best to take this drug on an empty stomach about 1 hour before a meal.
Adults: Up to 40 mg per day.
Lower doses are used in people with liver disease.
Forgotten doses: If you are scheduled to take the next dose within a few hours, do not take the forgotten dose. Otherwise take the forgotten dose as soon as you remember.

ALCOHOL, DRUG, HERB, AND SUPPLEMENT INTERACTIONS

Alcohol may increase some of the side effects from this drug, depending on the amount consumed. Ask your doctor about the risks caused by drinking alcohol with your condition.

Taking this drug with any of the ones listed below may change the effect of either drug with the possibility of causing toxicity or decreasing effectiveness:
amitriptyline, amoxicillin, carisoprodol, clarithromycin, clomipramine, diazepam, imipramine, lansoprazole, mephenytoin, omeprazole, pentamidine, warfarin

ALLERGIC REACTIONS AND SIDE EFFECTS

You should tell your doctor about all your allergies and any unexplained symptoms you may have while taking this drug.
MORE COMMON SIDE EFFECTS: Abdominal pain, diarrhea, headache
LESS COMMON SIDE EFFECTS: Constipation, dry mouth, gas, nausea, vomiting

PRECAUTIONS

Do not crush, break, or chew the extended-release products. The capsule

may be opened and the contents sprinkled in soft food to make it easier
to swallow. Do not chew the pellets.
This drug is typically not used for longer than 6 months.

PREGNANCY AND BREAST-FEEDING

Safety during pregnancy has not been established although there was no
evidence of harm during studies in animals.
Breast-feeding while taking this drug is not recommended.

HELPFUL COMMENTS

If needed, antacids may be used at any time while taking this drug.

ESTAZOLAM

Available since December 1990

COMMONLY USED TO TREAT

Sleeping difficulty, also known as insomnia

DRUG CATEGORY

sedative-hypnotic
Class: benzodiazepine

PRODUCTS

Brand-Name Products with Generic Alternatives
ProSom 1 mg tablet ($)
  Generic: estazolam 1 mg tablet (¢¢¢¢¢)
ProSom 2 mg tablet ($)
  Generic: estazolam 2 mg tablet (¢¢¢¢¢)

DOSING AND FOOD

Doses are taken once a day.
This drug may be taken with or without food.
Adults: Up to 2 mg per day.
Lower doses are used in people over age 65.

ALCOHOL, DRUG, HERB, AND SUPPLEMENT INTERACTIONS

Alcohol should not be used while taking this drug.
Catnip, kava, lady's slipper, lemon balm, passion flower, sassafras, skullcap,

---

and valerian should not be used while taking this drug due to an increased sedative effect.

Taking this drug with any of the ones listed below may change the effect of either drug with the possibility of causing toxicity or decreasing effectiveness: aminophylline, caffeine, cimetidine, digoxin, disulfiram, fluvoxamine, haloperidol, isoniazid, itraconazole, ketoconazole, levodopa, nefazodone, oral contraceptives, probenecid, rifampin, theophylline

Severe reactions are possible when this drug is taken with those listed below: antidepressants†, antihistamines†, barbiturates†, anesthetics†, monoamine oxidase inhibitors†, narcotics†, phenothiazines†

ALLERGIC REACTIONS AND SIDE EFFECTS

If you are allergic to any benzodiazepines†, you may also be allergic to this drug. You should tell your doctor about all your allergies and any unexplained symptoms you may have while taking this drug.

MORE COMMON SIDE EFFECTS: Clumsiness, drowsiness, lightheadedness

LESS COMMON SIDE EFFECTS: Anxiety*, confusion*, constipation, depression*, diarrhea, difficulty urinating, disorientation*, dizziness, dry mouth, headache, irregular heartbeat*, memory loss*, muscle spasm, nausea, sexual dysfunction, slurry speech, stomach cramps, thirst, trembling, vision changes, vomiting, watery mouth

RARE SIDE EFFECTS: Agitation*, behavior changes*, bleeding*, bruising*, chills*, delusions*, excitement*, eye movement*, fever*, hallucinations*, irritability*, low blood pressure*, mouth sores*, muscle weakness*, nervousness*, seizures*, skin irritation*, sleeping difficulty*, sore throat*, spastic movements*, tiredness*, weakness*, yellow eyes or skin*

PRECAUTIONS

This drug may be habit forming and will cause severe withdrawal symptoms if stopped abruptly. If you wish to stop taking this drug, ask your doctor for specific instructions.

You need to wait 2 weeks after stopping a monoamine oxidase inhibitor† before starting this drug.

If you have difficulty swallowing, emphysema, asthma, bronchitis, glaucoma, hyperactivity, mental depression, mental illness, myasthenia gravis, porphyria, or sleep apnea, this drug may make those conditions worse.

Heavy smoking may cause this drug to be less effective.

Be careful driving or handling equipment while taking this drug because the drug may cause dizziness and drowsiness.

PREGNANCY AND BREAST-FEEDING

This drug may cause birth defects and should not be used during pregnancy.
Breast-feeding while taking this drug is not recommended.

HELPFUL COMMENTS

Dangling your legs over the side of the bed for a few minutes may help
  reduce dizziness when first waking up.

ESTRADIOL

Available for over 20 years

COMMONLY USED TO TREAT

Breast cancer
Inflammation of the vagina, also known as atrophic vaginitis
Menopausal symptoms
Ovarian failure
Postmenopausal women at risk for bone loss, also known as osteoporosis
Prostate cancer
Women of childbearing age (when used in combination with another
  female hormone—see list of birth control pills below in **Combination
  Products That Contain This Drug**)

DRUG CATEGORY

antineoplastic
estrogen replacement
Class: estrogen hormone

PRODUCTS

Brand-Name Products with No Generic Alternative
Estinyl 0.02 mg tablet§ (¢¢¢)
Estinyl 0.05 mg tablet§ (¢¢¢¢)
Estinyl 0.5 mg tablet§ (n/a)
Estrace 0.01% vaginal cream (¢¢¢)
Estring 0.0075 mg/24 hours vaginal insert ($$$$$)
Vagifem 25 mcg vaginal tablet ($$$)
Brand-Name Products with Generic Alternatives
Estrace 0.5 mg tablet (¢¢¢)
  Generic: estradiol 0.5 mg tablet (¢¢)

---

†See page 52.   *See page 53.   § See "Precautions" in this entry.

Estrace 1 mg tablet (¢¢¢¢)
  Generic: estradiol 1 mg tablet (¢¢¢)
Estrace 2 mg tablet (¢¢¢¢)
  Generic: estradiol 2 mg tablet (¢¢¢)
Vivelle 0.025 mg/24 hours patch ($$$)
  Generic: estradiol 0.025 mg/24 hours patch ($$$)
Vivelle 0.0375 mg/24 hours patch ($$$)
  Generic: estradiol 0.0375 mg/24 hours patch ($$$)
Vivelle 0.05 mg/24 hours patch ($$$)
  Generic: estradiol 0.05 mg/24 hours patch ($$$)
Vivelle 0.075 mg/24 hours patch ($$$)
  Generic: estradiol 0.075 mg/24 hours patch ($$$)
Vivelle 0.1 mg/24 hours patch ($$$)
  Generic: estradiol 0.1 mg/24 hours patch ($$$)

Products Only Available as Generics
estradiol 1.5 mg tablet (¢¢¢)

Other Generic Product Names
Alora, Climara, Esclim, Estraderm, Gynodiol, Innofem, Vivelle-Dot

Combination Products That Contain This Drug
Activella tablet (¢¢¢¢¢)
Alesse tablet ($)
Aviane tablet ($)
Brevicon tablet (¢¢¢¢¢)
CombiPatch 24 hours patch ($$$)
Crysselle tablet (n/a)
Cyclessa tablet ($)
Demulen tablet ($$)
Desogen tablet ($)
Enpresse tablet (n/a)
Estrostep FE tablet ($)
Femhrt tablet (¢¢¢¢¢)
Gencept tablet (n/a)
Kariva tablet (n/a)
Lessina tablet (n/a)
Levlite tablet ($)
Levora tablet ($)
Lo/Ovral tablet ($$)
Loestrin tablet ($$)
Low-Ogestrel tablet (n/a)
Microgestin tablet ($)

Mircette tablet ($)
Modicon tablet ($)
Norcept tablet (n/a)
Nordette tablet ($$)
Norethin tablet (n/a)
Norinyl tablet ($)
Nortrel tablet ($)
Nuvaring vaginal insert (n/a)
Ogestrel tablet ($$)
Ortho Evra extended-release patch (n/a)
Ortho-Cept tablet ($)
Ortho-Cyclen tablet ($)
Ortho-Novum tablet ($)
Ortho Tricyclen tablet (n/a)
Ovcon tablet ($)
Ovral tablet ($$)
Portia tablet (n/a)
Preven tablet ($$$)
Prefest tablet (¢¢¢¢¢)
Sprintec tablet (n/a)
Tri-Norinyl tablet ($)
Triphasil tablet ($)
Trivora tablet (¢¢¢¢¢)
Yasmin tablet ($)
Zovia tablet ($)

DOSING AND FOOD

Oral products are taken 1 to 3 times a day with a drug-free rest period each
month when not used for cancer. Patches are applied from 1 to 7 times a
week depending on the brand. Vaginal insert is removed after 3 months.

Taking the oral form of this drug with food may avoid the stomach upset
that some people suffer. Do NOT drink grapefruit juice when taking this
drug.

Adults: Up to 30 mg per day in divided doses.

Forgotten doses: *Oral:* If you are scheduled to take the next dose within a
few hours, do not take the forgotten dose. Otherwise take the forgotten
dose as soon as you remember. *Transdermal:* Replace the patch as soon as
you remember and adjust your schedule for future doses based on the
instructions on your prescription.

---

†See page 52.   *See page 53.

ALCOHOL, DRUG, HERB, AND SUPPLEMENT INTERACTIONS

Alcohol may increase some of the side effects from this drug, depending on the amount consumed. Ask your doctor about the risks caused by drinking alcohol with your condition.

Red clover may interfere with the effects of this drug and should not be used.

Taking caffeine at the same time as this drug may increase the amount of caffeine in your body.

Several antibiotics may cause birth control pills to be ineffective.

Taking this drug with any of the ones listed below may change the effect of either drug with the possibility of causing toxicity or decreasing effectiveness: anticoagulants†, antidiabetics†, corticosteroids†, cyclosporine, insulin, protease inhibitors†, tamoxifen

Increased side effects are possible when this drug is taken with those listed below: acetaminophen, amiodarone, anabolic steroids†, androgens†, antibiotics†, antithyroid drugs†, barbiturates†, carbamazepine, carmustine, chloroquine, dantrolene, daunorubicin, disulfiram, divalproex, etretinate, gold salts†, hydroxychloroquine, isoniazid, mercaptopurine, methotrexate, methyldopa, naltrexone, phenothiazines†, phenytoin, plicamycin, primidone, rifampin, valproic acid

ALLERGIC REACTIONS AND SIDE EFFECTS

You should tell your doctor about all your allergies and any unexplained symptoms you may have while taking this drug.

MORE COMMON SIDE EFFECTS: Bloating, blood clots*, breast enlargement*, breast pain*, loss of appetite, nausea, seizures*, shortness of breath*, stomach cramps, swelling*, unconsciousness*, weight gain*

LESS COMMON SIDE EFFECTS: Abdominal pain, breast discharge*, breast lumps*, depression, diarrhea, dizziness, gum changes*, hair loss, headache, high cholesterol, high triglycerides, increased blood sugar*, irregular vaginal bleeding*, mood swings*, sexual dysfunction, skin rash, vaginal discharge*, vaginal itch*, vomiting, yellow eyes or skin*

RARE SIDE EFFECTS: Enlarged testicles, headache*, lack of coordination*, numbness*, pain*, speech disorders*, vision changes*, weakness*

PRECAUTIONS

§The strength of these products may appear to be the same as other products, but the form of the drug is different. These products may not be substituted without a new prescription.

Women have an increased risk of developing endometrial cancer and possibly breast cancer after taking this drug for a long period of time.

This drug may cause an increase in blood sugar. Diabetics should monitor their blood sugar frequently and may need a change in the dose of insulin or antidiabetic drug†.

Smoking may increase the risk of serious heart-related side effects including heart attack and stroke.

If you are taking an anticoagulant, the dose may need to be adjusted when taking this drug.

People with a history of developing blood clots may not be able to take this drug.

If you have endometriosis, high cholesterol, high triglycerides, gallbladder disease, pancreatitis, or liver disease, this drug may make those conditions worse.

This drug may cause changes to your gums and mouth. Your dentist may recommend that you clean your teeth and mouth differently to avoid infection.

Patches should be applied to the abdominal area, never near the breasts. The site for placement should be rotated making sure that the same area of skin is not used more frequently than once a week.

The precautions and warnings in this summary also apply to people taking birth control pills, although there may be additional side effects and interactions. St. John's wort may decrease the effectiveness of birth control pills and should not be used. Birth control pills may be associated with a change in thyroid hormone levels.

PREGNANCY AND BREAST-FEEDING

This drug may cause birth defects and should not be used during pregnancy. Breast-feeding while taking this drug is not recommended.

HELPFUL COMMENTS

The nausea that is often noticed when taking an oral dose of this drug will usually go away after several weeks of treatment.

Walking, running, and taking calcium and vitamin D supplements may reduce the advancement of osteoporosis.

See your doctor every 3 to 6 months while taking this drug to adjust the dose if necessary and possibly reduce the risk of side effects.

---

†See page 52.   *See page 53.

ESTRAMUSTINE PHOSPHATE SODIUM

Available for over 20 years

COMMONLY USED TO TREAT

Prostate cancer

DRUG CATEGORY

antineoplastic
Class: alkylating agent: estrogen

PRODUCTS

Brand-Name Products with No Generic Alternative
Emcyt 140 mg capsule ($$$)
No generics available.
No patents, no exclusivity.

DOSING AND FOOD

Doses are taken 3 to 4 times a day.
Taking this drug with food may avoid the nausea that many people suffer.
  Do not consume milk or dairy products within 2 hours of taking this drug.
Adults: Up to 16 mg/kg per day in divided doses.
Forgotten doses: Do not take a forgotten dose. Just go back to your usual
  schedule with the next dose. If you vomit within 2 hours of taking a dose,
  call your doctor to find out if the dose should be repeated.

ALCOHOL, DRUG, HERB, AND SUPPLEMENT INTERACTIONS

Alcohol may increase some of the side effects from this drug, depending
  on the amount consumed. Ask your doctor about the risks caused by
  drinking alcohol with your condition.

Taking this drug with any of the ones listed below may change the effect of
either drug with the possibility of causing toxicity or decreasing effectiveness:
antacids, anticoagulants†

Increased side effects are possible when this drug is taken with those listed below:
acetaminophen, amiodarone, anabolic steroids†, androgens†, antibiotics†,
  antithyroid drugs†, carbamazepine, carmustine, chloroquine, dantrolene,
  disulfiram, divalproex, estrogens†, etretinate, gold salts†, hydroxychloro-
  quine, mercaptopurine, methotrexate, methyldopa, naltrexone, oral con-
  traceptives, phenothiazines†, phenytoin, plicamycin, valproic acid

ALLERGIC REACTIONS AND SIDE EFFECTS

If you are allergic to estrogens† or mechlorethamine, you may also be allergic to this drug. You should tell your doctor about all your allergies and any unexplained symptoms you may have while taking this drug.

MORE COMMON SIDE EFFECTS: Breast englargement, breast tenderness, diarrhea, nausea, sexual dysfunction, swelling*, vomiting

LESS COMMON SIDE EFFECTS: Anxiety, flushing, gas, hair loss, itching, sleep disorders, thirst

RARE SIDE EFFECTS: Back pain*, black stools*, bleeding*, bloody urine*, bruising*, chest pain*, chills*, cough*, fever*, headache*, hoarseness*, leg pain*, numbness*, poor coordination*, shortness of breath*, skin irritation*, slurry speech*, tiredness*, urinary difficulty*, vision changes*, weakness*

PRECAUTIONS

Smoking while taking this drug may cause serious side effects that could lead to stroke or heart attack.

If you have a history of seizures, asthma, gallbladder disease, stomach ulcers, hepatitis, jaundice, depression, kidney disease, or migraine headaches, this drug may make those conditions worse.

Avoid contact with anyone who has the chickenpox, measles, or other communicable disease since it may be easier to catch the infection while taking this drug.

Exposure to skin tests, immunizations, and people who have received immunizations may put you at a greater risk of developing the disease when you are taking this drug.

If you are diabetic, you may need a change in the dose of your antidiabetic drug† or insulin, since this drug may cause changes in blood sugar.

This drug must be stored in the refrigerator.

Record your weight daily when taking this drug. Any weight gain, especially if more than 2 pounds per day, should be reported to your doctor.

This drug may cause high blood pressure.

PREGNANCY AND BREAST-FEEDING

This drug may cause birth defects and should not be used during pregnancy. This drug may also cause permanent sterility, so let your doctor know if you ever wish to have children.

Breast-feeding while taking this drug is not recommended.

---

†See page 52.   *See page 53.

HELPFUL COMMENTS

It takes about 3 months for the effects of this drug to be noticed.

If you need to take an antacid, take it either 2 hours before or after taking this drug.

It is very important to continue taking this drug as ordered by the doctor even if the side effects make you feel ill.

ESTROGEN

Available for over 20 years

COMMONLY USED TO TREAT

Breast cancer
Inflammation of the vagina, also known as atrophic vaginitis
Menopausal symptoms
Ovarian failure
Postmenopausal women at risk of bone loss, also known as osteoporosis
Prostate cancer

DRUG CATEGORY

antineoplastic
antiosteoporotic
estrogen replacement
Class: estrogen hormone

PRODUCTS

Brand-Name Products with No Generic Alternative
Cenestin 0.3 mg tablet§ (n/a)
Cenestin 0.625 mg tablet§ (¢¢¢¢)
Cenestin 0.9 mg tablet§ (¢¢¢¢¢)
Cenestin 1.25 mg tablet§ (¢¢¢¢¢)
Premarin 0.3 mg tablet§ (¢¢¢¢)
Premarin 0.625 mg tablet§ (¢¢¢¢)
Premarin 0.9 mg tablet§ (¢¢¢¢¢)
Premarin 1.25 mg tablet§ ($)
Premarin 2.5 mg tablet§ ($$)
Menest 0.3 mg tablet§ (¢¢¢)
Menest 0.625 mg tablet§ (¢¢¢)
Menest 1.25 mg tablet§ (¢¢¢¢)
Menest 2.5 mg tablet§ ($)

§ *See "Precautions" in this entry.*

Premarin 0.625 mg/gm vaginal cream (¢¢¢)

No generics available.

No patents, no exclusivity on Menest. Patent on Premarin expires in 2012. Patent on Cenestin expires in 2015.

Combination Products That Contain This Drug

Prempro tablet ($)

Premphase 14/14 tablet ($)

DOSING AND FOOD

Doses are taken 1 to 3 times a day with a drug-free rest period each month, unless used for cancer.

Taking this drug with a little food may avoid the stomach upset that some people suffer.

Adults: Up to 30 mg per day in divided doses.

Forgotten doses: If you are scheduled to take the next dose within a few hours, do not take the forgotten dose. Otherwise take the forgotten dose as soon as you remember.

ALCOHOL, DRUG, HERB, AND SUPPLEMENT INTERACTIONS

Alcohol may increase some of the side effects from this drug, depending on the amount consumed. Ask your doctor about the risks caused by drinking alcohol with your condition.

Red clover may interfere with the effects of this drug and should not be used.

Taking caffeine at the same time as this drug may increase the amount of caffeine in your body.

Taking this drug with any of the ones listed below may change the effect of either drug with the possibility of causing toxicity or decreasing effectiveness: anticoagulants†, antidiabetics†, corticosteroids†, cyclosporine, insulin, protease inhibitors†, tamoxifen

Increased side effects are possible when this drug is taken with those listed below: acetaminophen, amiodarone, anabolic steroids†, androgens†, antibiotics†, antithyroid drugs†, barbiturates†, carbamazepine, carmustine, chloroquine, dantrolene, daunorubicin, disulfiram, divalproex, etretinate, gold salts†, hydroxychloroquine, isoniazid, mercaptopurine, methotrexate, methyldopa, naltrexone, phenothiazines†, phenytoin, plicamycin, primidone, rifampin, valproic acid

ALLERGIC REACTIONS AND SIDE EFFECTS

You should tell your doctor about all your allergies and any unexplained symptoms you may have while taking this drug.

† See page 52.   * See page 53.

MORE COMMON SIDE EFFECTS: Bloating, blood clots*, breast enlargement*, breast pain*, loss of appetite, nausea, seizures*, shortness of breath*, stomach cramps, swelling*, unconsciousness*, weight gain*

LESS COMMON SIDE EFFECTS: Abdominal pain, breast discharge*, breast lumps*, depression, diarrhea, dizziness, gum changes*, hair loss, headache*, high cholesterol, high triglycerides, increased blood sugar*, mood swings*, sexual dysfunction, skin rash, vaginal bleeding*, vaginal discharge*, vaginal itch*, vomiting, yellow eyes or skin*

RARE SIDE EFFECTS: Enlarged testicles, lack of coordination*, numbness*, pain*, speech disorders*, vision changes*, weakness*

PRECAUTIONS

§The strength of these products may appear to be the same as other products, but the form of the drug is different. These products may not be substituted without a new prescription.

Women have an increased risk of developing endometrial cancer and possibly breast cancer after taking this drug for a long period of time.

This drug may cause an increase in blood sugar. Diabetics should monitor their blood sugar frequently and may need a change in the dose of insulin or antidiabetic drug†.

Smoking may increase the risk of serious heart-related side effects including heart attack and stroke.

If you are taking an anticoagulant†, the dose may need to be adjusted when taking this drug.

People with a history of developing blood clots may not be able to take this drug.

If you have endometriosis, high cholesterol, high triglycerides, gallbladder disease, pancreatitis, or liver disease, this drug may make those conditions worse.

This drug may cause changes to your gums and mouth. Your dentist may recommend that you clean your teeth and mouth differently to avoid infection.

PREGNANCY AND BREAST-FEEDING

This drug may cause birth defects and should not be used during pregnancy. Breast-feeding while taking this drug is not recommended.

HELPFUL COMMENTS

The nausea that is often noticed when taking a dose of this drug will usually go away after several weeks of treatment.

Walking, running, and taking calcium and vitamin D supplements may reduce the advancement of osteoporosis.

See your doctor every 3 to 6 months while taking this drug to adjust the dose if necessary and possibly reduce the risk of side effects.

ESTROPIPATE

Available for over 20 years

COMMONLY USED TO TREAT

Inflammation of the vagina, also known as atrophic vaginitis
Menopausal symptoms
Ovarian failure
Postmenopausal women at risk of bone loss, also known as osteoporosis

DRUG CATEGORY

antineoplastic
estrogen replacement
Class: estrogen hormone

PRODUCTS

Brand-Name Products with No Generic Alternative
Ogen vaginal cream (¢¢¢)
Brand-Name Products with Generic Alternatives
Ogen .625 (0.75 mg) tablet (¢¢¢¢¢)
  Generic: estropipate 0.75 mg tablet (¢¢¢)
Ogen 1.25 (1.5 mg) tablet ($)
  Generic: estropipate 1.5 mg tablet (¢¢¢¢)
Ogen 2.5 (3 mg) tablet ($$)
  Generic: estropipate 3 mg tablet ($)
Ogen 5 (6 mg) tablet (n/a)
  Generic: estropipate 6 mg tablet (n/a)
Other Generic Product Names
Ortho-Est

DOSING AND FOOD

Doses are taken once a day with a drug-free rest period each month.
This drug may be taken with or without food.
Adults: Up to 9 mg per day.

† See page 52.   * See page 53.

Forgotten doses: If you are scheduled to take the next dose within a few hours, do not take the forgotten dose. Otherwise take the forgotten dose as soon as you remember.

ALCOHOL, DRUG, HERB, AND SUPPLEMENT INTERACTIONS

Alcohol may increase some of the side effects from this drug, depending on the amount consumed. Ask your doctor about the risks caused by drinking alcohol with your condition.

Red clover may interfere with the effects of this drug and should not be used. Taking caffeine at the same time as this drug may increase the amount of caffeine in your body.

Taking this drug with any of the ones listed below may change the effect of either drug with the possibility of causing toxicity or decreasing effectiveness: anticoagulants†, antidiabetics†, corticosteroids†, cyclosporine, insulin, protease inhibitors†, tamoxifen

Increased side effects are possible when this drug is taken with those listed below: acetaminophen, amiodarone, anabolic steroids†, androgens†, antibiotics†, antithyroid drugs†, barbiturates†, carbamazepine, carmustine, chloroquine, dantrolene, daunorubicin, disulfiram, divalproex, etretinate, gold salts†, hydroxychloroquine, isoniazid, mercaptopurine, methotrexate, methyldopa, naltrexone, phenothiazines†, phenytoin, plicamycin, primidone, rifampin, valproic acid

ALLERGIC REACTIONS AND SIDE EFFECTS

You should tell your doctor about all your allergies and any unexplained symptoms you may have while taking this drug.

MORE COMMON SIDE EFFECTS: Bloating, blood clots*, breast enlargement*, breast pain*, loss of appetite, seizures*, shortness of breath*, stomach cramps, swelling*, unconsciousness*, weight gain*

LESS COMMON SIDE EFFECTS: Abdominal pain, breast discharge*, breast lumps*, depression, diarrhea, dizziness, gum changes*, hair loss, headaches, high cholesterol, high triglycerides, increased blood sugar*, mood swings*, PMS (premenstrual syndrome), sexual dysfunction, skin rash, vaginal bleeding*, vaginal discharge*, vaginal itch*, vomiting, yellow eyes or skin*

PRECAUTIONS

Women have an increased risk of developing endometrial cancer and possibly breast cancer after taking this drug for a long period of time.

This drug may cause an increase in blood sugar. Diabetics should monitor their blood sugar frequently and may need a change in the dose of insulin or antidiabetic drug†.

Smoking may increase the risk of serious heart-related side effects including heart attack and stroke.

If you are taking an anticoagulant, the dose may need to be adjusted when taking this drug.

People with a history of developing blood clots may not be able to take this drug.

If you have endometriosis, high cholesterol, high triglycerides, gallbladder disease, pancreatitis, or liver disease, this drug may make those conditions worse.

This drug may cause changes to your gums and mouth. Your dentist may recommend that you clean your teeth and mouth differently to avoid infection.

PREGNANCY AND BREAST-FEEDING

This drug may cause birth defects and should not be used during pregnancy. Breast-feeding while taking this drug is not recommended.

HELPFUL COMMENTS

Walking, running, and taking calcium and vitamin D supplements may reduce the advancement of osteoporosis.

See your doctor every 3 to 6 months while taking this drug to adjust the dose if necessary and possibly reduce the risk of side effects.

ETHACRYNIC ACID

Available for over 20 years

COMMONLY USED TO TREAT

Fluid retention, also known as edema
High blood pressure, also known as hypertension
High calcium levels, also known as hypercalcemia

DRUG CATEGORY

antihypercalcemic
antihypertensive
Class: loop diuretic

---

†*See page 52.* **See page 53.*

PRODUCTS

Brand-Name Products with No Generic Alternative
Edecrin 25 mg tablet (¢¢¢)
Edecrin 50 mg tablet (¢¢¢¢)
No generics available.
No patents, no exclusivity.

DOSING AND FOOD

Doses are given 1 to 2 times a day.
Taking this drug with a little food may avoid the stomach upset that some
  people suffer.
Adults: Up to 200 mg per day in divided doses.
Lower doses are used in children
Forgotten doses: If you are scheduled to take the next dose within a few
  hours, do not take the forgotten dose. Otherwise take the forgotten dose
  as soon as you remember.

ALCOHOL, DRUG, HERB, AND SUPPLEMENT INTERACTIONS

Alcohol may increase some of the side effects from this drug, depending
  on the amount consumed. Ask your doctor about the risks caused by
  drinking alcohol with your condition.
Several OTC drugs used for appetite control, asthma, colds, cough, hay
  fever, or sinus problems may cause an increase in blood pressure when
  taken with this drug. Check with your pharmacist when selecting OTC
  products.
Dandelion and licorice root may both interfere with this drug.
**Taking this drug with any of the ones listed below may change the effect of
either drug with the possibility of causing toxicity or decreasing effectiveness:**
amiloride, amphotericin B, antihypertensives†, cardiac glycosides†, corti-
  costeroids†, diuretics†, lithium, nonsteroidal antiinflammatories†, probenecid, spironolactone, triamterene, warfarin
Severe reactions are possible when this drug is taken with those listed below:
aminoglycosides†, cephalosporins†, cisplatin

ALLERGIC REACTIONS AND SIDE EFFECTS

You should tell your doctor about all your allergies and any unexplained
  symptoms you may have while taking this drug.
MORE COMMON SIDE EFFECTS: Diarrhea, dizziness, lightheadedness, loss of
  appetite

LESS COMMON SIDE EFFECTS: Blurry vision, confusion, headache, hearing loss*, nervousness, stomach pain*

RARE SIDE EFFECTS: Back pain*, black stools*, bleeding*, bloody urine, bruising*, chills*, cough*, dry mouth*, fever*, hives*, hoarseness*, increased thirst*, irregular heartbeat*, joint pain*, mood swings*, muscle cramps*, nausea*, painful urination*, ringing in ears*, skin rash*, tiredness*, vomiting*, weak pulse*, weakness*, yellow eyes or skin*

PRECAUTIONS

If you are diabetic, you may need a change in the dose of your antidiabetic drug or insulin, since this drug may cause changes in blood sugar.

Your body may lose potassium while taking this drug, which may cause severe side effects. Potassium levels should be monitored periodically and may need to be supplemented while taking this drug. Eat food rich in potassium, such as apricots, bananas, citrus fruit, dates, and tomatoes, if you are not taking a potassium supplement or potassium-sparing diuretic†.

If you have gout, hearing problems, or pancreatitis, this drug may make those conditions worse.

Record your weight twice a day, when first getting up in the morning and after the drug causes urination. A weight gain or loss of more than 2 pounds per day should be reported to your doctor.

Be careful driving or handling equipment while taking this drug because the drug may cause drowsiness.

Drink plenty of fluids to avoid dehydration when sweating, such as in hot weather and during exercise.

PREGNANCY AND BREAST-FEEDING

Safety during pregnancy has not been established although the drug is known to harm animal fetuses.

Breast-feeding while taking this drug is not recommended.

HELPFUL COMMENTS

This drug will cause you to urinate. The effect should start about 30 minutes after taking the dose and will peak at about 2 hours.

This drug should be taken in the morning to reduce the chance of having to urinate during the night.

It is very important to have your hearing checked regularly when taking this drug.

---

†See page 52.   *See page 53.

If you do not treat high blood pressure, you may develop more serious problems such as heart failure, blood vessel disease, stroke, or kidney disease. Losing weight, exercising, eating more fruits and vegetables, and avoiding salty foods, such as lunchmeat and pickles, may help make drug treatment more successful.

ETHAMBUTOL HYDROCHLORIDE

Available for over 20 years

COMMONLY USED TO TREAT

Tuberculosis

DRUG CATEGORY

antibiotic
Class: antimycobacterial

PRODUCTS

Brand-Name Products with Generic Alternatives
Myambutol 100 mg tablet (¢¢¢¢)
 Generic: ethambutol hydrochloride 100 mg tablet (¢¢¢¢)
Myambutol 400 mg tablet ($$)
 Generic: ethambutol hydrochloride 400 mg tablet ($$)

DOSING AND FOOD

Doses are taken anywhere from once a day to twice a week.
Taking this drug with a little food may avoid the stomach upset that some people suffer.
Adults: Up to 25 mg/kg per day.
Children age 6 and older: Up to 15 mg/kg per day.
Lower doses are used in people with kidney disease.
Forgotten doses: If you are scheduled to take the next dose within a few hours, do not take the forgotten dose. Otherwise take the forgotten dose as soon as you remember.

ALCOHOL, DRUG, HERB, AND SUPPLEMENT INTERACTIONS

Alcohol may increase some of the side effects from this drug, depending on the amount consumed. Ask your doctor about the risks caused by drinking alcohol with your condition.

aking this drug with any of the ones listed below may change the effect of
ither drug with the possibility of causing toxicity or decreasing effectiveness:
ntacids

ALLERGIC REACTIONS AND SIDE EFFECTS

ou should tell your doctor about all your allergies and any unexplained
symptoms you may have while taking this drug.

MORE COMMON SIDE EFFECTS: Allergy*, fever*, shortness of breath*, skin
rash*

LESS COMMON SIDE EFFECTS: Abdominal pain, chills*, confusion, headache, joint pain*, loss of appetite, nausea, swelling*, vomiting

RARE SIDE EFFECTS: Blurry vision*, burning sensation*, color blindness*,
eye pain*, loss of vision*, numbness*, tingling*, weakness*

PRECAUTIONS

f you have gout, kidney disease, or eye disorders, this drug may make
those conditions worse.

Be careful driving or handling equipment while taking this drug because
it may cause vision changes.

PREGNANCY AND BREAST-FEEDING

There is evidence that this drug may harm the fetus, but the drug may be
necessary to the health of the mother.

This drug passes into breast milk, but does not appear to harm the baby.
Talk to your doctor about the risks associated with breast-feeding while
taking this drug.

HELPFUL COMMENTS

The visual changes that affect many people taking this drug will return
to normal about 4 to 12 weeks after the drug is stopped.

Contact your doctor if your symptoms do not improve after 2 to 3 weeks.

Do not stop treatment early if you start to feel better. It may take years
for this drug to work completely.

If you need to take an antacid, take it either 2 hours before or after taking
this drug.

---

† See page 52.   * See page 53.

ETHOSUXIMIDE

Available for over 20 years

COMMONLY USED TO TREAT

Seizures

DRUG CATEGORY

Anticonvulsant
Class: Succinimide Derivative

PRODUCTS

Brand-Name Products with Generic Alternatives
Zarontin 250 mg capsule ($)
  Generic: ethosuximide 250 mg capsule (n/a)
Zarontin 250 mg/5 ml oral syrup ($)
  Generic: ethosuximide 250 mg/5 ml oral syrup (¢¢¢¢¢)

DOSING AND FOOD

Doses are taken twice a day.
Taking this drug with a little food may avoid the stomach upset that some
  people suffer.
Adults and children over age 6: Up to 1,500 mg per day in divided doses.
Children age 3 to 6: Up to 20 mg/kg (maximum 1,000 mg) per day in divided doses.
Forgotten doses: If you are scheduled to take the next dose within 4
  hours, do not take the forgotten dose. Otherwise take the forgotten dose
  as soon as you remember.

ALCOHOL, DRUG, HERB, AND SUPPLEMENT INTERACTIONS

Alcohol should not be used while taking this drug.
Several OTC drugs used for appetite control, asthma, colds, cough, hay
  fever, pain, or sinus problems may seriously increase the effects of this
  drug. Check with your pharmacist when selecting OTC products.
Taking this drug with any of the ones listed below may change the effect of
either drug with the possibility of causing toxicity or decreasing effectiveness:
phenytoin, valproic acid
Severe reactions are possible when this drug is taken with those listed below:
haloperidol

Increased side effects are possible when this drug is taken with those listed below: anticonvulsants†, antidepressants†, antipsychotics†, anxiolytics†, narcotics†

ALLERGIC REACTIONS AND SIDE EFFECTS

If you are allergic to any anticonvulsant†, you may also be allergic to this drug. You should tell your doctor about all your allergies and any unexplained symptoms you may have while taking this drug.

MORE COMMON SIDE EFFECTS: Clumsiness, dizziness, drowsiness*, fever*, headache, hiccups, itching*, loss of appetite, muscle pain*, nausea*, skin rash*, sore throat*, stomach cramps, swollen glands*, vomiting*

LESS COMMON SIDE EFFECTS: Aggressive behavior*, depression*, irritability, nightmares*, poor concentration*

RARE SIDE EFFECTS: Bleeding*, breathing difficulty*, bruising*, chest tightness*, chills*, mood swings*, mouth sores*, nosebleeds*, seizures*, shortness of breath*, tiredness*, weakness*, wheezing*

PRECAUTIONS

Be careful driving or handling equipment while taking this drug because the drug may cause drowsiness.

Stopping this drug suddenly may cause you to have a seizure. If you wish to stop taking this drug, ask your doctor for specific instructions.

This drug may cause the urine to turn pink or reddish in color.

PREGNANCY AND BREAST-FEEDING

Safety during pregnancy has not been established although the drug is known to harm animal fetuses.

Breast-feeding while taking this drug is not recommended.

HELPFUL COMMENTS

It takes 4 to 7 days for the full effect of this drug to be noticed.

Avoid quick movements to minimize dizziness. Dangling your legs over the side of the bed for a few minutes may help reduce dizziness when first waking up.

---

† See page 52.   * See page 53.

ETIDRONATE DISODIUM

Available for over 20 years

COMMONLY USED TO TREAT

Bone disease, specifically Paget's disease
High calcium levels associated with cancer

DRUG CATEGORY

antihypercalcemic
antiosteoporotic
Class: bisphosphonate

PRODUCTS

Brand-Name Products with Generic Alternatives
Didronel 200 mg tablet ($$$)
  Generic: etidronate disodium 200 mg tablet (n/a)
Didronel 400 mg tablet ($$$$)
  Generic: etidronate disodium 400 mg tablet (n/a)

DOSING AND FOOD

Doses are taken once a day usually at bedtime.
It is best to take this drug with a full glass of water on an empty stomach.
  Do not eat food, especially dairy products, or drink milk within 2 hours
  of taking a dose.

Adults: Up to 20 mg/kg per day.

Lower doses may be used in children.

Forgotten doses: If you are scheduled to take the next dose within a few
  hours, do not take the forgotten dose. Otherwise take the forgotten dose
  as soon as you remember.

ALCOHOL, DRUG, HERB, AND SUPPLEMENT INTERACTIONS

Alcohol may increase some of the side effects from this drug, depending
  on the amount consumed. Ask your doctor about the risks caused by
  drinking alcohol with your condition.

Taking this drug with any of the ones listed below may change the effect of
either drug with the possibility of causing toxicity or decreasing effectiveness:
antacids, iron supplements, mineral supplements

ALLERGIC REACTIONS AND SIDE EFFECTS

You should tell your doctor about all your allergies and any unexplained symptoms you may have while taking this drug.

MORE COMMON SIDE EFFECTS: Bone pain*, diarrhea, nausea

LESS COMMON SIDE EFFECTS: Broken bones*, taste changes

RARE SIDE EFFECTS: Hives*, itching*, skin rash*, swelling*

PRECAUTIONS

People with a history of intestinal disease may be at greater risk of developing diarrhea while taking this drug.

Tell your doctor if your bone pain gets worse while taking this drug.

PREGNANCY AND BREAST-FEEDING

Safety during pregnancy has not been established although the drug is known to harm animal fetuses.

This drug may pass into breast milk, but does not appear to harm the baby. Talk to your doctor about the risks associated with breast-feeding while taking this drug.

HELPFUL COMMENTS

This drug is also called by the generic name EHDP.

If you need to take an antacid, iron supplement, or multivitamin with minerals, take it either 2 hours before or after taking this drug.

It may take up to 3 months before you begin to notice the effects of this drug.

ETODOLAC

Available since January 1991

COMMONLY USED TO TREAT

Arthritis
Pain

DRUG CATEGORY

analgesic
antiarthritic
antigout
Class: nonsteroidal antiinflammatory

---

†*See page 52.*   **See page 53.*

PRODUCTS

Brand-Name Products with Generic Alternatives

Lodine 200 mg capsule ($)
   Generic: etodolac 200 mg capsule ($)
Lodine 300 mg capsule ($$)
   Generic: etodolac 300 mg capsule ($)
Lodine 400 mg tablet ($$)
   Generic: etodolac 400 mg tablet (¢¢¢)
Lodine 500 mg tablet ($$)
   Generic: etodolac 500 mg tablet (¢¢¢¢)
Lodine XL 400 mg extended-release tablet ($$)
   Generic: etodolac 400 mg extended-release tablet ($)
Lodine XL 500 mg extended-release tablet ($$)
   Generic: etodolac 500 mg extended-release tablet ($)
Lodine XL 600 mg extended-release tablet ($$$)
   Generic: etodolac 600 mg extended-release tablet ($$$)

DOSING AND FOOD

Doses are taken 3 to 4 times a day.
It is best to take this drug with food.
Adults: Up to 1,000 mg per day in divided doses.
Forgotten doses: If you are scheduled to take the next dose within a few
   hours, do not take the forgotten dose. Otherwise take the forgotten dose
   as soon as you remember.

ALCOHOL, DRUG, HERB, AND SUPPLEMENT INTERACTIONS

Alcohol may increase the risk of serious side effects from this drug. Ask your
   doctor about the risks caused by drinking alcohol with your condition.
Do not use dong quai, feverfew, garlic, ginger, horse chestnut, red clover,
   or St. John's wort while taking this drug since they may increase the risk
   of serious side effects.

**Taking this drug with any of the ones listed below may change the effect of
either drug with the possibility of causing toxicity or decreasing effectiveness:**
acetaminophen, antihypertensives†, beta blockers†, digoxin, diuretics†,
   furosemide, hydrochlorothiazide, nifedipine, lithium, methotrexate,
   phenytoin, probenecid, sulfonylureas†, sulindac, verapamil

Severe reactions are possible when this drug is taken with those listed below:
antibiotics†, anticoagulants†, aspirin, cefamandole, cefoperazone, cefote-
   tan, corticosteroids†, cyclosporine, gold salts†, heparin, nonsteroidal an-

tiinflammatories†, penicillamine, plicamycin, salicylates†, valproic acid, warfarin

ALLERGIC REACTIONS AND SIDE EFFECTS

If you are allergic to aspirin, zomepirac, salicylates†, or other nonsteroidal antiinflammatories†, you may also be allergic to this drug. You should tell your doctor about all your allergies and any unexplained symptoms you may have while taking this drug.

This drug promotes the effect of sunlight on the body and may cause severe sunburn and increased sensitivity of the eyes.

MORE COMMON SIDE EFFECTS: Abdominal pain, diarrhea, dizziness, drowsiness, gas, headache, heartburn*, indigestion*, itching*, mouth sores*, nausea*, skin rash*, swelling*, weight gain*

LESS COMMON SIDE EFFECTS: Black stools*, bloody urine*, bloody vomit, bruising*, constipation, high blood pressure*, sweating, vomiting

RARE SIDE EFFECTS: Back pain*, blue fingernails*, blue lips*, breathing difficulty*, chest pain*, chest tightness*, chills*, confusion*, cough*, dark urine*, fainting*, fever*, hallucinations*, hearing loss*, hives*, hoarseness*, lip sores*, loss of appetite*, low blood pressure*, mood swings*, muscle cramps*, nosebleeds*, pain*, pale skin*, pale stools*, puffy eyes*, rectal bleeding*, restlessness*, ringing in ears*, runny nose*, seizures*, shortness of breath*, sore throat*, stiff neck*, swollen glands*, swollen tongue*, thirst*, tiredness*, urinary changes*, vision changes*, weakness*, wheezing*, yellow eyes or skin*

PRECAUTIONS

This drug may cause serious stomach problems and possibly ulcers. Be careful to take this drug as directed with food, and let your doctor know if you develop any stomach-related symptoms.

Do not crush, break, or chew the extended-release products.

Be careful driving or handling equipment while taking this drug because the drug may cause drowsiness.

Do not lie down for about 30 minutes after taking this drug to help reduce the risk of heartburn and throat irritation.

If you use tobacco or have a history of alcohol abuse, stomach problems, intestinal problems, hemorrhoids, diabetes mellitus, severe fluid retention, or systemic lupus erythematosus, there may be an increased risk that you will develop side effects while taking this drug.

---

† See page 52.   * See page 53.

PREGNANCY AND BREAST-FEEDING

Safety during pregnancy has not been established although the drug is known to harm animal fetuses.

Breast-feeding while taking this drug is not recommended.

HELPFUL COMMENTS

People with arthritis usually notice the effects of this drug within 2 weeks.

Avoid quick movements to minimize dizziness.

Several nonsteroidal antiinflammatories† are available without a prescription in lower, nonprescription strengths, including ibuprofen, ketoprofen, and naproxen.

If you need to take an antacid, take it no sooner than 2 hours after taking this drug.

ETOPOSIDE

Available since November 1983

COMMONLY USED TO TREAT

Lung cancer

DRUG CATEGORY

antineoplastic
Class: podophyllotoxin

PRODUCTS

Brand-Name Products with Generic Alternatives
VePesid 50 mg capsule ($$$$$)
  Generic: etoposide 50 mg capsule ($$$$$)

DOSING AND FOOD

Doses are taken once a day for 4 to 5 days with a 3-to-4-week drug-free period before the next treatment.

This drug may be taken with or without food. Do not eat raw oysters or other raw shellfish at any time while taking this drug. If you vomit within 2 hours of taking a dose, call your doctor to find out if the dose should be repeated.

Adults: Up to 100 mg/m^2 per day in divided doses.

Lower doses are used in people with kidney disease.

Forgotten doses: Do not take a forgotten dose. Just go back to your usual schedule with the next dose.

ALCOHOL, DRUG, HERB, AND SUPPLEMENT INTERACTIONS

Alcohol may increase some of the side effects from this drug, depending on the amount consumed. Ask your doctor about the risks caused by drinking alcohol with your condition.

Taking this drug with any of the ones listed below may change the effect of either drug with the possibility of causing toxicity or decreasing effectiveness: amphotericin B, antithyroid drugs†, azathioprine, chloramphenicol, cisplatin, colchicine, ganciclovir, glucytosine, interferon, plicamycin, warfarin, zidovudine

ALLERGIC REACTIONS AND SIDE EFFECTS

You should tell your doctor about all your allergies and any unexplained symptoms you may have while taking this drug.

MORE COMMON SIDE EFFECTS: Allergy*, diarrhea, hair loss, loss of appetite, mouth sores*, nausea, tiredness*, vomiting, weakness*

LESS COMMON SIDE EFFECTS: Back pain*, black stools*, bleeding*, bloody urine*, bruising*, chills*, cough*, fever*, hoarseness*, skin irritation*, urinary changes

RARE SIDE EFFECTS: Fast heartbeat*, itching*, numbness*, shortness of breath*, skin rash*, sweating*, swelling*, throat tightness*, tingling*, unconsciousness*, wheezing*

PRECAUTIONS

Avoid contact with anyone who has the chickenpox, measles, or other communicable disease since it may be easier to catch the infection while taking this drug.

Exposure to skin tests, immunizations, and people who have received immunizations may put you at a greater risk of developing the disease when you are taking this drug.

This drug causes changes in your blood that put you at greater risk of getting an infection. Be careful not to cut yourself or get bruised. Tell your doctor if you develop signs of infection, such as fever or sore throat. Your dentist may recommend that you clean your teeth and mouth differently to avoid infection.

PREGNANCY AND BREAST-FEEDING

There is evidence that this drug may harm the fetus, but the drug may be necessary to the health of the mother.

Breast-feeding while taking this drug is not recommended.

---

† *See page 52.*   * *See page 53.*

HELPFUL COMMENTS

This drug is also called by the generic name VP-16.
It is very important to continue taking this drug as ordered by the doctor even if the side effects make you feel ill.

EXEMESTANE

Available since October 1999

COMMONLY USED TO TREAT

Breast cancer

DRUG CATEGORY

antineoplastic
Class: aromatase inactivator

PRODUCTS

Brand-Name Products with No Generic Alternative
Aromasin 25 mg tablet (n/a)
No generics available.
Multiple patents that expire in 2006. Exclusivity until 2006.

DOSING AND FOOD

Doses are taken once a day.
It is best to take this drug after a meal.
Women: Up to 25 mg per day.
Forgotten doses: Do not take a forgotten dose. Just go back to your usual schedule with the next dose.

ALCOHOL, DRUG, HERB, AND SUPPLEMENT INTERACTIONS

Alcohol may increase some of the side effects from this drug, depending on the amount consumed. Ask your doctor about the risks caused by drinking alcohol with your condition.

Taking this drug with any of the ones listed below may change the effect of either drug with the possibility of causing toxicity or decreasing effectiveness: estrogens†

ALLERGIC REACTIONS AND SIDE EFFECTS

You should tell your doctor about all your allergies and any unexplained symptoms you may have while taking this drug.

MORE COMMON SIDE EFFECTS: Abdominal pain, anxiety, back pain*, breathing difficulty*, chest tightness*, chills*, constipation, cough*, depression*, diarrhea, dizziness, fever*, hoarseness*, hot flashes, increased blood pressure*, loss of appetite, nausea, shortness of breath*, sleeping difficulty*, sweating, swelling*, tiredness, vomiting, weakness

LESS COMMON SIDE EFFECTS: Bone pain, broken bones*, chest pain*, confusion, hair loss, headache*, increased appetite, itching, joint pain, rash, runny nose, sore throat*, tingling, upset stomach, urinary changes*, wheezing*

PRECAUTIONS

This drug should only be used in postmenopausal women.
Be careful driving or handling equipment while taking this drug because it may cause dizziness.

PREGNANCY AND BREAST-FEEDING

There is evidence that this drug may harm the fetus.
Breast-feeding while taking this drug is not recommended.

HELPFUL COMMENTS

Drug absorption increases after a high-fat meal.

EZETIMIBE

Available since October 2002

COMMONLY USED TO TREAT

High blood cholesterol, also known as hypercholesterolemia

DRUG CATEGORY

antilipemic
Class: cholesterol absorption inhibitor

PRODUCTS

Brand-Name Products with No Generic Alternative
Zetia 10 mg tablet (n/a)
No generics available.
Multiple patents that begin to expire in 2013. Exclusivity until 2007.

---

† *See page 52.*   * *See page 53.*

DOSING AND FOOD

Doses are taken once a day.

This drug may be taken with or without food.

Adults: Up to 10 mg per day.

Forgotten doses: If you are scheduled to take the next dose within a few hours, do not take the forgotten dose. Otherwise take the forgotten dose as soon as you remember.

ALCOHOL, DRUG, HERB, AND SUPPLEMENT INTERACTIONS

Alcohol may increase some of the side effects from this drug, depending on the amount consumed. Ask your doctor about the risks caused by drinking alcohol with your condition.

Taking this drug with any of the ones listed below may change the effect of either drug with the possibility of causing toxicity or decreasing effectiveness: cholestyramine, cyclosporine, fenofibrate, gemfibrozil

ALLERGIC REACTIONS AND SIDE EFFECTS

You should tell your doctor about all your allergies and any unexplained symptoms you may have while taking this drug.

MORE COMMON SIDE EFFECTS: Abdominal pain, back pain, cough, diarrhea, muscle pain, runny nose, sore throat, tiredness

LESS COMMON SIDE EFFECTS: Breathing difficulty*, rash*, swelling*

PRECAUTIONS

People with liver disease may not be able to take this drug.

This drug is often used in combination with another cholesterol-lowering drug (statins), unless you have liver disease.

PREGNANCY AND BREAST-FEEDING

Safety during pregnancy has not been established although the drug is known to harm animal fetuses.

Breast-feeding while taking this drug is not recommended.

HELPFUL COMMENTS

It takes about 2 weeks for the effects of this drug to be noticed.

FAMCICLOVIR

Available since April 1996

COMMONLY USED TO TREAT

Herpes infections
Shingles, also known as herpes zoster

DRUG CATEGORY

antiviral
Class: synthetic acyclic guanine derivative

PRODUCTS

Brand-Name Products with No Generic Alternative
Famvir 125 mg tablet ($$$)
Famvir 250 mg tablet ($$$)
Famvir 500 mg tablet ($$$$)
No generics available.
Patent expires in 2010.

DOSING AND FOOD

Doses are taken 2 to 3 times a day.
This drug may be taken with or without food.
Adults: Up to 1,500 mg per day in divided doses.
Lower doses are used in people with kidney disease.
Forgotten doses: If you are scheduled to take the next dose within a few
hours, do not take the forgotten dose. Otherwise take the forgotten dose
as soon as you remember.

ALCOHOL, DRUG, HERB, AND SUPPLEMENT INTERACTIONS

Alcohol may increase some of the side effects from this drug, depending
on the amount consumed. Ask your doctor about the risks caused by
drinking alcohol with your condition.

**Taking this drug with any of the ones listed below may change the effect of
either drug with the possibility of causing toxicity or decreasing effectiveness:**
probenecid

ALLERGIC REACTIONS AND SIDE EFFECTS

You should tell your doctor about all your allergies and any unexplained
symptoms you may have while taking this drug.

---

† See page 52.   * See page 53.

MORE COMMON SIDE EFFECTS: Headache

LESS COMMON SIDE EFFECTS: Abdominal pain, back pain, constipation, diarrhea, dizziness, drowsiness, gas, fever, joint pain, loss of appetite, nausea, rash, stuffy nose, tiredness, vomiting, weakness

PRECAUTIONS

This drug works best when started within 6 hours of the development of pain and blisters associated with genital herpes, or within 48 hours of the development of pain, burning, and blisters associated with shingles. If started too late, this drug may not be effective.

The affected area should be kept clean and as dry as possible.

This drug does not prevent sexually transmitted disease, so intercourse should be avoided when infected with genital herpes.

This drug is only effective in treating the pain and discomfort caused by the disease and to help the sores heal more quickly.

PREGNANCY AND BREAST-FEEDING

Safety in pregnancy has not been established although there was no evidence of harm during studies in animals.

Breast-feeding while taking this drug is not recommended.

HELPFUL COMMENTS

Do not stop treatment early if you start to feel better. It takes the full prescription for this drug to work completely.

Contact your doctor if your symptoms do not improve after a couple of days.

Wear clothes that fit loosely and will not rub against the blisters.

FAMOTIDINE

Available since October 1986

COMMONLY USED TO TREAT

Heartburn
Stomach ulcers, specifically duodenal ulcers and gastric ulcers

DRUG CATEGORY

antiulcer
Class: H2 receptor antagonist

PRODUCTS

Brand-Name Products with No Generic Alternative
Pepcid 40 mg/5 ml oral suspension ($$$$$)
Brand-Name Products with Generic Alternatives
Pepcid 20 mg tablet ($$)
 Generic: famotidine 20 mg tablet (¢¢¢)
Pepcid 40 mg tablet ($$$)
 Generic: famotidine 40 mg tablet ($$$)

DOSING AND FOOD

Doses are taken 1 to 4 times a day.
It is best to take this drug with food or milk or within 1 hour before meals.
Adults: Up to 80 mg per day in divided doses.
Children more than 10 kg: Up to 2 mg/kg per day in divided doses.
Lower doses are used in people with kidney disease.
Forgotten doses: If you are scheduled to take the next dose within a few
 hours, do not take the forgotten dose. Otherwise take the forgotten dose
 as soon as you remember.

ALCOHOL, DRUG, HERB, AND SUPPLEMENT INTERACTIONS

Alcohol may increase some of the side effects from this drug, depending
 on the amount consumed. Ask your doctor about the risks caused by
 drinking alcohol with your condition.
Do not use guarana while taking this drug since the combination may lead
 to serious reactions.
**Taking this drug with any of the ones listed below may change the effect of
either drug with the possibility of causing toxicity or decreasing effectiveness:**
ketoconazole

ALLERGIC REACTIONS AND SIDE EFFECTS

If you are allergic to any H2 receptor antagonists†, you may also be allergic
 to this drug. You should tell your doctor about all your allergies and any
 unexplained symptoms you may have while taking this drug.
MORE COMMON SIDE EFFECTS: Headache
LESS COMMON SIDE EFFECTS: Constipation, diarrhea, dizziness*, drowsiness,
 dry mouth, ringing in ears
RARE SIDE EFFECTS: Abdominal pain*, agitation*, anxiety*, back pain*,
 bleeding*, blisters*, breathing difficulty*, bruising*, chest tightness*,

---

† See page 52.   * See page 53.

chills*, confusion*, cough*, dark urine*, depression*, fainting*, fever*, hallucinations*, hives*, irregular heartbeat*, itching*, joint pain*, leg pain*, loss of appetite*, mood swings*, muscle cramps*, nausea*, nervousness*, pain*, pale stools*, shallow breathing*, shortness of breath*, skin irritation*, sore eyes*, sore lips*, sore throat*, swallowing difficulty*, swelling*, tiredness*, vision changes*, vomiting*, weakness*, wheezing*, yellow eyes or skin*

PRECAUTIONS

This drug may cause false results from diagnostic skin tests.

Nonprescription strengths of this drug should not be taken for longer than 2 weeks unless recommended by your doctor.

Chewable tablets, available without a prescription, contain aspartame and should not be used in people with phenylketonuria.

PREGNANCY AND BREAST-FEEDING

Safety in pregnancy has not been established although there was no evidence of harm during studies in animals.

Breast-feeding while taking this drug is not recommended.

HELPFUL COMMENTS

Once-a-day doses should be taken at bedtime.

If you need to take an antacid, it may be taken at the same time as this drug.

Smoking may increase stomach acids, making your condition worse.

This drug is available without a prescription in 10 mg tablets as generic or brand-name products. Chewable 10 mg tablets are only available under the brand Pepcid AC. This drug is also sold without a prescription in a combinations product called Pepcid Complete that contains calcium carbonate.

FELBAMATE

Available since July 1993

COMMONLY USED TO TREAT

Seizures

DRUG CATEGORY

anticonvulsant
Class: carbamate

PRODUCTS

Brand-Name Products with No Generic Alternative
Felbatol 400 mg tablet ($)
Felbatol 600 mg tablet ($$)
Felbatol 600 mg/5 ml oral suspension ($$$)
No generics available.
Multiple patents that expire in 2009.

DOSING AND FOOD

Doses are taken 3 to 4 times a day.
This drug may be taken with or without food but is best taken with food to reduce the stomach upset that some people suffer.

Adults: Up to 3,600 mg per day in divided doses.

Children age 2 to 14: Up to 45 mg/kg (maximum 3,600 mg) per day in divided doses.

Forgotten doses: If you are scheduled to take the next dose within a few hours, do not take the forgotten dose. Otherwise take the forgotten dose as soon as you remember.

ALCOHOL, DRUG, HERB, AND SUPPLEMENT INTERACTIONS

Alcohol may increase the risk of liver damage from this drug. Ask your doctor about the risks caused by drinking alcohol with your condition.

Taking this drug with any of the ones listed below may change the effect of either drug with the possibility of causing toxicity or decreasing effectiveness: carbamazepine, phenobarbital, phenytoin, valproic acid

ALLERGIC REACTIONS AND SIDE EFFECTS

If you are allergic to carbromal, carisoprodol, mebutamate, meprobamate, or tybamate, you may also be allergic to this drug. You should tell your doctor about all your allergies and any unexplained symptoms you may have while taking this drug.

This drug promotes the effect of sunlight on the body and may cause severe sunburn and increased sensitivity of the eyes.

MORE COMMON SIDE EFFECTS: Constipation, dizziness, fever*, headache, indigestion, loss of appetite, nausea, shuffling walk*, skin spots*, sleep disorders, stomach pain, taste changes, vomiting

LESS COMMON SIDE EFFECTS: Aggression*, agitation*, blurry vision, clumsiness*, cough, diarrhea, drowsiness, ear pain, mood swings*, runny nose, sneezing, shaking*, skin rash*, trembling*, unsteadiness*, weight loss

† See page 52.   * See page 53.

RARE SIDE EFFECTS: Black stools*, bleeding*, bloody urine*, breathing difficulty*, bruising*, chest pain*, chest tightness*, chills*, congestion*, dark urine*, headache*, hives*, itching*, mouth sores*, muscle cramps*, nosebleeds*, pale stools*, shortness of breath*, sore throat*, stomachache*, swelling*, swollen glands*, vomiting*, wheezing*, yellow eyes or skin*

PRECAUTIONS

This drug may cause a serious side effect called aplastic anemia that may develop months after starting treatment. This condition is associated with complications and death but does not have symptoms until it is advanced. Make sure to have your blood tested regularly to detect this condition early.

Liver function should be tested periodically while taking this drug.

If you have anemia, liver disease, or blood disorders, this drug may make those conditions worse.

Stopping this drug suddenly may cause an increase in seizure activity. If you wish to stop taking this drug, ask your doctor for specific instructions.

Be careful driving or handling equipment while taking this drug because it may cause dizziness.

PREGNANCY AND BREAST-FEEDING

Safety during pregnancy has not been established although the drug is known to harm animal fetuses.

This drug passes into breast milk, but does not appear to harm the baby. Talk to your doctor about the risks associated with breast-feeding while taking this drug.

HELPFUL COMMENTS

This drug is also called by the generic name FBM.

Do not measure doses of the oral suspension with anything but a measuring cup intended for use with prescription drugs. Slight inaccuracy from other measuring spoons may result in over- or under-dosing.

Avoid quick movements to minimize dizziness.

FELODIPINE

Available since July 1991

COMMONLY USED TO TREAT

Chest pain, also known as angina
High blood pressure, also known as hypertension

DRUG CATEGORY

antianginal
antihypertensive
Class: calcium channel blocker

PRODUCTS

Brand-Name Products with No Generic Alternative
Plendil 2.5 mg extended-release tablet ($)
Plendil 5 mg extended-release tablet ($)
Plendil 10 mg extended-release tablet ($$)
No generics available.
Multiple patents that begin to expire in 2007.
Combination Products That Contain This Drug
Lexxel extended-release tablet ($)

DOSING AND FOOD

Doses are taken once a day.

This drug may be taken with or without food. Do not eat grapefruit or drink grapefruit juice while taking this drug.

Adults: Up to 10 mg per day.

Forgotten doses: If you are scheduled to take the next dose in less than 5 hours, do not take the forgotten dose. Otherwise take the forgotten dose as soon as you remember.

ALCOHOL, DRUG, HERB, AND SUPPLEMENT INTERACTIONS

Alcohol may increase some of the side effects from this drug, depending on the amount consumed. Ask your doctor about the risks caused by drinking alcohol with your condition.

Several OTC drugs used for appetite control, asthma, colds, cough, hay fever, or sinus problems may cause an increase in blood pressure when taken with this drug. Check with your pharmacist when selecting OTC products.

Taking this drug with any of the ones listed below may change the effect of either drug with the possibility of causing toxicity or decreasing effectiveness: anticonvulsants†, benzodiazepines†, carbamazepine, cimetidine, cyclosporine, digoxin, erythromycin, itraconazole, ketoconazole, lovastatin, rifampin, theophylline

Severe reactions are possible when this drug is taken with those listed below: beta blockers†

---

†See page 52. *See page 53.

ALLERGIC REACTIONS AND SIDE EFFECTS

If you are allergic to any other calcium channel blocker†, you may also be allergic to this drug. You should tell your doctor about all your allergies and any unexplained symptoms you may have while taking this drug.

MORE COMMON SIDE EFFECTS: Fluid retention, flushing, headache, swelling*

LESS COMMON SIDE EFFECTS: Abdominal pain, back pain, breathing difficulty*, constipation, cough*, diarrhea, dizziness, fever*, irregular heartbeat*, nausea, skin rash*, shortness of breath*, tiredness, weakness, wheezing*

RARE SIDE EFFECTS: Chest pain*, fainting*, tender gums*

PRECAUTIONS

Do not crush, break, or chew the extended-release products.

This drug may cause changes to your gums and mouth. Your dentist may recommend that you clean your teeth and mouth differently to avoid infection.

PREGNANCY AND BREAST-FEEDING

Safety in pregnancy has not been established although the drug is known to harm animal fetuses.

Breast-feeding while taking this drug is not recommended.

HELPFUL COMMENTS

Many people get a headache shortly after taking a dose of this drug. This side effect becomes less noticeable as you continue taking the drug over time.

FENOFIBRATE

Available since February 1998

COMMONLY USED TO TREAT

High levels of triglycerides in the blood, also known as hypertriglyceridemia

DRUG CATEGORY

antilipemic
Class: fibrotic acid derivative

PRODUCTS

Brand-Name Products with No Generic Alternative
Tricor 54 mg tablet§ (¢¢¢¢¢)
Tricor 160 mg tablet§ ($$$)

Brand-Name Products with Generic Alternatives
Tricor Micronized 67 mg capsule (¢¢¢¢¢)
   Generic: fenofibrate micronized 67 mg capsule (n/a)
Tricor Micronized 134 mg capsule (n/a)
   Generic: fenofibrate micronized 134 mg capsule (n/a)
Tricor Micronized 200 mg capsule ($$$)
   Generic: fenofibrate micronized 200 mg capsule (n/a)

DOSING AND FOOD

Doses are taken once a day.
It is best to take this drug with food or milk to improve absorption.
Adults: Up to 160 mg of plain drug or 200 mg of micronized drug per day.
Lower doses are used in people with kidney disease and adults over age 65.
Forgotten doses: If you are scheduled to take the next dose within a few
   hours, do not take the forgotten dose. Otherwise take the forgotten dose
   as soon as you remember.

ALCOHOL, DRUG, HERB, AND SUPPLEMENT INTERACTIONS

Alcohol may increase some of the side effects from this drug, depending
   on the amount consumed. Ask your doctor about the risks caused by
   drinking alcohol with your condition.
Several drugs increase triglyceride blood levels, including beta blockers†,
   estrogens†, and thiazide diuretics†, and may interfere with the ability of
   this drug to work effectively.
**Taking this drug with any of the ones listed below may change the effect of
either drug with the possibility of causing toxicity or decreasing effectiveness:**
cholestyramine, colesevelam, colestipol, cyclosporine, dicumerol, warfarin
Severe reactions are possible when this drug is taken with those listed below:
atrovastatin, cerivastatin, fluvastatin, lovastatin, pravastatin, simvastatin

ALLERGIC REACTIONS AND SIDE EFFECTS

You should tell your doctor about all your allergies and any unexplained
   symptoms you may have while taking this drug.
This drug promotes the effect of sunlight on the body and may cause
   severe sunburn and increased sensitivity of the eyes.
MORE COMMON SIDE EFFECTS: Irregular heartbeat*

† *See page 52.*   * *See page 53.*   § *See "Precautions" in this entry.*

LESS COMMON SIDE EFFECTS: Belching, blurry vision, chills*, constipation, diarrhea, dizziness, earache, eye irritation, fever*, gas, heartburn, hives*, itching*, joint pain, muscle aches*, nausea*, sexual dysfunction, sleep disorders, skin rash*, stuffy nose, vomiting*

RARE SIDE EFFECTS: Bleeding*, bloating*, breathing difficulty*, bruising*, cough*, dark urine*, indigestion*, loss of appetite*, pain*, shortness of breath*, sore throat*, stiffness*, stomach pain*, swelling*, tiredness*, weakness*, yellow eyes or skin*

PRECAUTIONS

§The tablet products are not the same as the capsule products and should not be substituted without a new prescription.

This drug may increase the risk of cancer, pancreatitis, pancreatic tumors, and gallstones. Talk to your doctor about the risks associated with taking this drug instead of other treatment.

If you have gallbladder disease, gallstones, or liver disease, this drug may make those conditions worse.

PREGNANCY AND BREAST-FEEDING

Safety in pregnancy has not been established although the drug is known to harm animal fetuses.

Breast-feeding while taking this drug is not recommended.

HELPFUL COMMENTS

It takes 4 to 8 weeks for the full effects of this drug to be noticed. If your triglyceride level has not gone down to the expected level in 2 months, the drug should be stopped.

FENOPROFEN CALCIUM

Available for over 20 years

COMMONLY USED TO TREAT

Arthritis
Pain

DRUG CATEGORY

analgesic
antiarthritic
antigout
antipyretic

Class: nonsteroidal antiinflammatory

PRODUCTS

Brand-Name Products with Generic Alternatives

Nalfon 200 mg capsule (¢¢¢¢)
   Generic: fenoprofen calcium 200 mg capsule (n/a)
Nalfon 300 mg capsule (¢¢¢)
   Generic: fenoprofen calcium 300 mg capsule (n/a)
Nalfon 600 mg capsule ($)
   Generic: fenoprofen calcium 600 mg capsule (¢¢¢)

DOSING AND FOOD

Doses are taken 3 to 6 times a day.
It is best to take this drug with food.
Adults: Up to 3,200 mg per day in divided doses.
Forgotten doses: If you are scheduled to take the next dose within a few hours, do not take the forgotten dose. Otherwise take the forgotten dose as soon as you remember.

ALCOHOL, DRUG, HERB, AND SUPPLEMENT INTERACTIONS

Alcohol may increase the risk of serious side effects from this drug. Ask your doctor about the risks caused by drinking alcohol with your condition.
Do not use dong quai, feverfew, garlic, ginger, horse chestnut, red clover, or St. John's wort while taking this drug since they may increase the risk of serious side effects.
Taking this drug with any of the ones listed below may change the effect of either drug with the possibility of causing toxicity or decreasing effectiveness: acetaminophen, antihypertensives†, digoxin, diuretics†, furosemide, hydrochlorothiazide, nifedipine, lithium, methotrexate, phenytoin, probenecid, sulfonylureas†, sulindac, verapamil
Severe reactions are possible when this drug is taken with those listed below: antibiotics†, anticoagulants†, aspirin, cefamandole, cefoperazone, cefotetan, corticosteroids†, cyclosporine, dipyridamole, gold salts, heparin, mezlocillin, nonsteroidal antiinflammatories†, penicillamine, piperacillin, plicamycin, salicylates†, sulfinpyrazone, ticarcillin, valproic acid, warfarin

ALLERGIC REACTIONS AND SIDE EFFECTS

If you are allergic to aspirin, zomepirac, salicylates†, or other nonsteroidal antiinflammatories†, you may also be allergic to this drug. You should tell your doctor about all your allergies and any unexplained symptoms you may have while taking this drug.

---

†See page 52.   *See page 53.

This drug promotes the effect of sunlight on the body and may cause severe sunburn and increased sensitivity of the eyes.

MORE COMMON SIDE EFFECTS: Abdominal pain, breathing difficulty*, diarrhea, drowsiness, headache, heartburn*, indigestion*, itching*, nausea*, skin rash*, swelling*, weight gain*

LESS COMMON SIDE EFFECTS: Bruising*, constipation, dizziness, gas, high blood pressure*, mouth sores*, sweating, vomiting

RARE SIDE EFFECTS: Back pain*, black stools*, bloody urine*, bloody vomit, blue fingernails*, blue lips*, chest pain*, chest tightness*, chills*, confusion*, cough*, dark urine*, fainting*, fever*, hallucinations*, hearing loss*, hives*, hoarseness*, lip sores*, loss of appetite*, low blood pressure*, mood swings*, muscle cramps*, nosebleeds*, pain*, pale skin*, pale stools*, puffy eyes*, rectal bleeding*, restlessness*, ringing in ears*, runny nose*, seizures*, shortness of breath*, sore throat*, stiff neck*, swollen glands*, swollen tongue*, thirst*, tiredness*, urinary changes*, vision changes*, weakness*, wheezing*, yellow eyes or skin*

PRECAUTIONS

This drug may cause serious stomach problems and possibly ulcers. Be careful to take this drug as directed with food, and let your doctor know if you develop any stomach-related symptoms.

Be careful driving or handling equipment while taking this drug because the drug may cause drowsiness.

Do not lie down for about 30 minutes after taking this drug to help reduce the risk of heartburn and throat irritation.

If you use tobacco or have a history of alcohol abuse, stomach problems, intestinal problems, hemorrhoids, diabetes mellitus, severe fluid retention, or systemic lupus erythematosus, there is an increased risk that you will develop side effects while taking this drug.

PREGNANCY AND BREAST-FEEDING

Safety in pregnancy has not been established although the drug is known to harm animal fetuses.

Breast-feeding while taking this drug is not recommended.

HELPFUL COMMENTS

Several nonsteroidal antiinflammatories† are available without a prescription in lower, nonprescription strengths, including ibuprofen, ketoprofen, and naproxen.

FEXOFENADINE

Available since February 2000

COMMONLY USED TO TREAT

Allergies

DRUG CATEGORY

antihistamine
Class: H1 receptor blocker: piperidine

PRODUCTS

Brand-Name Products with No Generic Alternative
Allegra 30 mg tablet (¢¢¢¢)
Allegra 60 mg tablet ($)
Allegra 60 mg capsule ($)
Allegra 180 mg tablet ($$)
No generics available.
Multiple patents that begin to expire in 2012.
Combination Products That Contain This Drug
Allegra-D extended-release tablet ($)

DOSING AND FOOD

Doses are taken 1 to 2 times a day.
This drug may be taken with or without food.
Adults and children over age 12: Up to 180 mg per day in divided doses.
Children age 6 to 11: Up to 60 mg per day in divided doses.
Lower doses may be used in people with kidney disease.
Forgotten doses: This drug should be taken no more often than is labeled on the prescription. If you have forgotten a dose and are having symptoms, take the dose right away. Then wait a full dosing interval (12 or 24 hours depending on the prescription label) before taking the next dose.

ALCOHOL, DRUG, HERB, AND SUPPLEMENT INTERACTIONS

Alcohol may increase some of the side effects from this drug, depending on the amount consumed. Ask your doctor about the risks caused by drinking alcohol with your condition.
Several OTC drugs used for appetite control, asthma, colds, cough, hay fever, pain, or sinus problems may seriously increase the effects of this drug. Check with your pharmacist when selecting OTC products.

Taking this drug with any of the ones listed below may change the effect of either drug with the possibility of causing toxicity or decreasing effectiveness:

antacids, anesthetics, anticholinergics†, antihistamines†, anxiolytics†, barbiturates†, erythromycin, ketoconazole, narcotics†, tricyclic antidepressants†

Severe reactions are possible when this drug is taken with those listed below: monoamine oxidase inhibitors†

Increased side effects are possible when this drug is taken with those listed below: alcohol, antihistamines†

ALLERGIC REACTIONS AND SIDE EFFECTS

If you are allergic to other antihistamines†, you may also be allergic to this drug. You should tell your doctor about all your allergies and any unexplained symptoms you may have while taking this drug.

This drug promotes the effect of sunlight on the body and may cause severe sunburn and increased sensitivity of the eyes.

LESS COMMON SIDE EFFECTS: Appetite changes, belching, bleeding*, body aches, bruising*, clumsiness, confusion, congestion, constipation, cough, diarrhea*, drowsiness, dry mouth, early menstruation, excitement, fatigue, fever*, headache*, heartburn, hoarseness, indigestion, irregular heartbeat*, irritability, joint pain, muscle cramps, nausea, nervousness, nightmares, painful menstruation, restlessness, ringing in ears, runny nose, skin rash, sore throat*, stiffness, stomachache, sweating, swelling*, thick mucus, tremor, urinary changes, vision changes, vomiting, weight gain

RARE SIDE EFFECTS: Abdominal pain*, chest tightness*, chills*, cough*, dark urine*, diarrhea*, dizziness*, hives*, itching*, pale stools*, seizures*, shortness of breath*, skin irritation*, swallowing difficulty*, tingling*, tiredness*, weakness*, wheezing*

PRECAUTIONS

If you have glaucoma, an enlarged prostate, or difficulty urinating, this drug may make those conditions worse.

This drug may interfere with skin tests used to diagnose allergies and should be stopped for at least 4 days before the test.

Be careful driving or handling equipment while taking this drug because the drug may cause drowsiness.

You need to wait 2 weeks after stopping a monoamine oxidase inhibitor† before starting this drug.

PREGNANCY AND BREAST-FEEDING

Safety in pregnancy has not been established although there was no evidence of harm during studies in animals.

Breast-feeding while taking this drug is not recommended.

HELPFUL COMMENTS

Sucking on hard sugarless candy or chewing sugarless gum may help relieve dry mouth caused by this drug.

Several antihistamines are sold without a prescription by the following generic names: brompheniramine, chlorpheniramine, clemastine, diphenhydramine, doxylamine, loratadine. Ask your pharmacist about specific products that contain these drugs.

If you need to take an antacid, take it either 2 hours before or after taking this drug.

FINASTERIDE

Available since June 1992

COMMONLY USED TO TREAT

Enlarged prostate, also known as benign (noncancerous) prostatic hyperplasia or BPH

Male-pattern baldness, also known as alopecia androgenetica

DRUG CATEGORY

androgen synthesis inhibitor
Class: steroid derivative

PRODUCTS

Brand-Name Products with No Generic Alternative
Propecia 1 mg tablet ($$)
Proscar 5 mg tablet ($$$)
No generics available.
Multiple patents that begin to expire in 2006.

DOSING AND FOOD

Doses are taken once a day.
This drug may be taken with or without food.
Adult men: Up to 5 mg per day.

---

†See page 52.   * See page 53.

Forgotten doses: If you are scheduled to take the next dose within a few hours, do not take the forgotten dose. Otherwise take the forgotten dose as soon as you remember.

ALCOHOL, DRUG, HERB, AND SUPPLEMENT INTERACTIONS

Taking this drug with any of the ones listed below may change the effect of either drug with the possibility of causing toxicity or decreasing effectiveness: theophylline

ALLERGIC REACTIONS AND SIDE EFFECTS

You should tell your doctor about all your allergies and any unexplained symptoms you may have while taking this drug.

LESS COMMON SIDE EFFECTS: Breast enlargement*, breast tenderness*, lip swelling*, skin rash*

RARE SIDE EFFECTS: Abdominal pain, back pain, diarrhea, dizziness, erectile dysfunction, headache, sexual dysfunction, testicular pain

PRECAUTIONS

Pregnant women and women of childbearing age need to avoid all exposure to this drug because of the risk of birth defects. Do not handle damaged tablets. Pregnant women should not have intercourse with men taking this drug since drug-containing semen may cause birth defects.

PREGNANCY AND BREAST-FEEDING

This drug may cause birth defects and should not be used during pregnancy. Any exposure to the drug, including touching broken tablets or having intercourse with a man taking the drug, may also be associated with birth defects.

This drug is not indicated for use in women; therefore, breast-feeding while taking this drug is not recommended.

HELPFUL COMMENTS

It takes about 6 to 12 months to see any difference in prostate size and about 3 months to see a change in hair growth when taking this drug.

Hair loss starts again within 12 months after this drug is discontinued.

FLECAINIDE ACETATE

Available since October 1985

COMMONLY USED TO TREAT

Irregular heartbeat, also known as arrhythmias

DRUG CATEGORY

antiarrhythmic
Class: benzamide derivative

PRODUCTS

Brand-Name Products with Generic Alternatives
Tambocor 50 mg tablet ($$)
  Generic: flecainide acetate 50 mg tablet (n/a)
Tambocor 100 mg tablet ($$$)
  Generic: flecainide acetate 100 mg tablet (n/a)
Tambocor 150 mg tablet ($$$)
  Generic: flecainide acetate 150 mg tablet (n/a)

DOSING AND FOOD

Doses are taken twice a day.
This drug may be taken with or without food.
Adults: Up to 400 mg per day in divided doses.
Lower doses are used in people with kidney disease.
Forgotten doses: If you are scheduled to take the next dose within 6 hours, do not take the forgotten dose. Otherwise take the forgotten dose as soon as you remember.

ALCOHOL, DRUG, HERB, AND SUPPLEMENT INTERACTIONS

Alcohol may increase some of the side effects from this drug, depending on the amount consumed. Ask your doctor about the risks caused by drinking alcohol with your condition.

Taking this drug with any of the ones listed below may change the effect of either drug with the possibility of causing toxicity or decreasing effectiveness: antacids, beta blockers†, carbonic anhydrase inhibitors†, cimetidine, digoxin, sodium bicarbonate

Severe reactions are possible when this drug is taken with those listed below: antiarrhythmics†

† See page 52.   * See page 53.

ALLERGIC REACTIONS AND SIDE EFFECTS

If you are allergic to lidocaine, tocainide, or any anesthetics, you may also be allergic to this drug. You should tell your doctor about all your allergies and any unexplained symptoms you may have while taking this drug.

MORE COMMON SIDE EFFECTS: Blurry vision*, dizziness*, headache, irregular heartbeat*, lightheadedness*, shortness of breath*, vision changes*

LESS COMMON SIDE EFFECTS: Anxiety, chest pain*, constipation, depression, flushing, loss of appetite, nausea, shaking*, skin rash, stomach pain, swelling*, tiredness, trembling*, vomiting, weakness

RARE SIDE EFFECTS: Yellow eyes or skin*

PRECAUTIONS

This drug may increase the risk of irregular heartbeats, especially in people with a recent history of heart attack.

If you have heart failure, this drug may make that condition worse.

Be careful driving or handling equipment while taking this drug because it may cause dizziness and blurry vision.

Smoking may cause this drug to be less effective.

This drug may interfere with a pacemaker, causing more-frequent visits to the doctor.

PREGNANCY AND BREAST-FEEDING

Safety in pregnancy has not been established although the drug is known to harm animal fetuses.

Breast-feeding while taking this drug is not recommended.

HELPFUL COMMENTS

It may take 3 to 5 days before the full effects of this drug are noticed.

Although antacids may interfere with this drug, the interaction is typically related to frequent use. Taking an antacid once in a while may be acceptable. Let your doctor know if you need to take an antacid often.

FLUCONAZOLE

Available since January 1990

COMMONLY USED TO TREAT

Fungal infections

DRUG CATEGORY

antifungal
Class: azole derivative

PRODUCTS

Brand-Name Products with No Generic Alternative
Diflucan 50 mg tablet ($$$$)
Diflucan 100 mg tablet ($$$$)
Diflucan 150 mg tablet ($$$$$)
Diflucan 200 mg tablet ($$$$$)
Diflucan 50 mg/5 ml oral suspension ($$$)
Diflucan 200 mg/5 ml oral suspension (n/a)
No generics available.
Patent expires in 2004.

DOSING AND FOOD

Doses are taken once a day.
This drug may be taken with or without food.
Adults: Up to 400 mg per day.
Children: Up to 8 mg/kg per day.
Lower doses are used in people with kidney disease.
Forgotten doses: If you are scheduled to take the next dose within a few
hours, do not take the forgotten dose. Otherwise take the forgotten dose
as soon as you remember.

ALCOHOL, DRUG, HERB, AND SUPPLEMENT INTERACTIONS

Alcohol may increase some of the side effects from this drug, depending
on the amount consumed. Ask your doctor about the risks caused by
drinking alcohol with your condition.
The effects of caffeine may be increased when taken with this drug.

**Taking this drug with any of the ones listed below may change the effect of
either drug with the possibility of causing toxicity or decreasing effectiveness:**
cimetidine, cyclosporine, digoxin, glipizide, glyburide, hydrochloroth-
iazide, isoniazid, phenytoin, rifampin, sulfonylureas†, tacrolimus, theo-
phylline, tolbutamide, warfarin, zidovudine

Severe reactions are possible when this drug is taken with those listed below:
astemizole, dofetilide, terfenadine

Increased side effects are possible when this drug is taken with those listed below:
acetaminophen, amiodarone, anabolic steroids†, androgens†, antibiotics†,

---

†See page 52.   *See page 53.

antithyroid drugs†, carmustine, chloroquine, dantrolene, daunorubicin, disulfiram, divalproex, estrogens†, etretinate, felodipine, gold salts†, hydroxychloroquine, mercaptopurine, methotrexate, methyldopa, naltrexone, nifedipine, oral contraceptives, phenothiazines†, plicamycin, valproic acid, verapamil

ALLERGIC REACTIONS AND SIDE EFFECTS

If you are allergic to any azole derivatives†, you may also be allergic to this drug. You should tell your doctor about all your allergies and any unexplained symptoms you may have while taking this drug.

MORE COMMON SIDE EFFECTS: Allergy, nausea, shortness of breath*, skin rash*, yellow eyes or skin*

LESS COMMON SIDE EFFECTS: Chills*, constipation, diarrhea, dizziness, drowsiness, eye sensitivity, fever*, headache, itching*, breast enlargement in men, menstrual dysfunction, sexual dysfunction, vomiting

RARE SIDE EFFECTS: Bleeding*, bruising*, dark urine*, loss of appetite*, pale stools*, skin irritation*, sore throat*, stomach pain*, tiredness*, weakness*

PRECAUTIONS

Be careful driving or handling equipment while taking this drug because it may cause dizziness and drowsiness.

People with a history of liver disease or alcohol abuse may not be able to take this drug.

PREGNANCY AND BREAST-FEEDING

Safety in pregnancy has not been established although the drug is known to harm animal fetuses.

Breast-feeding while taking this drug is not recommended.

HELPFUL COMMENTS

Contact your doctor if your symptoms do not improve after a few weeks.

Do not stop treatment early if you start to feel better. Treatment may last 6 months or longer. It takes the full prescription for this drug to work completely.

Do not measure doses of the oral suspension with anything but a measuring cup intended for use with prescription drugs. Slight inaccuracy from other measuring spoons may result in over- or under-dosing.

FLUCYTOSINE

Available for over 20 years

COMMONLY USED TO TREAT

Fungal infections

DRUG CATEGORY

antifungal
Class: fluorinated pyrimidine

PRODUCTS

Brand-Name Products with No Generic Alternative
Ancobon 250 mg capsule ($$$)
Ancobon 500 mg capsule ($$$$$)
No generics available.
No patents, no exclusivity.

DOSING AND FOOD

Doses are taken 4 times a day.
It is best to take this drug on an empty stomach. Do not eat raw oysters or
other raw shellfish at any time while taking this drug.
Adults: Up to 150 mg/kg per day in divided doses.
Lower doses are used in people with kidney disease.
Forgotten doses: If you are scheduled to take the next dose within a few
hours, do not take the forgotten dose. Otherwise take the forgotten dose
as soon as you remember.

ALCOHOL, DRUG, HERB, AND SUPPLEMENT INTERACTIONS

Alcohol may increase some of the side effects from this drug, depending
on the amount consumed. Ask your doctor about the risks caused by
drinking alcohol with your condition.

**Taking this drug with any of the ones listed below may change the effect of
either drug with the possibility of causing toxicity or decreasing effectiveness:**
amphotericin B

Increased side effects are possible when this drug is taken with those listed below:
antineoplastic†, antithyroid drugs†, azathioprine, chloramphenicol, colchi-
cine, cyclophosphamide, ganciclovir, interferon, mercaptopurine, metho-
trexate, plicamycin, zidovudine

---

†See page 52.   *See page 53.

ALLERGIC REACTIONS AND SIDE EFFECTS

You should tell your doctor about all your allergies and any unexplained symptoms you may have while taking this drug.

This drug promotes the effect of sunlight on the body and may cause severe sunburn and increased sensitivity of the eyes.

MORE COMMON SIDE EFFECTS: Abdominal pain, bleeding*, breathing difficulty*, bruising*, chest pain*, diarrhea, fever*, irregular heartbeat*, itching*, loss of appetite, nausea, skin rash*, sore throat*, tiredness*, vomiting, weakness*, yellow eyes or skin*

LESS COMMON SIDE EFFECTS: Confusion*, dizziness, drowsiness, hallucinations*, headache, hearing loss, lightheadedness, numbness, tingling

PRECAUTIONS

Let your dentist know if you are taking this drug since x-rays may increase the risk of serious side effects.

People with blood disease, kidney disease, or liver disease may not be able to take this drug because of the increased risk of developing serious side effects.

This drug causes changes in your blood that put you at greater risk of getting an infection. Be careful not to cut yourself or get bruised. Tell your doctor if you develop signs of infection, such as fever or sore throat. Your dentist may recommend that you clean your teeth and mouth differently to avoid infection.

Be careful driving or handling equipment while taking this drug because the drug may cause drowsiness.

PREGNANCY AND BREAST-FEEDING

Safety in pregnancy has not been established although the drug is known to harm animal fetuses.

Breast-feeding while taking this drug is not recommended.

HELPFUL COMMENTS

This drug also goes by the generic names 5-FC and 5-fluorocytosine.

Most people take more than 1 capsule to make up each dose. You may be able to reduce the nausea and stomach upset after a dose by waiting 2 to 3 minutes between each capsule.

Contact your doctor if symptoms do not improve after a week of treatment.

Do not stop treatment early if you start to feel better. It takes the full prescription for this drug to work completely.

FLUDROCORTISONE ACETATE

Available for over 20 years

COMMONLY USED TO TREAT

Adrenal gland disorders
Low blood pressure, also known as hypotension

DRUG CATEGORY

antihypotensive
mineralocorticoid replacement
Class: corticosteroid

PRODUCTS

Brand-Name Products with Generic Alternatives
Florinef 0.1 mg tablet (¢¢¢¢¢)
 Generic: fludrocortisone acetate 0.1 mg tablet (n/a)

DOSING AND FOOD

Doses are taken once a day.
This drug may be taken with or without food. Do not eat foods that contain a lot of sodium since they may increase the risk of side effects while taking this drug.

Adults: Up to 0.4 mg per day.

Children: Up to 0.1 mg per day.

Forgotten doses: If you are scheduled to take the next dose within a few hours, do not take the forgotten dose. Otherwise take the forgotten dose as soon as you remember.

ALCOHOL, DRUG, HERB, AND SUPPLEMENT INTERACTIONS

Alcohol may increase some of the side effects from this drug, depending on the amount consumed. Ask your doctor about the risks caused by drinking alcohol with your condition.

Do not take aspirin while on this drug since it may increase the risk of developing severe bleeding problems.

Taking this drug with any of the ones listed below may change the effect of either drug with the possibility of causing toxicity or decreasing effectiveness:
barbiturates†, carbamazepine, corticosteroids†, efavirenz, griseofulvin, isoniazid, modafinil, nevirapine, phenylbutazone, phenytoin, primidone, rifabutin, rifampin, rifapentine, salicylates†

---

†See page 52.   *See page 53.

Severe reactions are possible when this drug is taken with those listed below: acetazolamide, alcohol, amphotericin B, azlocillin, bronchodilators†, capreomycin, carbenicillin, corticotropin, dichlorphenamide, digoxin, diuretics†, insulin, laxatives, methazolamide, mezlocillin, piperacillin, sirolimus, sodium bicarbonate, sodium polystyrene sulfonate, ticarcillin

ALLERGIC REACTIONS AND SIDE EFFECTS

You should tell your doctor about all your allergies and any unexplained symptoms you may have while taking this drug.

MORE COMMON SIDE EFFECTS: Salt retention*, water retention*

LESS COMMON SIDE EFFECTS: Abdominal pain*, acne, agitation*, anxiety*, back pain*, black stools*, blindness*, bloating*, bloody sputum*, blurry vision*, breath odor*, breathing difficulty*, broken bones*, bruising, bulging eyes*, chest pain*, chills*, combativeness*, confusion*, constipation*, convulsions*, cough*, dark urine*, depression*, dizziness*, dry mouth*, dry skin*, eye pain*, fainting*, fat deposits in skin*, fever*, hair growth, hallucinations*, headache*, heartburn*, height loss*, hives*, hunger*, indigestion*, irregular heartbeat*, itching*, joint pain*, leg pain*, lightheadedness*, limp*, loss of appetite*, menstrual changes, muscle cramps*, nausea*, nervousness*, pimples, poor wound healing*, pounding in the ears, red eyes*, red face*, shortness of breath*, skin discoloration*, skin irritation*, sleeping difficulty*, stomachache*, sweating*, swelling*, tears*, thin skin, thirst*, throat disorders*, tiredness*, unconsciousness*, urinary changes*, vision changes*, vomiting*, weakness*, weight gain*, weight loss*, wheezing*, yellow eyes or skin*

PRECAUTIONS

This drug may cause the body to lose calcium and increase the risk of bone disease such as osteoporosis.

If you have high blood pressure, leg swelling, heart disease, or kidney disease, this drug may make those conditions worse.

This drug causes changes in your blood that put you at greater risk of getting an infection. Be careful not to cut yourself or get bruised. Tell your doctor if you develop signs of infection, such as fever or sore throat. Your dentist may recommend that you clean your teeth and mouth differently to avoid infection.

If you have myasthenia gravis, tuberculosis, stomach or intestinal disease, or recent surgery, and develop an infection while taking this drug, those conditions may become worse.

Be careful driving or handling equipment while taking this drug because the drug may cause dizziness.

PREGNANCY AND BREAST-FEEDING

Safety in pregnancy has not been established although the drug is known to harm animal fetuses.

Breast-feeding while taking this drug is not recommended.

HELPFUL COMMENTS

Sucking on hard sugarless candy or chewing sugarless gum may help relieve dry mouth caused by this drug.

Short-term changes in your weight are a direct indication of how much salt and water you are retaining. A weight gain or loss of more than 2 pounds per day or 5 pounds per week should be reported to your doctor.

FLUOXETINE HYDROCHLORIDE

Available since December 1987

COMMONLY USED TO TREAT

Bulimia
Depression

DRUG CATEGORY

antidepressant
Class: selective serotonin reuptake inhibitor (SSRI)

PRODUCTS

Brand-Name Products with No Generic Alternative
Prozac Weekly 90 mg delayed-release capsule ($$$$$)

Brand-Name Products with Generic Alternatives
Sarafem 10 mg capsule ($$$)
Prozac 10 mg capsule ($$$)
  Generic: fluoxetine hydrochloride 10 mg capsule ($$$)
Sarafem 20 mg capsule ($$$)
Prozac 20 mg capsule ($$$)
  Generic: fluoxetine hydrochloride 20 mg capsule ($$$)
Prozac 40 mg capsule ($$$$)
  Generic: fluoxetine hydrochloride 40 mg capsule ($$$$)

† See page 52.   * See page 53.

Prozac 20 mg/5 ml oral solution ($$$$)
  Generic: fluoxetine hydrochloride 20 mg/5 ml oral solution ($$$)

DOSING AND FOOD

Doses of the regular capsules are taken once-a-day. Delayed-release cap-
sules are taken once a week.

It is best to take this drug on an empty stomach, but taking this drug with
a little food may avoid the stomach upset that some people suffer.

Adults: Up to 80 mg per day.

Children age 7 to 18: Up to 20 mg per day.

Lower doses are used in people with liver or kidney disease.

Forgotten doses: Do not take a forgotten dose. Just go back to your usual
schedule with the next dose.

ALCOHOL, DRUG, HERB, AND SUPPLEMENT INTERACTIONS

Alcohol should not be used while taking this drug.

St. John's wort may interact with this drug, leading to possible toxicity,
and should not be used within 2 weeks of taking this drug.

Many OTC drugs used for appetite control, asthma, colds, cough, hay
fever, pain, or sinus problems affect the central nervous system and may
seriously increase the side effects of this drug. Check with your pharma-
cist for products to avoid.

**Taking this drug with any of the ones listed below may change the effect of
either drug with the possibility of causing toxicity or decreasing effectiveness:**
alprazolam, anticoagulants†, aspirin, astemizole, carbamazepine, clonaze-
pine, cyproheptadine, digitoxin, digoxin, flecainide, phenytoin, thiorida-
zine, vinblastine, warfarin

Severe reactions are possible when this drug is taken with those listed below:
amitriptyline, beta blockers†, bromocriptine, buspirone, citalopram, clo-
mipramine, dextromethorphan, fluvoxamine, imipramine, levodopa,
lithium, LSD, marijuana, MDMA (ecstasy), meclobemide, meperidine,
monoamine oxidase inhibitors†, nefazodone, paroxetine, pentazocine,
sertraline, sumatriptan, tramadol, trazodone, tricyclic antidepressants†,
tryptophan, venlafaxine

Increased side effects are possible when this drug is taken with those listed below:
haloperidol

ALLERGIC REACTIONS AND SIDE EFFECTS

You should tell your doctor about all your allergies and any unexplained
symptoms you may have while taking this drug.

This drug promotes the effect of sunlight on the body and may cause severe sunburn and increased sensitivity of the eyes.

MORE COMMON SIDE EFFECTS: Anxiety*, diarrhea*, dizziness, drowsiness*, dry mouth*, heartburn, headache*, hives*, itching*, loss of appetite, nausea*, nervousness, restlessness*, sexual dysfunction*, shaking*, skin rash*, sleeping difficulty*, stomach upset*, sweating*, tiredness, trembling, weakness

LESS COMMON SIDE EFFECTS: Abnormal dreams, chest pain, chills*, constipation, fever*, flushing, frequent urination, gas, hair loss, increased appetite, joint pain*, lightheadedness, menstrual pain, muscle pain*, skin irritation*, stomach cramps, taste changes, vision changes, vomiting*, weight loss*, yawning

RARE SIDE EFFECTS: Body twitches*, breast enlargement*, breast-milk secretion*, breathing difficulty*, confusion*, excitement*, facial movements*, hunger*, irregular heartbeat*, low blood sodium*, low blood sugar*, mood swings*, pale skin*, poor concentration*, seizures*, shivering*, skin spots*, thirst*, unsteadiness*

PRECAUTIONS

You need to wait 2 weeks after stopping a monoamine oxidase inhibitor† before starting this drug.

If you are a diabetic, you may need a change in the dose of your antidiabetic drug† or insulin, since this drug may cause changes in blood sugar.

Be careful driving or handling equipment while taking this drug because it may cause dizziness and drowsiness.

Do not open, crush, break, or chew the extended-release products.

People with a history of seizures, brain disease, or mental retardation, have an increased risk of developing a seizure while taking this drug.

If you have Parkinson's disease, this drug may make that condition worse.

If you develop a skin rash or hives, you should stop taking this drug and call your doctor right away.

Side effects may continue for several weeks after this drug is stopped.

This drug may cause dry mouth, which is associated with a greater risk of cavities. Your dentist may recommend that you clean your teeth and mouth differently to avoid infection.

PREGNANCY AND BREAST-FEEDING

Safety in pregnancy has not been established although the drug is known to harm animal fetuses.

Breast-feeding while taking this drug is not recommended.

† See page 52.　　* See page 53.

HELPFUL COMMENTS

Sucking on hard sugarless candy or chewing sugarless gum may help relieve dry mouth caused by this drug.

Avoid quick movements to minimize dizziness. Dangling your legs over the side of the bed for a few minutes may help reduce dizziness when first waking up.

Even a small weight loss should be reported to your doctor.

It may take up to 5 weeks or longer for the effects of this drug to be noticed, depending on the condition being treated.

FLUOXYMESTERONE

Available for over 20 years

COMMONLY USED TO TREAT

Breast cancer in women
Delayed puberty
Testosterone deficiency

DRUG CATEGORY

antineoplastic
male hormone replacement
Class: androgen

PRODUCTS

Brand-Name Products with No Generic Alternative
Halotestin 2 mg tablet (¢¢¢¢¢)
Halotestin 5 mg tablet ($$)

Brand-Name Products with Generic Alternatives
Halotestin 10 mg tablet ($$$)
  Generic: fluoxymesterone 10 mg tablet ($$)

DOSING AND FOOD

Doses are taken 1 to 4 times a day.
It is best to take this drug at mealtime.
Adult men: Up to 20 mg per day in divided doses.
Adult women: Up to 40 mg per day in divided doses.
Boys: Up to 10 mg per day in divided doses.
Forgotten doses: If more than half the time between doses has passed, do

not take the forgotten dose. Just return to your normal schedule with the next dose. If less than half the time between doses has passed, take the forgotten dose as soon as you remember.

ALCOHOL, DRUG, HERB, AND SUPPLEMENT INTERACTIONS

Alcohol may increase the risk of liver damage from this drug. Ask your doctor about the risks caused by drinking alcohol with your condition.

Taking this drug with any of the ones listed below may change the effect of either drug with the possibility of causing toxicity or decreasing effectiveness: anticoagulants†, oxyphenbutazone

Increased side effects are possible when this drug is taken with those listed below: acetaminophen, amiodarone, anabolic steroids†, antibiotics†, antithyroid drugs†, carmustine, chloroquine, dantrolene, daunorubicin, disulfiram, divalproex, estrogens†, etretinate, gold salts†, hydroxychloroquine, mercaptopurine, methotrexate, methyldopa, naltrexone, oral contraceptives, phenothiazines†, phenytoin, plicamycin, valproic acid

ALLERGIC REACTIONS AND SIDE EFFECTS

If you are allergic to any androgens† or anabolic steroids†, you may also be allergic to this drug. You should tell your doctor about all your allergies and any unexplained symptoms you may have while taking this drug.

MORE COMMON SIDE EFFECTS: Acne*, breast size change*, masculine characteristics in women*, menstrual irregularities*, penile erection*, urinary changes*

LESS COMMON SIDE EFFECTS: Black stools*, bleeding*, bloody vomit*, chills*, confusion*, constipation*, decreased testicle size, depression*, diarrhea, dizziness*, flushing*, hair loss, headache*, itching*, mood swings*, nausea*, nervousness, paranoia*, pubic-hair growth, sexual dysfunction, skin irritation*, sleep disorders, stomach pain, swelling*, thirst*, tiredness*, vomiting*, weakness*, weight gain*, yellow eyes or skin*

RARE SIDE EFFECTS: Abdominal pain*, bad breath*, dark urine*, fever*, hives*, loss of appetite*, mouth sores*, pain*, sore throat*

PRECAUTIONS

Men have a risk of developing painful, prolonged erection of the penis, which requires treatment by a doctor. If this happens, go to your doctor or the nearest emergency room immediately.

If you are a diabetic, you may need a change in the dose of your antidiabetic drug† or insulin, since this drug may cause changes in blood sugar.

---

†See page 52.   *See page 53.

If you have an enlarged prostate, this drug may make the condition worse. This drug may cause the body to retain water. If you have a history of headaches, seizures, heart disease, liver disease, or kidney disease, make sure your doctor knows about these conditions before this drug is prescribed. Report any swelling of your face, feet, hands, or legs right away. High-dose treatment in men may temporarily decrease sperm production. Talk to your doctor if you are planning to have children.

PREGNANCY AND BREAST-FEEDING

This drug may cause birth defects and should not be used during pregnancy. Breast-feeding while taking this drug is not recommended.

HELPFUL COMMENTS

Treatment with this drug should be re-evaluated at least every 6 months. This drug has been used to increase athletic performance without adequate safety information and is classified by the FDA as a controlled substance. The International Olympic Committee and World Anti-Doping Agency have banned this drug from use in competitive sports.

FLUPHENAZINE HYDROCHLORIDE
Available for over 20 years

COMMONLY USED TO TREAT

Mental illness, also known as psychosis

DRUG CATEGORY

antineuralgic
antipsychotic
Class: phenothiazine: piperazine derivative

PRODUCTS

Brand-Name Products with Generic Alternatives
Prolixin 1 mg tablet ($)
  Generic: fluphenazine hydrochloride 1 mg tablet (¢¢)
Prolixin 2.5 mg tablet (n/a)
  Generic: fluphenazine hydrochloride 2.5 mg tablet (¢¢¢)
Prolixin 5 mg tablet ($$)
  Generic: fluphenazine hydrochloride 5 mg tablet (¢¢¢)
Prolixin 10 mg tablet ($$$)

Generic: fluphenazine hydrochloride 10 mg tablet ($)
Prolixin 2.5 mg/5 ml oral elixir ($$)
Generic: fluphenazine hydrochloride 2.5 mg/5 ml oral elixir ($)
Prolixin 5 mg/ml oral concentrate ($$$$)
Generic: fluphenazine hydrochloride 5 mg/ml oral concentrate ($$$)

Other Generic Product Names
Permitil

DOSING AND FOOD

Doses are taken 3 to 4 times a day.
Taking this drug with food or a full glass of milk or water may avoid the stomach upset that some people suffer.

Adults: Up to 20 mg per day in divided doses.

Children: Up to 4 mg per day in divided doses.

Lower doses are used in people over age 65.

Forgotten doses: If you are scheduled to take the next dose within a few hours, do not take the forgotten dose. Otherwise take the forgotten dose as soon as you remember.

ALCOHOL, DRUG, HERB, AND SUPPLEMENT INTERACTIONS

Alcohol should not be used while taking this drug.

Do not use caffeine, kava, or yohimbe while taking this drug since the drug effects may be decreased and severe reactions may occur.

Several OTC drugs used for appetite control, asthma, colds, cough, hay fever, pain, or sinus problems may seriously increase the effects and side effects of this drug. Check with your pharmacist when selecting OTC products.

Taking this drug with any of the ones listed below may change the effect of either drug with the possibility of causing toxicity or decreasing effectiveness: antacids, antidepressants†, antihypertensives†, caffeine, beta blockers†, bromocriptine, dopamine, levodopa, lithium, phenobarbital, phenytoin, warfarin

Severe reactions are possible when this drug is taken with those listed below: alcohol, amantadine, anesthetics, antiarrhythmics†, anticholinergics†, antihistamines†, antithyroid drugs†, anxiolytics†, astemizole, barbiturates†, bromocriptine, cisapride, deferoxamine, disopyramide, diuretics†, epinephrine, erythromycin, levobunolol, lithium, metipranolol, metrizamide, monoamine oxidase inhibitors†, nabilone, narcotics†, pentamidine, phenothiazines†, probucol, procainamide, promethazine, propylthiouracil, quinidine, sympathomimetics†, tricyclic antidepressants†

† *See page 52.*   * *See page 53.*

Increased side effects are possible when this drug is taken with those listed below: antipsychotics†, metoclopramide, metyrosine, pemoline, pimozide, rauwalfia alkaloids†, trimeprazine

ALLERGIC REACTIONS AND SIDE EFFECTS

If you are allergic to any phenothiazines†, you may also be allergic to this drug. You should tell your doctor about all your allergies and any unexplained symptoms you may have while taking this drug.

This drug promotes the effect of sunlight on the body and may cause severe sunburn and increased sensitivity of the eyes.

MORE COMMON SIDE EFFECTS: Breathing difficulty*, chewing action*, congestion, constipation, decreased sweating*, dizziness, drowsiness, dry mouth, eye stare*, eyelid movement*, fainting*, lip smacking*, loss of balance*, muscle spasms*, muscle stiffness*, puffy cheeks*, restlessness*, seizures*, shuffling walk*, tongue movements*, trembling*, twitching*, vision changes*

LESS COMMON SIDE EFFECTS: Breast-milk secretion, breast swelling, dark urine*, menstrual changes, rough tongue, sexual dysfunction, skin rash*, urinary difficulty*, watery mouth, weight gain

RARE SIDE EFFECTS: Abdominal pain*, agitation*, bleeding*, blood pressure change*, bruising*, chest pain*, chills*, clumsiness*, coma*, confusion*, diarrhea*, dreams*, drooling*, excitement*, fast heartbeat*, fever*, hair loss*, headache*, irregular heartbeat*, itching*, joint pain*, loss of bladder control*, mouth sores*, muscle stiffness*, nausea*, penile erection*, red hands*, shivering*, skin discoloration*, sleep disorders*, sore throat*, speaking difficulty*, sweating*, tiredness*, vomiting*, weakness*, yellow eyes or skin*

PRECAUTIONS

If you have a history of enlarged prostate, glaucoma, ulcers, seizures, heart disease, urinary difficulty, or Parkinson's disease, this drug may make those conditions worse.

This drug may decrease the cough reflex, putting people with lung disease at greater risk of developing pneumonia.

Heavy smoking may cause this drug to be less effective.

This drug may cause false results from several diagnostic tests including pregnancy tests and should be stopped for at least 4 days before the test.

This drug should not be stopped suddenly, due to an increased risk of side effects. If you wish to stop taking this drug, ask your doctor for specific instructions.

Be careful driving or handling equipment while taking this drug because the drug may cause drowsiness.

You are more likely to overheat when taking this drug and should avoid exercising in hot weather and using a sauna or hot tub.

This drug may make you more sensitive to cold temperatures.

Touching the liquid form of this drug may cause skin irritation. Make sure you do not spill the liquid, and wash your hands immediately after taking the dose.

This drug may cause dry mouth, which is associated with a greater risk of cavities. Your dentist may recommend that you clean your teeth and mouth differently to avoid infection.

PREGNANCY AND BREAST-FEEDING

Safety in pregnancy has not been established although the drug is known to harm animal fetuses.

Breast-feeding while taking this drug is not recommended.

HELPFUL COMMENTS

If you need to take an antacid, take it either 2 hours before or after taking this drug.

Sucking on hard sugarless candy or chewing sugarless gum may help relieve dry mouth caused by this drug.

FLURAZEPAM

Available for over 20 years

COMMONLY USED TO TREAT

Sleeping difficulty, also known as insomnia

DRUG CATEGORY

sedative-hypnotic
Class: benzodiazepine

PRODUCTS

Brand-Name Products with Generic Alternatives
Dalmane 15 mg capsule ($)
  Generic: flurazepam 15 mg capsule (¢¢)
Dalmane 30 mg capsule ($$)
  Generic: flurazepam 30 mg capsule (¢¢)

---

† See page 52.   * See page 53.

DOSING AND FOOD

Doses are taken once a day.

This drug may be taken with or without food.

Adults: Up to 30 mg per day.

Lower doses are used in people over age 65.

ALCOHOL, DRUG, HERB, AND SUPPLEMENT INTERACTIONS

Alcohol should not be used while taking this drug.

Catnip, kava, lady's slipper, lemon balm, passion flower, sassafras, skullcap, and valerian should not be used while taking this drug due to an increased sedative effect.

Taking this drug with any of the ones listed below may change the effect of either drug with the possibility of causing toxicity or decreasing effectiveness: cimetidine, digoxin, disulfiram, fluvoxamine, haloperidol, itraconazole, ketoconazole, levodopa, nefazodone, oral contraceptives, phenytoin, rifampin, ritonavir

Severe reactions are possible when this drug is taken with those listed below: anesthetics†, antidepressants†, antihistamines†, barbiturates†, monoamine oxidase inhibitors†, narcotics†, phenothiazines†

Increased side effects are possible when this drug is taken with those listed below: aminophylline, theophylline

ALLERGIC REACTIONS AND SIDE EFFECTS

If you are allergic to any benzodiazepines†, you may also be allergic to this drug. You should tell your doctor about all your allergies and any unexplained symptoms you may have while taking this drug.

MORE COMMON SIDE EFFECTS: Clumsiness, delusions*, disorientation*, dizziness, drowsiness, headache, unconsciousness

LESS COMMON SIDE EFFECTS: Anxiety*, confusion*, constipation, depression*, diarrhea, difficulty urinating, dry mouth, irregular heartbeat*, lightheadedness, memory loss*, muscle spasm, nausea, sexual dysfunction, slurry speech, stomach cramps, thirst, trembling, vision changes, vomiting, watery mouth

RARE SIDE EFFECTS: Agitation*, behavior changes*, bleeding*, bruising*, chills*, excitement*, eye movement*, fever*, hallucinations*, irritability*, low blood pressure*, mouth sores*, nervousness*, seizures*, skin irritation*, sore throat*, spastic movements*, tiredness*, weakness*, yellow eyes or skin*

PRECAUTIONS

This drug may be habit forming and will cause severe withdrawal symptoms if stopped abruptly. If you wish to stop taking this drug, ask your doctor for specific instructions.

You need to wait 2 weeks after stopping a monoamine oxidase inhibitor† before starting this drug.

If you have difficulty swallowing, emphysema, asthma, bronchitis, glaucoma, hyperactivity, mental depression, mental illness, myasthenia gravis, porphyria, or sleep apnea, this drug may make those conditions worse.

Heavy smoking may cause this drug to be less effective.

Be careful driving or handling equipment while taking this drug because the drug may cause dizziness and drowsiness.

PREGNANCY AND BREAST-FEEDING

This drug may cause birth defects and should not be used during pregnancy. Breast-feeding while taking this drug is not recommended.

HELPFUL COMMENTS

This drug becomes more effective after 3 to 4 days of use.

Dangling your legs over the side of the bed for a few minutes may help reduce dizziness when first waking up.

FLURBIPROFEN

Available since October 1988

COMMONLY USED TO TREAT

Arthritis

DRUG CATEGORY

antiarthritic
antidysmenorrheal
antiinflammatory
Class: nonsteroidal antiinflammatory

PRODUCTS

Brand-Name Products with Generic Alternatives
Ansaid 50 mg tablet ($)
  Generic: flurbiprofen 50 mg tablet (¢¢¢¢¢)

---

† See page 52.   * See page 53.

Ansaid 100 mg tablet ($$)
  Generic: flurbiprofen 100 mg tablet (¢¢¢)
Ocufen 0.03% ophthalmic solution ($$$$$)
  Generic: flurbiprofen sodium 0.03% ophthalmic solution ($$$$$)

DOSING AND FOOD

Doses are taken 2 to 4 times a day.

It is best to take this drug on an empty stomach, but taking this drug with a little food may avoid the stomach upset that some people suffer.

Adults: Up to 300 mg per day in divided doses.

Lower doses may be used in people with kidney disease.

Forgotten doses: If you are scheduled to take the next dose within a few hours, do not take the forgotten dose. Otherwise take the forgotten dose as soon as you remember.

ALCOHOL, DRUG, HERB, AND SUPPLEMENT INTERACTIONS

Alcohol may increase the risk of serious side effects from this drug. Ask your doctor about the risks caused by drinking alcohol with your condition.

Do not use dong quai, feverfew, garlic, ginger, horse chestnut, red clover, or St. John's wort while taking this drug since they may increase the risk of serious side effects.

Taking this drug with any of the ones listed below may change the effect of either drug with the possibility of causing toxicity or decreasing effectiveness: acetaminophen, antihypertensives†, beta blockers†, digoxin, diuretics†, furosemide, hydrochlorothiazide, lithium, methotrexate, nifedipine, probenecid, sulfonylureas†, sulindac, verapamil

Severe reactions are possible when this drug is taken with those listed below: antibiotics†, anticoagulants†, aspirin, cefamandole, cefoperazone, cefotetan, corticosteroids†, cyclosporine, gold salts†, heparin, nonsteroidal antiinflammatories†, penicillamine, plicamycin, salicylates†, valproic acid, warfarin

ALLERGIC REACTIONS AND SIDE EFFECTS

If you are allergic to aspirin, zomepirac, salicylates†, or other nonsteroidal antiinflammatories†, you may also be allergic to this drug. You should tell your doctor about all your allergies and any unexplained symptoms you may have while taking this drug.

This drug promotes the effect of sunlight on the body and may cause severe sunburn and increased sensitivity of the eyes.

MORE COMMON SIDE EFFECTS: Abdominal pain, diarrhea, headache, heartburn*, indigestion*, itching*, mouth sores*, nausea*, skin rash*, swelling*, weight gain*

LESS COMMON SIDE EFFECTS: Bruising*, constipation, dizziness, drowsiness, gas, high blood pressure*, sweating, vomiting

RARE SIDE EFFECTS: Back pain*, black stools*, bloody urine*, bloody vomit*, blue fingernails*, blue lips*, breathing difficulty*, chest pain*, chest tightness*, chills*, confusion*, cough*, dark urine*, fainting*, fever*, hallucinations*, hearing loss*, hives*, hoarseness*, lip sores*, loss of appetite*, low blood pressure*, mood swings*, muscle cramps*, nosebleeds*, pain*, pale skin*, pale stools*, puffy eyes*, rectal bleeding*, restlessness*, ringing in ears*, runny nose*, seizures*, shortness of breath*, sore throat*, stiff neck*, swollen glands*, swollen tongue*, thirst*, tiredness*, urinary changes*, vision changes*, weakness*, wheezing*, yellow eyes or skin*

PRECAUTIONS

This drug may cause serious stomach problems and possibly ulcers. Be careful to take this drug as directed with food, and let your doctor know if you develop any stomach-related symptoms.

If you use tobacco or have a history of alcohol abuse, stomach problems, intestinal problems, hemorrhoids, diabetes mellitus, severe fluid retention, or systemic lupus erythematosus, there is an increased risk that you will develop side effects while taking this drug.

PREGNANCY AND BREAST-FEEDING

Safety in pregnancy has not been established although the drug is known to harm animal fetuses.

Breast-feeding while taking this drug is not recommended.

HELPFUL COMMENTS

Avoid quick movements to minimize dizziness.

Several nonsteroidal antiinflammatories are available without a prescription in lower, nonprescription strengths, including ibuprofen, ketoprofen, and naproxen.

---

† See page 52.   * See page 53.

FLUTAMIDE

Available since January 1989

COMMONLY USED TO TREAT

Prostate cancer

DRUG CATEGORY

antineoplastic
Class: nonsteroidal antiandrogen

PRODUCTS

Brand-Name Products with Generic Alternatives
Eulexin 125 mg capsule ($$$)
  Generic: flutamide 125 mg capsule ($$)

DOSING AND FOOD

Doses are taken 3 times a day.
This drug may be taken with or without food.
Men: Up to 1,500 mg per day in divided doses.
Forgotten doses: If you are scheduled to take the next dose within a few
hours, do not take the forgotten dose. Otherwise take the forgotten dose
as soon as you remember. If you vomit shortly after taking a dose, call
your doctor to find out if the dose should be repeated.

ALCOHOL, DRUG, HERB, AND SUPPLEMENT INTERACTIONS

Alcohol may increase some of the side effects from this drug, depending
on the amount consumed. Ask your doctor about the risks caused by
drinking alcohol with your condition.

**Taking this drug with any of the ones listed below may change the effect of
either drug with the possibility of causing toxicity or decreasing effectiveness:**
anticoagulants†

ALLERGIC REACTIONS AND SIDE EFFECTS

If you are allergic to bicalutamide or nilutamide, you may also be allergic
to this drug. You should tell your doctor about all your allergies and any
unexplained symptoms you may have while taking this drug.

MORE COMMON SIDE EFFECTS: Breast swelling, breast tenderness, breathing difficulty*, chest tightness*, constipation, cough*, diarrhea, dizziness*, fever*,
headache, hoarseness*, loss of appetite, nausea, runny nose*, sexual dysfunction, sleep disorders, sneezing*, sore throat*, urinary difficulty, wheezing*

LESS COMMON SIDE EFFECTS: Back pain*, bloating, bloody stools*, breathing difficulty*, chest pain*, chills*, confusion, depression*, drowsiness, dry mouth, gas, indigestion, itching*, nervousness, numbness*, pain*, shortness of breath*, skin rash*, swelling*, tingling*, tiredness*, vomiting, weakness*

RARE SIDE EFFECTS: Abdominal pain*, bleeding*, blue fingers*, blue lips*, bruising*, dark urine*, fainting*, head pressure*, skin irritation*, yellow eyes or skin*

PRECAUTIONS

If you have severe liver disease, you may not be able to take this drug.

Smoking tobacco may increase the risk of developing some rare but serious side effects.

Be careful driving or handling equipment while taking this drug because it may cause dizziness.

PREGNANCY AND BREAST-FEEDING

This drug should not be used in women, but if necessary, it should not be used during pregnancy. This drug may interfere with the normal development of a male fetus.

Breast-feeding while taking this drug is not recommended.

HELPFUL COMMENTS

It is very important to continue taking this drug as ordered by the doctor even if the side effects make you feel ill.

Avoid quick movements to minimize dizziness. Dangling your legs over the side of the bed for a few minutes may help reduce dizziness when first waking up.

FLUVASTATIN SODIUM

Available since December 1993

COMMONLY USED TO TREAT

High blood cholesterol and lipids, also known as hyperlipidemia

DRUG CATEGORY

antilipemic
Class: HMG CoA reductase inhibitor (statin)

---

† See page 52.   * See page 53.

PRODUCTS

Brand-Name Products with No Generic Alternative
Lescol 20 mg capsule ($)
Lescol 40 mg capsule ($)
Lescol XL 80 mg extended-release tablet ($$)
No generics available.
Multiple patents that begin to expire in 2011.

DOSING AND FOOD

Doses are taken once a day in the evening.
This drug may be taken with or without food.

Adults: Up to 80 mg per day.

Forgotten doses: If you are scheduled to take the next dose within a few hours, do not take the forgotten dose. Otherwise take the forgotten dose as soon as you remember.

ALCOHOL, DRUG, HERB, AND SUPPLEMENT INTERACTIONS

Alcohol should not be used while taking this drug.
Red yeast rice, banned from sale in the U.S. since 2001, contains a nutrient similar to this class of drugs and may cause toxicity if used while taking this prescription.

Taking this drug with any of the ones listed below may change the effect of either drug with the possibility of causing toxicity or decreasing effectiveness: cholestyramine, cimetidine, colestipol, digoxin, omeprazole, ranitidine, rifampin, warfarin

Severe reactions are possible when this drug is taken with those listed below: clofibrate, cyclosporine, erythromycin, fenofibrate, gemfibrozil, immuno-suppressants†, niacin

Increased side effects are possible when this drug is taken with those listed below: acetaminophen, amiodarone, anabolic steroids†, androgens†, antibiotics†, antithyroid drugs†, carbamazepine, carmustine, chloroquine, dantrolene, daunorubicin, disulfiram, divalproex, etetinate, gold salts†, hydroxy-chloroquine, isoniazid, mercaptopurine, methotrexate, naltrexone, oral contraceptives, phenothiazines†, phenytoin, plicamycin, valproic acid

ALLERGIC REACTIONS AND SIDE EFFECTS

If you are allergic to any HMG-CoA reductase inhibitors (statin)†, you may also be allergic to this drug. You should tell your doctor about all your allergies and any unexplained symptoms you may have while taking this drug.

MORE COMMON SIDE EFFECTS: Chest congestion*, fever*, infection*

LESS COMMON SIDE EFFECTS: Constipation, cough, diarrhea, dizziness, gas, headache, heartburn, itching*, muscle cramps*, nausea, skin rash*, sleeping difficulty, stomach pain*, stuffy nose, tiredness*, toothache, wheezing

RARE SIDE EFFECTS: Sexual dysfunction, weakness*

PRECAUTIONS

This drug should not be used in people with active liver disease.
Liver function should be tested every 1 to 6 months while taking this drug.

PREGNANCY AND BREAST-FEEDING

This drug may cause birth defects and should not be used during pregnancy.
Breast-feeding while taking this drug is not recommended.

HELPFUL COMMENTS

You need to continue with a low-cholesterol diet even after this drug is started.
This drug works best if taken at bedtime.

FLUVOXAMINE MALEATE

Available since December 1994

COMMONLY USED TO TREAT

Obsessive-compulsive disorder

DRUG CATEGORY

behavioral agent
Class: selective serotonin reuptake inhibitor (SSRI)

PRODUCTS

Products Only Available as Generics
fluvoxamine maleate 25 mg tablet ($$)
fluvoxamine maleate 50 mg tablet ($$$)
fluvoxamine maleate 100 mg tablet ($$$)

DOSING AND FOOD

Doses are taken 1 to 2 times a day.
This drug may be taken with or without food.

---

† See page 52.   * See page 53.

Adults: Up to 300 mg per day in divided doses.

Lower doses are used in people with liver disease and adults over age 65.

Forgotten doses: If more than 4 hours have passed since the forgotten dose, do not take the dose. Otherwise take the forgotten dose as soon as you remember.

ALCOHOL, DRUG, HERB, AND SUPPLEMENT INTERACTIONS

Alcohol should not be used while taking this drug.

St. John's wort should not be used while taking this drug since the combination may cause serious side effects.

Many OTC drugs used for appetite control, asthma, colds, cough, hay fever, pain, or sinus problems affect the central nervous system and may result in side effects when taken with this drug. Check with your pharmacist for products to avoid.

Taking this drug with any of the ones listed below may change the effect of either drug with the possibility of causing toxicity or decreasing effectiveness: alprazolam, benzodiazepines†, bromazepam, carbamazepine, clozapine, diazepam, methadone, metoprolol, midazolam, propranolol, theophylline, triazolam, tricyclic antidepressants†, warfarin

Severe reactions are possible when this drug is taken with those listed below: astemizole, cisapride, diltiazem, monoamine oxidase inhibitors†, terfenadine

Increased side effects are possible when this drug is taken with those listed below: bromocriptine, buspirone, dexfenfluramine, dextromethorphan, dihydroergotamine, fenfluramine, levodopa, lithium, LSD, marijuana, meperidine, moclobemide, MDMA (ecstasy), nefazodone, pentazocine, SSRIs†, sumatriptan, tramadol, trazodone, tryptophan, venlafaxine

ALLERGIC REACTIONS AND SIDE EFFECTS

You should tell your doctor about all your allergies and any unexplained symptoms you may have while taking this drug.

MORE COMMON SIDE EFFECTS: Constipation, diarrhea*, dizziness*, drowsiness*, dry mouth*, headache, nausea*, sexual dysfunction*, shortness of breath*, sleep disorders, tiredness, vomiting*

LESS COMMON SIDE EFFECTS: Abdominal pain, behavior changes*, breathing difficulty*, decreased appetite, heartburn, irregular heartbeat*, mood swings*, shaking*, sweating, taste changes, trembling*, twitching*, urinary difficulty*, weight change

RARE SIDE EFFECTS: Agitation*, blurry vision*, breast-milk secretion*, bruising*, chills*, clumsiness*, coma*, confusion*, dilated pupils*, eye irritation*, eye stillness*, facial movements*, fever*, low blood pressure*, menstrual changes*, nosebleeds*, poor coordination*, restlessness*, seizures*, shivering*, skin irritation*, skin rash*, sore throat*, spastic movements*, unsteadiness*, weakness*

PRECAUTIONS

Smoking may cause this drug to be less effective.

You need to wait 2 weeks after stopping a monoamine oxidase inhibitor† before starting this drug.

Be careful driving or handling equipment while taking this drug because it may cause dizziness and drowsiness.

People with a history of brain disease or seizures are at a greater risk of developing a seizure while taking this drug.

This drug may cause dry mouth, which is associated with a greater risk of cavities. Your dentist may recommend that you clean your teeth and mouth differently to avoid infection.

PREGNANCY AND BREAST-FEEDING

Safety in pregnancy has not been established although the drug is known to harm animal fetuses.

Breast-feeding while taking this drug is not recommended.

HELPFUL COMMENTS

It may take up to 3 months for the effects of this drug to be noticed.

Sucking on hard sugarless candy or chewing sugarless gum may help relieve dry mouth caused by this drug.

If switching from this drug to St. John's wort, you should wait about 2 weeks to avoid a drug interaction.

FOSFOMYCIN TROMETHAMINE

Available since December 1996

COMMONLY USED TO TREAT

Urinary tract and bladder infections in women

DRUG CATEGORY

antibiotic
Class: methenamine

---

† See page 52.   * See page 53.

PRODUCTS

Brand-Name Products with No Generic Alternative
Monurol 3 g powder for oral suspension ($$$$$)
No generics available.
No patents, no exclusivity.

DOSING AND FOOD

Only a single dose is taken.
This drug may be taken with or without food, but the powder must be mixed with $1/2$ cup of water.
Women over age 18: Up to 3 g.

ALCOHOL, DRUG, HERB, AND SUPPLEMENT INTERACTIONS

Alcohol may increase some of the side effects from this drug, depending on the amount consumed. Ask your doctor about the risks caused by drinking alcohol with your condition.

Taking this drug with any of the ones listed below may change the effect of either drug with the possibility of causing toxicity or decreasing effectiveness: metoclopramide

ALLERGIC REACTIONS AND SIDE EFFECTS

You should tell your doctor about all your allergies and any unexplained symptoms you may have while taking this drug.

MORE COMMON SIDE EFFECTS: Diarrhea, headache, nausea, vaginal discharge*

LESS COMMON SIDE EFFECTS: Abdominal pain, back pain, dizziness, heartburn, indigestion, menstrual pain, runny nose, skin rash, sore throat, weakness

PRECAUTIONS

Do not take the powdered drug without mixing it with water. Using hot water may destroy the drug.

PREGNANCY AND BREAST-FEEDING

Safety during pregnancy has not been established although there was no evidence of harm during studies in animals.
It is not known if this drug passes into breast milk. Talk to your doctor about the risks associated with breast-feeding while taking this drug.

HELPFUL COMMENTS

Contact your doctor if your symptoms do not improve after 2 to 3 days.

FOSINOPRIL

Available since May 1991

COMMONLY USED TO TREAT

Heart failure
High blood pressure, also known as hypertension

DRUG CATEGORY

antihypertensive
Class: ACE inhibitor

PRODUCTS

Brand-Name Products with No Generic Alternative
Monopril 10 mg tablet ($)
Monopril 20 mg tablet ($)
Monopril 40 mg tablet ($)
No generics available.
Multiple patents that began expiring in 2002.
Combination Products That Contain This Drug
Monopril-HCT tablet ($)

DOSING AND FOOD

Doses are taken once a day.
It is best to take this drug on an empty stomach at least 1 hour before meals.
Adults: Up to 80 mg per day.
This drug is rarely used in children.
Forgotten doses: If you are scheduled to take the next dose within a few hours, do not take the forgotten dose. Otherwise take the forgotten dose as soon as you remember.

ALCOHOL, DRUG, HERB, AND SUPPLEMENT INTERACTIONS

Alcohol may cause your blood pressure to rise, making this drug less effective. Ask your doctor about the risks caused by drinking alcohol with your condition.
Licorice may interfere with the effects of this drug.

† See page 52.   * See page 53.

Capsaicin and other foods or supplements, including hot peppers, sweet peppers, paprika, and chili powder, derived from the capsicum family of plants may increase the risk of developing a cough and should not be taken with this drug.

Several OTC drugs used for appetite control, asthma, colds, cough, hay fever, or sinus problems may cause an increase in blood pressure when taken with this drug. Check with your pharmacist when selecting OTC products.

Taking this drug with any of the ones listed below may change the effect of either drug with the possibility of causing toxicity or decreasing effectiveness: antacids, antidiabetics†, antihypertensives†, diuretics†, insulin, lithium, potassium supplements

ALLERGIC REACTIONS AND SIDE EFFECTS

If you are allergic to any ACE inhibitors†, you may also be allergic to this drug. You should tell your doctor about all your allergies and any unexplained symptoms you may have while taking this drug.

MORE COMMON SIDE EFFECTS: Breathing difficulty*, chest pain*, dry cough, headache, swallowing difficulty*, swelling*

LESS COMMON SIDE EFFECTS: Diarrhea, dizziness*, fainting*, fever*, joint pain*, lightheadedness*, loss of taste, nausea, skin rash*, tiredness

RARE SIDE EFFECTS: Abdominal pain*, chills*, confusion*, hoarseness*, irregular heartbeat*, itching*, nausea*, nervousness*, numbness*, stomach pain*, vomiting*, weakness*, yellow eyes or skin*

PRECAUTIONS

Be careful driving or handling equipment while taking this drug because the drug may cause drowsiness.

People with systemic lupus erythematosus may be at greater risk of developing blood problems while taking this drug.

Do not use potassium-containing products, including salt substitutes, while taking this drug.

Diuretics† should be stopped 2 to 3 days prior to starting this drug. If it is not possible to stop the diuretic, the dose of this drug should be lowered.

Drink plenty of fluids to avoid dehydration when sweating, such as in hot weather and during exercise.

PREGNANCY AND BREAST-FEEDING

Safety in pregnancy has not been established although the drug is known to harm animal fetuses.

Breast-feeding while taking this drug is not recommended.

HELPFUL COMMENTS

It may take several weeks before the full effects of this drug are noticed.

A persistent dry cough may appear while taking this drug, but it will go away when the drug is stopped.

If you need to take an antacid, take it either 2 hours before or after taking this drug.

FROVATRIPTAN SUCCINATE

Available since November 2001

COMMONLY USED TO TREAT

Migraine headache

DRUG CATEGORY

antimigraine
Class: triptan

PRODUCTS

Brand-Name Products with No Generic Alternative
Frova 2.5 mg tablet (n/a)
No generics available.
Multiple patents that begin to expire in 2012. Exclusivity until 2006.

DOSING AND FOOD

Doses are taken once and repeated two more times if instructed.
It is best to take this drug on an empty stomach with water.
Adults: Up to 7.5 mg per day in divided doses.

ALCOHOL, DRUG, HERB, AND SUPPLEMENT INTERACTIONS

Alcohol may make your headache worse. You should ask your doctor about drinking alcohol with your condition.

Taking this drug with any of the ones listed below may change the effect of either drug with the possibility of causing toxicity or decreasing effectiveness:
oral contraceptives, propranolol

Severe reactions are possible when this drug is taken with those listed below:
ergot alkaloids†, monoamine oxidase inhibitors†, naratriptan, rizatriptan, sumatriptan, zolmitriptan

Increased side effects are possible when this drug is taken with those listed below:
fluvoxamine, fluoxetine, paroxetine, sertraline

† See page 52.   * See page 53.

ALLERGIC REACTIONS AND SIDE EFFECTS

You should tell your doctor about all your allergies and any unexplained symptoms you may have while taking this drug.

MORE COMMON SIDE EFFECTS: Dizziness

LESS COMMON SIDE EFFECTS: Belching, bone pain, chest pain*, chills, drowsiness, dry mouth, flushing, heartburn, indigestion, nausea, sour stomach, stomach pain, tingling, tiredness, weakness

RARE SIDE EFFECTS: Chest tightness*

PRECAUTIONS

This drug is used to treat a headache that has already started, but is not used to prevent headaches from occurring.

If you have a history of stroke, blood vessel disease, heart disease, or high blood pressure, you may not be able to take this drug.

You need to wait 2 weeks after stopping a monoamine oxidase inhibitor† before starting this drug.

Be careful driving or handling equipment while taking this drug because it may cause dizziness.

Doses should not be taken more frequently than once every 2 hours.

PREGNANCY AND BREAST-FEEDING

Safety during pregnancy has not been established although the drug is known to harm animal fetuses.

Breast-feeding while taking this drug is not recommended.

HELPFUL COMMENTS

This drug works best if taken at the first sign that a migraine headache is about to start.

If the first dose of this drug does not relieve the headache pain, it is not likely that additional doses will work any better.

FUROSEMIDE

Available for over 20 years

COMMONLY USED TO TREAT

Fluid retention, also known as edema

High blood pressure, also known as hypertension

High calcium levels, also known as hypercalcemia

DRUG CATEGORY

antihypercalcemic
antihypertensive
Class: loop diuretic

PRODUCTS

Brand-Name Products with Generic Alternatives

Lasix 10 mg/ml oral solution (n/a)
  Generic: furosemide 10 mg/ml oral solution (¢¢¢¢¢)
Lasix 20 mg tablet (¢¢)
  Generic: furosemide 20 mg tablet (¢)
Lasix 40 mg tablet (¢¢¢)
  Generic: furosemide 40 mg tablet (¢)
Lasix 80 mg tablet (¢¢¢¢)
  Generic: furosemide 80 mg tablet (¢¢)

Products Only Available as Generics

furosemide 40 mg/5 ml oral solution (¢¢¢)

Other Generic Product Names

Furocot

DOSING AND FOOD

Doses are given 1 to 4 times a day.

It is better to take this drug on an empty stomach, but taking this drug with food or milk may avoid the stomach upset that some people suffer.

Adults: Up to 600 mg per day in divided doses.

Children: Up to 6 mg/kg per day in divided doses.

Forgotten doses: If you are scheduled to take the next dose within a few hours, do not take the forgotten dose. Otherwise take the forgotten dose as soon as you remember.

ALCOHOL, DRUG, HERB, AND SUPPLEMENT INTERACTIONS

Alcohol may increase some of the side effects from this drug, depending on the amount consumed. Ask your doctor about the risks caused by drinking alcohol with your condition.

Several OTC drugs used for appetite control, asthma, colds, cough, hay fever, or sinus problems may cause an increase in blood pressure when taken with this drug. Check with your pharmacist when selecting OTC products.

---

† See page 52.   * See page 53.

Aloe, dandelion, ginseng, and licorice root may all interfere with this drug.

Taking this drug with any of the ones listed below may change the effect of either drug with the possibility of causing toxicity or decreasing effectiveness: amiloride, amphotericin B, antihypertensives†, aspirin, cardiac glycosides†, corticosteroids†, corticotropin, diuretics†, indomethacin, lithium, metolazone, nonsteroidal antiinflammatories†, probenecid, spironolactone, sucralfate, triamterene

Severe reactions are possible when this drug is taken with those listed below: aminoglycosides†, cephalosporins†, cisplatin, ethacrynic acid

ALLERGIC REACTIONS AND SIDE EFFECTS

You should tell your doctor about all your allergies and any unexplained symptoms you may have while taking this drug.

This drug promotes the effect of sunlight on the body and may cause severe sunburn and increased sensitivity of the eyes.

MORE COMMON SIDE EFFECTS: Dizziness, lightheadedness

LESS COMMON SIDE EFFECTS: Blurry vision, diarrhea, headache, loss of appetite, sexual dysfunction, stomach cramps

RARE SIDE EFFECTS: Back pain*, black stools*, bleeding*, bloody urine, bruising*, chills*, cough*, dry mouth*, fever*, hearing loss*, hives*, hoarseness*, irregular heartbeat*, joint pain*, mood swings*, muscle cramps*, nausea*, painful urination*, ringing in ears*, skin rash*, stomach pain*, thirst*, tiredness*, vomiting*, weak pulse*, weakness*, yellow eyes or skin*

PRECAUTIONS

If you are diabetic, you may need a change in the dose of your antidiabetic drug or insulin, since this drug may cause changes in blood sugar.

Your body may lose potassium while taking this drug, which may cause severe side effects. Potassium levels should be monitored periodically and may need to be supplemented while taking this drug. Eat food rich in potassium, such as apricots, bananas, citrus fruit, dates, and tomatoes, if you are not taking a potassium supplement or potassium-sparing diuretic†.

If you have gout, hearing problems, or pancreatitis, this drug may make those conditions worse.

Be careful driving or handling equipment while taking this drug because the drug may cause drowsiness.

Drink plenty of fluids to avoid dehydration when sweating, such as in hot weather and during exercise.

PREGNANCY AND BREAST-FEEDING

Safety in pregnancy has not been established although the drug is known to harm animal fetuses.

Breast-feeding while taking this drug is not recommended.

HELPFUL COMMENTS

This drug will cause you to urinate. The effect should start about 30 minutes after taking the dose and will peak at about 2 hours.

This drug should be taken in the morning to reduce the chance of having to urinate during the night.

Short-term changes in your weight are a direct indication of how much fluid you are retaining. A weight gain or loss of more than 2 pounds per day or 5 pounds per week should be reported to your doctor.

The oral-solution products should be kept refrigerated.

GABAPENTIN

Available since December 1993

COMMONLY USED TO TREAT

Seizures

DRUG CATEGORY

anticonvulsant
Class: 1-aminomethyl cyclohexoneacetic acid

PRODUCTS

Brand-Name Products with No Generic Alternative
Neurontin 100 mg capsule (¢¢¢¢)
Neurontin 300 mg capsule ($)
Neurontin 400 mg capsule ($$)
Neurontin 600 mg capsule ($$)
Neurontin 800 mg capsule ($$$)
Neurontin 250 mg/5 ml oral solution ($)
No generics available.
Multiple patents that begin to expire in 2008.

DOSING AND FOOD

Doses are taken 3 times a day.
This drug may be taken with or without food.

† See page 52.   * See page 53.

Adults and children over age 12: Up to 3,600 mg daily in divided doses.

Children age 5 to 12: Up to 35 mg/kg per day in divided doses.

Children age 3 to 4: Up to 40 mg/kg per day in divided doses.

Lower doses are used in people with kidney disease.

Forgotten doses: Take the forgotten dose as soon as you remember even if it is time for the next dose. If you are scheduled to take the next dose in less than 2 hours, adjust the schedule to take the next dose 1 to 2 hours late. Then return to your regular schedule.

ALCOHOL, DRUG, HERB, AND SUPPLEMENT INTERACTIONS

Alcohol should not be used while taking this drug.

Several OTC drugs used for appetite control, asthma, colds, cough, hay fever, pain, or sinus problems may seriously increase the side effects of this drug. Check with your pharmacist when selecting OTC products.

Taking this drug with any of the ones listed below may change the effect of either drug with the possibility of causing toxicity or decreasing effectiveness:
antacids

ALLERGIC REACTIONS AND SIDE EFFECTS

You should tell your doctor about all your allergies and any unexplained symptoms you may have while taking this drug.

MORE COMMON SIDE EFFECTS: Anxiety*, behavior changes*, blurry vision, clumsiness*, crying*, depression*, distrust*, dizziness*, double vision*, drowsiness*, elevated emotions*, eye movement*, hyperactivity*, mood swings*, muscle pain*, poor concentration*, restlessness*, shaking*, spastic movements*, swelling*, tiredness*, trembling*, unsteadiness*, weakness*

LESS COMMON SIDE EFFECTS: Back pain*, constipation, diarrhea*, dry mouth, headache, indigestion, irritability*, low blood pressure, memory loss*, nausea, ringing in the ears, runny nose, sexual dysfunction, sleep disorders, slurry speech, throat irritation, twitching, urinary changes*, vomiting, weight gain

RARE SIDE EFFECTS: Chills*, cough*, fever*, hoarseness*, sluggishness*, slurry speech*

PRECAUTIONS

For this drug to be most effective, no more than 12 hours should lapse between doses.

Capsules may be opened and the contents mixed with applesauce or juice for easier swallowing. Do not mix doses in advance.

Avoid contact with anyone who has the chickenpox, measles, or other communicable disease since it may be easier to catch the infection while taking this drug.

Be careful driving or handling equipment while taking this drug because it may cause vision change, dizziness, and drowsiness.

Stopping this drug suddenly may cause additional seizure activity. If you wish to stop taking this drug, ask your doctor for specific instructions.

PREGNANCY AND BREAST-FEEDING

Safety in pregnancy has not been established although the drug is known to harm animal fetuses.

Breast-feeding while taking this drug is not recommended.

HELPFUL COMMENTS

If you need to take an antacid, take it either 2 hours before or after taking this drug.

Take your first dose at bedtime so you do not notice the drowsiness and dizziness that may occur.

GALANTAMINE HYDROBROMIDE

Available since February 2001

COMMONLY USED TO TREAT

Alzheimer's disease

DRUG CATEGORY

antidementia
Class: cholinesterase inhibitor

PRODUCTS

Brand-Name Products with No Generic Alternative
Reminyl 4 mg tablet ($$)
Reminyl 8 mg tablet ($$)
Reminyl 12 mg tablet ($$)
Reminyl 4 mg/ml oral solution ($$$$)
No generics available.
Multiple patents that begin to expire in 2006. Exclusivity until 2006.

---

†See page 52.   * See page 53.

DOSING AND FOOD

Doses are taken twice a day.

It is best to take this drug with food and a full glass of water at the morning and evening meal. If vomiting occurs within 1 hour after a dose, contact your doctor to determine if the dose should be repeated.

Adults: Up to 24 mg per day in divided doses.

Lower doses are used in people with liver disease.

Forgotten doses: If more than 2 hours have passed since the forgotten dose, do not take the dose. Otherwise take the forgotten dose as soon as you remember.

ALCOHOL, DRUG, HERB, AND SUPPLEMENT INTERACTIONS

Alcohol may increase some of the side effects from this drug, depending on the amount consumed. Ask your doctor about the risks caused by drinking alcohol with your condition.

Several OTC drugs used for appetite control, asthma, colds, cough, hay fever, pain, or sinus problems may seriously increase the side effects of this drug. Check with your doctor or pharmacist when selecting OTC products.

Taking this drug with any of the ones listed below may change the effect of either drug with the possibility of causing toxicity or decreasing effectiveness: amitriptyline, anticholinergics†, bethanechol, cholinergics†, cimetidine, erythromycin, fluoxetine, fluvoxamine, ketoconazole, paroxetine, quinidine, succinylcholine

ALLERGIC REACTIONS AND SIDE EFFECTS

You should tell your doctor about all your allergies and any unexplained symptoms you may have while taking this drug.

MORE COMMON SIDE EFFECTS: Diarrhea, loss of appetite, nausea*, slow heart rate*, vomiting*, weight loss

LESS COMMON SIDE EFFECTS: Abdominal pain, back pain, bleeding, blood pressure changes*, bloody urine, breathing difficulty*, bruising, dizziness*, drowsiness, fainting*, headache, indigestion, irregular heartbeat*, lightheadedness, pale skin, sleep disorders, stuffy nose, tiredness, tremor, urinary pain, weakness*

RARE SIDE EFFECTS: Drooling*, frequent bowel movements*, frequent urination*, seizures*, stomach cramps*, sweating*, watery eyes*, watery mouth*

PRECAUTIONS

If you have a history of asthma, arrhythmias, urinary difficulty, or stomach ulcers, this drug may make those conditions worse.

People with a history of seizures are at greater risk of developing a seizure while taking this drug.

Learn how to measure your heart rate and call your doctor if it falls below 50 beats per minute.

PREGNANCY AND BREAST-FEEDING

Safety in pregnancy has not been established although there was no evidence of harm during studies in animals.

Breast-feeding while taking this drug is not recommended.

HELPFUL COMMENTS

It takes about 4 weeks for the full effects of this drug to be noticed.

Do not measure doses of the oral solution with anything but a measuring spoon intended for use with prescription drugs. Slight inaccuracy from other measuring spoons may result in over- or under-dosing.

GANCICLOVIR

Available since June 1989

COMMONLY USED TO TREAT

Viral infections, specifically cytomegalovirus in AIDS

DRUG CATEGORY

antiviral
Class: synthetic nucleoside

PRODUCTS

Brand-Name Products with No Generic Alternative

Cytovene 250 mg capsule ($$$)
Cytovene 500 mg capsule ($$$$)
No generics available.
Multiple patents that begin to expire in 2003.

DOSING AND FOOD

Doses are taken 3 to 6 times a day.

It is best to take this drug with food or milk. Do not eat raw oysters or other raw shellfish at any time while taking this drug.

Adults: Up to 3,000 mg per day in divided doses.

Lower doses are used in people with kidney disease.

Forgotten doses: If you are scheduled to take the next dose within a few hours, do not take the forgotten dose. Otherwise take the forgotten dose as soon as you remember.

ALCOHOL, DRUG, HERB, AND SUPPLEMENT INTERACTIONS

Alcohol may increase some of the side effects from this drug, depending on the amount consumed. Ask your doctor about the risks caused by drinking alcohol with your condition.

Taking this drug with any of the ones listed below may change the effect of either drug with the possibility of causing toxicity or decreasing effectiveness: didanosine, probenecid

Severe reactions are possible when this drug is taken with those listed below: amphotericin B, antineoplastics†, antithyroid drugs†, azathioprine, chloramphenicol, colchicine, cyclophosphamide, flucytosine, imipenem/cilsastatin, immunosuppressants†, interferon, mercaptopurine, zidovudine

Increased side effects are possible when this drug is taken with those listed below: acetaminophen, antibiotics†, carmustine, cisplatin, cyclosporine, deferoxamine, gold salts†, lithium, methotrexate, nonnarcotic antiinflammatories†, penicillamine, plicamycin, salicylates†, streptozocin, tiopronin, zidovudine

ALLERGIC REACTIONS AND SIDE EFFECTS

If you are allergic to acyclovir, you may also be allergic to this drug. You should tell your doctor about all your allergies and any unexplained symptoms you may have while taking this drug.

MORE COMMON SIDE EFFECTS: Abdominal pain, bleeding*, bruising*, diarrhea, fever*, loss of appetite, nausea, seizures*, skin rash*, sore throat*, sweating

LESS COMMON SIDE EFFECTS: Agitation, anxiety, confusion, dizziness, drowsiness, dry mouth, eye damage, gas, headache, heartburn, memory loss, mood swings*, nervousness*, numbness, tingling, tiredness*, tremor*, vivid dreams, vomiting, weakness*

PRECAUTIONS

This drug causes changes in your blood that put you at greater risk of getting an infection. Be careful not to cut yourself or get bruised. Tell your doctor if you develop signs of infection, such as fever or sore throat. Your dentist may recommend that you clean your teeth and mouth differently to avoid infection.

If you have a low platelet count or a low white blood cell count, this drug may make those conditions worse.

PREGNANCY AND BREAST-FEEDING

Safety in pregnancy has not been established although the drug is known to harm animal fetuses.

Breast-feeding while taking this drug is not recommended.

HELPFUL COMMENTS

This drug is also called by the generic name DHPG.

GATIFLOXACIN

Available since December 1999

COMMONLY USED TO TREAT

Infection

DRUG CATEGORY

antibiotic
Class: fluoroquinolone

PRODUCTS

Brand-Name Products with No Generic Alternative
Tequin 200 mg tablet ($$$$)
Tequin 400 mg tablet ($$$$)
No generics available.
Multiple patents that begin to expire in 2007.

DOSING AND FOOD

Doses are taken once a day.
It is best to take this drug on an empty stomach, 2 hours after a meal.
Adults: Up to 400 mg per day.
Lower doses are used in people with kidney disease.
This drug is rarely used in children under age 18 because it may interfere with bone development.

Forgotten doses: If you are scheduled to take the next dose within a few hours, do not take the forgotten dose. Otherwise take the forgotten dose as soon as you remember.

ALCOHOL, DRUG, HERB, AND SUPPLEMENT INTERACTIONS

Alcohol may increase some of the side effects from this drug, depending on the amount consumed. Ask your doctor about the risks caused by drinking alcohol with your condition.

Taking this drug with any of the ones listed below may change the effect of either drug with the possibility of causing toxicity or decreasing effectiveness: antacids, antidiabetics†, digoxin, iron, mineral supplements, probenecid, sucralfate, warfarin

Severe reactions are possible when this drug is taken with those listed below: amiodarone, antipsychotics†, astemizole, bepridil, cisapride, erythromycin, nonsteroidal antiinflammatories†, phenothiazines†, procainamide, quinidine, sotalol, tricyclic antidepressants†

ALLERGIC REACTIONS AND SIDE EFFECTS

If you are allergic to any fluoroquinolones†, you may also be allergic to this drug. You should tell your doctor about all your allergies and any unexplained symptoms you may have while taking this drug.

This drug promotes the effect of sunlight on the body and may cause severe sunburn and increased sensitivity of the eyes.

LESS COMMON SIDE EFFECTS: Back pain, blisters*, diarrhea*, dizziness, dreams, drowsiness, headache, lightheadedness, mouth sores, muscle pain, nausea, nervousness, rash, seizures*, skin irritation*, sleep disorders, stomachache, taste changes, urinary difficulty, vaginal discharge, vaginal pain, vision changes, vomiting

RARE SIDE EFFECTS: Abdominal pain*, agitation*, bloody urine*, confusion*, dark urine*, fever*, flushing*, hallucinations*, irregular heartbeat*, joint pain*, leg pain*, loss of appetite*, pale stools*, shakiness*, shortness of breath*, sweating*, swelling*, tiredness*, tremors*, weakness*, yellow eyes or skin*

PRECAUTIONS

If you are a diabetic, you may need a change in the dose of your antidiabetic drug† or insulin, since this drug may cause changes in blood sugar.

If you have a history of tendinitis, this drug may make that condition worse.

Be careful driving or handling equipment while taking this drug because the drug may cause drowsiness.

PREGNANCY AND BREAST-FEEDING

Safety in pregnancy has not been established although the drug is known to harm animal fetuses.

Breast-feeding while taking this drug is not recommended.

HELPFUL COMMENTS

Contact your doctor if your symptoms do not improve after a couple of days.

Do not stop treatment early if you start to feel better. It takes the full prescription for this drug to work completely.

If you need to take an antacid, minerals, or iron supplements, take them either 4 hours before or after taking this drug.

Drink a lot of water while taking this drug.

GEFITINIB

Available since May 2003

COMMONLY USED TO TREAT

Lung cancer

DRUG CATEGORY

antineoplastic
Class: anilinoquinazoline

PRODUCTS

Brand-Name Products with No Generic Alternative
Iressa 250 mg tablet (n/a)
No generics available.
Exclusivity until 2008.

DOSING AND FOOD

Doses are taken once a day.
This drug may be taken with or without food.
Adults: Up to 250 mg per day.
Forgotten doses: If you are scheduled to take the next dose in less than 7 hours, do not take the forgotten dose. Otherwise take the forgotten dose as soon as you remember.

---

† See page 52.   * See page 53.

ALCOHOL, DRUG, HERB, AND SUPPLEMENT INTERACTIONS

Alcohol may increase some of the side effects from this drug, depending on the amount consumed. Ask your doctor about the risks caused by drinking alcohol with your condition.

There may be additional drug interactions that have not yet been identified since this drug is relatively new. Check with your pharmacist for the current list of drug interactions.

Taking this drug with any of the ones listed below may change the effect of either drug with the possibility of causing toxicity or decreasing effectiveness: barbiturates†, carbamazepine, cimetidine, corticosteroids†, famotidine, griseofulvin, itraconzole, ketoconazole, nafcillin, nizatidine, phenytoin, ranitidine, rifampin, troglitazone

ALLERGIC REACTIONS AND SIDE EFFECTS

You should tell your doctor about all your allergies and any unexplained symptoms you may have while taking this drug.

MORE COMMON SIDE EFFECTS: Acne, diarrhea*, dry skin, itching, loss of appetite*, nausea*, skin rash, vomiting*, weakness, weight loss.

LESS COMMON SIDE EFFECTS: Cough*, eye irritation*, hives*, mouth sores*, shortness of breath*, swelling*, vision changes*

PRECAUTIONS

People with liver disease may not be able to take this drug.

Your treatment may need to be temporarily stopped if you develop too many side effects from this drug, especially those related to the lungs.

If you develop eye irritation, look for an eyelash in your eye since this drug may cause your eyelashes to grow.

Since this drug is still relatively new, ask your pharmacist about any additional precautions each time you get your prescription refilled.

This drug is only used after the disease has not responded to treatment with other drugs.

PREGNANCY AND BREAST-FEEDING

There is evidence that this drug may harm the fetus, but the drug may be necessary to the health of the mother.

Breast-feeding while taking this drug is not recommended.

HELPFUL COMMENTS

It takes about 10 days for this drug to reach a constant blood level and begin working.

Eye irritation caused by this drug may be reduced by wearing sunglasses when outside.

GEMFIBROZIL

Available since November 1986

COMMONLY USED TO TREAT

High blood cholesterol, triglycerides, and lipids, also known as hyperlipidemia

DRUG CATEGORY

antilipemic
Class: fibric acid derivative

PRODUCTS

Brand-Name Products with Generic Alternatives
Lopid 600 mg tablet ($$)
  Generic: gemfibrozil 600 mg tablet (¢¢¢)

DOSING AND FOOD

Doses are taken twice a day.
Take this drug about 30 minutes before breakfast and dinner.
Adults: Up to 1,200 mg per day in divided doses.
Forgotten doses: If you are scheduled to take the next dose within a few hours, do not take the forgotten dose. Otherwise take the forgotten dose as soon as you remember.

ALCOHOL, DRUG, HERB, AND SUPPLEMENT INTERACTIONS

Alcohol may increase the risk of liver damage from this drug. Ask your doctor about the risks caused by drinking alcohol with your condition.

Taking this drug with any of the ones listed below may change the effect of either drug with the possibility of causing toxicity or decreasing effectiveness: anticoagulants†, beta blockers†, estrogens†, thiazide diuretics†

Severe reactions are possible when this drug is taken with those listed below: atorvastatin, fluvastatin, lovastatin, pravastatin, simvastatin

ALLERGIC REACTIONS AND SIDE EFFECTS

If you are allergic to clofibrate, you may also be allergic to this drug. You should tell your doctor about all your allergies and any unexplained symptoms you may have while taking this drug.

---

† See page 52.   * See page 53.

MORE COMMON SIDE EFFECTS: Heartburn, gas, stomachache

LESS COMMON SIDE EFFECTS: Abdominal pain, constipation, diarrhea, fever*, itching, irregular heartbeat*, nausea*, skin rash, vomiting*

RARE SIDE EFFECTS: Back pain*, chills*, cough*, hoarseness*, muscle pain*, stomach pain*, tiredness*, urinary difficulty*, weakness*

PRECAUTIONS

There is research suggesting that this drug may be associated with a greater risk of cancer, although the studies are not conclusive.

If you have gallstones or gallbladder disease, this drug may make those conditions worse.

PREGNANCY AND BREAST-FEEDING

Safety in pregnancy has not been established although the drug is known to harm animal fetuses.

Breast-feeding while taking this drug is not recommended.

HELPFUL COMMENTS

You need to continue with a low-cholesterol diet even after this drug is started. Increasing the fiber in your diet may help relieve the constipation that some people suffer.

GLIMEPIRIDE

Available since November 1995

COMMONLY USED TO TREAT

High blood sugar, specifically type 2 diabetes

DRUG CATEGORY

antidiabetic
Class: sulfonylurea: second generation

PRODUCTS

Brand-Name Products with No Generic Alternative
Amaryl 1 mg tablet (¢¢¢)
Amaryl 2 mg tablet (¢¢¢)
Amaryl 4 mg tablet (¢¢¢¢¢)
No generics available.
Patent expires in 2005.

DOSING AND FOOD

Doses are taken once a day.

It is best to take this drug just before breakfast.

Adults: Up to 8 mg per day.

Lower doses are used in people over age 65.

People with kidney or liver disease may need lower doses.

Forgotten doses: If you are scheduled to take the next dose in less than 12 hours, do not take the forgotten dose. Otherwise take the forgotten dose as soon as you remember.

ALCOHOL, DRUG, HERB, AND SUPPLEMENT INTERACTIONS

Alcohol should not be used while taking this drug since the combination may cause a severe reaction.

Aloe, bilberry leaf, bitter melon, burdock, dandelion, fenugreek, garlic, ginkgo biloba, and ginseng may lower blood sugar and cause the need for a dose adjustment when taken with this drug. Tell your doctor if you are taking any of these supplements.

Several OTC drugs used for asthma, colds, cough, hay fever, sleep aid, or sinus problems may seriously change the effects of this drug. Check with your pharmacist when selecting OTC products.

Taking this drug with any of the ones listed below may change the effect of either drug with the possibility of causing toxicity or decreasing effectiveness: anticoagulants†, antihistamines†, aspirin, beta blockers†, calcium channel blockers†, chloramphenicol, cimetidine, corticosteroids†, cyclosporine, estrogens†, fluconazole, fluoroquinolones†, insulin, isoniazid, lithium, miconazole, nonsteroidal antiinflammatories†, oral contraceptives, phenothiazines†, probenecid, quinine, quinidine, ranitidine, salicylates†, sulfonamides†, sympathomimetics†, thiazide diuretics†, triamterene

Severe reactions are possible when this drug is taken with those listed below: guanethidine, monoamine oxidase inhibitors†, octreotide, pentamidine

ALLERGIC REACTIONS AND SIDE EFFECTS

If you are allergic to any sulfonylureas† or sulfonamides†, you may also be allergic to this drug. You should tell your doctor about all your allergies and any unexplained symptoms you may have while taking this drug.

This drug promotes the effect of sunlight on the body and may cause severe sunburn and increased sensitivity of the eyes.

MORE COMMON SIDE EFFECTS: Anxiety*, appetite changes, behavior change*, blurry vision*, chills*, confusion*, constipation, diarrhea,

---

†*See page 52.*   **See page 53.*

drowsiness*, fast heartbeat*, frequent urination, gas, heartburn, hunger*, low blood sugar*, nausea*, nervousness*, nightmares*, poor concentration*, shakiness*, sleep disorders*, slurry speech*, stomach pain, sweating*, taste changes, tiredness*, vomiting, weakness*, weight gain*

LESS COMMON SIDE EFFECTS: Dizziness, headache*, seizures*, skin irritation*, unconsciousness*

RARE SIDE EFFECTS: Bleeding*, bruising*, chest pain*, coughing up blood*, dark urine*, excess sputum*, fever*, hives*, pale skin*, pale stools*, shortness of breath*, sore throat*, yellow eyes or skin*

PRECAUTIONS

Burns, diarrhea, fever, hormonal changes, infection, malnourishment, severe stress, uncontrolled thyroid disease, and vomiting may cause changes in blood sugar that may make this drug less effective.

You need to wait 2 weeks after stopping a monoamine oxidase inhibitor† before starting this drug.

This drug is not effective in treating type 1 diabetes.

PREGNANCY AND BREAST-FEEDING

Safety in pregnancy has not been established although the drug is known to harm animal fetuses.

Breast-feeding while taking this drug is not recommended.

HELPFUL COMMENTS

Blood sugar level should be checked if you experience any side effects.

If you do not treat high blood sugar, you may develop more serious problems such as heart failure, blood vessel disease, eye disease, or kidney disease.

GLIPIZIDE

Available since May 1984

COMMONLY USED TO TREAT

High blood sugar, specifically type 2 diabetes

DRUG CATEGORY

antidiabetic

Class: sulfonylurea: second generation

PRODUCTS

Brand-Name Products with No Generic Alternative

Glucotrol XL 2.5 mg extended-release tablet (¢¢¢)
Glucotrol XL 5 mg extended-release tablet (¢¢¢)
Glucotrol XL 10 mg extended-release tablet (¢¢¢¢)
No generic extended-release products available.
Multiple patents that begin to expire in 2003.

Brand-Name Products with Generic Alternatives

Glucotrol 5 mg tablet (¢¢¢)
  Generic: glipizide 5 mg tablet (¢)
Glucotrol 10 mg tablet (¢¢¢¢¢)
  Generic: glipizide 10 mg tablet (¢¢)

Combination Products That Contain This Drug

Metaglip tablet (n/a)

DOSING AND FOOD

Doses are taken 1 to 2 times a day. Extended-release products are taken once a day.

It is best to take this drug about 30 minutes before a meal, starting with the first meal of the day.

Adults: Up to 40 mg per day.

Lower doses are used in people over age 65 and in people with kidney or liver disease.

Forgotten doses: If you are scheduled to take the next dose within a few hours, do not take the forgotten dose. Otherwise take the forgotten dose as soon as you remember.

ALCOHOL, DRUG, HERB, AND SUPPLEMENT INTERACTIONS

Alcohol should not be used while taking this drug since the combination may cause a severe reaction.

Aloe, bilberry leaf, bitter melon, burdock, dandelion, fenugreek, garlic, ginkgo biloba, and ginseng may lower blood sugar and cause the need for a dose adjustment when taken with this drug. Tell your doctor if you are taking any of these supplements.

Several OTC drugs used for asthma, colds, cough, hay fever, sleep aid, or sinus problems may seriously change the effects of this drug. Check with your pharmacist when selecting OTC products.

---

†See page 52.   *See page 53.

Taking this drug with any of the ones listed below may change the effect of either drug with the possibility of causing toxicity or decreasing effectiveness: anticoagulants†, antihistamines†, aspirin, beta blockers†, calcium channel blockers†, chloramphenicol, cimetidine, clofibrate, corticosteroids†, cyclosporine, estrogens†, fluconazole, fluoroquinolones†, furosemide, hydrantoins†, insulin, isoniazid, lithium, miconazole, nonsteroidal antiinflammatories†, oral contraceptives, phenothiazines†, probenecid, quinine, quinidine, ranitidine, rifampin, salicylates†, sulfonamides†, sympathomimetics†, thiazide diuretics†, triamterene

Severe reactions are possible when this drug is taken with those listed below: guanethidine, monoamine oxidase inhibitors†, octreotide, pentamidine

ALLERGIC REACTIONS AND SIDE EFFECTS

If you are allergic to any sulfonylureas† or sulfonamides†, you may also be allergic to this drug. You should tell your doctor about all your allergies and any unexplained symptoms you may have while taking this drug.

This drug promotes the effect of sunlight on the body and may cause severe sunburn and increased sensitivity of the eyes.

MORE COMMON SIDE EFFECTS: Anxiety*, appetite changes, behavior change*, blurry vision*, chills*, confusion*, constipation, diarrhea, fast heartbeat*, frequent urination, heartburn, hunger*, low blood sugar*, poor concentration*, slurry speech*, sweating*, taste changes, tiredness*, weakness*, weight gain*

LESS COMMON SIDE EFFECTS: Depression, dizziness, drowsiness*, gas, headache*, nausea*, nervousness*, nightmares*, seizures*, shakiness*, skin irritation*, sleep disorders*, stomach pain, unconsciousness*, vomiting

RARE SIDE EFFECTS: Bleeding*, bruising*, chest pain*, coughing up blood*, dark urine*, excess sputum*, fever*, hives*, pale skin*, pale stools*, shortness of breath*, sore throat*, yellow eyes or skin*

PRECAUTIONS

Do not crush, break, or chew the extended-release products.

Burns, diarrhea, fever, hormonal changes, infection, malnourishment, severe stress, uncontrolled thyroid disease, and vomiting may cause changes in blood sugar that may make this drug less effective.

You need to wait 2 weeks after stopping a monoamine oxidase inhibitor† before starting this drug.

This drug has a mild diuretic effect, which may cause urination a few hours after taking a dose.

PREGNANCY AND BREAST-FEEDING

Safety in pregnancy has not been established although the drug is known to harm animal fetuses.

Breast-feeding while taking this drug is not recommended.

HELPFUL COMMENTS

Blood sugar level should be checked if you experience any side effects.

* If you are a smoker and stop smoking while taking this drug, your dose may need to be reduced.

* If you do not treat high blood sugar, you may develop more serious problems such as heart failure, blood vessel disease, eye disease, or kidney disease.

GLYBURIDE

Available since May 1984

COMMONLY USED TO TREAT

High blood sugar, specifically type 2 diabetes

DRUG CATEGORY

antidiabetic
Class: sulfonylurea: second generation

PRODUCTS

Brand-Name Products with Generic Alternatives
Micronase 1.25 mg tablet (¢¢¢)
 Generic: glyburide 1.25 mg tablet (¢¢)
Micronase 2.5 mg tablet (¢¢¢¢)
 Generic: glyburide 2.5 mg tablet (¢¢)
Micronase 5 mg tablet (¢¢¢¢¢¢)
 Generic: glyburide 5 mg tablet (¢¢¢)
Glynase 1.5 mg tablet (¢¢¢)
 Generic: glyburide micronized 1.5 mg tablet (¢¢¢)
Glynase 3 mg tablet (¢¢¢¢¢)
 Generic: glyburide micronized 3 mg tablet (¢¢¢)
Glynase 6 mg tablet ($)
 Generic: glyburide micronized 6 mg tablet (¢¢¢¢¢)
Products Only Available as Generics
glyburide micronized 4.5 mg tablet (n/a)

† See page 52.   * See page 53.

Other Generic Product Names
Diabeta

Combination Products That Contain This Drug
Glucovance tablet (¢¢¢¢¢)

DOSING AND FOOD

Doses are taken 1 to 2 times a day.
It is best to take this drug just before a meal.

Adults: Up to 12 mg per day in divided doses when using micronized glyburide. Up to 20 mg per day in divided doses when using regular glyburide.

Lower doses are used in people over age 65 and in people with kidney or liver disease.

Forgotten doses: If you are scheduled to take the next dose within a few hours, do not take the forgotten dose. Otherwise take the forgotten dose as soon as you remember.

ALCOHOL, DRUG, HERB, AND SUPPLEMENT INTERACTIONS

Alcohol should not be used while taking this drug since the combination may cause a severe reaction.

Aloe, bilberry leaf, bitter melon, burdock, dandelion, fenugreek, garlic, ginkgo biloba, and ginseng may lower blood sugar and cause the need for a dose adjustment when taken with this drug. Tell your doctor if you are taking any of these supplements.

Several OTC drugs used for asthma, colds, cough, hay fever, sleep aid, or sinus problems may seriously change the effects of this drug. Check with your pharmacist when selecting OTC products.

Taking this drug with any of the ones listed below may change the effect of either drug with the possibility of causing toxicity or decreasing effectiveness:
anticoagulants†, antihistamines†, aspirin, baclofen, beta blockers†, calcium channel blockers†, chloramphenicol, cimetidine, corticosteroids†, cyclosporine, estrogens†, fluconazole, fluoroquinolones†, furosemide, insulin, isoniazid, lithium, miconazole, nonsteroidal antiinflammatories†, oral contraceptives, phenothiazines†, phenytoin, probenecid, quinine, quinidine, ranitidine, rifampin, salicylates†, sulfonamides†, sympatho-mimetics†, thiazide diuretics†, triamterene

Severe reactions are possible when this drug is taken with those listed below:
guanethidine, monoamine oxidase inhibitors†, octreotide, pentamidine

ALLERGIC REACTIONS AND SIDE EFFECTS

If you are allergic to any sulfonylureas† or sulfonamides†, you may also be allergic to this drug. You should tell your doctor about all your allergies and any unexplained symptoms you may have while taking this drug.

This drug promotes the effect of sunlight on the body and may cause severe sunburn and increased sensitivity of the eyes.

MORE COMMON SIDE EFFECTS: Anxiety*, behavior change*, chills*, confusion*, constipation, diarrhea, fast heartbeat*, frequent urination, low blood sugar*, poor concentration*, slurry speech*, sweating*, swelling*, tiredness*, weakness*,

LESS COMMON SIDE EFFECTS: Appetite changes, blurry vision*, dizziness, drowsiness*, gas, headache*, heartburn, hunger*, nausea*, nervousness*, seizures*, shakiness*, skin irritation*, stomach pain, taste changes, unconsciousness*, vomiting, weight gain*

RARE SIDE EFFECTS: Bleeding*, bruising*, chest pain*, coughing up blood*, dark urine*, excess sputum*, fever*, hives*, pale skin*, pale stools*, shortness of breath*, sore throat*, yellow eyes or skin*

PRECAUTIONS

Burns, diarrhea, fever, hormonal changes, infection, malnourishment, severe stress, uncontrolled thyroid disease, and vomiting may cause changes in blood sugar that may make this drug less effective.

You need to wait 2 weeks after stopping a monoamine oxidase inhibitor† before starting this drug.

Three milligrams (3 mg) of glyburide micronized has about the same effect as 5 mg of regular glyburide.

PREGNANCY AND BREAST-FEEDING

Safety in pregnancy has not been established although the drug is known to harm animal fetuses.

Breast-feeding while taking this drug is not recommended.

HELPFUL COMMENTS

Blood sugar level should be checked if you experience any side effects.

If you are a smoker and stop smoking while taking this drug, your dose may need to be reduced.

This drug stays in the body for about a week after each dose.

If you do not treat high blood sugar, you may develop more serious problems such as heart failure, blood vessel disease, eye disease, or kidney disease.

---

† See page 52.   * See page 53.

GLYCOPYRROLATE HYDROCHLORIDE

Available for over 20 years

COMMONLY USED TO TREAT

Intestinal disorders
Ulcers

DRUG CATEGORY

antidiarrheal
Class: anticholinergic

PRODUCTS

Brand-Name Products with No Generic Alternative
Robinul 1 mg tablet (¢¢¢¢)
Robinul 2 mg tablet ($)
No generics available.
No patents, no exclusivity.

DOSING AND FOOD

Doses are taken 2 to 3 times a day.
It is best to take this drug on an empty stomach at least 30 minutes before meals.
Adults: Up to 8 mg per day in divided doses.
Forgotten doses: If you are scheduled to take the next dose within a few hours, do not take the forgotten dose. Otherwise take the forgotten dose as soon as you remember.

ALCOHOL, DRUG, HERB, AND SUPPLEMENT INTERACTIONS

Alcohol may increase some of the side effects from this drug, depending on the amount consumed. Ask your doctor about the risks caused by drinking alcohol with your condition.
OTC drugs used to treat diarrhea may contain an ingredient that can interfere with the effects of this drug. Ask your pharmacist for help when selecting an OTC product.

Taking this drug with any of the ones listed below may change the effect of either drug with the possibility of causing toxicity or decreasing effectiveness:
antacids, anticholinergics†, attapulgite, digoxin, kaolin, ketoconazole, levodopa, tricyclic antidepressants†

Increased side effects are possible when this drug is taken with those listed below: amantadine, antihistamines†, antidyskinetics†, disopyramide, glutethimide, meperidine, phenothiazines†, potassium supplements, procainamide, quinidine

ALLERGIC REACTIONS AND SIDE EFFECTS

If you are allergic to any belladonna alkaloids†, you may also be allergic to this drug. You should tell your doctor about all your allergies and any unexplained symptoms you may have while taking this drug.

This drug may cause your eyes to be more sensitive to sunlight, but there are no special risks associated with sunburn while taking this drug.

MORE COMMON SIDE EFFECTS: Blurry vision, constipation, decreased sweating, dry mouth*, dry skin*, urinary difficulty

LESS COMMON SIDE EFFECTS: Bloated feeling, decreased breast milk, drowsiness*, headache, memory loss, nausea, swallowing difficulty, tiredness*, vomiting, weakness*

RARE SIDE EFFECTS: Breathing difficulty*, clumsiness*, confusion*, dizziness*, excitement*, eye pain*, fainting*, fast heartbeat*, fever*, flushing*, hallucinations, hives*, irritability*, lightheadedness*, nervousness*, restlessness*, seizures*, skin rash*, slurry speech*, unsteadiness*, vision changes*

PRECAUTIONS

Be careful driving or handling equipment while taking this drug because it may cause blurry vision and sensitivity of the eyes to light.

If you have colitis, enlarged prostate, fever, glaucoma, heart disease, hernia, high blood pressure, intestinal blockage, lung disease, myasthenia gravis, or urinary difficulty, this drug may make those conditions worse.

People with hyperthyroidism or Down's syndrome may feel an increase in heart rate from this drug.

You are more likely to overheat when taking this drug and should avoid exercising in hot weather and using a sauna or hot tub.

This drug may cause dry mouth, which is associated with a greater risk of cavities. Your dentist may recommend that you clean your teeth and mouth differently to avoid infection.

PREGNANCY AND BREAST-FEEDING

Safety in pregnancy has not been established although there was no evidence of harm during studies in animals.

Breast-feeding while taking this drug is not recommended.

† See page 52.   * See page 53.

HELPFUL COMMENTS

If you need to take an antacid, take it either 2 hours before or after taking this drug.

Eye irritation caused by the sun may be reduced by wearing sunglasses when outside.

Sucking on hard sugarless candy or chewing sugarless gum may help relieve dry mouth caused by this drug.

You may need to drink more water to reduce the constipation that many people suffer when taking this drug.

GRANISETRON HYDROCHLORIDE

Available since March 1994

COMMONLY USED TO TREAT

Nausea
Vomiting

DRUG CATEGORY

antiemetic
Class: selective 5-HT3 receptor antagonist

PRODUCTS

Brand-Name Products with No Generic Alternative
Kytril 1 mg tablet ($$$$$)
No generics available.
Patent expires in 2007.

DOSING AND FOOD

Doses are taken 1 to 2 times a day.
This drug may be taken with or without food.
Adults: Up to 2 mg per day in divided doses.

ALCOHOL, DRUG, HERB, AND SUPPLEMENT INTERACTIONS

Alcohol may increase some of the side effects from this drug, depending on the amount consumed. Ask your doctor about the risks caused by drinking alcohol with your condition.

Do not use horehound while taking this drug because of an increased risk of side effects.

ALLERGIC REACTIONS AND SIDE EFFECTS

If you are allergic to dolasetron or ondansetron, you may also be allergic to this drug. You should tell your doctor about all your allergies and any unexplained symptoms you may have while taking this drug.

MORE COMMON SIDE EFFECTS: Abdominal pain, constipation, headache, tiredness, weakness

LESS COMMON SIDE EFFECTS: Agitation, anxiety, diarrhea, dizziness, drowsiness, fever*, hair loss, heartburn, indigestion, loss of appetite, sleep disorders, sour stomach, taste changes, vomiting

RARE SIDE EFFECTS: Chest pain*, fainting*, hives*, irregular heartbeat*, itching*, shortness of breath*, skin rash*

PRECAUTIONS

Call your doctor immediately if you have hives, chest tightness, wheezing, and dizziness, which may be signs of an allergic reaction.

PREGNANCY AND BREAST-FEEDING

Safety in pregnancy has not been established although there was no evidence of harm during studies in animals.

It is not known if this drug passes into breast milk. Talk to your doctor about the risks of breast-feeding while taking this drug.

HELPFUL COMMENTS

Only 1 or 2 doses of this drug are taken with each chemotherapy or radiation session.

GRISEOFULVIN

Available for over 20 years

COMMONLY USED TO TREAT

Fungal infections

DRUG CATEGORY

antifungal
Class: penicillium antibiotic

PRODUCTS

Brand-Name Products with No Generic Alternative
Fulvicin P/G 165 mg tablet (¢¢¢¢¢)

---

† See page 52.   * See page 53.

Grifulvin V 125 mg/5 ml oral suspension ($)

Brand-Name Products with Generic Alternatives
Fulvicin P/G 125 mg tablet (¢¢¢¢)
   Generic: griseofulvin ultramicrocrystalline 125 mg tablet (¢¢¢)
Fulvicin P/G 250 mg tablet§ ($)
   Generic: griseofulvin ultramicrocrystalline 250 mg tablet§ (¢¢¢¢)
Fulvicin P/G 330 mg tablet ($$)
   Generic: griseofulvin ultramicrocrystalline 330 mg tablet (¢¢¢¢¢)
Grifulvin V 250 mg tablet§(n/a)
   Generic: griseofulvin microcrystalline 250 mg tablet§ ($)
Grifulvin V 500 mg tablet ($$)
   Generic: griseofulvin microcrystalline 500 mg tablet ($)

Other Generic Product Names
Fulvicin U/F, Griseofulvin Microsize, Gris-Peg

DOSING AND FOOD

Doses are taken once a day.

Taking the microcrystalline form of this drug with fatty foods will help increase absorption of the drug. Be careful not to eat too much fatty food. The ultramicrocrystalline form of this drug may be taken with or without food.

Adults: Up to 1,000 mg per day of microcrystalline products, or 660 mg per day of ultramicrocrystalline products.

Children over 23 kg: Up to 500 mg per day of microcrystalline products, or 330 mg per day of ultramicrocrystalline products.

Children 14 to 23 kg: Up to 250 mg per day of microcrystalline products, or 165 mg per day of ultramicrocrystalline products.

Forgotten doses: If you are scheduled to take the next dose within a few hours, do not take the forgotten dose. Otherwise take the forgotten dose as soon as you remember.

ALCOHOL, DRUG, HERB, AND SUPPLEMENT INTERACTIONS

Alcohol should not be used while taking this drug since it may increase the risk of serious side effects.

Taking this drug with any of the ones listed below may change the effect of either drug with the possibility of causing toxicity or decreasing effectiveness: anticoagulants†, barbiturates†, oral contraceptives

ALLERGIC REACTIONS AND SIDE EFFECTS

If you are allergic to penicillamine or any penicillins†, you may also be

§ *See "Precautions" in this entry.*

allergic to this drug. You should tell your doctor about all your allergies and any unexplained symptoms you may have while taking this drug.

This drug promotes the effect of sunlight on the body and may cause severe sunburn and increased sensitivity of the eyes.

MORE COMMON SIDE EFFECTS: Bleeding, headache, skin rash*

LESS COMMON SIDE EFFECTS: Abdominal pain, confusion*, diarrhea, dizziness, hearing loss, hives*, itching*, mouth irritation*, nausea, sleep disorders, tiredness, vomiting

RARE SIDE EFFECTS: Fever*, numbness*, sore throat*, tingling*, weakness*, yellow eyes or skin*

PRECAUTIONS

The strength of these products may appear to be the same as other products, but the form of the drug is different. These products may not be substituted for others without a new prescription.

If you have lupus erythematosus or a lupuslike disease, this drug may make those conditions worse.

People with porphyria, liver disease, or heart failure may not be able to take this drug.

Be careful driving or handling equipment while taking this drug because it may cause dizziness.

PREGNANCY AND BREAST-FEEDING

Safety in pregnancy has not been established although the drug is known to harm animal fetuses.

It is not known if this drug passes into breast milk. Talk to your doctor about the risks associated with breast-feeding while taking this drug.

HELPFUL COMMENTS

Oral contraceptives may not work properly when taken with this drug. You need to use a barrier contraceptive, such as a condom, or other nonhormonal contraceptive to prevent pregnancy.

Contact your doctor if your symptoms do not improve after a week.

Do not stop treatment early if you start to feel better. It takes the full prescription for this drug to work completely.

If treating athlete's feet, you may need to use both an oral and topical product.

Do not measure doses of the oral suspension with anything but a measuring cup intended for use with prescription drugs. Slight inaccuracy from other measuring spoons may result in over- or under-dosing.

---

†See page 52.   * See page 53.

GUANABENZ ACETATE

Available for over 20 years

COMMONLY USED TO TREAT

High blood pressure, also known as hypertension
Opiate withdrawal symptoms

DRUG CATEGORY

antihypertensive
Class: centrally acting antiadrenergic

PRODUCTS

Brand-Name Products with Generic Alternatives
Wytensin 4 mg tablet (n/a)
  Generic: guanabenz acetate 4 mg tablet (¢¢¢¢)
Wytensin 8 mg tablet (n/a)
  Generic: guanabenz acetate 8 mg tablet (¢¢¢¢¢)

DOSING AND FOOD

Doses are taken 2 to 4 times a day.
This drug may be taken with or without food.
Adults: Up to 64 mg per day in divided doses.
Children age 12 and older: Up to 24 mg per day in divided doses.
Lower doses may be needed in people with liver disease.
Forgotten doses: If you are scheduled to take the next dose within a few hours, do not take the forgotten dose. Otherwise take the forgotten dose as soon as you remember.

ALCOHOL, DRUG, HERB, AND SUPPLEMENT INTERACTIONS

Alcohol should not be used while taking this drug.
Several OTC drugs used for appetite control, asthma, colds, cough, hay fever, or sinus problems may cause an increase in blood pressure when taken with this drug and increase the risk of side effects from this drug. Check with your pharmacist when selecting OTC products.
Taking this drug with any of the ones listed below may change the effect of either drug with the possibility of causing toxicity or decreasing effectiveness: antihypertensives[†], beta blockers[†], diuretics[†], monoamine oxidase inhibitors[†], tricyclic antidepressants[†]

increased side effects are possible when this drug is taken with those listed below: barbiturates†, benzodiazepines†, phenothiazines†, sedative-hypnotics†

ALLERGIC REACTIONS AND SIDE EFFECTS

You should tell your doctor about all your allergies and any unexplained symptoms you may have while taking this drug.

MORE COMMON SIDE EFFECTS: Dizziness*, drowsiness, dry mouth, weakness*

LESS COMMON SIDE EFFECTS: Headache, nausea, sexual dysfunction

RARE SIDE EFFECTS: Irritability*, nervousness*, slow heartbeat*, small pupils*, tiredness*

PRECAUTIONS

This drug may cause severe high blood pressure if stopped quickly over less than 2 to 4 days. If you wish to stop taking this drug, ask your doctor for specific instructions.

Be careful driving or handling equipment while taking this drug because it may cause dizziness and drowsiness.

This drug may cause dry mouth, which is associated with a greater risk of cavities. Your dentist may recommend that you clean your teeth and mouth differently to avoid infection.

PREGNANCY AND BREAST-FEEDING

Safety in pregnancy has not been established although the drug is known to harm animal fetuses.

It is not known if this drug passes into breast milk. Talk to your doctor about the risks associated with breast-feeding while taking this drug.

HELPFUL COMMENTS

The full effects of this drug should be noticed in 1 to 2 weeks.

Sucking on hard sugarless candy or chewing sugarless gum may help relieve dry mouth caused by this drug.

Taking the last daily dose at bedtime may help make side effects less noticeable.

If you do not treat high blood pressure, you may develop more serious problems such as heart failure, blood vessel disease, stroke, or kidney disease. Losing weight, exercising, eating more fruits and vegetables, and avoiding salty foods, such as lunchmeat and pickles, may help make drug treatment more successful.

---

† See page 52.   * See page 53.

GUANFACINE HYDROCHLORIDE

Available since October 1986

COMMONLY USED TO TREAT

High blood pressure, also known as hypertension

DRUG CATEGORY

antihypertensive
Class: centrally acting antiadrenergic

PRODUCTS

Brand-Name Products with Generic Alternatives
Tenex 1 mg tablet ($)
  Generic: guanfacine hydrochloride 1 mg tablet (¢¢¢¢)
Tenex 2 mg tablet ($$)
  Generic: guanfacine hydrochloride 2 mg tablet (¢¢¢¢¢)

DOSING AND FOOD

Doses are taken once a day at bedtime.
This drug may be taken with or without food.
Adults: Up to 3 mg per day in divided doses.
Lower doses are used in people with liver disease and people over age 65.
Forgotten doses: If you are scheduled to take the next dose within a few hours, do not take the forgotten dose. Otherwise take the forgotten dose as soon as you remember.

ALCOHOL, DRUG, HERB, AND SUPPLEMENT INTERACTIONS

Alcohol should not be used while taking this drug.
Many OTC drugs used for appetite control, asthma, colds, cough, hay fever, pain, or sinus problems affect the central nervous system and may cause a change in the effects or side effects of this drug. Check with your pharmacist for products to avoid.

Taking this drug with any of the ones listed below may change the effect of either drug with the possibility of causing toxicity or decreasing effectiveness: phenobarbital, phenytoin

Increased side effects are possible when this drug is taken with those listed below: anesthetics, antihistamines†, anxiolytics†, barbiturates†, phenothiazines†, tricyclic antidepressants†

ALLERGIC REACTIONS AND SIDE EFFECTS

You should tell your doctor about all your allergies and any unexplained symptoms you may have while taking this drug.

MORE COMMON SIDE EFFECTS: Constipation*, dizziness*, drowsiness, dry mouth

LESS COMMON SIDE EFFECTS: Confusion*, depression*, headache, itchy eyes, nausea, sexual dysfunction, sleeping difficulty, tiredness*, vomiting, weakness*

RARE SIDE EFFECTS: Breathing difficulty, fainting*, slow heartbeat*

PRECAUTIONS

This drug works best when given in combination with other antihypertensives†, especially a thiazide diuretic†.

Stopping this drug suddenly may cause dangerously high blood pressure. If you wish to stop taking this drug, ask your doctor for specific instructions.

Be careful driving or handling equipment while taking this drug because it may cause dizziness and drowsiness.

This drug may cause dry mouth, which is associated with a greater risk of cavities. Your dentist may recommend that you clean your teeth and mouth differently to avoid infection.

PREGNANCY AND BREAST-FEEDING

Safety during pregnancy has not been established although there was no evidence of harm during studies in animals.

It is not known if this drug passes into breast milk. Talk to your doctor about the risks associated with breast-feeding while taking this drug.

HELPFUL COMMENTS

If this drug causes constipation, you may need to add more fiber to your diet.

It takes 3 to 4 days before the effects of this drug are noticed.

If you do not treat high blood pressure, you may develop more serious problems such as heart failure, blood vessel disease, stroke, or kidney disease. Losing weight, exercising, eating more fruits and vegetables, and avoiding salty foods, such as lunchmeat and pickles, may help make drug treatment more successful.

Sucking on hard sugarless candy or chewing sugarless gum may help relieve dry mouth caused by this drug.

Avoid quick movements to minimize dizziness.

---

† See page 52.   * See page 53.

HALAZEPAM

Available for over 20 years

COMMONLY USED TO TREAT

Anxiety
Sleeping difficulty, also known as insomnia

DRUG CATEGORY

anxiolytic
sedative-hypnotic
Class: benzodiazepine

PRODUCTS

Brand-Name Products with No Generic Alternative
Paxipam 20 mg tablet (n/a)
Paxipam 40 mg tablet (n/a)
No generics available.
No patents, no exclusivity.

DOSING AND FOOD

Doses are taken 3 to 4 times a day.
This drug may be taken with or without food.
Adults: Up to 160 mg per day in divided doses.
Lower doses are used in people over age 65.
Forgotten doses: If you are scheduled to take the next dose within a few
hours, do not take the forgotten dose. Otherwise take the forgotten dose
as soon as you remember.

ALCOHOL, DRUG, HERB, AND SUPPLEMENT INTERACTIONS

Alcohol should not be used while taking this drug.
Catnip, kava, lady's slipper, lemon balm, passion flower, sassafras, skullcap,
and valerian should not be used while taking this drug due to an increased sedative effect.

Taking this drug with any of the ones listed below may change the effect of
either drug with the possibility of causing toxicity or decreasing effectiveness:
cimetidine, digoxin, disulfiram, fluvoxamine, haloperidol, itraconazole, ketoconazole, levodopa, nefazodone, oral contraceptives, rifampin

Severe reactions are possible when this drug is taken with those listed below:
antidepressants†, antihistamines†, barbiturates†, anesthetics†, monoamine
oxidase inhibitors†, narcotics†, phenothiazines†

Increased side effects are possible when this drug is taken with those listed below: aminophylline, theophylline

ALLERGIC REACTIONS AND SIDE EFFECTS

If you are allergic to any benzodiazepines†, you may also be allergic to this drug. You should tell your doctor about all your allergies and any unexplained symptoms you may have while taking this drug.

MORE COMMON SIDE EFFECTS: Clumsiness, dizziness, drowsiness, lightheadedness, slurry speech

LESS COMMON SIDE EFFECTS: Anxiety*, confusion*, constipation, depression*, diarrhea, difficulty urinating, dry mouth, headache, irregular heartbeat*, memory loss*, muscle spasm, nausea, sexual dysfunction, stomach cramps, thirst, trembling, vision changes, vomiting, watery mouth

RARE SIDE EFFECTS: Agitation*, behavior changes*, bleeding*, bruising*, chills*, delusions*, disorientation*, excitement*, eye movement*, fever*, hallucinations*, irritability*, low blood pressure*, mouth sores*, nervousness*, seizures*, skin irritation*, sleeping difficulty*, sore throat*, spastic movements*, tiredness*, weakness*, yellow eyes or skin*

PRECAUTIONS

This drug may be habit forming and will cause severe withdrawal symptoms if stopped abruptly. If you wish to stop taking this drug, ask your doctor for specific instructions.

You need to wait 2 weeks after stopping a monoamine oxidase inhibitor† before starting this drug.

If you have difficulty swallowing, emphysema, asthma, bronchitis, glaucoma, hyperactivity, depression, mental illness, myasthenia gravis, porphyria, or sleep apnea, this drug may make those conditions worse.

Heavy smoking may cause this drug to be less effective.

Be careful driving or handling equipment while taking this drug because the drug may cause dizziness and drowsiness.

PREGNANCY AND BREAST-FEEDING

There is evidence that this drug may harm the fetus, but the drug may be necessary to the health of the mother.

Breast-feeding while taking this drug is not recommended.

HELPFUL COMMENTS

Dangling your legs over the side of the bed for a few minutes may help reduce dizziness when first waking up.

---

†See page 52.   *See page 53.

HALOPERIDOL

Available for over 20 years

COMMONLY USED TO TREAT

Alcoholism
Mental illness, also known as psychosis
Muscle movements and speaking associated with Tourette's syndrome
Muscle movements associated with Huntington's chorea

DRUG CATEGORY

antipsychotic
Class: butyrophenone

PRODUCTS

Products Only Available as Generics
haloperidol 0.5 mg tablet (¢)
haloperidol 1 mg tablet (¢)
haloperidol 2 mg tablet (¢¢)
haloperidol 5 mg tablet (¢)
haloperidol 10 mg tablet (¢¢)
haloperidol 20 mg tablet ($)
haloperidol lactate 1 mg/ml oral solution (n/a)
haloperidol lactate 2 mg/ml oral concentrate ($)

DOSING AND FOOD

Doses are taken 2 to 3 times a day.
It is best to take this drug on an empty stomach, but taking this drug with
 a little food may avoid the stomach upset that some people suffer.
Adults: Up to 100 mg per day in divided doses.
Children age 3 to 12: Up to 0.225 mg/kg per day in divided doses.
Forgotten doses: If you are scheduled to take the next dose within a few
 hours, do not take the forgotten dose. Otherwise take the forgotten dose
 as soon as you remember.

ALCOHOL, DRUG, HERB, AND SUPPLEMENT INTERACTIONS

Alcohol should not be used while taking this drug.
Nutmeg may decrease the effects of this drug and should not be used.
Several OTC drugs used for asthma, colds, cough, hay fever, sleep aid, or
 sinus problems may seriously change the effects and side effects of this
 drug. Check with your pharmacist when selecting OTC products.

Taking this drug with any of the ones listed below may change the effect of either drug with the possibility of causing toxicity or decreasing effectiveness: antacids, antiarrhythmics†, beta blockers†, bromocriptine, clonidine, disopyramide, dopamine, ephedrine, epinephrine, guanabenz, guanadrel, guanethidine, levodopa, methyldopa, phenobarbital, phenylephrine, phenytoin, procainamide, quinidine, reserpine, rifampin

Severe reactions are possible when this drug is taken with those listed below: anticholinergics†, antidepressants†, antidyskinetics†, antihistamines†, atropine, lithium, meperidine, metrizamide, monoamine oxidase inhibitors†, nitrates†, phenothiazines†, propylthiouracil, tricyclic antidepressants†

Increased side effects are possible when this drug is taken with those listed below: alseroxylon, amoxapine, antipsychotics†, deserpidine, metoclopramide, metyrosine, pemoline, pimozide, promethazine, rauwolfia serpentine, reserpine, trimeprazine

ALLERGIC REACTIONS AND SIDE EFFECTS

You should tell your doctor about all your allergies and any unexplained symptoms you may have while taking this drug.

This drug promotes the effect of sunlight on the body and may cause severe sunburn and increased sensitivity of the eyes.

MORE COMMON SIDE EFFECTS: Blurry vision, breast-milk secretion, breast swelling, constipation, dry mouth, expressionless face*, loss of balance*, menstrual changes, muscle spasms*, restlessness*, seizures*, shaking*, shuffling walk*, spastic movements*, speech disorders*, stiffness*, still eyes*, swallowing disorder*, trembling*, weakness*, weight gain

LESS COMMON SIDE EFFECTS: Chewing action*, decreased thirst*, dizziness*, drowsiness*, fainting*, hallucinations, lightheadedness*, lip smacking*, nausea, sexual dysfunction, skin rash*, tongue movements*, urinary difficulty*, vomiting

RARE SIDE EFFECTS: Bleeding*, blinking*, blood pressure changes*, breathing changes*, bruising*, confusion*, dizziness*, dry skin*, eyelid spasms*, facial expressions*, fast heartbeat*, fever*, irregular pulse*, lack of sweat*, muscle jerks*, pale skin*, poor bladder control*, sore throat*, sweating*, tiredness*, yellow eyes or skin*

PRECAUTIONS

This drug may cause severe withdrawal symptoms if stopped suddenly. If you wish to stop taking this drug, ask your doctor for specific instructions.

If you have a history of seizure disorders, there may be an increased risk of developing a seizure while taking this drug.

† See page 52.,   * See page 53.

If you have glaucoma, urinary difficulty, heart disease, blood vessel disease, lung disease, or Parkinson's disease, this drug may make those conditions worse.

People with a history of alcohol abuse are at greater risk of having a stroke while taking this drug.

Be careful driving or handling equipment while taking this drug because it may cause blurry vision.

Heavy smoking may cause this drug to be less effective.

Drink plenty of fluids to avoid dehydration when sweating, such as in hot weather and during exercise.

Touching the liquid form of this drug may cause skin irritation. You should wash your hands immediately after taking the dose.

This drug may cause dry mouth, which is associated with a greater risk of cavities. Your dentist may recommend that you clean your teeth and mouth differently to avoid infection.

PREGNANCY AND BREAST-FEEDING

Safety during pregnancy has not been established although the drug is known to harm animal fetuses.

Breast-feeding while taking this drug is not recommended.

HELPFUL COMMENTS

It may take several days or weeks before the full effects of this drug are noticed.

If you need to take an antacid, take it either 2 hours before or after taking this drug.

Sucking on hard sugarless candy or chewing sugarless gum may help relieve dry mouth caused by this drug.

Do not measure doses of the oral liquids with anything but a measuring cup intended for use with prescription drugs. Slight inaccuracy from other measuring spoons may result in over- or under-dosing.

HYDRALAZINE HYDROCHLORIDE

Available for over 20 years

COMMONLY USED TO TREAT

Heart failure

High blood pressure, also known as hypertension

DRUG CATEGORY

antihypertensive
Class: peripheral vasodilator

PRODUCTS

Brand-Name Products with Generic Alternatives
Apresoline 10 mg tablet (n/a)
  Generic: hydralazine hydrochloride 10 mg tablet (¢)
Apresoline 25 mg tablet (n/a)
  Generic: hydralazine hydrochloride 25 mg tablet (¢)
Apresoline 50 mg tablet (¢¢¢¢)
  Generic: hydralazine hydrochloride 50 mg tablet (¢)
Apresoline 100 mg tablet (n/a)
  Generic: hydralazine hydrochloride 100 mg tablet (¢¢)
Combination Products That Contain This Drug
Apresazide capsule (n/a)

DOSING AND FOOD

Doses are taken 4 times a day.
It is best to take this drug with food or milk.
Adults: Up to 600 mg per day in divided doses.
Children: Up to 7.5 mg/kg per day in divided doses.
Lower doses may be needed in people with kidney disease.
Forgotten doses: If you are scheduled to take the next dose within a few
  hours, do not take the forgotten dose. Otherwise take the forgotten dose
  as soon as you remember.

ALCOHOL, DRUG, HERB, AND SUPPLEMENT INTERACTIONS

Alcohol may cause your blood pressure to rise, making this drug less effective. Ask your doctor about the risks caused by drinking alcohol with
  your condition.
Several OTC drugs used for appetite control, asthma, colds, cough, hay
  fever, or sinus problems may cause an increase in blood pressure when
  taken with this drug. Check with your pharmacist when selecting OTC
  products.
Taking this drug with any of the ones listed below may change the effect of
either drug with the possibility of causing toxicity or decreasing effectiveness:
antihypertensives†, diuretics†, epinephrine

---
†See page 52.   *See page 53.

Severe reactions are possible when this drug is taken with those listed below: diazoxide, monoamine oxidase inhibitors†

ALLERGIC REACTIONS AND SIDE EFFECTS

Some products contain tartrazine, which may cause an allergic reaction in people allergic to aspirin. If you are allergic to aspirin, ask your pharmacist to fill your prescription with a product that does not contain tartrazine. You should tell your doctor about all your allergies and any unexplained symptoms you may have while taking this drug.

MORE COMMON SIDE EFFECTS: Diarrhea, fever*, headache, irregular heartbeat, loss of appetite, nausea, vomiting

LESS COMMON SIDE EFFECTS: Blisters*, chest pain*, constipation, dizziness, flushing, foot pain*, hand pain*, itching*, joint pain*, lightheadedness, muscle pain*, numbness*, shortness of breath, skin rash*, sore throat*, stuffy nose, swelling*, tingling*, watery eyes, weakness*

PRECAUTIONS

Do not stop this drug suddenly since it may cause extreme elevation of your blood pressure. If you wish to stop taking this drug, ask your doctor for specific instructions.

Measure your weight daily and call your doctor if you gain more than 5 pounds in a week.

Headache and irregular heartbeat often occur 2 to 4 hours after taking the first dose of this drug. These effects should go away without additional treatment.

Be careful driving or handling equipment while taking this drug because it may cause headaches and dizziness.

PREGNANCY AND BREAST-FEEDING

Safety during pregnancy has not been established although the drug is known to harm animal fetuses.

Breast-feeding while taking this drug is not recommended.

HELPFUL COMMENTS

Plan to rest for at least 6 hours after the first dose of this drug.

If you do not treat high blood pressure, you may develop more serious problems such as heart failure, blood vessel disease, stroke, or kidney disease. Losing weight, exercising, eating more fruits and vegetables, and avoiding salty foods, such as lunchmeat and pickles, may help make drug treatment more successful.

HYDROCHLOROTHIAZIDE

Available for over 20 years

COMMONLY USED TO TREAT

Fluid retention, also known as edema
Frequent urination in people with diabetes
High blood pressure, also known as hypertension

DRUG CATEGORY

antihypertensive
Class: thiazide diuretic

PRODUCTS

Brand-Name Products with Generic Alternatives
Microzide 12.5 mg capsule (¢¢¢¢)
  Generic: hydrochlorothiazide 12.5 mg capsule (¢¢¢)
Oretic 50 mg tablet (¢)
  Generic: hydrochlorothiazide 50 mg tablet (¢)

Products Only Available as Generics
hydrochlorothiazide 25 mg tablet (¢)
hydrochlorothiazide 100 mg tablet (¢)
hydrochlorothiazide 50 mg/5 ml oral solution (¢¢)

Other Generic Product Names
Aquazide H, Ezide, Esidrix, Hydrocot

Combination Products That Contain This Drug

Accuretic tablet ($)
Aldactazide tablet (¢¢¢¢) to ($)
Aldoril tablet (¢¢¢¢) to ($)
Apresazide capsule (n/a)
Atamayd HCT tablet ($) to ($$)
Avalide tablet ($$)
Capozide tablet ($) to ($$)
Diovan HCT tablet ($$)
Dyazide capsule (¢¢¢¢)
Hyzaar tablet ($) to ($$)
Inderide tablet ($) to ($$)
Inderide LA tablet ($)
Lopressor HCT tablet (¢¢¢¢) to ($$)
Lotensin HCT tablet (¢¢¢¢¢)
Maxzide tablet (¢¢¢¢) to ($)
Micardis HCT tablet ($$)
Moduretic tablet (¢¢¢¢)
Monopril-HCT tablet ($)
Prinzide tablet ($)
Teveten HCT tablet ($)
Timolide tablet (¢¢¢¢¢)
Uniretic tablet (¢¢¢¢¢)
Vaseretic tablet ($)
Zestoretic tablet ($)
Ziac tablet ($)

---

† *See page 52.*   * *See page 53.*

DOSING AND FOOD

Doses are taken 1 to 2 times a day but may be taken as little as 3 times a week.

It is best to take this drug on an empty stomach, but taking this drug with a little food may avoid the stomach upset that some people suffer. Avoid food with excess salt.

Adults: Up to 200 mg per day in divided doses.

Lower doses may be used in children.

Forgotten doses: If you are scheduled to take the next dose within a few hours, do not take the forgotten dose. Otherwise take the forgotten dose as soon as you remember.

ALCOHOL, DRUG, HERB, AND SUPPLEMENT INTERACTIONS

Alcohol may cause your blood pressure to rise, making this drug less effective. Ask your doctor about the risks caused by drinking alcohol with your condition.

Dandelion may interfere with the effect of this drug and should not be used. Tell your doctor if you are taking any of these supplements.

Licorice root may increase potassium loss and should not be used while taking this drug.

Several OTC drugs used for appetite control, asthma, colds, cough, hay fever, or sinus problems may cause an increase in blood pressure when taken with this drug. Check with your pharmacist when selecting OTC products.

Taking this drug with any of the ones listed below may change the effect of either drug with the possibility of causing toxicity or decreasing effectiveness: amphetamines†, antidiabetics†, antihypertensive†, cholestyramine, colestipol, digoxin, insulin, lithium, methenamine, quinidine

Severe reactions are possible when this drug is taken with those listed below: diazoxide

ALLERGIC REACTIONS AND SIDE EFFECTS

If you are allergic to acetazolamide, bumetanide, dichlorphenamide, furosemide, methazolamide, sulfonamides† or thiazide diuretics†, you may also be allergic to this drug. You should tell your doctor about all your allergies and any unexplained symptoms you may have while taking this drug.

This drug promotes the effect of sunlight on the body and may cause severe sunburn and increased sensitivity of the eyes.

LESS COMMON SIDE EFFECTS: Diarrhea*, dizziness, lightheadedness, loss of appetite, sexual dysfunction, stomach upset

RARE SIDE EFFECTS: Back pain*, black stools*, bleeding*, bloody urine*, breathing difficulty*, bruising*, burning sensation*, chest pain*, chills*, confusion*, cough*, fatigue*, fever*, hives*, headache*, hoarseness*, irregular heartbeat*, joint pain*, leg pain*, muscle cramps*, nausea*, numbness*, painful urination*, shortness of breath*, skin rash*, stomach pain*, swelling*, vomiting*, weakness*, yellow eyes or skin*

PRECAUTIONS

This drug may cause your blood sugar level to rise and may lead to type 2 diabetes.

Your body may lose potassium while taking this drug, which may cause severe side effects. Potassium levels should be monitored periodically and may need to be supplemented while taking this drug. Eat food rich in potassium, such as apricots, bananas, citrus fruit, dates, and tomatoes, if you are not taking a potassium supplement or potassium-sparing diuretic.

People with kidney disease may not be able to take this drug.

This drug may increase the level of uric acid in the body, which may lead to gout or kidney stones.

If you have lupus erythematosus or pancreatitis, this drug may make those conditions worse.

Nicotine in cigarettes may increase blood pressure, making this drug less effective.

This drug may cause an increase in the levels of cholesterol or triglyceride in the blood.

PREGNANCY AND BREAST-FEEDING

Safety in pregnancy has not been established although the drug is known to harm animal fetuses.

Breast-feeding while taking this drug is not recommended.

HELPFUL COMMENTS

Take your last dose of the day no later than 6 P.M. to avoid urination during the night.

Avoid quick movements to minimize dizziness. Dangling your legs over the side of the bed for a few minutes may help reduce dizziness when first waking up.

Record your weight twice a day, when first getting up in the morning and after the drug causes urination. A weight gain or loss of more than 2 pounds per day should be reported to your doctor.

The antihypertensive effects of this drug will last about 1 week after it is stopped.

† See page 52.   * See page 53.

HYDROCORTISONE

Available for over 20 years

COMMONLY USED TO TREAT

Allergic reactions
Severe inflammation

DRUG CATEGORY

antiinflammatory
immunosuppressant
Class: corticosteroid

PRODUCTS

Brand-Name Products with No Generic Alternative
Cortef 5 mg tablet (¢¢)
Cortef 10 mg/5 ml oral suspension ($)
Cortifoam 10% rectal aerosol ($$$$$)
Locoid 0.1% topical cream (¢¢¢)
Locoid 0.1% topical ointment (¢¢¢)
Locoid 0.1% topical solution ($$$$$)
Mycort-HC 2% topical cream (n/a)
Pandel 0.1% topical cream (¢¢¢¢)
Texacort 2.5% topical solution ($$$)

Brand-Name Products with Generic Alternatives
Cortef 10 mg tablet (¢¢¢)
  Generic: hydrocortisone 10 mg tablet (n/a)
Cortef 20 mg tablet (¢¢¢¢)
  Generic: hydrocortisone 20 mg tablet (¢¢)
Cortenema 100 mg rectal enema (n/a)
  Generic: hydrocortisone 100 mg rectal enema (n/a)
Cortril 1% topical ointment (n/a)
  Generic: hydrocortisone 1% topical ointment (¢)
Cortril 2.5% topical ointment (n/a)
  Generic: hydrocortisone 2.5% topical ointment (¢)
Hytone 1% topical cream (n/a)
  Generic: hydrocortisone 1% topical cream (¢)
Hytone 2.5% topical cream (¢¢¢)
  Generic: hydrocortisone 2.5% topical cream (¢)
Hytone 1% topical lotion (n/a)

Generic: hydrocortisone 1% topical lotion (¢)

Hytone 2.5% topical lotion ($$$$)

Generic: hydrocortisone 2.5% topical lotion ($$$)

Mycort-HC 2.5% topical cream (n/a)

Generic: hydrocortisone acetate 2.5% topical cream (n/a)

Texacort 1% topical solution (¢¢¢¢)

Generic: hydrocortisone 1% topical solution (n/a)

Westcort 0.2% topical cream (¢¢¢)

Generic: hydrocortisone valerate 0.2% topical cream (¢¢)

Westcort 0.2% topical ointment (¢¢¢)

Generic: hydrocortisone 0.2% topical ointment (¢¢¢)

Other Generic Product Names

AlaCort, AlaScalp, Anusol HC, Cetacort, Colocort, Epicort, HiCor, Hydro-
cortone, Nutracort, Penecort, StieCort, Synacort

Combination Products That Contain This Drug

Carmol HC topical cream (¢¢)

Cipro HC ear suspension ($$$$$)

Coly-Mycin S ear suspension ($$$$$)

Cortisporin ear drops ($$$$$)

Cortisporin ear suspension ($$$$$)

Cortisporin ophthalmic ointment ($$$$$)

Cortisporin ophthalmic suspension ($$$$$)

Cortisporin topical cream ($$$$)

Cortisporin topical ointment ($$)

Epifoam topical aerosol (¢¢¢¢¢)

Neo-Cort-Dome ear suspension (n/a)

Neo-Cort-Dome topical cream (n/a)

Otobiotic ear drops (n/a)

Pramosone topical cream (¢¢¢)

Pramosone topical lotion ($$$)

Proctofoam HC topical aerosol ($$$$)

Terr-Cortril ophthalmic suspension (n/a)

DOSING AND FOOD

Doses are taken 1 to 4 times a day.

The oral form of this drug should be taken with food.

Adults: Up to 320 mg per day in divided doses.

Children: Up to 8 mg/kg per day in divided doses.

Topical preparations should be applied in a thin layer.

---

† See page 52.   * See page 53.

Forgotten doses: Determining when to take a forgotten dose will depend on your prescription schedule. If you remember the forgotten dose within a few hours of when it was due, you may take the dose immediately and continue with your regular schedule. If you are tapering the drug to avoid withdrawal symptoms, you may need to evaluate the time since the last dose and the interval between the next doses. A complete change in schedule may be needed. Talk to your doctor or pharmacist for more help.

ALCOHOL, DRUG, HERB, AND SUPPLEMENT INTERACTIONS

Alcohol may increase the risk of side effects from this drug, especially stomach problems. Ask your doctor about the risks caused by drinking alcohol with your condition.

Taking this drug with any of the ones listed below may change the effect of either drug with the possibility of causing toxicity or decreasing effectiveness: aminoglutethimide, antacids, anticoagulants†, antidiabetics†, barbiturates†, carbamazepine, cholestyramine, colestipol, diuretics†, estrogens†, griseofulvin, insulin, isoniazid, mitotane, phenylbutazone, phenytoin, primidone, rifampin, salicylates†, somatrem, somatropin

Severe reactions are possible when this drug is taken with those listed below: aspirin, amphotericin B, cardiac glycosides†, immunizations, nonsteroidal antiinflammatories†, ritodrine

ALLERGIC REACTIONS AND SIDE EFFECTS

If you are allergic to any corticosteroids†, you may also be allergic to this drug. You should tell your doctor about all your allergies and any unexplained symptoms you may have while taking this drug.

This drug may cause your eyes to be more sensitive to sunlight, but there are no special risks associated with sunburn while taking this drug.

MORE COMMON SIDE EFFECTS: Excitement*, indigestion, irregular heartbeat*, leg pain*, nervousness, restlessness*, sleep disorders, seizures*, stomach pain*, swelling*

LESS COMMON SIDE EFFECTS: Acne*, bloody stools*, bruising*, dizziness, eye pain*, flushing, frequent urination*, headache*, hiccups, increased appetite, increased hair growth*, lightheadedness, menstrual problems*, muscle cramps*, nausea*, pain*, red eyes*, rounding of the face*, skin discoloration, skin irritation*, sleeping difficulty*, spinning sensation, stunted growth*, sweating, tearing eyes*, thirst*, tiredness*, vision changes*, vomiting*, weakness*, weight gain*, wounds that will not heal*

RARE SIDE EFFECTS: Confusion*, depression*, hallucinations*, hives*, mood swings*, skin rash*

PRECAUTIONS

This drug may cause severe and possibly fatal withdrawal symptoms if stopped abruptly. If you wish to stop taking this drug, ask your doctor for specific instructions.

This drug may cause an increase in blood sugar or cholesterol level, calcium loss, and/or retention of fluid.

Avoid contact with anyone who has the chickenpox, measles, or other communicable disease since it may be easier to catch the infection while taking this drug.

Exposure to skin tests, immunizations, and people who have received immunizations may put you at a greater risk of developing the disease when you are taking this drug.

This drug causes changes in your blood that put you at greater risk of getting an infection. Be careful not to cut yourself or get bruised. Tell your doctor if you develop signs of infection, such as fever or sore throat. Your dentist may recommend that you clean your teeth and mouth differently to avoid infection.

The topical form of this drug is absorbed through the skin and may carry the same warnings as the oral product if it is used for a long time, covers a large area, or is used on broken or irritated skin.

The eye ointment works only on the eye and is not absorbed very well into the body. Most of the interactions and warnings in this summary do not apply to the eye ointment.

PREGNANCY AND BREAST-FEEDING

Safety in pregnancy has not been established although the drug is known to harm animal fetuses.

This drug passes into breast milk and may cause growth problems in the baby. The risk is related to the dose and route of the drug. Small amounts the drug are absorbed into the body from topical products.

HELPFUL COMMENTS

The topical form of this drug is available at low strengths without a prescription. In some cases, the same strengths are available in both OTC and prescription-only products depending on the drug manufacturer. Check with your pharmacist for more-specific details.

If you need to take an antacid, take it either 2 hours before or after taking this drug.

---

†*See page 52.*   **See page 53.*

HYDROFLUMETHIAZIDE

Available for over 20 years

COMMONLY USED TO TREAT

Fluid retention, also known as edema
Frequent urination in people with diabetes
High blood pressure, also known as hypertension

DRUG CATEGORY

antihypertensive
Class: thiazide diuretic

PRODUCTS

Brand-Name Products with Generic Alternatives
Saluron 50 mg tablet (n/a)
  Generic: hydroflumethiazide 50 mg tablet (n/a)
Other Generic Product Names
Diucardin
Combination Products That Contain This Drug
Salutensin tablet (n/a)

DOSING AND FOOD

Doses are taken 1 to 2 times a day but may be taken as little as 3 times a week.
Adults: Up to 200 mg per day in divided doses.
Lower doses may be used in children.
It is best to take this drug on an empty stomach, but taking this drug with a little food may avoid the stomach upset that some people suffer. Avoid food with excess salt.
Forgotten doses: If you are scheduled to take the next dose within a few hours, do not take the forgotten dose. Otherwise take the forgotten dose as soon as you remember.

ALCOHOL, DRUG, HERB, AND SUPPLEMENT INTERACTIONS

Alcohol may cause your blood pressure to rise, making this drug less effective. Ask your doctor about the risks caused by drinking alcohol with your condition.
Licorice root may increase potassium loss and should not be used while taking this drug.

Several OTC drugs used for appetite control, asthma, colds, cough, hay fever, or sinus problems may cause an increase in blood pressure when taken with this drug. Check with your pharmacist when selecting OTC products.

Taking this drug with any of the ones listed below may change the effect of either drug with the possibility of causing toxicity or decreasing effectiveness: antidiabetics†, cholestyramine, colestipol, digoxin, insulin, lithium

ALLERGIC REACTIONS AND SIDE EFFECTS

If you are allergic to acetazolamide, bumetanide, dichlorphenamide, furosemide, methazolamide, sulfonamides†, or thiazide diuretics†, you may also be allergic to this drug. You should tell your doctor about all your allergies and any unexplained symptoms you may have while taking this drug.

This drug promotes the effect of sunlight on the body and may cause severe sunburn and increased sensitivity of the eyes.

LESS COMMON SIDE EFFECTS: Diarrhea*, dizziness, lightheadedness, loss of appetite, sexual dysfunction, stomachache

RARE SIDE EFFECTS: Back pain*, black stools*, bleeding*, bloody urine*, breathing difficulty*, bruising*, burning sensation*, chest pain*, chills*, confusion*, cough*, fatigue*, fever*, hives*, headache*, hoarseness*, irregular heartbeat*, joint pain*, leg pain*, muscle cramps*, nausea*, numbness*, painful urination*, shortness of breath*, skin rash*, stomach pain*, swelling*, vomiting*, weakness*, yellow eyes or skin*

PRECAUTIONS

This drug may cause your blood sugar level to rise and may lead to type 2 diabetes.

Your body may lose potassium while taking this drug, which may cause severe side effects. Potassium levels should be monitored periodically and may need to be supplemented while taking this drug. Eat food rich in potassium, such as apricots, bananas, citrus fruit, dates, and tomatoes, if you are not taking a potassium supplement or potassium-sparing diuretic.

People with kidney disease may not be able to take this drug.

This drug may increase the level of uric acid in the body, which may lead to gout or kidney stones.

If you have lupus erythematosus or pancreatitis, this drug may make those conditions worse.

Nicotine in cigarettes may increase blood pressure, making this drug less effective.

---

† *See page 52.*   * *See page 53.*

This drug may cause an increase in the levels of cholesterol or triglyceride in the blood.

PREGNANCY AND BREAST-FEEDING

Safety in pregnancy has not been established although the drug is known to harm animal fetuses.

Breast-feeding while taking this drug is not recommended.

HELPFUL COMMENTS

Take your last dose of the day no later than 6 P.M. to avoid urination during the night.

Avoid quick movements to minimize dizziness. Dangling your legs over the side of the bed for a few minutes may help reduce dizziness when first waking up.

Record your weight twice a day, when first getting up in the morning and after the drug causes urination. A weight gain or loss of more than 2 pounds per day should be reported to your doctor.

The antihypertensive effects of this drug will last about 1 week after it is stopped.

HYDROMORPHONE HYDROCHLORIDE

Available for over 20 years

COMMONLY USED TO TREAT

Pain

DRUG CATEGORY

analgesic
antitussive
Class: narcotic analgesic/opioid

PRODUCTS

Brand-Name Products with Generic Alternatives
Dilaudid 2 mg tablet (¢¢¢)
  Generic: hydromorphone hydrochloride 2 mg tablet (¢¢¢)
Dilaudid 4 mg tablet (¢¢¢¢¢)
  Generic: hydromorphone hydrochloride 4 mg tablet (¢¢¢)
Dilaudid 8 mg tablet ($)
  Generic: hydromorphone hydrochloride 8 mg tablet ($)

Dilaudid 5 mg/5 ml oral solution (¢¢¢¢¢)
   Generic: hydromorphone hydrochloride 5 mg/5 ml oral solution (¢¢¢¢¢)

DOSING AND FOOD

Doses are taken 4 to 8 times a day.

It is best to take this drug on an empty stomach, but taking this drug with a little food may avoid the stomach upset that some people suffer.

Adults: Up to 80 mg per day in divided doses.

Children age 6 to 12: Up to 4 mg per day in divided doses.

Forgotten doses: If you are scheduled to take the next dose within a few hours, do not take the forgotten dose. Otherwise take the forgotten dose as soon as you remember.

ALCOHOL, DRUG, HERB, AND SUPPLEMENT INTERACTIONS

Alcohol should not be used while taking this drug.

Several OTC drugs used for asthma, colds, cough, hay fever, sleep aid, or sinus problems may seriously change the effects and side effects of this drug. Check with your pharmacist when selecting OTC products.

Taking this drug with any of the ones listed below may change the effect of either drug with the possibility of causing toxicity or decreasing effectiveness: natrexone, rifampin

Severe reactions are possible when this drug is taken with those listed below: analgesics†, anesthetics, anticholinergics†, antihistamines†, barbiturates†, benzodiazepines†, cimetidine, monoamine oxidase inhibitors†, naloxone, narcotics†, phenothiazines†, sedative-hypnotics†, skeletal muscle relaxants†, tricyclic antidepressants†

ALLERGIC REACTIONS AND SIDE EFFECTS

If you are allergic to any narcotics†, you may also be allergic to this drug. You should tell your doctor about all your allergies and any unexplained symptoms you may have while taking this drug.

MORE COMMON SIDE EFFECTS: Dizziness*, drowsiness*, fainting, lightheadedness, nausea, vomiting

LESS COMMON SIDE EFFECTS: Blurry vision, breathing difficulty*, constipation, depression*, dry mouth, excitement*, flushing*, hallucinations*, headache, hives*, irregular breathing*, irregular heartbeat*, itching*, loss of appetite, mood swings*, nervousness*, restlessness*, ringing in ears*, shortness of breath*, skin rash*, sleep disorders, spastic movements*, stomach cramps, sweating*, swelling*, tiredness, trembling*, urinary changes, vision changes, weakness*, wheezing*

---

†*See page 52.*   ** See page 53.*

RARE SIDE EFFECTS: Body aches, clammy skin*, confusion*, diarrhea, fever, goosebumps, irritability, low blood pressure*, runny nose, seizures*, shivering, small pupils*, sneezing, yawning

PRECAUTIONS

Be careful driving or handling equipment while taking this drug because it may cause dizziness and drowsiness.

If you have a history of head injury, brain disease, emphysema, asthma, lung disease, enlarged prostate, urinary disorders, gallbladder disease, or gallstones, you may not be able to take this drug.

People with colitis, heart disease, kidney disease, liver disease, and thyroid disease are at increased risk of developing side effects.

If you have a history of seizures, there may be an increased risk of developing a seizure while taking this drug.

This drug may cause withdrawal symptoms if stopped suddenly. If you wish to stop taking this drug, ask your doctor for specific instructions.

Side effects may continue to develop even after the drug is stopped.

Because this drug has a high abuse potential, your prescription quantity may be limited.

PREGNANCY AND BREAST-FEEDING

Safety during pregnancy has not been established although the drug is known to harm animal fetuses.

Breast-feeding while taking this drug is not recommended.

HELPFUL COMMENTS

If the drug does not seem to be working properly, an increase in dose may not help. Talk to your doctor about other drugs and treatment options.

Sucking on hard sugarless candy or chewing sugarless gum may help relieve dry mouth caused by this drug.

Lie down for a while after taking a dose of this drug to help reduce the nausea.

Avoid quick movements to minimize dizziness. Dangling your legs over the side of the bed for a few minutes may help reduce dizziness when first waking up.

If being used for pain, this drug works best when taken before the pain gets too severe.

Add more fiber to your diet to help minimize the constipation that occurs with this drug. If severe, constipation may need to be treated with a stool softener. Ask your doctor or pharmacist for recommendations.

HYDROXYCHLOROQUINE SULFATE

Available for over 20 years

COMMONLY USED TO TREAT

Malaria
Lupus erythematosus
Rheumatoid arthritis

DRUG CATEGORY

antiinflammatory
antimalarial
Class: 4-amino-quinoline

PRODUCTS

Brand-Name Products with Generic Alternatives
Plaquenil 200 mg tablet ($$)
   Generic: hydroxychloroquine sulfate 200 mg tablet (¢¢¢)

DOSING AND FOOD

Doses are taken twice a day to once a week.
Taking this drug with food, usually just before or after a meal, may avoid
   the stomach upset that some people suffer.

Adults: Up to 800 mg per day in divided doses.

Lower doses are used in infants and children to treat and prevent malaria.

Forgotten doses: Have your doctor tell you what to do about forgotten
   doses when you first get the prescription. It is very important to take this
   drug exactly on schedule for the drug to work properly.

ALCOHOL, DRUG, HERB, AND SUPPLEMENT INTERACTIONS

Alcohol may increase some of the side effects from this drug, depending
   on the amount consumed. Ask your doctor about the risks caused by
   drinking alcohol with your condition.

Several antacids and antidiarrheal drugs may interfere with this drug.
   Check with your pharmacist when selecting OTC products.

**Taking this drug with any of the ones listed below may change the effect of
either drug with the possibility of causing toxicity or decreasing effectiveness:**
digoxin, kaolin, magnesium trisilicate

---

† See page 52.   * See page 53.

ALLERGIC REACTIONS AND SIDE EFFECTS

If you are allergic to chloroquine, you may also be allergic to this drug. You should tell your doctor about all your allergies and any unexplained symptoms you may have while taking this drug.

This drug promotes the effect of sunlight on the body and may cause severe sunburn and increased sensitivity of the eyes.

MORE COMMON SIDE EFFECTS: Diarrhea, headache*, itching, loss of appetite, nausea, seizures*, stomach pain, vision changes*, vomiting

LESS COMMON SIDE EFFECTS: Blue fingernails, blue mouth, blurry vision*, dizziness, hair color change, hair loss, lightheadedness, nervousness, restlessness, skin discoloration, skin rash

RARE SIDE EFFECTS: Bleeding*, bruising*, drowsiness*, excitability*, fever*, hearing loss*, mood swings*, ringing in ears*, sore throat*, tiredness*, weakness*

PRECAUTIONS

Vision changes that occur while taking this drug may begin after the drug is stopped or continue to get worse for a month or longer.

Itching is more common in African Americans.

If you have difficulty swallowing, the tablets may be crushed and mixed with food such as jelly, jam, or jello. Make sure to eat all the mixture to get the entire dose.

If you have a history of stomach or intestinal disorders, psoriasis, or porphyria, this drug may make those conditions worse.

People with glucose-6-phosphate dehydrogenase deficiency (G6PD) may not be able to take this drug.

Tell your doctor if you take large doses of aspirin on a regular basis since this drug may mask the symptoms of aspirin toxicity.

The dose of this drug may be stated in two different ways. Two hundred (200) mg of the salt is equivalent to 150 mg of base. Talk to your pharmacist if your prescription is labeled differently than discussed with your doctor.

Be careful driving or handling equipment while taking this drug because it may cause vision changes.

PREGNANCY AND BREAST-FEEDING

Safety during pregnancy has not been established although the drug is known to harm animal fetuses.

This drug passes into breast milk, but does not appear to harm the baby.

Talk to your doctor about the risks associated with breast-feeding while taking this drug.

HELPFUL COMMENTS

Eye irritation caused by the sun may be reduced by wearing sunglasses when outside.

If you are using the drug to prevent malaria, it should be started 2 weeks before traveling, and for 8 weeks after leaving the infected area. You should also use a DEET-containing mosquito repellent and use other precautions when traveling.

HYDROXYUREA

Available for over 20 years

COMMONLY USED TO TREAT

Cancer
Leukemia
Tumors

DRUG CATEGORY

antineoplastic
Class: urea

PRODUCTS

Brand-Name Products with No Generic Alternative
Droxia 200 mg capsule (¢¢¢¢¢)
Droxia 300 mg capsule (¢¢¢¢¢)
Droxia 400 mg capsule (¢¢¢¢¢)

Brand-Name Products with Generic Alternatives
Hydrea 500 mg capsule ($)
  Generic: hydroxyurea 500 mg capsule ($)

Products Only Available as Generics
hydroxyurea 250 mg capsule (n/a)
hydroxyurea 1,000 mg capsule (n/a)

DOSING AND FOOD

Doses are taken once a day for 3 days.

This drug may be taken with or without food. Do not eat raw oysters or other raw shellfish at any time while taking this drug.

---

† See page 52.   * See page 53.

Taking this drug with food may avoid the stomach upset that many people suffer.

Adults: Up to 30 mg/kg per day.

Forgotten doses: Do not take a forgotten dose unless told to do so by your doctor. Just go back to your usual schedule with the next dose. If you vomit shortly after taking a dose, call your doctor to find out if the dose should be repeated.

ALCOHOL, DRUG, HERB, AND SUPPLEMENT INTERACTIONS

Alcohol may increase some of the side effects from this drug, depending on the amount consumed. Ask your doctor about the risks caused by drinking alcohol with your condition.

Taking this drug with any of the ones listed below may change the effect of either drug with the possibility of causing toxicity or decreasing effectiveness: amphotericin B, antithyroid drugs†, azathioprine, chloramphenicol, colchicine, cyclophosphamide, flucytosine, ganciclovir, interferon, mercaptopurine, methotrexate, plicamycin, probenecid, sulfinpyrazone, zidovudine

Severe reactions are possible when this drug is taken with those listed below: didanosine, fluorouracil, indinavir, stavudine

Increased side effects are possible when this drug is taken with those listed below: abacavir, amprenavir, delavirdine, efavirenz, lamivudine, nelfinavir, nevirapine, ritonavir, saquinavir, zalcitavine, zidovudine

ALLERGIC REACTIONS AND SIDE EFFECTS

You should tell your doctor about all your allergies and any unexplained symptoms you may have while taking this drug.

MORE COMMON SIDE EFFECTS: Back pain*, chills*, cough*, diarrhea, drowsiness, fever*, hoarseness*, loss of appetite, nausea, urinary difficulty*, vomiting

LESS COMMON SIDE EFFECTS: Black fingernails and toenails*, black stools*, bleeding*, bloody urine*, bruising*, constipation, itching, mouth sores*, skin irritation*, skin rash

RARE SIDE EFFECTS: Confusion*, dizziness*, flushing*, hallucinations*, headache*, joint pain*, scaly skin*, seizures*, skin discoloration*, swelling*

PRECAUTIONS

This drug causes changes in your blood that put you at greater risk of getting an infection. Be careful not to cut yourself or get bruised. Tell your doctor if you develop signs of infection, such as fever or sore throat. Your dentist may recommend that you clean your teeth and mouth differently to avoid infection.

Avoid contact with anyone who has the chickenpox, measles, or other communicable disease since it may be easier to catch the infection while taking this drug.

Exposure to skin tests, immunizations, and people who have received immunizations may put you at a greater risk of developing the disease when you are taking this drug.

People with a history of gout or kidney stones may not be able to take this drug.

If you experience changes in your blood count, including anemia, you may not be able to take this drug.

If you cannot swallow the capsules, they may be opened and mixed with water. The powder that floats on the top of the water does not contain the active drug, and you do not need to worry about mixing it all together before drinking.

This drug may cause skin irritation if capsules are broken or opened. You should wash your hands immediately after any contact with the drug powder.

PREGNANCY AND BREAST-FEEDING

There is evidence that this drug may harm the fetus, but the drug may be necessary to the health of the mother.

Breast-feeding while taking this drug is not recommended.

HELPFUL COMMENTS

It is very important to continue taking this drug as ordered by the doctor even if the side effects make you feel ill.

Drinking 10 to 12 glasses of water each day will help reduce the risk of developing kidney stones.

HYDROXYZINE

Available for over 20 years

COMMONLY USED TO TREAT

Itching caused by allergies
Nervous disorders, such as anxiety and tension

---

† See page 52.   * See page 53.

DRUG CATEGORY

antihistamine
antipruritic
anxiolytic
Class: H1 receptor blocker: piperazine

PRODUCTS

Brand-Name Products with No Generic Alternative
Vistaril 25 mg/5 ml oral suspension ($$)

Brand-Name Products with Generic Alternatives
Atarax 10 mg tablet (¢¢¢¢)
  Generic: hydroxyzine hydrochloride 10 mg tablet (¢)
Atarax 25 mg tablet ($)
  Generic: hydroxyzine hydrochloride 25 mg tablet (¢)
Atarax 50 mg tablet ($)
  Generic: hydroxyzine hydrochloride 50 mg tablet (¢)
Atarax 100 mg tablet ($$)
  Generic: hydroxyzine hydrochloride 100 mg tablet (¢¢)
Atarax 10 mg/5 ml oral syrup (¢¢¢¢)
  Generic: hydroxyzine hydrochloride 10 mg/5 ml oral syrup (¢¢)
Vistaril 25 mg capsule ($)
  Generic: hydroxyzine pamoate 25 mg capsule (¢)
Vistaril 50 mg capsule ($)
  Generic: hydroxyzine pamoate 50 mg capsule (¢¢)
Vistaril 100 mg capsule ($$)
  Generic: hydroxyzine pamoate 100 mg capsule (¢¢)

DOSING AND FOOD

Doses are taken 3 to 4 times a day.
This drug may be taken with or without food.
Adults: Up to 400 mg per day in divided doses.
Children over age 6: Up to 100 mg per day in divided doses.
Children under age 6: Up to 50 mg per day in divided doses.
Forgotten doses: If you are scheduled to take the next dose within a few
  hours, do not take the forgotten dose. Otherwise take the forgotten dose
  as soon as you remember.

ALCOHOL, DRUG, HERB, AND SUPPLEMENT INTERACTIONS

Alcohol may increase some of the side effects from this drug, depending

on the amount consumed. Ask your doctor about the risks caused by drinking alcohol with your condition.

Several OTC drugs used for appetite control, asthma, colds, cough, hay fever, pain, or sinus problems may seriously increase the effects of this drug. Check with your pharmacist when selecting OTC products.

Taking this drug with any of the ones listed below may change the effect of either drug with the possibility of causing toxicity or decreasing effectiveness: anesthetics, anticholinergics†, antihistamines†, anxiolytics†, barbiturates†, epinephrine, narcotics†, tricyclic antidepressants†

Severe reactions are possible when this drug is taken with those listed below: monoamine oxidase inhibitors†

Increased side effects are possible when this drug is taken with those listed below: alcohol, antihistamines†

ALLERGIC REACTIONS AND SIDE EFFECTS

If you are allergic to other antihistamines†, you may also be allergic to this drug. You should tell your doctor about all your allergies and any unexplained symptoms you may have while taking this drug.

This drug promotes the effect of sunlight on the body and may cause severe sunburn and increased sensitivity of the eyes.

MORE COMMON SIDE EFFECTS: Drowsiness, dry mouth, headache*

LESS COMMON SIDE EFFECTS: Body aches, clumsiness, chest tightness*, confusion, congestion, constipation, cough, diarrhea*, early menstruation, excitement, fatigue, fever*, heartburn, hoarseness, indigestion, irregular heartbeat*, irritability, joint pain, menstrual pain, muscle cramps, nervousness, nightmares, restlessness, ringing in ears, runny nose, skin rash, shortness of breath*, sore throat*, stiffness, sweating, swelling*, tingling*, tremor, urinary difficulty, vision changes, vomiting

RARE SIDE EFFECTS: Abdominal pain*, bleeding*, bruising*, chills*, cough*, dark urine*, dizziness*, hives*, itching*, nausea, pale stools*, seizures*, skin irritation*, stomachache, swallowing difficulty*, tiredness*, weakness*, wheezing*

PRECAUTIONS

If you have glaucoma, an enlarged prostate, or difficulty urinating, this drug may make those conditions worse.

This drug may interfere with skin tests used to diagnose allergies and should be stopped for at least 4 days before the test.

---

†See page 52.   *See page 53.

You should wait 2 weeks after stopping a monoamine oxidase inhibitor†
before starting this drug to avoid an increase in side effects.

Be careful driving or handling equipment while taking this drug because
the drug may cause drowsiness.

This drug may cause dry mouth, which is associated with a greater risk of
cavities. Your dentist may recommend that you clean your teeth and
mouth differently to avoid infection.

PREGNANCY AND BREAST-FEEDING

Safety in pregnancy has not been established although there was no evidence of harm during studies in animals.

Breast-feeding while taking this drug is not recommended.

HELPFUL COMMENTS

Sucking on hard sugarless candy or chewing sugarless gum may help relieve dry mouth caused by this drug.

Several antihistamines are sold without a prescription by the following
generic names: brompheniramine, chlorpheniramine, clemastine, diphenhydramine, doxylamine, loratadine. Ask your pharmacist about specific
products that contain these drugs.

IBUPROFEN

Available for over 20 years

COMMONLY USED TO TREAT

Arthritis
Fever
Gout
Menstrual pain
Pain

DRUG CATEGORY

analgesic
antiarthritic
antidysmenorrheal
antigout
antipyretic
Class: nonsteroidal antiinflammatory

PRODUCTS

Brand-Name Products with Generic Alternatives
Motrin 300 mg tablet (n/a)
  Generic: ibuprofen 300 mg tablet (n/a)
Motrin 400 mg tablet (¢¢)
  Generic: ibuprofen 400 mg tablet (¢)
Motrin 600 mg tablet (¢¢¢)
  Generic: ibuprofen 600 mg tablet (¢)
Motrin 800 mg tablet (¢¢¢)
  Generic: ibuprofen 800 mg tablet (¢)
Motrin 100 mg/5 ml oral suspension (¢¢¢)
  Generic: ibuprofen 100 mg/5 ml oral suspension (¢¢)

Other Generic Product Names
Advil, Cap-Profen, Ibu, Ibuprohm, Ibu-tab, Medipren, Profen
Other Products That Contain This Drug
Vicoprofen tablet ($)
Sine-Aid IB tablet (n/a)

DOSING AND FOOD

Doses are taken 3 to 6 times a day.
It is better to take this drug on an empty stomach, but taking this drug with food may avoid the stomach upset that some people suffer.

Adults: Up to 3,200 mg per day in divided doses.

Children: Up to 40 mg/kg per day in divided doses.

Forgotten doses: If you are scheduled to take the next dose within a few hours, do not take the forgotten dose. Otherwise take the forgotten dose as soon as you remember.

ALCOHOL, DRUG, HERB, AND SUPPLEMENT INTERACTIONS

Alcohol may increase some of the side effects from this drug, depending on the amount consumed. Ask your doctor about the risks caused by drinking alcohol with your condition.

Do not use dong quai, feverfew, garlic, ginger, horse chestnut, red clover, or St. John's wort while taking this drug since they may increase the risk of serious side effects.

Taking this drug with any of the ones listed below may change the effect of either drug with the possibility of causing toxicity or decreasing effectiveness:
ACE inhibitors†, acetaminophen, antacids, antihypertensives†, digoxin, di-

†_See page 52._   *_See page 53._

ureticst, furosemide, hydrochlorothiazide, nifedipine, lithium, methotrexate, phenytoin, probenecid, sulfonylureast, sulindac, verapamil

Severe reactions are possible when this drug is taken with those listed below:
antibioticst, anticoagulantst, aspirin, cefamandole, cefoperazone, cefotetan, corticosteroidst, cyclosporine, dipyridamole, gold saltst, heparin,
mezlocillin, nonsteroidal antiinflammatoriest, penicillamine, piperacillin,
plicamycin, salicylatest, sulfinpyrazone, ticarcillin, valproic acid, warfarin

ALLERGIC REACTIONS AND SIDE EFFECTS

If you are allergic to aspirin, zomepirac, salicylatest, or other nonsteroidal
antiinflammatoriest, you may also be allergic to this drug. You should
tell your doctor about all your allergies and any unexplained symptoms
you may have while taking this drug.

This drug promotes the effect of sunlight on the body and may cause
severe sunburn and increased sensitivity of the eyes.

MORE COMMON SIDE EFFECTS: Black stools*, dizziness, headache, heartburn*, indigestion*, itching*, mouth sores*, nausea*, skin rash*,
swelling*, weight gain*

LESS COMMON SIDE EFFECTS: Abdominal pain, bruising*, constipation,
diarrhea, gas, high blood pressure*, sweating, vomiting

RARE SIDE EFFECTS: Back pain*, bloody urine*, bloody vomit, blue fingernails*, blue lips*, breathing difficulty*, chest pain*, chest tightness*,
chills*, confusion*, cough*, dark urine*, drowsiness, fainting*, fever*, hallucinations*, hearing loss*, hives*, hoarseness*, lip sores*, loss of appetite*, low blood pressure*, mood swings*, muscle cramps*,
nosebleeds*, pain*, pale skin*, pale stools*, puffy eyes*, rectal bleeding*,
restlessness*, ringing in ears*, runny nose*, seizures*, shortness of
breath*, sore throat*, stiff neck*, swollen glands*, swollen tongue*,
thirst*, tiredness*, urinary changes*, vision changes*, weakness*, wheezing*, yellow eyes or skin*

PRECAUTIONS

This drug may cause serious stomach problems and possibly ulcers. Be
careful to take this drug as directed with food, and let your doctor know
if you develop any stomach-related symptoms.

Do not lie down for about 30 minutes after taking this drug to help reduce
the risk of heartburn and throat irritation.

Be careful driving or handling equipment while taking this drug because it
may cause dizziness.

If you use tobacco or have a history of alcohol abuse, stomach problems, intestinal problems, hemorrhoids, diabetes mellitus, severe fluid retention, or systemic lupus erythematosus, there is an increased risk that you will develop side effects while taking this drug.

PREGNANCY AND BREAST-FEEDING

Safety in pregnancy has not been established although the drug is known to harm animal fetuses.

Breast-feeding while taking this drug is not recommended.

HELPFUL COMMENTS

Do not mix the oral suspension with anything before taking the dose.

It may take 1 to 2 weeks before the effects of this drug are noticed.

Avoid quick movements to minimize dizziness.

If you need to take an antacid, take it either 2 hours before or after taking this drug.

Several nonsteroidal antiinflammatories† are available without a prescription in lower, nonprescription strengths, including ibuprofen, ketoprofen, and naproxen.

If you are taking the OTC form of this drug for more than 10 days, you should talk to your doctor to verify your diagnosis and consider higher doses or another drug.

IMATINIB MESYLATE

Available since May 2001

COMMONLY USED TO TREAT

Cancer
Tumors

DRUG CATEGORY

antineoplastic
Class: protein-tyrosine kinase inhibitor

PRODUCTS

Brand-Name Products with No Generic Alternative
Gleevac 50 mg capsule (n/a)
Gleevac 100 mg capsule ($$$$$)
No generics available.

---

†See page 52.   *See page 53.

Patent expires in 2013. Multiple exclusivity restrictions that begin to expire in 2005.

DOSING AND FOOD

Doses are taken 1 to 2 times a day.

Take this drug with food and a full glass of water. Do not drink grapefruit juice or eat grapefruit while taking this drug.

Adults: Up to 800 mg per day in divided doses.

Forgotten doses: Do not take a forgotten dose unless told to do so by your doctor. Just go back to your usual schedule with the next dose.

ALCOHOL, DRUG, HERB, AND SUPPLEMENT INTERACTIONS

Alcohol may increase some of the side effects from this drug, depending on the amount consumed. Ask your doctor about the risks caused by drinking alcohol with your condition.

St. John's wort may decrease the effect of this drug and should not be used while taking this drug.

Taking this drug with any of the ones listed below may change the effect of either drug with the possibility of causing toxicity or decreasing effectiveness: bezodiazepines†, calcium channel blockers†, carbamazepine, clarithromycin, cyclosporine, dexamethasone, dihydropyridine, erythromycin, HMG-CoA reductase inhibitors†, itraconazole, ketoconazole, phenobarbital, phenytoin, pimozide, rifampin, warfarin

Increased side effects are possible when this drug is taken with those listed below: amphotericin B, antineoplastics†, antithyroid drugs†, azathioprine, chloramphenicol, colchicine, cyclophosphamide, flucytosine, ganciclovir, interferon, mercaptopurine, methotrexate, plicamycin, zidovudine

ALLERGIC REACTIONS AND SIDE EFFECTS

You should tell your doctor about all your allergies and any unexplained symptoms you may have while taking this drug.

MORE COMMON SIDE EFFECTS: Black stools*, bleeding*, bone pain, breathing difficulty*, bruising*, chest pain*, chills*, cough*, diarrhea, fever*, frequent bowel movements, joint pain, mouth sores*, pale skin*, shortness of breath*, skin rash, sore throat*, stomach pain, swelling*, swollen glands*, tiredness*, urinary changes*, weakness*, weight gain*

LESS COMMON SIDE EFFECTS: Back pain, bloody nose, body aches*, chest tightness*, clogged ears*, dizziness, dry mouth*, gas, headache*, irregular heartbeat*, itching, loss of appetite*, loss of voice*, mood swings*, muscle pain*, nausea*, night sweats, numbness*, runny nose*, seizures*, shivering*, skin irritation*, sleep disorders, sneezing*, stomach upset, stuffy nose*, sweating*, taste changes, thirst*, tingling*, vomiting*, watery eyes, weight loss, wheezing*

RARE SIDE EFFECTS: Blindness (temporary)*, bloody stools*, bloody vomit*, blurry vision*, muteness*, slurry speech*

PRECAUTIONS

This drug causes changes in your blood that put you at greater risk of getting an infection. Be careful not to cut yourself or get bruised. Tell your doctor if you develop signs of infection, such as fever or sore throat. Your dentist may recommend that you clean your teeth and mouth differently to avoid infection.

Avoid contact with anyone who has the chickenpox, measles, or other communicable disease since it may be easier to catch the infection while taking this drug.

Exposure to skin tests, immunizations, and people who have received immunizations may put you at a greater risk of developing the disease when you are taking this drug.

If you experience changes in your blood count, including anemia, you may not be able to take this drug.

PREGNANCY AND BREAST-FEEDING

There is evidence that this drug may harm the fetus, but the drug may be necessary to the health of the mother.

Breast-feeding while taking this drug is not recommended.

HELPFUL COMMENTS

It is very important to continue taking this drug as ordered by the doctor even if the side effects make you feel ill.

You will need to have your blood count, kidney function, and liver function tested regularly while taking this drug.

IMIPRAMINE

Available for over 20 years

COMMONLY USED TO TREAT

Bed-wetting
Depression

---

†*See page 52.* **See page 53.*

DRUG CATEGORY

antibulemic
anticataplectic
antidepressant
antienuretic
antineuralgic
antipanic
Class: tricyclic antidepressant

PRODUCTS

Brand-Name Products with No Generic Alternative
Tofranil PM 75 mg capsule ($$)
Tofranil PM 100 mg capsule ($$$)
Tofranil PM 125 mg capsule ($$$)
Tofranil PM 150 mg capsule ($$$)

Brand-Name Products with Generic Alternatives
Tofranil 10 mg tablet (¢¢¢¢)
   Generic: imipramine hydrochloride 10 mg tablet (¢)
Tofranil 25 mg tablet (¢¢¢¢¢)
   Generic: imipramine hydrochloride 25 mg tablet (¢)
Tofranil 50 mg tablet ($$)
   Generic: imipramine hydrochloride 50 mg tablet (¢)

Products Only Available as Generics
imipramine hydrochloride 25 mg/ml oral concentrate (n/a)

DOSING AND FOOD

Doses are taken 3 to 4 times a day.
Taking this drug with food or milk may avoid the stomach upset that some
   people suffer.

Adults: Up to 300 mg per day in divided doses.

Children age 6 and older: Up to 5 mg/kg per day in divided doses.

Forgotten doses: If you have forgotten a bedtime dose, do not take the
   forgotten dose. Just go back to your usual schedule with the next dose. If
   you have forgotten a daytime dose and are scheduled to take the next
   dose within a few hours, do not take the forgotten dose. Otherwise take
   the forgotten dose as soon as you remember.

ALCOHOL, DRUG, HERB, AND SUPPLEMENT INTERACTIONS

Alcohol should not be used while taking this drug.

Evening primrose oil, SAMe, St. John's wort, and yohimbe may cause serious reactions when taken with this drug. Notify your doctor if you are
taking any of these supplements.

Several OTC drugs used for asthma, colds, cough, hay fever, sleep aid, or sinus problems may seriously change the effects and side effects of this
drug. Check with your pharmacist when selecting OTC products.

**Taking this drug with any of the ones listed below may change the effect of
either drug with the possibility of causing toxicity or decreasing effectiveness:**
anesthetics, antipsychotics†, barbiturates†, beta blockers†, cimetidine,
clonidine, fluoxetine, guanabenz, guanadrel, guanethidine, haloperidol,
methyldopa, methylphenidate, oral contraceptives, phenothiazines†,
propoxyphene, reserpine

Severe reactions are possible when this drug is taken with those listed below:
amphetamines†, anesthetics, antiarrhythmics†, anticholinergics†, antidysk-
inetics†, antihistamines†, antithyroid drug†, anxiolytics†, appetite suppressants, barbiturates†, disopyramide, disulfiram, ephedrine, epinephrine,
ethchlorvynol, isoproterenol, meperidine, metrizamide, monoamine oxidase inhibitors†, narcotics†, phenylephrine, pimozide, procainamide,
quinidine, tricyclic antidepressants†, warfarin

Increased side effects are possible when this drug is taken with those listed below:
alseroxylon, deserpidine, metoclopramide, metyrosine, pemoline, promethazine, rauwolfia serpentine, trimeprazine

ALLERGIC REACTIONS AND SIDE EFFECTS

If you are allergic to carbamazepine, maprotiline, trazodone, or any tricyclic antidepressants†, you may also be allergic to this drug. You should
tell your doctor about all your allergies and any unexplained symptoms
you may have while taking this drug.

This drug promotes the effect of sunlight on the body and may cause
severe sunburn and increased sensitivity of the eyes.

MORE COMMON SIDE EFFECTS: Constipation*, dizziness, drowsiness, dry
mouth, fainting*, headache*, irregular heartbeat*, seizures*, sweating,
tiredness, urinary changes*

LESS COMMON SIDE EFFECTS: Blurry vision*, confusion*, diarrhea, expressionless face*, eye pain*, hallucinations*, heartburn, increased appetite,
loss of balance*, nausea, nervousness*, restlessness*, shakiness*, shuffling
walk*, sleeping difficulty, slowed movements*, stiffness*, swallowing difficulty*, taste changes, trembling*, vomiting, weakness*, weight gain

RARE SIDE EFFECTS: Anxiety*, breast enlargement*, hair loss, irritability*,

---

†*See page 52.*   **See page 53.*

muscle twitching*, ringing in ears*, skin rash*, sore throat*, fever*, swelling*, teeth or gum problems*, yellow eyes or skin*

PRECAUTIONS

You need to wait 2 weeks after stopping a monoamine oxidase inhibitor† before starting this drug.

Be careful driving or handling equipment while taking this drug because it may cause drowsiness and dizziness.

Stopping this drug abruptly may result in withdrawal symptoms that include nausea, headache, and general discomfort. If you wish to stop taking this drug, ask your doctor for specific instructions.

This drug may cause dry mouth, which is associated with a greater risk of cavities. Your dentist may recommend that you clean your teeth and mouth differently to avoid infection.

If you have a history of asthma, blood disorders, seizures, enlarged prostate, glaucoma, heart disease, high blood pressure, urinary difficulty, schizophrenia, or manic depression, this drug may make those conditions worse.

PREGNANCY AND BREAST-FEEDING

Safety in pregnancy has not been established although there was no evidence of harm during studies in animals.

Breast-feeding while taking this drug is not recommended.

HELPFUL COMMENTS

Heavy smoking may decrease the effectiveness of this drug.

You may need to take this drug for 4 to 6 weeks before you notice the effects.

Sucking on hard sugarless candy or chewing sugarless gum may help relieve dry mouth caused by this drug.

Avoid quick movements to minimize dizziness. Dangling your legs over the side of the bed for a few minutes may help reduce dizziness when first waking up.

INDAPAMIDE

Available for over 20 years

COMMONLY USED TO TREAT

Fluid retention, also known as edema
High blood pressure, also known as hypertension

DRUG CATEGORY

antihypertensive
Class: thiazidelike diuretic

PRODUCTS

Brand-Name Products with Generic Alternatives
Lozol 1.25 mg tablet (¢¢¢¢¢)
  Generic: indapamide 1.25 mg tablet (¢)
Lozol 2.5 mg tablet ($)
  Generic: indapamide 2.5 mg tablet (¢¢)

DOSING AND FOOD

Doses are taken once a day.

Adults: Up to 5 mg per day in divided doses.

This drug is not used in children.

Taking this drug with a little food may avoid the stomach upset that some
  people suffer. Avoid food with excess salt.

Forgotten doses: If you are scheduled to take the next dose within a few
  hours, do not take the forgotten dose. Otherwise take the forgotten dose
  as soon as you remember.

ALCOHOL, DRUG, HERB, AND SUPPLEMENT INTERACTIONS

Alcohol may cause your blood pressure to rise, making this drug less effective. Ask your doctor about the risks caused by drinking alcohol with
  your condition.

Licorice root may increase potassium loss and should not be used while
  taking this drug.

Several OTC drugs used for appetite control, asthma, colds, cough, hay
  fever, or sinus problems may cause an increase in blood pressure when
  taken with this drug. Check with your pharmacist when selecting OTC
  products.

**Taking this drug with any of the ones listed below may change the effect of
either drug with the possibility of causing toxicity or decreasing effectiveness:**
amphetamines, antidiabetics†, antihypertensives†, cholestyramine, colestipol,
digoxin, insulin, lithium, methenamine, quinidine

Severe reactions are possible when this drug is taken with those listed below:
diazoxide

†*See page 52.*   * *See page 53.*

ALLERGIC REACTIONS AND SIDE EFFECTS

If you are allergic to acetazolamide, bumetanide, dichlorphenamide, furosemide, methazolamide, sulfonamides†, or thiazide diuretics†, you may also be allergic to this drug. You should tell your doctor about all your allergies and any unexplained symptoms you may have while taking this drug.

This drug promotes the effect of sunlight on the body and may cause severe sunburn and increased sensitivity of the eyes.

LESS COMMON SIDE EFFECTS: Diarrhea*, dizziness, lightheadedness, loss of appetite, sleep disorders, stomach upset

RARE SIDE EFFECTS: Back pain*, black stools*, bleeding*, bloody urine*, breathing difficulty*, bruising*, burning sensation*, chest pain*, chills*, confusion*, cough*, fatigue*, fever*, hives*, headache*, hoarseness*, irregular heartbeat*, joint pain*, leg pain*, muscle cramps*, nausea*, numbness*, painful urination*, shortness of breath*, skin rash*, stomach pain*, swelling*, vomiting*, weakness*, yellow eyes or skin*

PRECAUTIONS

This drug may cause your blood sugar level to rise and lead to type 2 diabetes.

Your body may lose potassium while taking this drug, which may cause severe side effects. Potassium levels should be monitored periodically and may need to be supplemented while taking this drug. Eat food rich in potassium, such as apricots, bananas, citrus fruit, dates, and tomatoes, if you are not taking a potassium supplement or potassium-sparing diuretic†.

People with kidney disease may not be able to take this drug.

This drug may increase the level of uric acid in the body which may lead to gout or kidney stones.

Nicotine in cigarettes may increase blood pressure, making this drug less effective.

This drug may cause an increase in the levels of cholesterol or triglyceride in the blood.

PREGNANCY AND BREAST-FEEDING

Safety in pregnancy has not been established although the drug is known to harm animal fetuses.

Breast-feeding while taking this drug is not recommended.

HELPFUL COMMENTS

Take your last dose of the day no later than 6 P.M. to avoid urination during the night.

Avoid quick movements to minimize dizziness. Dangling your legs over the side of the bed for a few minutes may help reduce dizziness when first waking up.

Record your weight twice a day, when first getting up in the morning and after the drug causes urination. A weight gain or loss of more than 2 pounds per day should be reported to your doctor.

The antihypertensive effects of this drug will last about 1 week after stopping this drug.

INDINAVIR SULFATE

Available since March 1996

COMMONLY USED TO TREAT

HIV infections

DRUG CATEGORY

antiretroviral
Class: protease inhibitor (PI)

PRODUCTS

Brand-Name Products with No Generic Alternative
Crixivan 100 mg capsule (¢¢¢¢)
Crixivan 200 mg capsule ($)
Crixivan 333 mg capsule ($$)
Crixivan 400 mg capsule ($$$)
No generics available.
Patent expires in 2012.

DOSING AND FOOD

Doses are taken 3 times a day.

It is best to take this drug on an empty stomach with a full glass of water at least 1 hour before or 2 hours after a meal. Do not drink grapefruit juice while taking this drug. If this drug causes nausea, a little food may be eaten.

Adults: Up to 800 mg per day in divided doses.

---

† See page 52.   * See page 53.

Lower doses may be used in people with liver disease.

Forgotten doses: Do not take a forgotten dose. Just go back to your usual schedule with the next dose.

ALCOHOL, DRUG, HERB, AND SUPPLEMENT INTERACTIONS

Alcohol may increase some of the side effects from this drug, depending on the amount consumed. Ask your doctor about the risks caused by drinking alcohol with your condition.

St. John's wort may reduce the effectiveness of this drug and should not be used.

Taking this drug with any of the ones listed below may change the effect of either drug with the possibility of causing toxicity or decreasing effectiveness: amprenavir, carbamazepine, clarithromycin, delavirdine, didanosine, efavirenz, ergot alkaloids†, HMG CoA reductase inhibitors†, itraconazole, ketoconazole, lopinavir/ritonavir combination, midazolam, nelfinavir, nevirapine, pimozide, rifabutin, rifampin, saquinavir, sildenafil, triazolam

ALLERGIC REACTIONS AND SIDE EFFECTS

You should tell your doctor about all your allergies and any unexplained symptoms you may have while taking this drug.

MORE COMMON SIDE EFFECTS: Back pain*, bloody urine*, diarrhea, sleep disorders, taste changes

LESS COMMON SIDE EFFECTS: Abdominal pain*, appetite changes*, bad breath*, belching, bloody vomit*, chills*, cough, dark urine*, dizziness*, fever*, headache*, heartburn, indigestion, itching*, nausea*, pale stools*, rash*, regurgitation, sleepiness, sour stomach, tiredness*, weakness*, yellow eyes or skin*

RARE SIDE EFFECTS: Bleeding*, breathing difficulty*, bruising*, confusion*, dehydration*, dry skin*, fatigue*, frequent urination*, hunger*, pale skin*, thirst*, vomiting*, weight loss*

PRECAUTIONS

Drinking at least 7 large glasses of water each day while taking this drug may reduce the risk of developing kidney stones.

If you have hemophilia or hepatitis, this drug may make those conditions worse.

This drug is usually prescribed in combination with another antiretroviral drug. Ask your pharmacist about the type of drug interaction that may occur between antiretroviral drugs† to coordinate the administration times of multiple drugs.

HIV precautions should be followed since the infection may still be passed to others while taking this drug.

PREGNANCY AND BREAST-FEEDING

Safety during pregnancy has not been established although the drug is known to harm animal fetuses.

Breast-feeding while taking this drug is not recommended.

HELPFUL COMMENTS

Do not stop treatment early if you start to feel better. It takes the full prescription for this drug to work completely.

INDOMETHACIN

Available for over 20 years

COMMONLY USED TO TREAT

Arthritis
Gout pain
Menstrual pain
Pain

DRUG CATEGORY

antiarthritic
antidysmenorrheal
antigout
antiinflammatory
antipyretic
Class: nonsteroidal antiinflammatory

PRODUCTS

Brand-Name Products with No Generic Alternative
Indomethegan 50 mg rectal suppository (n/a)

Brand-Name Products with Generic Alternatives
Indocin 25 mg capsule (¢¢¢¢)
  Generic: indomethacin 25 mg capsule (¢)
Indocin 50 mg capsule ($)
  Generic: indomethacin 50 mg capsule (¢)
Indocin SR 75 mg extended-release capsule ($)
  Generic: indomethacin 75 mg extended-release capsule (¢¢¢¢)

---

† See page 52.   * See page 53.

Indocin 25 mg/5 ml oral suspension ($)
  Generic: indomethacin 25 mg/5 ml oral suspension (n/a)

Other Generic Product Names
Indo-Lemmon

DOSING AND FOOD

Doses are taken 2 to 4 times a day.
It is best to take this drug with food or antacids.

Adults: Up to 200 mg per day in divided doses.

Children: Up to 4 mg/kg (maximum 200 mg) per day in divided doses.

Forgotten doses: If you are scheduled to take the next dose within a few hours, do not take the forgotten dose. Otherwise take the forgotten dose as soon as you remember.

ALCOHOL, DRUG, HERB, AND SUPPLEMENT INTERACTIONS

Alcohol may increase the risk of serious side effects from this drug. Ask your doctor about the risks caused by drinking alcohol with your condition.

Do not use dong quai, feverfew, garlic, ginger, horse chestnut, red clover, senna, or St. John's wort while taking this drug since they may increase the risk of serious side effects.

Taking this drug with any of the ones listed below may change the effect of either drug with the possibility of causing toxicity or decreasing effectiveness: ACE inhibitors†, acetaminophen, antihypertensives†, digoxin, diuretics†, furosemide, hydrochlorothiazide, nifedipine, lithium, methotrexate, phenytoin, probenecid, sulfonylureas†, sulindac, verapamil

Severe reactions are possible when this drug is taken with those listed below: antibiotics†, anticoagulants†, aspirin, cefamandole, cefoperazone, cefotetan, corticosteroids†, cyclosporine, dipyridamole, gold salts†, heparin, mezlocillin, nonsteroidal antiinflammatories†, penicillamine, piperacillin, plicamycin, salicylates†, sulfinpyrazone, ticarcillin, valproic acid, warfarin

ALLERGIC REACTIONS AND SIDE EFFECTS

If you are allergic to aspirin, zomepirac, salicylates†, or other nonsteroidal antiinflammatories†, you may also be allergic to this drug. You should tell your doctor about all your allergies and any unexplained symptoms you may have while taking this drug.

This drug promotes the effect of sunlight on the body and may cause severe sunburn and increased sensitivity of the eyes.

MORE COMMON SIDE EFFECTS: Diarrhea, dizziness, headache, indigestion*, itching*, mouth sores*, nausea*, seizures*, skin rash*, swelling*, weight gain*

LESS COMMON SIDE EFFECTS: Abdominal pain, bruising*, constipation, drowsiness, gas, heartburn*, high blood pressure*, sweating, vomiting

RARE SIDE EFFECTS: Back pain*, black stools*, bloody urine*, bloody vomit, blue fingernails*, blue lips*, breathing difficulty*, chest pain*, chest tightness*, chills*, confusion*, cough*, dark urine*, fainting*, fever*, hallucinations*, hearing loss*, hives*, hoarseness*, lip sores*, loss of appetite*, low blood pressure*, mood swings*, muscle cramps*, nosebleeds*, pain*, pale skin*, pale stools*, puffy eyes*, rectal bleeding*, restlessness*, ringing in ears*, runny nose*, seizures*, shortness of breath*, sore throat*, stiff neck*, swollen glands*, swollen tongue*, thirst*, tiredness*, urinary changes*, vision changes*, weakness*, wheezing*, yellow eyes or skin*

PRECAUTIONS

This drug may cause serious stomach problems and possibly ulcers. Be careful to take this drug as directed with food, and let your doctor know if you develop any stomach-related symptoms.

Do not open, crush, break, or chew the extended-release products.

Be careful driving or handling equipment while taking this drug because it may cause dizziness.

Do not lie down for about 30 minutes after taking this drug to help reduce the risk of heartburn and throat irritation.

If you use tobacco or have a history of alcohol abuse, stomach problems, intestinal problems, hemorrhoids, diabetes mellitus, severe fluid retention, or systemic lupus erythematosus, there is an increased risk that you will develop side effects while taking this drug.

People over age 60 are at greater risk of developing fluid retention and swelling when taking this drug.

PREGNANCY AND BREAST-FEEDING

Safety in pregnancy has not been established although the drug is known to harm animal fetuses.

Breast-feeding while taking this drug is not recommended.

HELPFUL COMMENTS

Do not mix the oral suspension with anything before taking the dose.

---

† See page 52.   * See page 53.

Avoid quick movements to minimize dizziness. Dangling your legs over the side of the bed for a few minutes may help reduce dizziness when first waking up.

If using a suppository, remove the foil and run under cold water before inserting. Try to keep the suppositories in for at least 1 hour to make sure the full dose is absorbed.

Several nonsteroidal antiinflammatories† are available without a prescription in lower, nonprescription strengths, including ibuprofen, ketoprofen, and naproxen.

IRBESARTAN

Available since September 1997

COMMONLY USED TO TREAT

High blood pressure, also known as hypertension

DRUG CATEGORY

antihypertensive
Class: angiotensin II receptor antagonist

PRODUCTS

Brand-Name Products with No Generic Alternative
Avapro 75 mg tablet ($)
Avapro 150 mg tablet ($)
Avapro 300 mg tablet ($$)
No generics available.
Multiple patents that begin to expire in 2011.
Combination Products That Contain This Drug
Avalide tablet ($$)

DOSING AND FOOD

Doses are taken once a day.
This drug may be taken with or without food.
Adults: Up to 300 mg per day in divided doses.
Children age 6 to 12: Up to 75 mg per day.
Forgotten doses: If you are scheduled to take the next dose within a few hours, do not take the forgotten dose. Otherwise take the forgotten dose as soon as you remember.

ALCOHOL, DRUG, HERB, AND SUPPLEMENT INTERACTIONS

Alcohol may increase some of the side effects from this drug, depending on the amount consumed. Ask your doctor about the risks caused by drinking alcohol with your condition.

Several OTC drugs used for appetite control, asthma, colds, cough, hay fever, or sinus problems may cause an increase in blood pressure when taken with this drug. Check with your pharmacist when selecting OTC products.

Taking this drug with any of the ones listed below may change the effect of either drug with the possibility of causing toxicity or decreasing effectiveness: diuretics†

ALLERGIC REACTIONS AND SIDE EFFECTS

You should tell your doctor about all your allergies and any unexplained symptoms you may have while taking this drug.

LESS COMMON SIDE EFFECTS: Anxiety, belching, bone pain, cough, diarrhea, headache, heartburn, muscle pain, nervousness, runny nose, stomachache, tiredness

RARE SIDE EFFECTS: Breathing difficulty*, confusion*, dark urine*, dizziness*, fainting*, hives*, irregular heartbeat*, itching*, lightheadedness*, loss of appetite*, pale stools*, shortness of breath*, skin irritation, stomach pain*, tingling*, weakness*, yellow eyes or skin*

PRECAUTIONS

If you are dehydrated, the blood-pressure-lowering effect of this drug may be increased. Drink plenty of fluids to avoid dehydration when sweating, such as in hot weather and during exercise.

Be careful driving or handling equipment while taking this drug because the drug may cause dizziness.

PREGNANCY AND BREAST-FEEDING

There is evidence that this drug may harm the fetus, but the drug may be necessary to the health of the mother.

Breast-feeding while taking this drug is not recommended.

HELPFUL COMMENTS

Doses higher than 300 mg per day do not appear to have any additional effect on lowering the blood pressure.

---

† See page 52.   * See page 53.

ISONIAZID

Available for over 20 years

COMMONLY USED TO TREAT

Tuberculosis

DRUG CATEGORY

antibiotic
Class: antimycobacterial

PRODUCTS

Brand-Name Products with No Generic Alternative
Laniazid 50 mg tablet (n/a)
Products Only Available as Generics
isoniazid 100 mg tablet (¢)
isoniazid 300 mg tablet (¢)
isoniazid 50 mg/5 ml oral syrup (¢¢)
Other Generic Product Names
Laniazid
Combination Products That Contain This Drug
Rifater tablet ($$)
Rifamate capsule ($$$)

DOSING AND FOOD

Doses are taken once a day.
It is best to take this drug on an empty stomach, but taking this drug with
   a little food may avoid the stomach upset that some people suffer.
Adults and children: Up to 300 mg per day.
Forgotten doses: If you are scheduled to take the next dose within a few
   hours, do not take the forgotten dose. Otherwise take the forgotten dose
   as soon as you remember.

ALCOHOL, DRUG, HERB, AND SUPPLEMENT INTERACTIONS

Alcohol should not be used while taking this drug.

**Taking this drug with any of the ones listed below may change the effect of
either drug with the possibility of causing toxicity or decreasing effectiveness:**
antacids, anticoagulants†, benzodiazepines†, carbamazepine, corticos-
   teroids†, ketoconazole, phenytoin, rifampin

Severe reactions are possible when this drug is taken with those listed below: cycloserine

Increased side effects are possible when this drug is taken with those listed below: acetaminophen, alfentanil, amiodarone, anabolic steroids†, androgens†, antithyroid drugs†, carmustine, chloroquine, dantrolene, daunorubicin, disulfiram, divalproex, estrogens†, etretinate, gold salts†, hydroxychloroquine, mercaptopurine, methotrexate, methyldopa, naltrexone, oral contraceptives, phenothiazines†, plicamycin, valproic acid

ALLERGIC REACTIONS AND SIDE EFFECTS

If you are allergic to ethionamide, pyrazinamide, or niacin, you may also be allergic to this drug. You should tell your doctor about all your allergies and any unexplained symptoms you may have while taking this drug.

MORE COMMON SIDE EFFECTS: Burning*, clumsiness*, dark urine*, diarrhea, fever*, loss of appetite*, nausea*, numbness*, stomach pain, tiredness*, unsteadiness*, vomiting*, weakness*, yellow eyes or skin*

RARE SIDE EFFECTS: Bleeding*, blurry vision*, bruising*, depression*, eye pain*, joint pain*, mood swings*, seizures*, skin rash*, sore throat*, vision loss*

PRECAUTIONS

People with a history of alcoholism, kidney disease, or liver disease may not be able to take this drug.

This drug may cause liver damage, which is more likely to occur in people over age 50.

Diabetics may notice changes in their blood sugar while taking this drug.

This drug may interfere with several diagnostic tests including some urine glucose tests. Diabetics should use glucose oxidase tests or glucose enzyme test strips.

People with a history of seizures may be at greater risk of developing a seizure while taking this drug.

There are some foods that may cause people taking this drug to have a reaction. Do not eat swiss cheese, cheshire cheese, tuna fish, skipjack fish, or sardinella fish.

PREGNANCY AND BREAST-FEEDING

Safety during pregnancy has not been established although the drug is known to harm animal fetuses.

This drug passes into breast milk, but does not appear to harm the baby.

†See page 52.   *See page 53.

The amount taken in by the baby is not enough to prevent the infant from getting tuberculosis. The baby should be monitored for signs of toxicity.

HELPFUL COMMENTS

This drug is also called by the generic name INH.

If you need to take an antacid, take it either 2 hours before or after taking this drug.

Vitamin B_6 is often taken with this drug in people who have numbness and tingling in their hands or feet.

Do not measure doses of the oral syrup with anything but a specially marked prescription measuring cup. Slight inaccuracy from other measuring spoons may result in over- or under-dosing.

Contact your doctor if your symptoms do not improve after 2 to 3 weeks of treatment.

Do not stop treatment early if you start to feel better. It takes the full prescription for this drug to work completely.

ISOSORBIDE

Available for over 20 years

COMMONLY USED TO TREAT

Chest pain, also known as angina
People at risk of developing chest pain

DRUG CATEGORY

antianginal
Class: nitrate

PRODUCTS

Brand-Name Products with No Generic Alternative
Isordil 10 mg sublingual tablet (¢¢¢)
Sorbitrate 10 mg chewable tablet (n/a)
Brand-Name Products with Generic Alternatives
Isordil 5 mg tablet (¢¢¢)
  Generic: isosorbide dinitrate 5 mg tablet (¢)
Isordil 10 mg tablet (¢¢¢)
  Generic: isosorbide dinitrate 10 mg tablet (¢)

Isordil 20 mg tablet (¢¢¢¢)
 Generic: isosorbide dinitrate 20 mg tablet (¢)
Isordil 30 mg tablet (¢¢¢¢)
 Generic: isosorbide dinitrate 30 mg tablet (¢)
Isordil 40 mg tablet (¢¢¢¢)
 Generic: isosorbide dinitrate 40 mg tablet (n/a)
Isordil 40 mg extended-release capsule (n/a)
 Generic: isosorbide dinitrate 40 mg extended-release capsule (¢¢)
Isordil 2.5 mg sublingual tablet (¢¢¢)
 Generic: isosorbide dinitrate 2.5 mg sublingual tablet (¢)
Isordil 5 mg sublingual tablet (¢¢¢)
 Generic: isosorbide dinitrate 5 mg sublingual tablet (¢)
Imdur 30 mg extended-release tablet ($$)
 Generic: isosorbide mononitrate 30 mg extended-release tablet (¢¢¢¢)
Imdur 60 mg extended-release tablet ($$)
 Generic: isosorbide mononitrate 60 mg extended-release tablet (¢¢¢)
Imdur 120 mg extended-release tablet ($$)
 Generic: isosorbide mononitrate 120 mg extended-release tablet ($$)
Monoket 10 mg tablet (¢¢¢¢¢)
 Generic: isosorbide mononitrate 10 mg tablet (¢¢¢)
Monoket 20 mg tablet ($)
 Generic: isosorbide mononitrate 20 mg tablet (¢¢¢)

Other Generic Product Names
Dilatrate-SR, Ismo, Sorbitrate

DOSING AND FOOD

Oral regular-release doses are taken 2 to 4 times a day. Extended-release products are taken once a day. Sublingual doses are taken up to 3 times within 15 to 30 minutes.

It is best to take this drug on an empty stomach, 1 hour before or 2 hours after meals.

Adults: Up to 160 mg per day for isosorbide dinitrate, or 120 mg per day for isosorbide mononitrate, in divided doses.

Forgotten doses: If you are scheduled to take the next dose within 2 hours (6 hours if taking an extended-release product), do not take the forgotten dose. Otherwise take the forgotten dose as soon as you remember.

ALCOHOL, DRUG, HERB, AND SUPPLEMENT INTERACTIONS

Alcohol should not be used while taking this drug.

Taking this drug with any of the ones listed below may change the effect of either drug with the possibility of causing toxicity or decreasing effectiveness: antihypertensives†, calcium channel blockers†, phenothiazines†, vaso-dilators†

Severe reactions are possible when this drug is taken with those listed below: silfenafil

ALLERGIC REACTIONS AND SIDE EFFECTS

You should tell your doctor about all your allergies and any unexplained symptoms while taking this drug.

MORE COMMON SIDE EFFECTS: Dizziness*, fast pulse, flushing, headache*, lightheadedness, nausea, restlessness, swelling*, vomiting

RARE SIDE EFFECTS: Blue hands*, blue lips*, blurry vision*, dry mouth*, fainting*, fever*, head pressure*, irregular heartbeat*, seizures*, short-ness of breath*, skin rash*, tiredness*, weakness*

PRECAUTIONS

Most products are used to prevent chest pain from occurring, but sublin-gual or chewable tablets are used to stop the pain once it starts.

Sublingual tablets should be moistened with saliva when placed under the tongue and allowed to dissolve without chewing, sucking, or swallowing.

Be careful driving or handling equipment while taking this drug because it may cause dizziness and blurry vision.

This drug should not be stopped suddenly after it has been taken for a while since severe chest pains may occur. If you wish to stop taking this drug, ask your doctor for specific instructions.

Do not open, crush, break, or chew the extended-release products.

This drug may interfere with cholesterol tests, resulting in a cholesterol level reported to be lower than actual.

The effect of sublingual tablets should be noticed in about 3 minutes. If chest pain continues, go to the hospital.

If you have a history of head injury, stroke, anemia, or glaucoma, this drug may make those conditions worse.

If taken too often, it is possible for this drug to become less effective over time. Make sure you follow the prescription exactly as written, and tell your doctor how often you have chest pain.

Some people notice partially dissolved extended-release products in their stools. Tell your doctor if this happens since you are not getting the com-plete dose.

PREGNANCY AND BREAST-FEEDING

Safety during pregnancy has not been established although the drug is known to harm animal fetuses.

Breast-feeding while taking this drug is not recommended.

HELPFUL COMMENTS

Aspirin or acetaminophen may be used to relieve headache pain that many people suffer.

Avoid quick movements to minimize dizziness. Dangling your legs over the side of the bed for a few minutes may help reduce dizziness when first waking up.

People should always be sitting down while taking a sublingual dose or chewable tablets.

Sucking on hard sugarless candy or chewing sugarless gum may help relieve dry mouth caused by this drug.

Keep sublingual tablets with you at all times.

ISOTRETINOIN

Available for over 20 years

COMMONLY USED TO TREAT

Acne
Cancer of the head and neck
People at risk of developing skin cancer

DRUG CATEGORY

antiacne
Class: retinoid

PRODUCTS

Brand-Name Products with Generic Alternatives

Accutane 10 mg capsule ($$$$)
  Generic: isotretinoin 10 mg capsule (n/a)
Accutane 20 mg capsule ($$$$)
  Generic: isotretinoin 20 mg capsule (n/a)
Accutane 40 mg capsule ($$$$)
  Generic: isotretinoin 40 mg capsule (n/a)

Other Generic Product Names

Amnesteem

---

† See page 52.   * See page 53.

DOSING AND FOOD

Doses are taken twice a day.

This drug may be taken with or without food but is best taken with food to reduce the stomach upset that some people suffer.

Adults: Up to 4 mg/kg per day in divided doses.

Adolescents: Up to 2 mg/kg per day in divided doses.

Forgotten doses: If you are scheduled to take the next dose within a few hours, do not take the forgotten dose. Otherwise take the forgotten dose as soon as you remember.

ALCOHOL, DRUG, HERB, AND SUPPLEMENT INTERACTIONS

Alcohol should not be used while taking this drug.

Taking this drug with any of the ones listed below may change the effect of either drug with the possibility of causing toxicity or decreasing effectiveness: carbamazepine, vitamin A

Severe reactions are possible when this drug is taken with those listed below: tetracycline

Increased side effects are possible when this drug is taken with those listed below: acitretin, tretinoin

ALLERGIC REACTIONS AND SIDE EFFECTS

If you are allergic to acitretin, tretinoin, or vitamin A, you may also be allergic to this drug. You should tell your doctor about all your allergies and any unexplained symptoms you may have while taking this drug.

This drug promotes the effect of sunlight on the body and may cause severe sunburn and increased sensitivity of the eyes.

MORE COMMON SIDE EFFECTS: Abdominal pain*, bone pain*, dry mouth, dry skin, eye irritation*, hair loss, headache*, itching*, joint pain*, lip irritation*, muscles aches*, nausea*, nosebleeds*, poor night vision, rash*, skin irritation*, tiredness, upset stomach, vomiting*

RARE SIDE EFFECTS: Back pain*, behavior changes, blurry vision*, depression*, diarrhea*, gum irritation*, rectal bleeding*, suicidal thoughts*, vision changes*, yellow eyes or skin*

PRECAUTIONS

This drug is taken for 3 to 5 months followed by at least an 8-week drug-free period.

Be careful driving or handling equipment while taking this drug because it may cause blurry vision and eye irritation.

This drug is derived from vitamin A and may cause serious side effects if taken with multivitamins that contain vitamin A or any other forms of vitamin A.

Side effects may begin up to 1 month after this drug is stopped.

If you have high triglyceride levels, this drug may make the condition worse.

People with diabetes may notice a change in blood sugar while taking this drug; the dose of the antidiabetic drug† or insulin may need to be adjusted.

Because of the risk of birth defects, women should use 2 forms of contraception while taking this drug and for 1 month after the drug is stopped.

This drug may cause changes to your gums and mouth. Your dentist may recommend that you clean your teeth and mouth differently to avoid infection.

Do not donate blood while taking this drug and for 1 month after the drug is stopped.

PREGNANCY AND BREAST-FEEDING

This drug may cause birth defects and should not be used during pregnancy.

Breast-feeding while taking this drug is not recommended.

HELPFUL COMMENTS

Sucking on hard sugarless candy or chewing sugarless gum may help relieve dry mouth caused by this drug.

Protect your eyes with sunglasses when outside. Use lubricating eyedrops to help reduce eye irritation.

You should begin to notice the effects of this drug in 1 to 2 months.

This drug may continue to work for about 1 month after it is stopped.

ISRADIPINE

Available since December 1990

COMMONLY USED TO TREAT

Chest pain, also known as angina

High blood pressure, also known as hypertension

DRUG CATEGORY

antianginal

antihypertensive

Class: calcium channel blocker

---

† See page 52.   * See page 53.

PRODUCTS

Brand-Name Products with No Generic Alternative
DynaCirc 2.5 mg capsule ($)
DynaCirc 5 mg capsule ($$)
DynaCirc CR 5 mg extended-release tablet ($)
DynaCirc CR 10 mg extended-release tablet ($$)
No generics available.
Multiple patents that begin to expire in 2003.

DOSING AND FOOD

Doses are taken twice a day. Extended-release products are taken once a day.

This drug may be taken with or without food.

Adults: Up to 20 mg per day in divided doses.

Forgotten doses: If you are scheduled to take the next dose within a few hours, do not take the forgotten dose. Otherwise take the forgotten dose as soon as you remember.

ALCOHOL, DRUG, HERB, AND SUPPLEMENT INTERACTIONS

Alcohol may increase some of the side effects from this drug, depending on the amount consumed. Ask your doctor about the risks caused by drinking alcohol with your condition.

Several OTC drugs used for appetite control, asthma, colds, cough, hay fever, or sinus problems may cause an increase in blood pressure when taken with this drug. Check with your pharmacist when selecting OTC products.

Taking this drug with any of the ones listed below may change the effect of either drug with the possibility of causing toxicity or decreasing effectiveness: anesthetics, carbamazepine, cyclosporine, digoxin, procainamide, quinidine

Severe reactions are possible when this drug is taken with those listed below: beta blockers†

ALLERGIC REACTIONS AND SIDE EFFECTS

If you are allergic to any other calcium channel blocker†, you may also be allergic to this drug. You should tell your doctor about all your allergies and any unexplained symptoms you may have while taking this drug.

MORE COMMON SIDE EFFECTS: Headache

LESS COMMON SIDE EFFECTS: Abdominal pain, breathing difficulty*, cough*, diarrhea, dizziness, fluid retention, flushing, nausea, shortness of breath*, skin rash*, swelling*, tiredness, weakness, wheezing*

RARE SIDE EFFECTS: Chest pain*, fainting*, tender gums*

PRECAUTIONS

Do not crush, break, or chew the extended-release products.

This drug may cause changes to your gums and mouth. Your dentist may recommend that you clean your teeth and mouth differently to avoid infection.

People with heart failure or liver disease may not be able to use this drug.

PREGNANCY AND BREAST-FEEDING

Safety in pregnancy has not been established although the drug is known to harm animal fetuses.

Breast-feeding while taking this drug is not recommended.

HELPFUL COMMENTS

It takes 2 to 4 weeks before the full effects of this drug are noticed.

ITRACONAZOLE

Available since September 1992

COMMONLY USED TO TREAT

Fungal infections

DRUG CATEGORY

antifungal
Class: azole derivative

PRODUCTS

Brand-Name Products with No Generic Alternative
Sporanox 100 mg capsule ($$$$)
Sporanox 10 mg/ml oral solution ($$$)
No generics available.
Patent expires in 2014.

DOSING AND FOOD

Doses are taken 1 to 2 times a day.

---

†See page 52.   * See page 53.

Taking this drug with food will help increase absorption of the drug. Do not drink grapefruit juice or eat grapefruit when taking this drug.

Adults: Up to 400 mg per day.

Forgotten doses: If you are scheduled to take the next dose within a few hours, do not take the forgotten dose. Otherwise take the forgotten dose as soon as you remember.

ALCOHOL, DRUG, HERB, AND SUPPLEMENT INTERACTIONS

Alcohol may increase some of the side effects from this drug, depending on the amount consumed. Ask your doctor about the risks caused by drinking alcohol with your condition.

Antihistamines†, found in OTC allergy, cough, and cold products, may cause serious side effects when taken with this drug. Talk to your doctor before you take any OTC products.

Several OTC products used for stomach upset and heartburn may interfere with the absorption of this drug and should not be used for 2 hours before or after taking a dose of this drug.

Taking this drug with any of the ones listed below may change the effect of either drug with the possibility of causing toxicity or decreasing effectiveness:
amantadine, antacids, anticholinergics†, antidepressants†, antidyskinetics†, antihistamines†, antipsychotics†, atorvastatin, buclizine, busulfan, carbamazepine, cerivastatin, cimetidine, clarithromycin, cyclizine, cyclobenzaprine, cyclosporine, didanosine, digoxin, disopyramide, do-cetaxel, erythromycin, famotidine, flavoxate, glipizide, glyburide, H2 antagonists†, indinavir, ipratropium, isoniazid, lovastatin, meclizine, methylphenidate, nevirapine, nizatidine, omeprazole, orphenadrine, oxybutynin, phenobarbital, phenytoin, procainamide, promethazine, ranitidine, rifampin, ritonavir, saquinivir, simvastatin, sucralfate, sulfonylureas†, tacrolimus, tolbutamide, trimeprazine, vinblastine, vincristine, warfarin

Severe reactions are possible when this drug is taken with those listed below:
astemizole, dofetilide, pimizole, quinidine, terfenadine

Increased side effects are possible when this drug is taken with those listed below:
acetaminophen, alprazolam, amiodarone, anabolic steroids†, androgens†, antibiotics†, antithyroid drugs†, carmustine, chloroquine, dantrolene, daunorubicin, diazepam, disulfiram, divalproex, estrogens†, etretinate, felodipine, gold salts†, hydroxychloroquine, mercaptopurine, methotrexate, methyldopa, midazolam, naltrexone, nifedipine, oral contraceptives, phenothiazines†, plicamycin, triazolam, valproic acid, verapamil

ALLERGIC REACTIONS AND SIDE EFFECTS

If you are allergic to any azole derivative†, you may also be allergic to this drug. You should tell your doctor about all your allergies and any unexplained symptoms you may have while taking this drug.

MORE COMMON SIDE EFFECTS: Nausea

LESS COMMON SIDE EFFECTS: Abdominal pain, diarrhea, dizziness, drowsiness, fever*, headache, high blood pressure*, itching*, loss of appetite*, sexual dysfunction, swelling*, vomiting

RARE SIDE EFFECTS: Bleeding*, bruising*, chills*, constipation, dark urine*, male breast enlargement, menstrual dysfunction, pale stools*, skin irritation*, skin rash*, sore throat*, stomach pain*, tiredness*, weakness*, yellow eyes or skin*

PRECAUTIONS

People with kidney disease may not be able to take this drug.

The oral-solution products should be swished in the mouth before swallowing.

Do not measure doses of the oral solution with anything but a measuring cup intended for use with prescription drugs. Slight inaccuracy from other measuring spoons may result in over- or under-dosing.

PREGNANCY AND BREAST-FEEDING

Safety in pregnancy has not been established although the drug is known to harm animal fetuses.

Breast-feeding while taking this drug is not recommended.

HELPFUL COMMENTS

Contact your doctor if your symptoms do not improve after a few weeks.

Do not stop treatment early if you start to feel better. Treatment may last 6 months or longer. It takes the full prescription for this drug to work completely.

KANAMYCIN SULFATE

Available for over 20 years

COMMONLY USED TO TREAT

Coma from liver disease

Infection

People preparing for intestinal surgery

† *See page 52.*   * *See page 53.*

DRUG CATEGORY

antibiotic
Class: aminoglycoside

PRODUCTS

Brand-Name Products with No Generic Alternative
Kantrex 500 mg capsule (n/a)
No generics available.
No patents, no exclusivity.

DOSING AND FOOD

Doses are taken 4 times a day.
This drug may be taken with or without food.
Adults and children: Up to 1,200 mg per day in divided doses.
Forgotten doses: If you are scheduled to take the next dose within a few
hours, do not take the forgotten dose. Otherwise take the forgotten dose
as soon as you remember.

ALCOHOL, DRUG, HERB, AND SUPPLEMENT INTERACTIONS

Alcohol may increase some of the side effects from this drug, depending
on the amount consumed. Ask your doctor about the risks caused by
drinking alcohol with your condition.

Taking this drug with any of the ones listed below may change the effect of
either drug with the possibility of causing toxicity or decreasing effectiveness:
anesthetics, antibiotics†, indomethacin

ALLERGIC REACTIONS AND SIDE EFFECTS

If you are allergic to any aminoglycosides†, you may also be allergic to this
drug. You should tell your doctor about all your allergies and any unexplained symptoms you may have while taking this drug.
MORE COMMON SIDE EFFECTS: Diarrhea, nausea, vomiting
RARE SIDE EFFECTS: Clumsiness*, dizziness*, gas, hearing loss*, pale stools,
ringing in ears*, thirst*, unsteadiness*, urinary changes*

PRECAUTIONS

If you have a history of intestinal obstruction, you may not be able to take
this drug.
People with kidney disease or ulcers are at increased risk of developing
side effects when taking this drug.

If you have hearing or balance problems, this drug may make those conditions worse.

Tell your doctor if you take large doses of aspirin on a regular basis since this drug may mask the symptoms of aspirin toxicity.

PREGNANCY AND BREAST-FEEDING

There is evidence that this drug may harm the fetus, but the drug may be necessary to the health of the mother.

Breast-feeding while taking this drug is not recommended.

HELPFUL COMMENTS

Drink a lot of water while taking this drug to help move the drug quickly through the kidneys.

KETOCONAZOLE

Available for over 20 years

COMMONLY USED TO TREAT

Athlete's foot
Dandruff
Fungal infections
Ringworm
Yeast infections on the skin

DRUG CATEGORY

antifungal
Class: azole derivative

PRODUCTS

Brand-Name Products with No Generic Alternative
Nizoral 2% topical shampoo (¢)
Brand-Name Products with Generic Alternatives
Nizoral 200 mg tablet ($$$)
  Generic: ketoconazole 200 mg tablet ($$$)
Nizoral 2% topical cream (¢¢¢)
  Generic: ketoconazole 2% topical cream (¢¢¢)

DOSING AND FOOD

Doses are taken once a day.

† See page 52.   * See page 53.

This drug is absorbed best when there is acid in the stomach, so it should be taken with citrus juice or a full meal.

Adults: Up to 400 mg per day.

Children over age 2: Up to 6.6 mg/kg per day.

Forgotten doses: If you are scheduled to take the next dose within a few hours, do not take the forgotten dose. Otherwise take the forgotten dose as soon as you remember.

ALCOHOL, DRUG, HERB, AND SUPPLEMENT INTERACTIONS

Alcohol should not be used while taking this drug.

Do not use yew supplements when taking this drug since there is a risk of developing toxicity.

Antihistamines, found in OTC allergy, cough, and cold products, may cause serious side effects when taken with this drug. Talk to your doctor before you take any OTC products.

Several OTC products used for stomach upset and heartburn may interfere with the absorption of this drug and should not be used for 2 hours before or after taking a dose of this drug.

Taking this drug with any of the ones listed below may change the effect of either drug with the possibility of causing toxicity or decreasing effectiveness: amantadine, antacids, anticholinergics†, antidepressants†, antidyskinetics†, antihistamines†, antimuscarinics†, antipsychotics†, atorvastatin, buclizine, cerivastatin, cimetidine, corticosteroids†, cyclizine, cyclobenzaprine, cyclosporine, didanosine, digoxin, disopyramide, famotidine, flavoxate, glipizide, glyburide, H2 antagonists†, indinavir, ipratropium, isoniazid, lovastatin, meclizine, methylphenidate, nevirapine, nizatidine, omeprazole, orphenadrine, oxybutynin, phenytoin, procainamide, promethazine, ranitidine, rifampin, ritonavir, saquinivir, simvastatin, sucralfate, sulfonylureas†, tacrolimus, tolbutamide, trimeprazine, warfarin

Increased side effects are possible when this drug is taken with those listed below: acetaminophen, alprazolam, amiodarone, anabolic steroids†, androgens†, antibiotics†, antithyroid drugs†, carmustine, chloroquine, dantrolene, daunorubicin, diazepam, disulfiram, divalproex, estrogens†, etretinate, felodipine, gold salts†, hydroxychloroquine, mercaptopurine, methotrexate, methyldopa, midazolam, naltrexone, nifedipine, oral contraceptives, phenothiazines†, plicamycin, triazolam, valproic acid, verapamil

ALLERGIC REACTIONS AND SIDE EFFECTS

If you are allergic to any azole derivative or sulfites†, you may also be allergic to this drug. You should tell your doctor about all your allergies

and any unexplained symptoms you may have while taking this drug.
This drug may cause your eyes to be more sensitive to sunlight, but there are no special risks associated with sunburn while taking this drug.

MORE COMMON SIDE EFFECTS: Nausea, suicidal thoughts, vomiting

LESS COMMON SIDE EFFECTS: Abdominal pain, breast enlargement, chills*, depression, diarrhea, dizziness, drowsiness, eye sensitivity, fever*, headache, itching*, nervousness, sexual dysfunction, skin irritation*, yellow eyes or skin*

RARE SIDE EFFECTS: Bleeding*, bruising*, constipation, dark urine*, loss of appetite*, menstrual dysfunction, pale stools*, skin rash*, sore throat*, tiredness*, weakness*

PRECAUTIONS

Be careful driving or handling equipment while taking this drug because the drug may cause dizziness and drowsiness.
Most of the precautions and warnings in the summary do not apply to the topical cream and shampoo products since very small amounts of the drug are absorbed into the body. Contact your doctor if you notice itching, stinging, or skin rash that was not there before treatment with topical products.

PREGNANCY AND BREAST-FEEDING

Safety in pregnancy has not been established although the drug is known to harm animal fetuses.
Breast-feeding while taking this drug is not recommended.

HELPFUL COMMENTS

Contact your doctor if your symptoms do not improve after a few weeks.
Do not stop treatment early if you start to feel better. Treatment may last 6 months or longer. It takes the full prescription for this drug to work completely.

KETOPROFEN

Available since July 1987

COMMONLY USED TO TREAT

Menstrual cramps
Pain
Swelling

---

† See page 52.   * See page 53.

DRUG CATEGORY

analgesic
antiarthritic
antidysmenorrheal
antigout
Class: nonsteroidal antiinflammatory

PRODUCTS

Brand-Name Products with Generic Alternatives
Orudis 25 mg capsule (n/a)
  Generic: ketoprofen 25 mg capsule (n/a)
Orudis 50 mg capsule ($)
  Generic: ketoprofen 50 mg capsule (¢¢)
Orudis 75 mg capsule ($$)
  Generic: ketoprofen 75 mg capsule (¢¢¢)
Oruvail 100 mg extended-release capsule ($$)
  Generic: ketoprofen 100 mg extended-release capsule ($$)
Oruvail 150 mg extended-release capsule ($$$)
  Generic: ketoprofen 150 mg extended-release capsule ($$)
Oruvail 200 mg extended-release capsule ($$$)
  Generic: ketoprofen 200 mg extended-release capsule ($$$)

DOSING AND FOOD

Doses are taken 3 to 4 times a day. Extended-release products are taken once a day.

It is best to take this drug with food.

Adults: Up to 200 mg per day in divided doses.

Lower doses are used in adults over age 65.

Forgotten doses: If you are scheduled to take the next dose within a few hours, do not take the forgotten dose. Otherwise take the forgotten dose as soon as you remember.

ALCOHOL, DRUG, HERB, AND SUPPLEMENT INTERACTIONS

Alcohol may increase the risk of serious side effects from this drug. Ask your doctor about the risks caused by drinking alcohol with your condition.

Do not use dong quai, feverfew, garlic, ginger, horse chestnut, red clover, or St. John's wort while taking this drug since they may increase the risk of serious side effects.

Taking this drug with any of the ones listed below may change the effect of either drug with the possibility of causing toxicity or decreasing effectiveness: antihypertensives†, digoxin, diuretics†, furosemide, hydrochlorothiazide, nifedipine, lithium, methotrexate, phenytoin, probenecid, sulfonylureas†, sulindac, verapamil

Severe reactions are possible when this drug is taken with those listed below: antibiotics†, anticoagulants†, aspirin, cefamandole, cefoperazone, cefotetan, corticosteroids†, cyclosporine, dipyridamole, gold salts†, heparin, mezlocillin, nonsteroidal antiinflammatories†, penicillamine, piperacillin, plicamycin, salicylates†, sulfinpyrazone, ticarcillin

ALLERGIC REACTIONS AND SIDE EFFECTS

If you are allergic to aspirin, zomepirac, salicylates†, or other nonsteroidal antiinflammatories†, you may also be allergic to this drug. You should tell your doctor about all your allergies and any unexplained symptoms you may have while taking this drug.

This drug promotes the effect of sunlight on the body and may cause severe sunburn and increased sensitivity of the eyes.

MORE COMMON SIDE EFFECTS: Abdominal pain, constipation, diarrhea, dizziness, drowsiness, excitement, gas, headache, heartburn*, indigestion*, irregular heartbeat*, itching*, nausea*, shortness of breath*, swelling*, swollen tongue*, weight gain*

LESS COMMON SIDE EFFECTS: Bruising*, high blood pressure*, skin rash*, sweating, vomiting

RARE SIDE EFFECTS: Back pain*, black stools*, bloody urine*, bloody vomit, blue fingernails*, blue lips*, breathing difficulty*, chest pain*, chest tightness*, chills*, confusion*, cough*, dark urine*, fainting*, fever*, hallucinations*, hearing loss*, hives*, hoarseness*, lip sores*, loss of appetite*, low blood pressure*, mood swings*, mouth sores*, muscle cramps*, nosebleeds*, pain*, pale skin*, pale stools*, puffy eyes*, rectal bleeding*, restlessness*, ringing in ears*, runny nose*, seizures*, sore throat*, stiff neck*, swollen glands*, thirst*, tiredness*, urinary changes*, vision changes*, weakness*, wheezing*, yellow eyes or skin*

PRECAUTIONS

This drug may cause serious stomach problems and possibly ulcers. Be careful to take this drug as directed with food, and let your doctor know if you develop any stomach-related symptoms.

Do not open, crush, break, or chew the extended-release products.

---

† See page 52.   * See page 53.

Be careful driving or handling equipment while taking this drug because it may cause dizziness and drowsiness.

Do not lie down for about 30 minutes after taking this drug to help reduce the risk of heartburn and throat irritation.

If you use tobacco or have a history of alcohol abuse, stomach problems, intestinal problems, hemorrhoids, diabetes mellitus, severe fluid retention, or systemic lupus erythematosus, there is an increased risk that you will develop side effects while taking this drug.

PREGNANCY AND BREAST-FEEDING

Safety in pregnancy has not been established although the drug is known to harm animal fetuses.

Breast-feeding while taking this drug is not recommended.

HELPFUL COMMENTS

Avoid quick movements to minimize dizziness.

Several nonsteroidal antiinflammatories are available without a prescription in lower, nonprescription strengths, including ibuprofen, ketoprofen, and naproxen.

If you are taking the OTC form of this drug for more than 10 days, you should talk to your doctor to verify your diagnosis and consider higher doses or another drug.

KETOROLAC TROMETHAMINE

Available since November 1989

COMMONLY USED TO TREAT

Pain

DRUG CATEGORY

analgesic
Class: nonsteroidal antiinflammatory

PRODUCTS

Brand-Name Products with No Generic Alternative
Acular 0.5% ophthalmic solution ($$$$$)
Acular 0.5% preservative-free ophthalmic solution ($$$$$)
Brand-Name Products with Generic Alternatives
Toradol 10 mg tablet ($)
  Generic: ketorolac tromethamine 10 mg tablet (¢¢¢¢)

DOSING AND FOOD

Doses are taken 4 times a day.

It is best to take this drug with food.

Adults: Up to 40 mg per day in divided doses.

Lower doses are used in people with kidney disease and adults over age 65.

Forgotten doses: If you are scheduled to take the next dose within a few hours, do not take the forgotten dose. Otherwise take the forgotten dose as soon as you remember.

ALCOHOL, DRUG, HERB, AND SUPPLEMENT INTERACTIONS

Alcohol should not be used while taking this drug.

Do not use dong quai, feverfew, garlic, ginger, horse chestnut, red clover, or St. John's wort while taking this drug since they may increase the risk of serious side effects.

Taking this drug with any of the ones listed below may change the effect of either drug with the possibility of causing toxicity or decreasing effectiveness: diuretics†, lithium, methotrexate, probenecid

Severe reactions are possible when this drug is taken with those listed below: anticoagulants†, aspirin, cefamandole, cefoperazone, cefotetan, heparin, nonsteroidal antiinflammatories†, plicamycin, salicylates†, valproic acid, warfarin

ALLERGIC REACTIONS AND SIDE EFFECTS

If you are allergic to aspirin, salicylates†, or other nonsteroidal antiinflammatories†, you may also be allergic to this drug. You should tell your doctor about all your allergies and any unexplained symptoms you may have while taking this drug.

This drug promotes the effect of sunlight on the body and may cause severe sunburn and increased sensitivity of the eyes.

MORE COMMON SIDE EFFECTS: Abdominal pain, diarrhea, dizziness, drowsiness, headache, heartburn*, indigestion*, irregular heartbeat*, nausea*, swelling*, weight gain*

LESS COMMON SIDE EFFECTS: Bruising*, constipation, gas, high blood pressure*, itching*, mouth sores*, skin rash*, sweating, vomiting

RARE SIDE EFFECTS: Back pain*, black stools*, bloody urine*, bloody vomit, blue fingernails*, blue lips*, breathing difficulty*, chest pain*, chest tightness*, chills*, confusion*, cough*, dark urine*, fainting*, fever*, hallucinations*, hearing loss*, hives*, hoarseness*, lip sores*, loss of appe-

---

† See page 52.   * See page 53.

tite*, low blood pressure*, mood swings*, muscle cramps*, nosebleeds*, pain*, pale skin*, pale stools*, puffy eyes*, rectal bleeding*, restlessness*, ringing in ears*, runny nose*, seizures*, shortness of breath*, skin irritation*, sore throat*, stiff neck*, swollen glands*, swollen tongue*, thirst*, tiredness*, urinary changes*, vision changes*, weakness*, wheezing*, yellow eyes or skin*

PRECAUTIONS

This drug may cause serious stomach problems and possibly ulcers. Be careful to take this drug as directed with food, and let your doctor know if you develop any stomach-related symptoms.

If you have a history of alcohol abuse, diabetes mellitus, severe fluid retention, or systemic lupus erythematosus, there is an increased risk that you will develop side effects while taking this drug.

This drug should not be used in people with bleeding disorders such as hemophilia, peptic ulcers, or bleeding in the brain.

If you have asthma, heart disease, or high blood pressure, this drug may make those conditions worse.

Do not lie down for about 30 minutes after taking this drug to help reduce the risk of heartburn and throat irritation.

Be careful driving or handling equipment while taking this drug because the drug may cause dizziness and drowsiness.

Eyedrops are irritating to the eye and surrounding area, but most of the other warnings and precautions in this drug summary do not apply.

PREGNANCY AND BREAST-FEEDING

Safety in pregnancy has not been established although the drug is known to harm animal fetuses.

Breast-feeding while taking this drug is not recommended.

HELPFUL COMMENTS

This drug may be taken with an antacid to reduce stomach upset.

The oral form of this drug is not used for more than 5 days.

Avoid quick movements to minimize dizziness. Dangling your legs over the side of the bed for a few minutes may help reduce dizziness when first waking up.

Several nonsteroidal antiinflammatories† are available without a prescription in lower, nonprescription strengths, including ibuprofen, ketoprofen, and naproxen.

LABETALOL HYDROCHLORIDE

Available since August 1984

COMMONLY USED TO TREAT

High blood pressure, also known as hypertension

DRUG CATEGORY

Antihypertensive
Class: Alpha Adrenergic Blocker and Beta Blocker

PRODUCTS

Brand-Name Products with Generic Alternatives
Normodyne 100 mg tablet (¢¢¢¢)
  Generic: labetalol 100 mg tablet (¢¢¢)
Normodyne 200 mg tablet (¢¢¢¢¢)
  Generic: labetalol 200 mg tablet (¢¢¢¢)
Normodyne 300 mg tablet ($)
  Generic: labetalol 300 mg tablet (¢¢¢¢¢)
Other Generic Product Names
Trandate

DOSING AND FOOD

Doses are taken twice a day.
This drug may be taken with or without food.
Adults: Up to 2,400 mg per day in divided doses.
Lower doses are used in people with renal disease and liver disease.
This drug is rarely used in children.
Forgotten doses: If you are scheduled to take the next dose in less than 8
  hours, do not take the forgotten dose. Otherwise take the forgotten dose
  as soon as you remember.

ALCOHOL, DRUG, HERB, AND SUPPLEMENT INTERACTIONS

Alcohol may increase some of the side effects from this drug, depending
  on the amount consumed. Ask your doctor about the risks caused by
  drinking alcohol with your condition.
Several OTC drugs used for appetite control, asthma, colds, cough, hay fever,
  or sinus problems may cause an increase in blood pressure when taken
  with this drug. Check with your pharmacist when selecting OTC products.

†*See page 52.*   **See page 53.*

Taking this drug with any of the ones listed below may change the effect of either drug with the possibility of causing toxicity or decreasing effectiveness:

adrenergics†, aminophylline, anesthetics, antidiabetics†, caffeine, calcium channel blockers†, carbonic anhydrase inhibitors†, cimetidine, clonidine, diuretics†, dyphylline, epinephrine, guanabenz, guanethidine, lidocaine, nitroglycerin, nonsteroidal antiinflammatories†, oxtriphylline, pilocarpine, reserpine, theophylline

Severe reactions are possible when this drug is taken with those listed below:

allergy shots, beta blockers†, cocaine, halothane, monoamine oxidase inhibitors†, tricyclic antidepressants†

Increased effects or side effects are possible when this drug is taken with those listed below:

antihypertensives†

ALLERGIC REACTIONS AND SIDE EFFECTS

If you are allergic to any other beta blockers†, you may also be allergic to this drug.

This drug may exaggerate the reaction from your current allergies. You should tell your doctor about all your allergies that you have as well as the severity of the allergic reaction before starting this drug.

MORE COMMON SIDE EFFECTS: Dizziness, drowsiness, lightheadedness*, tiredness, sexual dysfunction*, sleeping difficulty, weakness

LESS COMMON SIDE EFFECTS: Anxiety, breathing difficulty*, cold hands and feet*, constipation, depression*, diarrhea, itching, nausea, nervousness, numbness, shortness of breath*, slow heartbeat*, sore eyes, stomachache, stuffy nose, swelling, taste changes, tingling, vivid dreams, vomiting, wheezing

RARE SIDE EFFECTS: Back pain*, bleeding*, bruising*, chest pain*, confusion*, dark urine*, dizziness*, fever*, hallucinations*, irregular heartbeat*, joint pain*, rash*, scaly skin*, sore throat*, yellow eyes or skin*

PRECAUTIONS

Stopping this drug suddenly may cause chest pain or heart attack. If you wish to stop taking this drug, ask your doctor for specific instructions.

You need to wait 2 weeks after stopping a monoamine oxidase inhibitor† before starting this drug.

People with asthma may not be able to take this drug.

Be careful driving or handling equipment while taking this drug because the drug may cause dizziness and drowsiness.

f you are diabetic, this drug may increase blood sugar levels or make the symptoms of low blood sugar less noticeable.

This drug may cause nondiabetics to develop type 2 diabetes.

f you have psoriasis or myasthenia gravis, this drug may make those conditions worse.

PREGNANCY AND BREAST-FEEDING

Safety in pregnancy has not been established although the drug is known to harm animal fetuses. This drug has been used to treat hypertension in pregnancy and to prevent eclampsia, and side effects are rarely seen in the baby.

This drug passes into breast milk and may affect the baby.

HELPFUL COMMENTS

This drug may make you more sensitive to cold temperatures.

You may get a tingling feeling on your scalp when the drug is first started, but this should go away quickly.

If you do not treat high blood pressure, you may develop more serious problems such as heart failure, blood vessel disease, stroke, or kidney disease. Losing weight, exercising, eating more fruits and vegetables, and avoiding salty foods, such as lunchmeat and pickles, may help make drug treatment more successful.

LAMIVUDINE

Available since November 1995

COMMONLY USED TO TREAT

Hepatitis B infection
HIV infection
People at risk of getting an HIV infection

DRUG CATEGORY

antiretroviral
Class: nucleoside reverse transcriptase inhibitor (NsRTI)

PRODUCTS

Brand-Name Products with No Generic Alternative
Epivir-HBV 100 mg tablet ($$$$)
Epivir 150 mg tablet ($$$$)

Epivir-HBV 5 mg/ml oral solution ($)
Epivir 10 mg/ml oral solution ($$)
No generics available.
Multiple patents that begin to expire in 2009. Exclusivity until 2005.

Combination Products That Contain This Drug
Combivir tablet
Trizivir tablet

DOSING AND FOOD

Doses are taken 1 to 3 times a day.
This drug may be taken with or without food but is best taken with food to reduce the stomach upset that some people suffer.
Adults and children over 3 months: Up to 300 mg per day in divided doses.
Lower doses are used in babies and in people with kidney disease.
Forgotten doses: If you are scheduled to take the next dose within a few hours, do not take the forgotten dose. Otherwise take the forgotten dose as soon as you remember.

ALCOHOL, DRUG, HERB, AND SUPPLEMENT INTERACTIONS

Alcohol may increase some of the side effects from this drug, depending on the amount consumed. Ask your doctor about the risks caused by drinking alcohol with your condition.

Taking this drug with any of the ones listed below may change the effect of either drug with the possibility of causing toxicity or decreasing effectiveness:
co-trimoxazole

ALLERGIC REACTIONS AND SIDE EFFECTS

You should tell your doctor about all your allergies and any unexplained symptoms you may have while taking this drug.
MORE COMMON SIDE EFFECTS: Abdominal pain*, ear discharge, ear swelling, mouth sores, nausea*, numbness*, runny nose, skin irritation, swollen glands, tingling*, vomiting*
LESS COMMON SIDE EFFECTS: Cough, dizziness, headache, sleeping difficulty
RARE SIDE EFFECTS: Chills*, diarrhea*, fever*, hair loss, irregular breathing*, loss of appetite*, muscle cramps*, shortness of breath*, skin rash*, sore throat*, tiredness*, weakness*

PRECAUTIONS

This drug does not prevent transmission of the HIV virus.

If you have a history of nerve damage or pancreatitis, this drug may make those conditions worse.

This drug is usually prescribed in combination with another antiretroviral† drug. Ask your pharmacist about the type of drug interaction that may occur between antiretroviral drugs† to coordinate the administration times of multiple drugs.

Your skin may feel warm to the touch even if you do not have a fever.

PREGNANCY AND BREAST-FEEDING

Safety during pregnancy has not been established although the drug is known to harm animal fetuses.

Breast-feeding while taking this drug is not recommended.

HELPFUL COMMENTS

This drug is also called by the generic name 3TC.

Do not stop treatment early if you start to feel better. It takes the full prescription for this drug to work completely.

Do not measure doses of the oral solution with anything but a measuring cup intended for use with prescription drugs. Slight inaccuracy from other measuring spoons may result in over- or under-dosing.

LAMOTRIGINE

Available since December 1994

COMMONLY USED TO TREAT

Seizures

DRUG CATEGORY

anticonvulsant
Class: phenyltriazine

PRODUCTS

Brand-Name Products with No Generic Alternative
Lamictal 25 mg tablet ($$$)
Lamictal 100 mg tablet ($$$)
Lamictal 150 mg tablet ($$$)
Lamictal 200 mg tablet ($$$)
Lamictal CD 2 mg chewable tablet (n/a)
Lamictal CD 5 mg chewable tablet ($$)

---

†See page 52.   *See page 53.

Lamictal CD 25 mg chewable tablet ($$)
No generics available.
Patent expires in 2008. Exclusivity until 2005.

DOSING AND FOOD

Doses are taken 1 to 2 times a day.
This drug may be taken with or without food.
Adults: Up to 500 mg per day in divided doses.
Lower doses are used in children.
Forgotten doses: If you are scheduled to take the next dose within a few hours, do not take the forgotten dose. Otherwise take the forgotten dose as soon as you remember.

ALCOHOL, DRUG, HERB, AND SUPPLEMENT INTERACTIONS

Alcohol may increase some of the side effects from this drug, depending on the amount consumed. Ask your doctor about the risks caused by drinking alcohol with your condition.

Many OTC drugs used for appetite control, asthma, colds, cough, hay fever, pain, or sinus problems affect the central nervous system and may interfere with this drug. Check with your pharmacist for products to avoid.

Taking this drug with any of the ones listed below may change the effect of either drug with the possibility of causing toxicity or decreasing effectiveness: carbamazepine, co-trimoxazole, methotrexate, phenobarbital, phenytoin, primidone, valproic acid

Increased side effects are possible when this drug is taken with those listed below: alcohol, anesthetics, antihistamines†, barbiturates†; narcotics†, skeletal muscle relaxants†

ALLERGIC REACTIONS AND SIDE EFFECTS

You should tell your doctor about all your allergies and any unexplained symptoms you may have while taking this drug.

This drug promotes the effect of sunlight on the body and may cause severe sunburn and increased sensitivity of the eyes.

MORE COMMON SIDE EFFECTS: Blurry vision*, clumsiness*, dizziness, drowsiness, headache, nausea, poor coordination*, skin rash*, unsteadiness*, vision changes*, vomiting

LESS COMMON SIDE EFFECTS: Anxiety*, chest pain*, confusion*, constipation, depression*, diarrhea, dry mouth, eye movement*, fever*, indigestion, irritability*, menstrual pain, mood swings*, runny nose, seizures*, shaking, sleeping difficulty, slurry speech, trembling, weakness*, weight loss

RARE SIDE EFFECTS: Bleeding*, blistering*, breathing difficulty*, bruising*, chills*, coma*, dark urine*, eye irrItation*, increased heart rate*, itching*, memory loss*, mouth sores*, muscle pain*, skin irritation*, sore throat*, suicidal thoughts*, swelling*, swollen glands*, tiredness*, yellow eyes or skin*

PRECAUTIONS

People with a type of anemia called thalassemia may not be able to take this drug.

Be careful driving or handling equipment while taking this drug because it may cause dizziness, drowsiness, and blurry vision.

Stopping this drug suddenly may cause seizures to occur. If you wish to stop taking this drug, ask your doctor for specific instructions.

If you have Parkinson's disease, this drug may make that condition worse.

Call your doctor right away if you get a skin rash since it may be the start of a serious side effect.

PREGNANCY AND BREAST-FEEDING

Safety during pregnancy has not been established although the drug is known to harm animal fetuses.

Breast-feeding while taking this drug is not recommended.

HELPFUL COMMENTS

Contact your doctor if your seizure activity appears to increase.

It is okay for the chewable tablets to be swallowed whole.

Eye irritation caused by the sun may be reduced by wearing sunglasses when outside.

LANSOPRAZOLE

Available since May 1995

COMMONLY USED TO TREAT

Heartburn, specifically gastroesophageal reflux disease (GERD)
Stomach ulcers

DRUG CATEGORY

antiulcer
Class: proton pump inhibitor

---

† See page 52.   * See page 53.

PRODUCTS

Brand-Name Products with No Generic Alternative
Prevacid 15 mg delayed-release capsule ($$$)
Prevacid 30 mg delayed-release capsule ($$$)
Prevacid 15 mg delayed-release packet ($$$)
Prevacid 30 mg delayed-release packet ($$$)
Prevacid 15 mg disintegrating tablet (n/a)
Prevacid 30 mg disintegrating tablet(n/a)
No generics available.
Multiple patents that begin to expire in 2009. Exclusivity until 2005.

Combination Products That Contain This Drug
Prevpac extended-release capsule ($$$$$)

DOSING AND FOOD

Doses are taken once a day.
It is best to take this drug just before breakfast.
Adults: Up to 120 mg per day.
Lower doses may be used in people with liver disease.
Forgotten doses: If you are scheduled to take the next dose within a few
   hours, do not take the forgotten dose. Otherwise take the forgotten dose
   as soon as you remember.

ALCOHOL, DRUG, HERB, AND SUPPLEMENT INTERACTIONS

Alcohol may increase some of the side effects from this drug, depending
   on the amount consumed. Ask your doctor about the risks caused by
   drinking alcohol with your condition.
The herb male fern is not effective when taken with this drug.

**Taking this drug with any of the ones listed below may change the effect of
either drug with the possibility of causing toxicity or decreasing effectiveness:**
ampicillin, iron supplements, ketoconazole, sucralfate, theophylline

ALLERGIC REACTIONS AND SIDE EFFECTS

You should tell your doctor about all your allergies and any unexplained
   symptoms you may have while taking this drug.
MORE COMMON SIDE EFFECTS: Abdominal pain*, diarrhea*, dizziness,
   headache, nausea*, itching*, skin rash*
LESS COMMON SIDE EFFECTS: Appetite changes*, joint pain*, vomiting*
RARE SIDE EFFECTS: Anxiety*, bleeding*, bruising*, constipation*, cough*,
   depression*, muscle pain*, rectal bleeding*, runny nose*

PRECAUTIONS

Do not crush, break, or chew the delayed-release products. Capsules may be opened and the pellets sprinkled in applesauce, pudding, fruit juice, or vegetable juice. Be careful not to chew the pellets.

If taking another drug in the morning, it should be taken about 30 minutes prior to taking this drug.

PREGNANCY AND BREAST-FEEDING

Safety during pregnancy has not been established although there was no evidence of harm during studies in animals.

Breast-feeding while taking this drug is not recommended.

HELPFUL COMMENTS

This drug is usually used for short-term treatment that lasts 1 to 2 months.

If mixing the drug pellets with food or juice, make sure to rinse the container and drink to get the entire dose. Do not mix doses in advance.

LEFLUNOMIDE

Available since September 1998

COMMONLY USED TO TREAT

Arthritis

DRUG CATEGORY

antirheumatic
Class: pyrimidine synthesis inhibitor

PRODUCTS

Brand-Name Products with No Generic Alternative
Arava 10 mg tablet (n/a)
Arava 20 mg tablet (n/a)
Arava 100 mg tablet (n/a)
No generics available.
No patents. Exclusivity expires in 2003.

DOSING AND FOOD

Doses are taken once a day.
This drug may be taken with or without food.
Adults: Up to 20 mg per day. Higher doses are used for the first 3 days.

---

†See page 52.   *See page 53.

Forgotten doses: If you are scheduled to take the next dose in less than 6 hours, do not take the forgotten dose. Otherwise take the forgotten dose as soon as you remember.

ALCOHOL, DRUG, HERB, AND SUPPLEMENT INTERACTIONS

Alcohol may increase the risk of liver damage from this drug. Ask your doctor about the risks caused by drinking alcohol with your condition.

Taking this drug with any of the ones listed below may change the effect of either drug with the possibility of causing toxicity or decreasing effectiveness: activated charcoal, cholestyramine, rifampin

Increased side effects are possible when this drug is taken with those listed below: acetaminophen, amiodarone, anabolic steroids†, androgens†, antibiotics†, antithyroid drugs†, carmustine, chloroquine, dantrolene, daunorubicin, disulfiram, divalproex, estrogens†, etretinate, felodipine, gold salts†, hydroxychloroquine, mercaptopurine, methotrexate, methyldopa, naltrexone, nifedipine, oral contraceptives, phenothiazines†, plicamycin, valproic acid, verapamil

ALLERGIC REACTIONS AND SIDE EFFECTS

You should tell your doctor about all your allergies and any unexplained symptoms you may have while taking this drug.

MORE COMMON SIDE EFFECTS: Back pain, bloody urine*, breathing difficulty*, congestion*, cough*, dizziness*, fever*, hair loss, headache*, heartburn, loss of appetite*, nausea*, skin rash, sneezing*, sore throat*, stomach pain*, urinary changes*, vomiting*, weight loss, yellow eyes or skin*

LESS COMMON SIDE EFFECTS: Acne, anxiety, burning sensation*, chest pain*, constipation, diarrhea*, dry mouth, eye irritation, gas, indigestion*, irregular heartbeat*, itching, joint pain*, muscle pain*, runny nose, shortness of breath*, sore mouth, tiredness*, weakness*

PRECAUTIONS

Pregnant women and women of childbearing age need to avoid all exposure to this drug because of the risk of birth defects. Do not handle damaged tablets. Pregnant women should not have intercourse with men taking this drug since drug-containing semen may cause birth defects.

Men planning to have children need to discontinue this drug and take another prescription that will remove this drug from the body.

Blood tests to monitor liver function are needed regularly while taking this drug.

People with a decreased immune system are at higher risk of getting an infection while taking this drug.

Exposure to skin tests, immunizations, and people who have received immunizations may put you at a greater risk of developing the disease when you are taking this drug.

PREGNANCY AND BREAST-FEEDING

This drug may cause birth defects and should not be used during pregnancy. Any exposure to the drug including touching broken tablets or having intercourse with a man taking the drug may also be associated with birth defects.

Breast-feeding while taking this drug is not recommended.

HELPFUL COMMENTS

Low doses of this drug are taken for the first 3 days to avoid side effects. It may take 2 months for the effects to be noticed.

Men taking this drug who have sexual intercourse with women of child-bearing age should use 2 forms of contraception while taking this drug and for at least 2 months after the drug is stopped.

LETROZOLE

Available since July 1997

COMMONLY USED TO TREAT

Breast cancer

DRUG CATEGORY

antineoplastic
Class: aromatase inhibitor

PRODUCTS

Brand-Name Products with No Generic Alternative
Femara 2.5 mg tablet ($$$$)
No generics available.
Patent expires in 2011. Exclusivity until 2004.

DOSING AND FOOD

Doses are taken once a day.
This drug may be taken with or without food.

---

†See page 52.   * See page 53.

Adults: Up to 2.5 mg per day.

Forgotten doses: If you are scheduled to take the next dose within a few hours, do not take the forgotten dose. Otherwise take the forgotten dose as soon as you remember.

ALCOHOL, DRUG, HERB, AND SUPPLEMENT INTERACTIONS

Alcohol may increase some of the side effects from this drug, depending on the amount consumed. Ask your doctor about the risks caused by drinking alcohol with your condition.

Taking this drug with any of the ones listed below may change the effect of either drug with the possibility of causing toxicity or decreasing effectiveness: tamoxifen

ALLERGIC REACTIONS AND SIDE EFFECTS

You should tell your doctor about all your allergies and any unexplained symptoms you may have while taking this drug.

MORE COMMON SIDE EFFECTS: Back pain, bone pain, calf pain*, hot flashes, joint pain, muscle pain, nausea*, shortness of breath*

LESS COMMON SIDE EFFECTS: Anxiety, breast pain*, broken bones*, chest pain*, chills*, confusion, constipation, depression*, diarrhea, dry mouth, fever*, frequent urination, headache*, itching, loss of appetite, poor coordination*, runny nose*, skin rash, sleepiness, sleeping difficulty, spinning sensation, swelling*, taste changes, thirst, tiredness, vomiting, weakness*, weight gain, weight loss

RARE SIDE EFFECTS: Cough*, dizziness*, fainting*, fast heartbeat*, hair loss, heart attack*, lightheadedness*, nervousness*, numbness*, slurry speech*, sweating*, vaginal bleeding*, vision changes*

PRECAUTIONS

This drug decreases the amount of female hormone in the body and should only be used by postmenopausal women.

Avoid contact with anyone who has the chickenpox, measles, or other communicable disease since it may be easier to catch a viral infection while taking this drug.

People with a history of liver disease may not be able to take this drug.

PREGNANCY AND BREAST-FEEDING

There is evidence that this drug may harm the fetus, but the drug may be necessary to the health of the mother.

It is not known if this drug passes into breast milk. Talk to your doctor about the risks associated with breast-feeding while taking this drug.

HELPFUL COMMENTS

It takes about 2 to 6 weeks after starting this drug for it to reach the desired level in the body and begin working fully.

It is very important to continue taking this drug as ordered by the doctor even if the side effects make you feel ill.

LEVAMISOLE

Available since June 1990

COMMONLY USED TO TREAT

Colon cancer

DRUG CATEGORY

antineoplastic
Class: biological response modifier

PRODUCTS

Brand-Name Products with No Generic Alternative
Ergamisol 50 mg tablet ($$$$)
No generics available.
Patent expires in 2004.

DOSING AND FOOD

Doses are taken 3 times a day.

This drug may be taken with or without food. Do not eat raw oysters or other raw shellfish at any time while taking this drug.

Adults: Up to 150 mg per day in divided doses.

Forgotten doses: Do not take a forgotten dose. Just go back to your usual schedule with the next dose. If you vomit within 2 hours of taking a dose, call your doctor to find out if the dose should be repeated.

ALCOHOL, DRUG, HERB, AND SUPPLEMENT INTERACTIONS

Consuming any alcohol while on this drug will cause a severe reaction that includes anxiety, blurry vision, breathing difficulty, chest pain, confusion, dizziness, fainting, flushing, headache, irregular heartbeat, muscle

---

†See page 52.   *See page 53.

weakness, nausea, sweating, thirst, and vomiting. This reaction may also be triggered by the alcohol found in food, herbs, supplements, and OTC drugs.

Taking this drug with any of the ones listed below may change the effect of either drug with the possibility of causing toxicity or decreasing effectiveness: phenytoin, warfarin

ALLERGIC REACTIONS AND SIDE EFFECTS

You should tell your doctor about all your allergies and any unexplained symptoms you may have while taking this drug.

MORE COMMON SIDE EFFECTS: Diarrhea, metallic taste, nausea

LESS COMMON SIDE EFFECTS: Anxiety, chills*, depression, dizziness, fever*, headache, itching, joint pain, mouth sores*, nervousness, nightmares, skin rash, sleepiness, sleeping difficulty, tiredness, vomiting, weakness*

RARE SIDE EFFECTS: Back pain*, black stools*, bleeding*, bloody urine*, blurry vision*, bruising*, confusion*, cough*, hoarseness*, lip smacking*, numbness*, paranoia*, puffy cheeks*, seizures*, shaking*, skin irritation*, spastic movements*, tingling*, tongue movements*, trembling*, trouble walking*, urinary changes*

PRECAUTIONS

Avoid contact with anyone who has the chickenpox, measles, or other communicable disease since the infection may be worse for people on this drug.

Exposure to skin tests, immunizations, and people who have received immunizations may put you at a greater risk of developing the disease when you are taking this drug.

This drug causes changes in your blood that put you at greater risk of getting an infection. Be careful not to cut yourself or get bruised. Tell your doctor if you develop signs of infection, such as fever or sore throat. Your dentist may recommend that you clean your teeth and mouth differently to avoid infection.

For best results, this drug should be started 7 to 30 days after surgery.

This drug is given in combination with fluorouracil in a pattern that includes a drug-free rest period during which this drug is not taken.

PREGNANCY AND BREAST-FEEDING

Safety during pregnancy has not been established although the drug is known to harm animal fetuses.

It is not known if this drug passes into breast milk. Talk to your doctor about the risks associated with breast-feeding while taking this drug.

HELPFUL COMMENTS

It is very important to continue taking this drug as ordered by the doctor even if the side effects make you feel ill. Make sure to tell your doctor if you develop flulike symptoms or other notable side effects.

LEVETIRACETAM

Available since November 1999

COMMONLY USED TO TREAT

Seizures

DRUG CATEGORY

anticonvulsant
Class: unclassified

PRODUCTS

Brand-Name Products with No Generic Alternative
Keppra 250 mg tablet ($$)
Keppra 500 mg tablet ($$)
Keppra 750 mg tablet ($$$)
No generics available.
Multiple patents that expire in 2006. Exclusivity expires in 2004.

DOSING AND FOOD

Doses are taken twice a day.
This drug may be taken with or without food.
Adults: Up to 1,500 mg per day in divided doses.
Lower doses may be used in people with kidney disease.
Forgotten doses: Take the forgotten dose as soon as you remember even if it is time for the next dose. If the next dose is scheduled in less than 2 hours, delay the next dose for 1 to 2 hours. Take the forgotten dose on an empty stomach which makes it work a little quicker.

ALCOHOL, DRUG, HERB, AND SUPPLEMENT INTERACTIONS

Alcohol should not be used while taking this drug.

---

† See page 52.   * See page 53.

Several OTC drugs used for allergies, colds, cough, hay fever, pain, or sinus problems may cause excessive drowsiness when taken with this drug. Check with your pharmacist when selecting OTC products.

Severe reactions are possible when this drug is taken with those listed below: antihistamines†, benzodiazepines†, narcotics†, tricyclic antidepressants†

ALLERGIC REACTIONS AND SIDE EFFECTS

You should tell your doctor about all your allergies and any unexplained symptoms you may have while taking this drug.

MORE COMMON SIDE EFFECTS: Cough*, dizziness, drowsiness, fever*, hoarseness*, loss of energy*, muscle pain, runny nose*, sore throat, swallowing difficulty*, swollen glands, voice changes, weakness

LESS COMMON SIDE EFFECTS: Anger*, back pain*, breathing difficulty*, burning, chest tightness*, chills*, clumsiness*, crying*, depersonalization*, depression*, double vision*, eye pain*, headache*, itching, lightheadedness, loss of appetite, memory loss*, mood swings*, nervousness*, numbness, painful urination*, paranoia*, poor coordination*, shortness of breath*, stuffy nose*, tingling, unsteadiness*, weight loss, wheezing

PRECAUTIONS

Be careful driving or handling equipment while taking this drug because it may cause drowsiness and dizziness.

Stopping this drug suddenly may cause seizures to occur frequently. If you wish to stop taking this drug, ask your doctor for specific instructions.

PREGNANCY AND BREAST-FEEDING

Safety during pregnancy has not been established although the drug is known to harm animal fetuses.

It is not known if this drug passes into breast milk. Talk to your doctor about the risks associated with breast-feeding while taking this drug.

HELPFUL COMMENTS

Avoid quick movements to minimize dizziness. Dangling your legs over the side of the bed for a few minutes may help reduce dizziness when first waking up.

LEVODOPA/CARBIDOPA
(levodopa is only available in combination with carbidopa, which is the focus of this drug summary)

Available for over 20 years

COMMONLY USED TO TREAT

Parkinson's disease

DRUG CATEGORY

antidyskinetic
Class: decarboxylase inhibitor/dopamine precursor

PRODUCTS

Brand-Name Products with Generic Alternatives

Sinemet 10 mg/100 mg tablet (¢¢¢¢¢)
  Generic: carbidopa/levodopa 10 mg/100 mg tablet (¢¢¢¢)
Sinemet 25 mg/100 mg tablet (¢¢¢¢¢)
  Generic: carbidopa/levodopa 25 mg/100 mg tablet (¢¢¢)
Sinemet 25 mg/250 mg tablet ($)
  Generic: carbidopa/levodopa 25 mg/250 mg tablet (¢¢¢¢)
Sinemet CR 25 mg/100 mg extended-release tablet ($)
  Generic: carbidopa/levodopa 25 mg/100 mg extended-release
  tablet (¢¢¢¢¢)
Sinemet CR 50 mg/200 mg extended-release tablet ($$)
  Generic: carbidopa/levodopa 50 mg/200 mg extended-release
  tablet ($$)

DOSING AND FOOD

Doses are taken 3 to 4 times a day.
Eat a little food soon after taking this drug to reduce the stomach upset
  that some people suffer.
Adults: Up to 8 regular tablets per day or 5 extended-release tablets per
  day in divided doses.
Lower doses are used in children.
Forgotten doses: If you are scheduled to take the next dose in 2 hours or
  less, do not take the forgotten dose. Otherwise take the forgotten dose as
  soon as you remember.

†See page 52.   * See page 53.

ALCOHOL, DRUG, HERB, AND SUPPLEMENT INTERACTIONS

Alcohol may increase some of the side effects from this drug, depending on the amount consumed. Ask your doctor about the risks caused by drinking alcohol with your condition.

Kava may increase the symptoms of Parkinson's disease, making it appear that this drug is ineffective.

Jimsonweed and rauwolfia should not be used while taking this drug since they may decrease the effects or increase the side effects of the drug.

Several OTC drugs used for appetite control, asthma, colds, cough, hay fever, pain, or sinus problems may cause serious side effects when taken with this drug. Check with your pharmacist when selecting OTC products.

Taking this drug with any of the ones listed below may change the effect of either drug with the possibility of causing toxicity or decreasing effectiveness: antacids, anticonvulsants†, benzodiazepines†, bromocriptine, haloperidol, papaverine, phenothiazines†, rauwolfia alkaloids†, selegiline, thioxanthenes†

Severe reactions are possible when this drug is taken with those listed below: anesthetics, cocaine, methyldopa, molindone, monoamine oxidase inhibitors†, sympathomimetics†

Increased side effects are possible when this drug is taken with those listed below: antihypertensives†

ALLERGIC REACTIONS AND SIDE EFFECTS

You should tell your doctor about all your allergies and any unexplained symptoms you may have while taking this drug.

MORE COMMON SIDE EFFECTS: Abdominal pain, agitation*, anxiety*, clumsiness*, confusion*, dizziness*, dry mouth, fainting*, gas, hallucinations*, lightheadedness*, loss of appetite*, nausea*, nightmares, numbness*, spastic movements*, swallowing difficulty*, teeth clenching*, tiredness*, tremor*, unsteadiness*, vomiting*, watery mouth*, weakness*

LESS COMMON SIDE EFFECTS: Blurry vision*, constipation, depression*, diarrhea, double vision*, eyelid spasm*, headache, hiccups, hot flashes*, irregular heartbeat*, large pupils*, mood swings*, poor bladder control*, skin rash*, sleeping difficulty, suicidal thoughts*, sweating, twitching, urinary difficulty*, weight changes*

RARE SIDE EFFECTS: Back pain*, bloody stool*, bloody vomit, chills*, dark urine, eye stillness*, fever*, high blood pressure*, leg pain*, pale skin*, prolonged penile erection*, seizures*, sore throat*, stomach pain*, swelling*, yellow eyes or skin*

PRECAUTIONS

You need to wait 2 weeks after stopping a monoamine oxidase inhibitor†
  before starting this drug.

High-protein diets may interfere with the effects of this drug.

This drug has a bitter flavor and may irritate the tongue before swallowing.

Extended-release products may be broken in half, but should not be
  crushed or chewed.

Men have a small risk of developing painful, prolonged erection of the
  penis, which requires treatment by a doctor. If this happens, go to your
  doctor or the nearest emergency room immediately.

This drug may interfere with several tests including urine glucose tests,
  urine ketones, urine protein, and others, providing false results.

Be careful driving or handling equipment while taking this drug because
  it may cause dizziness.

If you are diabetic, you may need a change in the dose of your antidiabetic
  drug† or insulin while taking this drug.

If you have asthma, bronchitis, lung disease, glaucoma, heart disease, skin
  cancer, mental illness, or hormone problems, this drug may make those
  conditions worse.

People with a history of seizures may be at greater risk of having a seizure
  while taking this drug.

This drug may cause dry mouth, which is associated with a greater risk of
  cavities. Your dentist may recommend that you clean your teeth and
  mouth differently to avoid infection.

PREGNANCY AND BREAST-FEEDING

Safety during pregnancy has not been established although the drug is
  known to harm animal fetuses.

Breast-feeding while taking this drug is not recommended.

HELPFUL COMME, MNTS

It may take several weeks or months for the full effects of this drug to be
  noticed.

Sucking on hard sugarless candy or chewing sugarless gum may help
  relieve dry mouth caused by this drug.

Do not be alarmed if you notice a color change to your saliva, urine,
  or sweat.

This drug impairs movement and balance and may cause you to fall if
  you do too much physical activity. Avoid quick movements to minimize
  dizziness. Dangling your legs over the side of the bed for a few minutes
  may help reduce dizziness when first waking up.

† See page 52.   * See page 53.

LEVOFLOXACIN

Available since December 1996

COMMONLY USED TO TREAT

Infection

DRUG CATEGORY

antibiotic
Class: fluoroquinolone

PRODUCTS

Brand-Name Products with No Generic Alternative
Levaquin 250 mg tablet ($$$$)
Levaquin 500 mg tablet ($$$$)
Levaquin 750 mg tablet ($$$$$)
Quixin 0.5% ophthalmic solution ($$$$$)
No generics available.
Multiple patents that begin to expire in 2003.

DOSING AND FOOD

Doses are taken once a day.
It is best to take this drug on an empty stomach, 2 hours after a meal.
Adults: Up to 750 mg per day.
Lower doses are used in people with kidney disease.
Oral products are rarely used in children under age 18 because they may in-
terfere with bone development. Eyedrops are used in children over age 1.
Eyedrops: 1 to 2 drops per dose, 1 to 8 times per day.
Forgotten doses: If you are scheduled to take the next dose within a few
hours, do not take the forgotten dose. Otherwise take the forgotten dose
as soon as you remember.

ALCOHOL, DRUG, HERB, AND SUPPLEMENT INTERACTIONS

Alcohol may increase some of the side effects from this drug, depending
on the amount consumed. Ask your doctor about the risks caused by
drinking alcohol with your condition.

**Taking this drug with any of the ones listed below may change the effect of
either drug with the possibility of causing toxicity or decreasing effectiveness:**
antacids, antidiabetics†, digoxin, iron supplements, mineral supplements,
probenecid, sucralfate, theophylline, warfarin

Severe reactions are possible when this drug is taken with those listed below: amiodarone, antipsychotics†, astemizole, bepridil, cisapride, erythromycin, nonsteroidal antiinflammatories†, phenothiazines†, procainamide, quinidine, sotalol, tricyclic antidepressants†

ALLERGIC REACTIONS AND SIDE EFFECTS

If you are allergic to any fluoroquinolones†, you may also be allergic to this drug. You should tell your doctor about all your allergies and any unexplained symptoms you may have while taking this drug.

This drug promotes the effect of sunlight on the body and may cause severe sunburn and increased sensitivity of the eyes.

MORE COMMON SIDE EFFECTS: Nausea, nervousness, rash*, seizures*, severe diarrhea*, shortness of breath*, skin irritation*, swelling*, vomiting

LESS COMMON SIDE EFFECTS: Back pain, blisters*, dreams, dizziness, drowsiness, headache, lightheadedness, muscle pain, sleep disorders, sore mouth, stomachache, urinary difficulty, vaginal discharge, vaginal pain, taste changes, vision changes

RARE SIDE EFFECTS: Abdominal pain*, agitation*, bloody urine*, confusion*, dark urine*, fever*, flushing*, hallucinations*, irregular heartbeat*, joint pain*, leg pain*, loss of appetite*, pale stools*, shakiness*, sweating*, tiredness*, tremors*; weakness*, yellow eyes or skin*

PRECAUTIONS

Be careful driving or handling equipment while taking this drug because the drug may cause dizziness and drowsiness.

A rash may be the first symptom of an allergic reaction and should be reported to your doctor immediately.

If you have a history of tendinitis, this drug may make that condition worse.

If you are a diabetic, you may need a change in the dose of your antidiabetic drug† or insulin, since this drug may cause changes in blood sugar.

If you are using eyedrops, many of the side effects and warnings do not apply. Watch for burning and irritation when the drops are used and report any rash, itching, swelling, or redness around the eye to your doctor. Eyedrops may also cause throat irritation, runny nose, swollen glands, and voice changes, which should be reported to your doctor.

PREGNANCY AND BREAST-FEEDING

Safety in pregnancy has not been established although the drug is known to harm animal fetuses.

Breast-feeding while taking this drug is not recommended.

---

†See page 52.   *See page 53.

HELPFUL COMMENTS

Contact your doctor if your symptoms do not improve after a couple of days.

Do not stop treatment early if you start to feel better. It takes the full prescription for this drug to work completely.

If you need to take an antacid, minerals, or iron supplements, take them either 2 hours before or after taking this drug.

Drink a lot of water while taking this drug.

LEVORPHANOL TARTRATE

Available for over 20 years

COMMONLY USED TO TREAT

Pain

DRUG CATEGORY

analgesic
Class: narcotic analgesic/opioid

PRODUCTS

Products Only Available as Generics
levorphanol tartrate 2 mg tablet (¢¢¢¢¢)

DOSING AND FOOD

Doses are taken 3 to 4 times a day.

It is best to take this drug on an empty stomach, but taking this drug with a little food may avoid the stomach upset that some people suffer.

Adults: Up to 24 mg per day in divided doses.

Forgotten doses: If you are scheduled to take the next dose within a few hours, do not take the forgotten dose. Otherwise take the forgotten dose as soon as you remember.

ALCOHOL, DRUG, HERB, AND SUPPLEMENT INTERACTIONS

Alcohol should not be used while taking this drug.

Several OTC drugs used for asthma, colds, cough, hay fever, sleep aid, or sinus problems may seriously change the effects and side effects of this drug. Check with your pharmacist when selecting OTC products.

Taking this drug with any of the ones listed below may change the effect of either drug with the possibility of causing toxicity or decreasing effectiveness:
natrexone, rifampin

Severe reactions are possible when this drug is taken with those listed below: analgesics, anesthetics, anticholinergics†, antihistamines†, barbiturates†, benzodiazepines†, cimetidine, monoamine oxidase inhibitors†, naloxone, narcotics†, phenothiazines†, sedative-hypnotics†, skeletal muscle relaxants†, tricyclic antidepressants†

ALLERGIC REACTIONS AND SIDE EFFECTS

If you are allergic to any narcotics†, you may also be allergic to this drug. You should tell your doctor about all your allergies and any unexplained symptoms you may have while taking this drug.

MORE COMMON SIDE EFFECTS: Dizziness*, drowsiness*, fainting, lightheadedness, nausea, vomiting

LESS COMMON SIDE EFFECTS: Blurry vision, breathing difficulty*, constipation, depression*, dry mouth, excitement*, flushing*, hallucinations*, headache, hives*, irregular breathing*, irregular heartbeat*, itching*, loss of appetite, mood swings*, nervousness*, restlessness*, ringing in ears*, shortness of breath*, skin rash*, sleep disorders, spastic movements*, stomach cramps, sweating*, swelling*, tiredness, trembling*, urinary changes, vision changes, weakness*, wheezing*

RARE SIDE EFFECTS: Body aches, clammy skin*, confusion*, diarrhea, fever, goosebumps, irritability, low blood pressure*, runny nose, seizures*, shivering, slow breathing*, slow heartbeat*, small pupils*, sneezing, yawning

PRECAUTIONS

Be careful driving or handling equipment while taking this drug because it may cause dizziness and drowsiness.

If you have a history of head injury, brain disease, emphysema, asthma, lung disease, enlarged prostate, urinary disorders, gallbladder disease, or gallstones, you may not be able to take this drug.

People with colitis, heart disease, kidney disease, liver disease, and thyroid disease are at increased risk of developing side effects.

If you have a history of seizures, this drug may make those conditions worse.

This drug may cause withdrawal symptoms if stopped suddenly. If you wish to stop taking this drug, ask your doctor for specific instructions.

Side effects may continue to develop for about a month after this drug is stopped.

Because this drug has a high abuse potential, your prescription quantity may be limited.

---

† See page 52.   * See page 53.

PREGNANCY AND BREAST-FEEDING

Safety during pregnancy has not been established although the drug is known to harm animal fetuses.

Breast-feeding while taking this drug is not recommended.

HELPFUL COMMENTS

If the drug does not seem to be working properly, an increase in dose may not help. Talk to your doctor about other drugs and treatment options.

Sucking on hard sugarless candy or chewing sugarless gum may help relieve dry mouth caused by this drug.

Lie down for a while after taking a dose of this drug to help reduce the nausea.

Avoid quick movements to minimize dizziness. Dangling your legs over the side of the bed for a few minutes may help reduce dizziness when first waking up.

This drug works best for treating pain when taken before the pain gets too severe.

LEVOTHYROXINE SODIUM

Available for over 20 years

COMMONLY USED TO TREAT

Low thyroid levels, also known as hypothyroidism

DRUG CATEGORY

thyroid replacement
Class: thyroid hormone

PRODUCTS

Brand-Name Products with Generic Alternatives§

Synthroid 0.025 mg tablet (¢¢¢)
  Generic: levothyroxine sodium 0.025 mg tablet (¢)

Synthroid 0.05 mg tablet (¢¢¢)
  Generic: levothyroxine sodium 0.05 mg tablet (¢)

Synthroid 0.075 mg tablet (¢¢¢)
  Generic: levothyroxine sodium 0.075 mg tablet (¢)

Synthroid 0.088 mg tablet (¢¢¢)
  Generic: levothyroxine sodium 0.088 mg tablet (¢¢)

§ *See "Precautions" in this entry.*

Synthroid 0.1 mg tablet (¢¢¢)
 Generic: levothyroxine sodium 0.1 mg tablet (¢)
Synthroid 0.112 mg tablet (¢¢¢)
 Generic: levothyroxine sodium 0.112 mg tablet (¢¢¢)
Synthroid 0.125 mg tablet (¢¢¢)
 Generic: levothyroxine sodium 0.125 mg tablet (¢)
Synthroid 0.137 mg tablet (n/a)
 Generic: levothyroxine sodium 0.137 mg tablet (¢¢¢)
Synthroid 0.15 mg tablet (¢¢¢)
 Generic: levothyroxine sodium 0.15 mg tablet (¢)
Synthroid 0.175 mg tablet (¢¢¢¢)
 Generic: levothyroxine sodium 0.175 mg tablet (¢¢)
Synthroid 0.2 mg tablet (¢¢¢¢)
 Generic: levothyroxine sodium 0.2 mg tablet (¢)
Synthroid 0.3 mg tablet (¢¢¢¢¢)
 Generic: levothyroxine sodium 0.3 mg tablet (¢¢)

Other Generic Product Names
Levo-T, Levothroid, Levoxyl, L-Thyroxine, Novothyrox, Thyro-tabs, Unithroid

DOSING AND FOOD

Doses are taken once a day before breakfast.
It is best to take this drug on an empty stomach at least 1 hour before a meal.

Adults: Up to 300 mcg per day.

Lower doses are used in children and in people with heart disease.

Forgotten doses: If you are scheduled to take the next dose within a few
hours, do not take the forgotten dose. Otherwise take the forgotten dose
as soon as you remember.

ALCOHOL, DRUG, HERB, AND SUPPLEMENT INTERACTIONS

Alcohol may increase some of the side effects from this drug, depending
on the amount consumed. Ask your doctor about the risks caused by
drinking alcohol with your condition.
Several OTC drugs used for appetite control, asthma, colds, cough, hay fever,
pain, or sinus problems may cause serious side effects when taken with
this drug. Check with your pharmacist when selecting OTC products.
Many OTC products, including antacids, iron supplements, and soy-based
infant formulas, may interfere with the absorption of this drug and
should be taken 2 hours before or after taking this drug.

---

†See page 52.   *See page 53.

Taking this drug with any of the ones listed below may change the effect of either drug with the possibility of causing toxicity or decreasing effectiveness: antacids, anticoagulants†, antidiabetics†, beta blockers†, cholestyramine, colestipol, corticosteroids†, corticotropin, estrogens†, insulin, iron supplements, phenytoin, sodium polystyrene sulfonate, sucralfate, theophylline

Severe reactions are possible when this drug is taken with those listed below: amphetamines†, appetite suppressants†, somatrem, sympathomimetics†, tricyclic antidepressants†

ALLERGIC REACTIONS AND SIDE EFFECTS

If you are allergic to any thyroid hormones†, you may also be allergic to this drug. Synthroid 100 mcg and 300 mcg tablets contain tartrazine dye, which may cause allergic reactions. You should tell your doctor about all your allergies and any unexplained symptoms you may have while taking this drug.

MORE COMMON SIDE EFFECTS: Chest pain*, irregular heartbeat*, nervousness, shakiness, sleep disorders

LESS COMMON SIDE EFFECTS: Appetite changes, diarrhea, fever, headache*, hives*, irritability, leg cramps, menstrual changes, skin rash*, sweating, vomiting, weight loss

RARE SIDE EFFECTS: Behavior changes*, confusion*, mood swings*, restlessness*, shortness of breath*, weakness*, yellow eyes or skin*

PRECAUTIONS

§The effectiveness of this drug may vary from product to product. Do not switch from one manufacturer to another when your prescription is refilled. Talk to your pharmacist to make sure you get the same product each time.

This drug may make you more sensitive to warm temperatures.

If you are a diabetic, you may need a change in the dose of your antidiabetic drug† or insulin, since this drug may cause changes in blood sugar.

People with diabetes, heart disease, high blood pressure, adrenal gland deficiency, pituitary gland deficiency, or atherosclerosis may not be able to take this drug.

The Levothroid products contain lactose, which may cause gastric upset in people who are lactose intolerant.

If your thyroid drug therapy is changed to liothyronine, this drug should be stopped as soon as the other is started.

PREGNANCY AND BREAST-FEEDING

Safety studies in pregnant women have not found a risk to the fetus.
This drug passes into breast milk, but does not appear to harm the baby.
Talk to your doctor about the risks associated with breast-feeding while
taking this drug.

HELPFUL COMMENTS

This drug is also called by the generic name T4.
It takes about 1 to 3 weeks before you begin to notice the effects of this drug.
Take your dose in the morning to help reduce the sleep disorders that
some people suffer.

LINEZOLID

Available since August 2000

COMMONLY USED TO TREAT

Infection

DRUG CATEGORY

antibiotic
Class: oxazolidinone derivative

PRODUCTS

Brand-Name Products with No Generic Alternative
Zyvox 600 mg tablet ($$$$$)
Zyvox 100 mg/5 ml oral suspension ($$$$)
No generics available.
Patent expires in 2014. Exclusivity until 2005.

DOSING AND FOOD

Doses are taken 2 times a day.
This drug may be taken with or without food. Do not eat raw oysters or
other raw shellfish at any time while taking this drug. Foods that are high
in tyramine may cause elevation in blood pressure while taking this drug.
Foods prepared by aging, fermentation, pickling, or smoking, such as
aged cheese, red wine, soy sauce, tap beer (including alcohol-free beer),
sauerkraut, bologna, pepperoni, salami, summer sausage, and dried
meats, are considered high in tyramine.
Adults: Up to 1,200 mg per day in divided doses.

---

†See page 52.   * See page 53.

Forgotten doses: If you are scheduled to take the next dose within a few hours, do not take the forgotten dose. Otherwise take the forgotten dose as soon as you remember.

ALCOHOL, DRUG, HERB, AND SUPPLEMENT INTERACTIONS

Alcohol may increase some of the side effects from this drug, depending on the amount consumed. Ask your doctor about the risks caused by drinking alcohol with your condition.

Several OTC drugs used for appetite control, asthma, colds, cough, hay fever, or sinus problems may cause an increase in blood pressure when taken with this drug. Check with your pharmacist when selecting OTC products.

Severe reactions are possible when this drug is taken with those listed below: citalopram, clomipramine, fluvoxamine, moclobemide, monoamine oxidase inhibitors†, nefazodone, paroxetine, sertraline, sibutramine, SSRI†, tryptophan, venlafaxine

ALLERGIC REACTIONS AND SIDE EFFECTS

You should tell your doctor about all your allergies and any unexplained symptoms you may have while taking this drug.

MORE COMMON SIDE EFFECTS: Diarrhea*, nausea

LESS COMMON SIDE EFFECTS: Abdominal pain*, back pain*, black stools*, bleeding*, bloody urine*, bruising*, chills*, cough*, dizziness, fever*, headache*, hoarseness*, mouth sores*, painful urination*, shortness of breath*, skin irritation*, taste changes, tiredness*, tongue discoloration, vaginal discharge*, vaginal itch*, vomiting, weakness*

PRECAUTIONS

Shaking the oral suspension product may damage the drug. Instead of shaking, the suspension should be mixed by gently inverting the bottle 3 to 5 times before each use.

The oral suspension product contains phenylalanine, which should not be used in people with phenylketonuria.

This drug causes changes in your blood that put you at greater risk of getting an infection. Be careful not to cut yourself or get bruised. Tell your doctor if you develop signs of infection, such as fever or sore throat. Your dentist may recommend that you clean your teeth and mouth differently to avoid infection.

Avoid contact with anyone who has the chickenpox, measles, or other communicable disease since the infection may be worse for people on this drug.

Exposure to skin tests, immunizations, and people who have received immunizations may put you at a greater risk of developing the disease when you are taking this drug.

PREGNANCY AND BREAST-FEEDING

Safety during pregnancy has not been established although the drug is known to harm animal fetuses.

It is not known if this drug passes into breast milk. Talk to your doctor about the risks associated with breast-feeding while taking this drug.

HELPFUL COMMENTS

Contact your doctor if your symptoms do not improve after a couple of days.

Do not stop treatment early if you start to feel better. It takes the full prescription for this drug to work completely.

Do not measure doses of the oral suspension with anything but a measuring cup intended for use with prescription drugs. Slight inaccuracy from other measuring spoons may result in over- or under-dosing.

LIOTHYRONINE SODIUM

Available for over 20 years

COMMONLY USED TO TREAT

Goiter
Low thyroid levels, also known as hypothyroidism

DRUG CATEGORY

thyroid replacement
Class: thyroid hormone

PRODUCTS

Brand-Name Products with No Generic Alternative
Cytomel 5 mcg tablet (¢¢¢¢)
Cytomel 25 mcg tablet (¢¢¢¢)
Cytomel 50 mcg tablet (¢¢¢¢¢)
No generics available.
No patents, no exclusivity.

DOSING AND FOOD

Doses are taken once a day in the morning.

This drug may be taken with or without food.

Adults: Up to 100 mcg per day.

Lower doses are used in children.

Forgotten doses: If you are scheduled to take the next dose within a few hours, do not take the forgotten dose. Otherwise take the forgotten dose as soon as you remember.

ALCOHOL, DRUG, HERB, AND SUPPLEMENT INTERACTIONS

Alcohol may increase some of the side effects from this drug, depending on the amount consumed. Ask your doctor about the risks caused by drinking alcohol with your condition.

Several OTC drugs used for appetite control, asthma, colds, cough, hay fever, pain, or sinus problems may cause serious side effects when taken with this drug. Check with your pharmacist when selecting OTC products.

Taking this drug with any of the ones listed below may change the effect of either drug with the possibility of causing toxicity or decreasing effectiveness: anticoagulants†, antidiabetics†, cholestyramine, colestipol, corticosteroids†, corticotropin, estrogens†, insulin, theophylline

Severe reactions are possible when this drug is taken with those listed below: amphetamines†, appetite suppressants†, sympathomimetics†, tricyclic antidepressants†

ALLERGIC REACTIONS AND SIDE EFFECTS

If you are allergic to any thyroid hormones†, you may also be allergic to this drug. You should tell your doctor about all your allergies and any unexplained symptoms you may have while taking this drug.

MORE COMMON SIDE EFFECTS: Irregular heartbeat*, nervousness, shakiness, sleep disorders

LESS COMMON SIDE EFFECTS: Appetite changes, diarrhea, fever, headache*, hives*, irritability, leg cramps, menstrual changes, skin rash*, sweating, vomiting, weight loss

RARE SIDE EFFECTS: Behavior changes*, chest pain*, confusion*, mood swings*, restlessness*, shortness of breath*, weakness*, yellow eyes or skin*

PRECAUTIONS

If you are a diabetic, you may need a change in the dose of your antidiabetic drug† or insulin, since this drug may cause changes in blood sugar.

This drug may make you more sensitive to warm temperatures.

People with diabetes, heart disease, high blood pressure, adrenal deficiency, pituitary deficiency, or atherosclerosis may not be able to take this drug.

If you are taking liothyronine sodium and you are switched to levothyroxine, continue taking liothyronine for several days while taking levothyroxine to reduce the risk of relapse.

PREGNANCY AND BREAST-FEEDING

Safety studies in pregnant women have not found a risk to the fetus.

This drug passes into breast milk, but does not appear to harm the baby. Talk to your doctor about the risks associated with breast-feeding while taking this drug.

HELPFUL COMMENTS

It takes about 2 weeks before you begin to notice the effects of this drug.

Take your dose in the morning to help reduce the sleep disorders that some people suffer.

This drug is also called by the generic name T3.

LIOTRIX

Available for over 20 years

COMMONLY USED TO TREAT

Low thyroid levels, also known as hypothyroidism

DRUG CATEGORY

thyroid replacement
Class: thyroid hormone

PRODUCTS

Brand-Name Products with No Generic Alternative
Thyrolar-0.25 tablet (¢¢¢)
Thyrolar-0.5 tablet (¢¢¢¢)
Thyrolar-1 tablet (¢¢¢¢)
Thyrolar-2 tablet (¢¢¢¢¢)
Thyrolar-3 tablet (¢¢¢¢¢)
No generics available.
No patents, no exclusivity.

---

† See page 52.   * See page 53.

DOSING AND FOOD

Doses are taken once a day before breakfast.

It is best to take this drug on an empty stomach at least 1 hour before a meal.

Adults: Up to 180 mg "thyroid equivalents" per day.§

Lower doses are used in children.

Forgotten doses: If you are scheduled to take the next dose within a few hours, do not take the forgotten dose. Otherwise take the forgotten dose as soon as you remember.

ALCOHOL, DRUG, HERB, AND SUPPLEMENT INTERACTIONS

Alcohol may increase some of the side effects from this drug, depending on the amount consumed. Ask your doctor about the risks caused by drinking alcohol with your condition.

Several OTC drugs used for appetite control, asthma, colds, cough, hay fever, pain, or sinus problems may cause serious side effects when taken with this drug. Check with your pharmacist when selecting OTC products.

Taking this drug with any of the ones listed below may change the effect of either drug with the possibility of causing toxicity or decreasing effectiveness: anticoagulants†, antidiabetics†, beta blockers†, cholestyramine, colestipol, corticosteroids†, corticotropin, estrogens†, insulin, phenytoin, theophylline

Severe reactions are possible when this drug is taken with those listed below: amphetamines†, appetite suppressants, sympathomimetics†, somatrem, tricyclic antidepressants†

ALLERGIC REACTIONS AND SIDE EFFECTS

If you are allergic to any thyroid hormones†, you may also be allergic to this drug. You should tell your doctor about all your allergies and any unexplained symptoms you may have while taking this drug.

MORE COMMON SIDE EFFECTS: Irregular heartbeat*

LESS COMMON SIDE EFFECTS: Appetite changes, diarrhea, fever, headache*, hives*, irritability, leg cramps, menstrual changes, nervousness, shakiness, skin rash*, sleep disorders, sweating, vomiting, weight loss

RARE SIDE EFFECTS: Behavior changes*, chest pain*, confusion*, mood swings*, restlessness*, shortness of breath*, weakness*, yellow eyes or skin*

§ See "Precautions" in this entry.

PRECAUTIONS

§This drug is a synthetic combination of 2 thyroid hormones (T3 and T4) in a fixed combination. Doses are compared to the natural thyroid hormone and called "thyroid equivalents." One hundred eighty (180) mg "thyroid equivalents" is the same as 1 Thyrolar-3 tablet.

People with diabetes, heart disease, high blood pressure, adrenal gland deficiency, pituitary gland deficiency, or atherosclerosis may not be able to take this drug.

This drug may make you more sensitive to warm temperatures.

If you are a diabetic, you may need a change in the dose of your antidiabetic drug† or insulin, since this drug may cause changes in blood sugar.

PREGNANCY AND BREAST-FEEDING

Safety studies in pregnant women have not found a risk to the fetus.

This drug passes into breast milk, but does not appear to harm the baby. Talk to your doctor about the risks associated with breast-feeding while taking this drug.

HELPFUL COMMENTS

It takes about 2 weeks before you begin to notice the effects of this drug.

Take your dose in the morning to help reduce the sleep disorders that some people suffer.

LISINOPRIL

Available since December 1987

COMMONLY USED TO TREAT

Heart failure

High blood pressure, also known as hypertension

DRUG CATEGORY

antihypertensive

Class: ACE inhibitor

PRODUCTS

Brand-Name Products with Generic Alternatives

Prinivil 2.5 mg tablet (¢¢¢¢)

Zestril 2.5 mg tablet (¢¢¢¢)

  Generic: lisinopril 2.5 mg tablet (n/a)

---

†See page 52.   * See page 53.

Prinivil 5 mg tablet (¢¢¢¢¢)
Zestril 5 mg tablet ($)
  Generic: lisinopril 5 mg tablet (n/a)
Prinivil 10 mg tablet ($)
Zestril 10 mg tablet ($)
  Generic: lisinopril 10 mg tablet (n/a)
Prinivil 20 mg tablet ($)
Zestril 20 mg tablet ($)
  Generic: lisinopril 20 mg tablet (n/a)
Zestril 30 mg tablet ($$)
  Generic: lisinopril 30 mg tablet (n/a)
Prinivil 40 mg tablet ($$)
Zestril 40 mg tablet ($$)
  Generic: lisinopril 40 mg tablet (n/a)
Other Products That Contain This Drug
Prinzide tablet ($)
Zestoretic tablet ($)

DOSING AND FOOD

Doses are taken once a day.
This drug may be taken with or without food.
Adults: Up to 80 mg per day.
Lower doses are used in people with kidney disease.
This drug is rarely used in children.
Forgotten doses: If you are scheduled to take the next dose within a few hours, do not take the forgotten dose. Otherwise take the forgotten dose as soon as you remember.

ALCOHOL, DRUG, HERB, AND SUPPLEMENT INTERACTIONS

Alcohol may cause your blood pressure to rise, making this drug less effective. Ask your doctor about the risks caused by drinking alcohol with your condition.
Licorice may interfere with the effects of this drug.
Capsaicin and other foods or supplements, including hot peppers, sweet peppers, paprika, and chili powder, derived from the capsicum family of plants may increase the risk of developing a cough and should not be taken with this drug.
Several OTC drugs used for appetite control, asthma, colds, cough, hay fever, or sinus problems may cause an increase in blood pressure when

taken with this drug. Check with your pharmacist when selecting OTC products.

Taking this drug with any of the ones listed below may change the effect of either drug with the possibility of causing toxicity or decreasing effectiveness: antacids, antidiabetics†, antihypertensives†, diuretics†, insulin, lithium, nonsteroidal antiinflammatories†, potassium supplements

ALLERGIC REACTIONS AND SIDE EFFECTS

If you are allergic to any ACE inhibitors†, you may also be allergic to this drug. You should tell your doctor about all your allergies and any unexplained symptoms you may have while taking this drug.

MORE COMMON SIDE EFFECTS: Breathing difficulty*, diarrhea, dizziness*, dry cough, fainting*, headache, stuffy nose, swallowing difficulty, swelling*

LESS COMMON SIDE EFFECTS: Fever*, joint pain*, lightheadedness*, loss of taste, nausea*, skin rash*, tiredness

RARE SIDE EFFECTS: Abdominal pain*, chest pain*, chills*, confusion*, hoarseness*, irregular heartbeat*, itching*, nervousness*, numbness*, stomach pain*, vomiting*, weakness*, yellow eyes or skin*

PRECAUTIONS

Be careful driving or handling equipment while taking this drug because the drug may cause dizziness.

People with systemic lupus erythematosus may be at greater risk of developing blood problems while taking this drug.

Do not use potassium-containing products, including salt substitutes, while taking this drug.

Diuretics† should be stopped 2 to 3 days prior to starting this drug. If not possible to stop the diuretic, the dose of this drug should be lowered.

Drink plenty of fluids to avoid dehydration when sweating, such as in hot weather and during exercise.

PREGNANCY AND BREAST-FEEDING

Safety in pregnancy has not been established although the drug is known to harm animal fetuses.

Breast-feeding while taking this drug is not recommended.

HELPFUL COMMENTS

A persistent dry cough may appear while taking this drug, but it will go away when the drug is stopped.

† See page 52.   * See page 53.

If you need to take an antacid, take it either 2 hours before or after taking this drug.

Avoid quick movements to minimize dizziness. Dangling your legs over the side of the bed for a few minutes may help reduce dizziness when first waking up.

LITHIUM

Available for over 20 years

COMMONLY USED TO TREAT

Manic-depressive illness

DRUG CATEGORY

behavioral agent
Class: alkali metal

PRODUCTS

Brand-Name Products with No Generic Alternative
Eskalith-CR 450 mg extended-release tablet (¢¢¢)
Brand-Name Products with Generic Alternatives
Eskalith 300 mg capsule (¢¢)
  Generic: lithium carbonate 300 mg capsule (¢¢)
Lithobid 300 mg extended-release tablet (¢¢¢)
  Generic: lithium carbonate 300 mg extended-release tablet (n/a)
Products Only Available as Generics
lithium carbonate 150 mg capsule (¢¢).
lithium carbonate 300 mg tablet (¢¢)
lithium carbonate 600 mg capsule (¢¢¢)
lithium citrate 300 mg/5 ml oral syrup (¢¢)

DOSING AND FOOD

Doses are taken 1 to 4 times a day.
It is best to take this drug with food or milk.
Adults: Up to 1,000 mg per day in divided doses.
Lower doses are used in children.
Forgotten doses: If you are scheduled to take the next dose in 6 hours or less, do not take the forgotten dose. Otherwise take the forgotten dose as soon as you remember.

ALCOHOL, DRUG, HERB, AND SUPPLEMENT INTERACTIONS

Alcohol may increase some of the side effects from this drug, depending on the amount consumed. Ask your doctor about the risks caused by drinking alcohol with your condition.

Parsley may trigger a serious reaction when taken with this drug and should not be used.

Psyllium seed decreases the absorption of this drug, making it less effective.

Caffeine may decrease the effectiveness of this drug.

Taking this drug with any of the ones listed below may change the effect of either drug with the possibility of causing toxicity or decreasing effectiveness:
ACE inhibitors†, acetazolamide, aminophylline, antacids, antipsychotics†, atracurium, caffeine, calcium, carbamazepine, fluoxetine, indomethacin, mazindol, methyldopa, metronidazole, nonsteroidal antiinflammatories†, pancuronium, phenylbutazone, phenytoin, piroxicam, sodium, SSRI†, succinylcholine, sympathomimetics†, tetracycline, theophylline, thiazide diuretics†

Severe reactions are possible when this drug is taken with those listed below:
calcium channel blockers†, haloperidol

Increased side effects are possible when this drug is taken with those listed below:
calcium iodide, iodinated glycerol, potassium iodide

ALLERGIC REACTIONS AND SIDE EFFECTS

You should tell your doctor about all your allergies and any unexplained symptoms you may have while taking this drug.

MORE COMMON SIDE EFFECTS: Nausea*, poor bladder control, thirst*, trembling*, urinary changes*

LESS COMMON SIDE EFFECTS: Acne, bloating, breathing difficulty, confusion*, fainting*, irregular heartbeat*, irregular pulse*, muscle twitch, poor memory*, skin rash, slurry speech*, stiffness*, tiredness*, weakness*, weight gain*

RARE SIDE EFFECTS: Blue fingers*, blue toes*, blurry vision*, clumsiness*, coldness*, coma*, confusion*, depression*, diarrhea*, dizziness*, drowsiness*, dry skin*, excitement*, eye pain*, hair loss*, headache*, hoarseness*, loss of appetite*, poor coordination*, ringing in ears*, seizures*, sensitivity to cold*, swelling*, trembling*, unsteadiness*, vision problems*, vomiting*

PRECAUTIONS

This drug may easily reach high, toxic levels in the body even with normal

† See page 52.　　* See page 53.

doses. Blood tests are required frequently for safety. Report any unusual symptoms to your doctor right away. Early warning signs of toxicity include diarrhea, vomiting, dehydration, drowsiness, weakness, fever, tremor, and poor coordination.

The amount of sodium in the diet may influence the amount of drug in the body. Do not make changes to your diet without telling the doctor in advance. Make sure to eat a balanced diet with a normal amount of salt, and drink 10 to 12 glasses of water each day. Drink plenty of fluids to avoid dehydration when sweating, such as in hot weather and during exercise.

People receiving electroconvulsive therapy are at greater risk of developing nerve toxicity while taking this drug. The drug should be stopped before therapy.

This drug may interfere with thyroid function tests, resulting in false results.

Do not open, crush, break, or chew the extended-release products.

If you are a diabetic, you may need a change in the dose of your antidiabetic drug† or insulin, since this drug may cause changes in blood sugar.

People with brain disease or schizophrenia may be more sensitive to the effects of this drug.

If you have a history of leukemia, seizures, goiter, thyroid disease, heart disease, Parkinson's disease, or psoriasis, this drug may make those conditions worse.

Be careful driving or handling equipment while taking this drug because it may cause dizziness, drowsiness, and blurry vision.

PREGNANCY AND BREAST-FEEDING

There is evidence that this drug may harm the fetus, but the drug may be necessary to the health of the mother.

Breast-feeding while taking this drug is not recommended.

HELPFUL COMMENTS

It takes about 1 to 3 weeks for the effects of this drug to be noticed.

Oral syrup products may be diluted in water or fruit juice to make them easier to swallow.

You should carry identification and emergency medical information with you while taking this drug.

If you need to take an antacid, take it either 2 hours before or after taking this drug.

LOMEFLOXACIN HYDROCHLORIDE

Available since February 1992

COMMONLY USED TO TREAT

Infection

DRUG CATEGORY

antibiotic
Class: fluoroquinolone

PRODUCTS

Brand-Name Products with No Generic Alternative
Maxaquin 400 mg tablet ($$$$)
No generics available.
Patent expires in 2006.

DOSING AND FOOD

Doses are taken once a day.
It is best to take this drug on an empty stomach, 2 hours after a meal.

Adults: Up to 400 mg per day.

Lower doses are used in people with kidney disease.

This drug is rarely used in children under age 18 because it may interfere with bone development.

Forgotten doses: If you are scheduled to take the next dose within a few hours, do not take the forgotten dose. Otherwise take the forgotten dose as soon as you remember.

ALCOHOL, DRUG, HERB, AND SUPPLEMENT INTERACTIONS

Alcohol may increase some of the side effects from this drug, depending on the amount consumed. Ask your doctor about the risks caused by drinking alcohol with your condition.

Taking this drug with any of the ones listed below may change the effect of either drug with the possibility of causing toxicity or decreasing effectiveness:
antacids, cimetidine, cyclosporine, didanosine, iron supplements, mineral supplements, phenytoin, probenecid, sucralfate

Severe reactions are possible when this drug is taken with those listed below:
aminophylline, oxtriphylline, theophylline

---

† See page 52.   * See page 53.

ALLERGIC REACTIONS AND SIDE EFFECTS

If you are allergic to any fluoroquinolones†, you may also be allergic to this drug. You should tell your doctor about all your allergies and any unexplained symptoms you may have while taking this drug.

This drug promotes the effect of sunlight on the body and may cause severe sunburn and increased sensitivity of the eyes.

MORE COMMON SIDE EFFECTS: Back pain*, chills*, coma*, dizziness, fever*, headache, irregular heartbeat*, diarrhea*, nausea, nervousness, rash*, seizures*, shortness of breath*, skin irritation*, swelling*, vomiting

LESS COMMON SIDE EFFECTS: Blisters*, dreams, drowsiness, lightheadedness, muscle pain, sleep disorders, sore mouth, stomachache, urinary difficulty, vaginal discharge, vaginal pain, taste changes, vision changes

RARE SIDE EFFECTS: Abdominal pain*, agitation*, bloody urine*, confusion*, dark urine*, flushing*, hallucinations*, joint pain*, leg pain*, loss of appetite*, pale stools*, shakiness*, sweating*, tiredness*, tremors*, weakness*, yellow eyes or skin*

PRECAUTIONS

Be careful driving or handling equipment while taking this drug because the drug may cause dizziness and drowsiness.

If you have a history of tendinitis, this drug may make that condition worse.

This drug may interfere with the results of urine opiate tests. If you have a pre-employment drug-screening test, make sure the laboratory knows that you are taking this drug.

PREGNANCY AND BREAST-FEEDING

Safety in pregnancy has not been established although the drug is known to harm animal fetuses.

Breast-feeding while taking this drug is not recommended.

HELPFUL COMMENTS

Contact your doctor if your symptoms do not improve after a couple of days.

Do not stop treatment early if you start to feel better. It takes the full prescription for this drug to work completely.

If you need to take an antacid, minerals, or iron supplements, take them either 4 hours before or after taking this drug.

Drink a lot of water while taking this drug.

LOMUSTINE

Available for over 20 years

COMMONLY USED TO TREAT

Brain tumor
Cancer in the lymph tissue, also known as a lymphoma
Hodgkins' disease

DRUG CATEGORY

antineoplastic
Class: alkylating agent: nitrosurea

PRODUCTS

Brand-Name Products with No Generic Alternative
CeeNu 10 mg capsule ($$$$)
CeeNu 40 mg capsule ($$$$$)
CeeNu 100 mg capsule ($$$$$)
No generics available.
No patents, no exclusivity.

DOSING AND FOOD

A single dose is repeated every 6 weeks.
This drug should be taken 2 to 4 hours after a meal. Do not eat raw oysters
   or other raw shellfish at any time while taking this drug.
Adults and children: Up to 130 mg/m^2 per dose.
Lower doses are used in people with bone marrow depression.

ALCOHOL, DRUG, HERB, AND SUPPLEMENT INTERACTIONS

Alcohol may increase some of the side effects from this drug, depending
   on the amount consumed. Ask your doctor about the risks caused by
   drinking alcohol with your condition.
Do not take aspirin while taking this drug.

**Taking this drug with any of the ones listed below may change the effect of
either drug with the possibility of causing toxicity or decreasing effectiveness:**
amphotericin B, antithyroid drugs†, azathioprine, chloramphenicol, colchicine, flucytosine, ganciclovir, interferon, plicamycin, zidovudine

ALLERGIC REACTIONS AND SIDE EFFECTS

You should tell your doctor about all your allergies and any unexplained
   symptoms you may have while taking this drug.

† *See page 52.*   * *See page 53.*

MORE COMMON SIDE EFFECTS: Loss of appetite, nausea, pale skin, vomiting

LESS COMMON SIDE EFFECTS: Awkwardness*, back pain*, black stools*, bleeding*, bloody urine*, bruising*, chills*, confusion*, cough*, diarrhea, fever*, hair loss, hoarseness*, itching, mouth sores*, skin discoloration, skin irritation*, skin rash, slurry speech*, swelling*, tiredness*, urinary difficulty*, weakness*

RARE SIDE EFFECTS: Cough*, shortness of breath*

PRECAUTIONS

If vomiting occurs shortly after taking the dose, call your doctor to find out if the dose should be repeated.

Avoid contact with anyone who has the chickenpox, measles, or other communicable disease since it may be easier to catch the infection while taking this drug.

Exposure to skin tests, immunizations, and people who have received immunizations may put you at a greater risk of developing the disease when you are taking this drug.

This drug causes changes in your blood that put you at greater risk of getting an infection. Be careful not to cut yourself or get bruised. Tell your doctor if you develop signs of infection, such as fever or sore throat. Your dentist may recommend that you clean your teeth and mouth differently to avoid infection.

People with lung disease may be at greater risk of developing lung-related side effects from this drug.

PREGNANCY AND BREAST-FEEDING

There is evidence that this drug may harm the fetus, but the drug may be necessary to the health of the mother.

Breast-feeding while taking this drug is not recommended.

HELPFUL COMMENTS

This drug is also called by the generic name CCNU.

It is very important to continue taking this drug as ordered by the doctor even if the side effects make you feel ill.

Nausea and vomiting after a dose will usually stop in about 24 hours, although it may be 3 days before your appetite returns.

Many side effects do not start until weeks after the dose is taken and may last 6 weeks or longer.

To get the right dose of this drug, your prescription may contain capsules of different shapes and colors.

LORACARBEF

Available since December 1991

COMMONLY USED TO TREAT

Ear infection, also known as otitis media
Infections
Pneumonia
Sinus infection, also known as sinusitis
Strep throat
Tonsilitis

DRUG CATEGORY

antibiotic
Class: second generation cephalosporin

PRODUCTS

Brand-Name Products with No Generic Alternative
Lorabid 200 mg capsule ($$$)
Lorabid 400 mg capsule ($$$$)
Lorabid 100 mg/5 ml oral suspension ($$)
Lorabid 200 mg/5 ml oral suspension ($$$)
No generics available.
No patents, no exclusivity.

DOSING AND FOOD

Doses are taken 2 times a day.
It is best to take this drug on an empty stomach at least 1 hour before or 2 hours after a meal.
Adults: Up to 800 mg per day in divided doses.
Children age 13 and older: Up to 800 mg per day in divided doses.
Children age 6 months and older: Up to 30 mg/kg per day in divided doses.
Lower doses are used in people with kidney disease.
Forgotten doses: If you are scheduled to take the next dose within a few hours, do not take the forgotten dose. Otherwise take the forgotten dose as soon as you remember.

ALCOHOL, DRUG, HERB, AND SUPPLEMENT INTERACTIONS

Alcohol may increase some of the side effects from this drug, depending

---

† See page 52.   * See page 53.

on the amount consumed. Ask your doctor about the risks caused by drinking alcohol with your condition.

Taking this drug with any of the ones listed below may change the effect of either drug with the possibility of causing toxicity or decreasing effectiveness: probenecid

ALLERGIC REACTIONS AND SIDE EFFECTS

If you are allergic to any penicillins† or cephalosporins†, you may also be allergic to this drug. You should tell your doctor all your allergies and any unexplained symptoms you may have while taking this drug.

MORE COMMON SIDE EFFECTS: Diarrhea, itching*, loss of appetite, nausea, skin rash*, stomach pain, vomiting

RARE SIDE EFFECTS: Dizziness, drowsiness, headache, nervousness, sleeping difficulty, vaginal discharge, vaginal itch

PRECAUTIONS

The capsule products are absorbed differently than the oral suspension products and should not be substituted without a new prescription.

Diarrhea caused by this drug is often treated first with OTC products. Using the wrong OTC drug may make the diarrhea more severe or last longer. Take kaolin- or attapulgite-containing products such as Kaopectate or Di-asorb to treat mild diarrhea. Call your doctor if diarrhea gets severe or continues after using OTC drugs. You may need a prescription drug to keep your condition from getting worse.

PREGNANCY AND BREAST-FEEDING

Safety during pregnancy has not been established although there was no evidence of harm during studies in animals.

It is not known if this drug passes into breast milk. Talk to your doctor about the risks associated with breast-feeding while taking this drug.

HELPFUL COMMENTS

Contact your doctor if your symptoms do not improve after a couple of days.

Do not stop treatment early if you start to feel better. It takes the full prescription for this drug to work completely.

Oral suspension products may be stored at room temperature but begin to degrade after 14 days.

LORAZEPAM

Available for over 20 years

COMMONLY USED TO TREAT

Anxiety
Sleeping difficulty, also known as insomnia

DRUG CATEGORY

antipanic
antitremor
anxiolytic
sedative-hypnotic
skeletal muscle relaxant
Class: benzodiazepine

PRODUCTS

Brand-Name Products with Generic Alternatives
Ativan 0.5 mg tablet (¢¢¢¢¢)
  Generic: lorazepam 0.5 mg tablet (¢¢¢)
Ativan 1 mg tablet ($)
  Generic: lorazepam 1 mg tablet (¢¢¢)
Ativan 2 mg tablet ($$)
  Generic: lorazepam 2 mg tablet (¢¢¢¢)
Products Only Available as Generics
lorazepam 0.5 mg/5 ml oral solution (n/a)
lorazepam intensol 2 mg/ml oral concentrate ($$$$)

DOSING AND FOOD

Doses are taken 1 to 3 times a day.
This drug may be taken with or without food.
Adults: Up to 10 mg per day in divided doses.
Lower doses are used in people over age 65.
Forgotten doses: If you are scheduled to take the next dose within a few
  hours, do not take the forgotten dose. Otherwise take the forgotten dose
  as soon as you remember.

ALCOHOL, DRUG, HERB, AND SUPPLEMENT INTERACTIONS

Alcohol should not be used while taking this drug.
Catnip, kava, lady's slipper, lemon balm, passion flower, sassafras, skullcap,

---

† See page 52.   * See page 53.

and valerian should not be used while taking this drug due to an increased sedative effect.

Taking this drug with any of the ones listed below may change the effect of either drug with the possibility of causing toxicity or decreasing effectiveness: caffeine, cimetidine, disulfiram, fluvoxamine, itraconazole, ketoconazole, nefazodone

Severe reactions are possible when this drug is taken with those listed below: anesthetics†, antidepressants†, antihistamines†, barbiturates†, monoamine oxidase inhibitors†, narcotics†, phenothiazines†

Increased side effects are possible when this drug is taken with those listed below: aminophylline, scopolamine, theophylline

ALLERGIC REACTIONS AND SIDE EFFECTS

If you are allergic to any benzodiazepines†, you may also be allergic to this drug. You should tell your doctor about all your allergies and any unexplained symptoms you may have while taking this drug.

MORE COMMON SIDE EFFECTS: Drowsiness, lightheadedness, vivid dreams

LESS COMMON SIDE EFFECTS: Anxiety*, clumsiness, confusion*, constipation, depression*, diarrhea, difficulty urinating, dizziness, dry mouth, headache, irregular heartbeat*, memory loss*, muscle spasm, nausea, sexual dysfunction, slurry speech, stomach cramps, thirst, trembling, vision changes, vomiting, watery mouth

RARE SIDE EFFECTS: Agitation*, behavior changes*, bleeding*, bruising*, chills*, delusions*, disorientation*, excitement*, eye movement*, fever*, hallucinations*, irritability*, low blood pressure*, mouth sores*, nervousness*, skin irritation*, sore throat*, spastic movements*, tiredness*, weakness*, yellow eyes or skin*

PRECAUTIONS

This drug may be habit forming and will cause severe withdrawal symptoms if stopped abruptly.
You need to wait 2 weeks after stopping a monoamine oxidase inhibitor† before starting this drug.
If you have difficulty swallowing, emphysema, asthma, bronchitis, glaucoma, hyperactivity, mental depression, mental illness, myasthenia gravis, porphyria, or sleep apnea, this drug may make those conditions worse.
Heavy smoking may cause this drug to be less effective.
Be careful driving or handling equipment while taking this drug because the drug may cause dizziness and drowsiness.

PREGNANCY AND BREAST-FEEDING

There is evidence that this drug may harm the fetus, but the drug may be necessary to the health of the mother.

Breast-feeding while taking this drug is not recommended.

HELPFUL COMMENTS

Dangling your legs over the side of the bed for a few minutes may help reduce dizziness when first waking up.

LOSARTAN POTASSIUM

Available since April 1995

COMMONLY USED TO TREAT

High blood pressure, also known as hypertension

DRUG CATEGORY

antihypertensive
Class: angiotensin II receptor antagonist

PRODUCTS

Brand-Name Products with No Generic Alternative
Cozaar 25 mg tablet ($)
Cozaar 50 mg tablet ($)
Cozaar 100 mg tablet ($$)
No generics available.
Multiple patents that begin to expire in 2009.
Combination Products That Contain This Drug
Hyzaar tablet ($) to ($$)

DOSING AND FOOD

Doses are taken 1 to 2 times a day.
This drug may be taken with or without food.
Adults: Up to 100 mg per day.
Lower doses are used in people with kidney or liver disease.
This drug is rarely used in children.
Forgotten doses: If you are scheduled to take the next dose within a few hours, do not take the forgotten dose. Otherwise take the forgotten dose as soon as you remember.

---

† See page 52.   * See page 53.

ALCOHOL, DRUG, HERB, AND SUPPLEMENT INTERACTIONS

Alcohol may increase some of the side effects from this drug, depending on the amount consumed. Ask your doctor about the risks caused by drinking alcohol with your condition.

Several OTC drugs used for appetite control, asthma, colds, cough, hay fever, or sinus problems may cause an increase in blood pressure when taken with this drug. Check with your pharmacist when selecting OTC products.

Taking this drug with any of the ones listed below may change the effect of either drug with the possibility of causing toxicity or decreasing effectiveness: diuretics†

ALLERGIC REACTIONS AND SIDE EFFECTS

You should tell your doctor about all your allergies and any unexplained symptoms you may have while taking this drug.

MORE COMMON SIDE EFFECTS: Headache

LESS COMMON SIDE EFFECTS: Back pain, cough*, diarrhea, dizziness*, fatigue, fever*, sinus congestion, sore throat*

RARE SIDE EFFECTS: Breathing difficulty*, hoarseness*, leg pain, muscle pain, sleep disorders, swallowing difficulty*, swelling*

PRECAUTIONS

If you are dehydrated, the blood-pressure-lowering effect of this drug may be increased. Drink plenty of fluids to avoid dehydration when sweating, such as in hot weather and during exercise.

Be careful driving or handling equipment while taking this drug because the drug may cause dizziness.

This drug contains potassium, which may cause high potassium levels in the body. Do not add extra potassium to your diet or use salt substitutes that contain potassium while taking this drug.

PREGNANCY AND BREAST-FEEDING

There is evidence that this drug may harm the fetus, but the drug may be necessary to the health of the mother.

Breast-feeding while taking this drug is not recommended.

HELPFUL COMMENTS

If you are taking this drug once a day and still having difficulty with your blood pressure, talk to your doctor about taking the same dose twice a day.

LOVASTATIN

Available since August 1987

COMMONLY USED TO TREAT

High blood cholesterol and lipids, also known as hyperlipidemia

DRUG CATEGORY

antilipemic
Class: HMG-CoA reductase inhibitor (statin)

PRODUCTS

Brand-Name Products with No Generic Alternative
Altocor 10 mg extended-release tablet (n/a)
Altocor 20 mg extended-release tablet (n/a)
Altocor 40 mg extended-release tablet (n/a)
Altocor 60 mg extended-release tablet (n/a)
No generic extended-release products available.
Multiple patents that begin to expire in 2017.

Brand-Name Products with Generic Alternatives
Mevacor 10 mg tablet ($)
  Generic: lovastatin 10 mg tablet ($)
Mevacor 20 mg tablet ($$$)
  Generic: lovastatin 20 mg tablet ($$)
Mevacor 40 mg tablet ($$$)
  Generic: lovastatin 40 mg tablet ($$$)

Combination Products That Contain This Drug
Advicor extended-release tablet ($) to ($$)

DOSING AND FOOD

Doses are taken once a day with the evening meal.
It is best to take this drug with food to improve absorption. Do not drink
  grapefruit juice while taking this drug.
Adults: Up to 80 mg per day.
Forgotten doses: If you are scheduled to take the next dose within a few
  hours, do not take the forgotten dose. Otherwise take the forgotten dose
  as soon as you remember.

ALCOHOL, DRUG, HERB, AND SUPPLEMENT INTERACTIONS

Alcohol should not be used while taking this drug.

† See page 52.   * See page 53.

Red yeast rice, banned from sale in the U.S. since 2001, contains a nutrient similar to this class of drugs and may cause toxicity if used while taking this drug.

Taking this drug with any of the ones listed below may change the effect of either drug with the possibility of causing toxicity or decreasing effectiveness: cholestyramine, cimetidine, colestipol, isradipine, itraconazole, warfarin

Severe reactions are possible when this drug is taken with those listed below: clofibrate, cyclosporine, erythromycin, fenofibrate, gemfibrozil, immunosuppressants†, niacin

Increased side effects are possible when this drug is taken with those listed below: acetaminophen, amiodarone, anabolic steroids†, androgens†, antibiotics†, antithyroid drugs†, carbamazepine, carmustine, chloroquine, dantrolene, daunorubicin, disulfiram, divalproex, etetinate, gold salts†, hydroxychloroquine, isoniazid, mercaptopurine, methotrexate, naltrexone, oral contraceptives, phenothiazines†, phenytoin, plicamycin, valproic acid

ALLERGIC REACTIONS AND SIDE EFFECTS

If you are allergic to any HMG-CoA reductase inhibitors (statins)†, you may also be allergic to this drug. You should tell your doctor about all your allergies and any unexplained symptoms you may have while taking this drug.

This drug promotes the effect of sunlight on the body and may cause severe sunburn and increased sensitivity of the eyes.

MORE COMMON SIDE EFFECTS: Muscle cramps*

LESS COMMON SIDE EFFECTS: Blurry vision, chest pain*, constipation, diarrhea, dizziness, fever*, gas, hair loss, headache, heartburn, itching, nausea, numbness, skin rash, sleeping difficulty*, stomach pain*, tingling, tiredness*, vomiting, weakness*

RARE SIDE EFFECTS: Sexual dysfunction

PRECAUTIONS

People with liver disease may not be able to take this drug.

Liver function should be tested every 1 to 6 months while taking this drug.

Be careful driving or handling equipment while taking this drug because it may cause blurry vision and dizziness.

Do not break, crush, or chew the extended-release products.

PREGNANCY AND BREAST-FEEDING

This drug may cause birth defects and should not be used during pregnancy. Breast-feeding while taking this drug is not recommended.

HELPFUL COMMENTS

You need to continue with a low-cholesterol diet even after this drug is started.

It takes about 4 to 6 weeks for the effects of this drug to be noticed.

Wear sunglasses and sunscreen when outside to protect the eyes and skin from irritation and sunburn.

LOXAPINE SUCCINATE

Available for over 20 years

COMMONLY USED TO TREAT

Mental illness, also known as psychosis
Nervous disorders
Psychosis

DRUG CATEGORY

antipsychotic
Class: dibenzoxazepine

PRODUCTS

Brand-Name Products with Generic Alternatives

Loxitane 5 mg capsule ($)
  Generic: loxapine succinate 5 mg capsule (¢¢¢¢¢)
Loxitane 10 mg capsule ($)
  Generic: loxapine succinate 10 mg capsule (¢¢¢¢¢)
Loxitane 25 mg capsule ($$)
  Generic: loxapine succinate 25 mg capsule ($$)
Loxitane 50 mg capsule ($$$)
  Generic: loxapine succinate 50 mg capsule ($$)

DOSING AND FOOD

Doses are taken 2 to 4 times a day.
This drug may be taken with or without food.

Adults: Up to 100 mg per day in divided doses.

Forgotten doses: If you are scheduled to take the next dose within a few hours, do not take the forgotten dose. Otherwise take the forgotten dose as soon as you remember.

ALCOHOL, DRUG, HERB, AND SUPPLEMENT INTERACTIONS

Alcohol should not be used while taking this drug.

Several OTC drugs used for appetite control, asthma, colds, cough, hay fever, pain, or sinus problems may seriously increase the side effects of this drug. Check with your pharmacist when selecting OTC products.

Taking this drug with any of the ones listed below may change the effect of either drug with the possibility of causing toxicity or decreasing effectiveness: analgesics, anesthetics, antacids, antiarrhythmics†, antidiarrheals, anxiolytics†, barbiturates†, beta blockers†, bromocriptine, dopamine, levodopa, narcotics†, nitrates†, sympathomimetics†

Severe reactions are possible when this drug is taken with those listed below: anticholinergics†, antidepressants†, antidyskinetics†, antihistamines†, atropine, disopyramide, lithium, meperidine, monoamine oxidase inhibitors†, phenothiazines†, procainamide, quinidine

Increased side effects are possible when this drug is taken with those listed below: amoxapine, methyldopa, metoclopramide, metyrosine, pemoline, pimozide, promethazine, rauwolfia alkaloids†, trimeprazine

ALLERGIC REACTIONS AND SIDE EFFECTS

If you are allergic to amoxapine, you may also be allergic to this drug. You should tell your doctor about all your allergies and any unexplained symptoms you may have while taking this drug.

This drug promotes the effect of sunlight on the body and may cause severe sunburn and increased sensitivity of the eyes.

MORE COMMON SIDE EFFECTS: Blurry vision, chewing motion*, confusion, dizziness, drowsiness, dry mouth, expressionless face*, fainting, lightheadedness, lip smacking*, poor balance*, puffy cheeks*, restlessness*, shakiness*, shuffling walk*, spastic movements*, speaking difficulty*, stiffness*, swallowing difficulty*, tongue movement*, trembling*

LESS COMMON SIDE EFFECTS: Breast enlargement, breast-milk secretion, constipation*, eye stillness*, headache, menstrual dysfunction, muscle spasms*, nausea, sexual dysfunction, skin rash*, sleep disorders, urinary difficulty*, vomiting, weight gain

RARE SIDE EFFECTS: Bleeding*, blood pressure changes*, breathing difficulty*, bruising*, eyelid spasms*, facial movements*, fever*, irregular heartbeat*, jerking*, pale skin*, poor bladder control*, seizures*, sore throat*, sweating*, tiredness*, weakness*, yellow eyes or skin*

PRECAUTIONS

If you have a history of urinary problems, enlarged prostate, glaucoma, or Parkinson's disease, this drug may make those conditions worse.

People with a history of seizures are at greater risk of developing a seizure while taking this drug.

The oral solution product may be mixed with orange or grapefruit juice to make it easier to swallow.

Be careful driving or handling equipment while taking this drug because the drug may cause dizziness and drowsiness.

This drug may cause false results from several diagnostic tests including pregnancy tests.

Side effects may first appear months or years after the start of treatment.

This drug may cause dry mouth, which is associated with a greater risk of cavities. Your dentist may recommend that you clean your teeth and mouth differently to avoid infection.

PREGNANCY AND BREAST-FEEDING

Safety during pregnancy has not been established although the drug is known to harm animal fetuses.

Breast-feeding while taking this drug is not recommended.

HELPFUL COMMENTS

If you need to take an antacid or a drug for diarrhea, take it either 2 hours before or after taking this drug.

Sucking on hard sugarless candy or chewing sugarless gum may help relieve dry mouth caused by this drug.

Avoid quick movements to minimize dizziness. Dangling your legs over the side of the bed for a few minutes may help reduce dizziness when first waking up.

Eye irritation caused by the sun may be reduced by wearing sunglasses when outside.

MEBENDAZOLE

Available for over 20 years

COMMONLY USED TO TREAT

Hookworm infection
Pinworm infection
Trichinosis

---

† See page 52. * See page 53.

DRUG CATEGORY

antihelminic
Class: benzimidazole

PRODUCTS

Brand-Name Products with Generic Alternatives
Vermox 100 mg chewable tablet ($$$$)
  Generic: mebendazole 100 mg chewable tablet (¢)

DOSING AND FOOD

Doses are taken 1 to 3 times a day.
Taking this drug with fatty foods will help increase absorption of this drug.
  Be careful not to eat too much fatty food.
Adults and children over age 2: Up to 1,500 mg per day in divided doses.
Forgotten doses: If you are scheduled to take the next dose within a few
  hours, do not take the forgotten dose. Otherwise take the forgotten dose
  as soon as you remember.

ALCOHOL, DRUG, HERB, AND SUPPLEMENT INTERACTIONS

Alcohol may increase some of the side effects from this drug, depending
  on the amount consumed. Ask your doctor about the risks caused by
  drinking alcohol with your condition.

Taking this drug with any of the ones listed below may change the effect of
either drug with the possibility of causing toxicity or decreasing effectiveness:
anticonvulsants†, carbamazepine, cimetidine, phenytoin

ALLERGIC REACTIONS AND SIDE EFFECTS

You should tell your doctor about all your allergies and any unexplained
  symptoms you may have while taking this drug.
LESS COMMON SIDE EFFECTS: Abdominal pain, diarrhea, stomach upset,
  vomiting
RARE SIDE EFFECTS: Dizziness, fever*, hair loss, headache, itching*, skin
  rash*, sore throat*, tiredness*, weakness*

PRECAUTIONS

People with Crohn's disease, liver disease, or ulcerative colitis are at greater
  risk of developing side effects while taking this drug.
Make sure your doctor or pharmacist has advised you of all the actions that
  should be taken to prevent the spread or recurrence of infections treated

with this drug. Shaking clothes or bedding may release eggs into the air, promoting the spread of airborne infection.

PREGNANCY AND BREAST-FEEDING

Safety during pregnancy has not been established although the drug is known to harm animal fetuses.

It is not known if this drug passes into breast milk. Talk to your doctor about the risks associated with breast-feeding while taking this drug.

HELPFUL COMMENTS

Tablets may be broken, chewed, crushed, mixed with food, or swallowed whole:

Contact your doctor if your symptoms do not improve after a couple of days.

Do not stop treatment early if you start to feel better. It takes the full prescription for this drug to work completely.

Pinworm infections may easily return. Washing all bedding, linens, and clothes may reduce the risk of recurrence.

Iron supplements may be needed in people with hookworm or whipworm infections.

MECLIZINE HYDROCHLORIDE

Available for over 20 years

COMMONLY USED TO TREAT

Dizziness
Motion sickness
Nausea
Vertigo
Vomiting

DRUG CATEGORY

antiemetic
antivertigo
Class: piperazine-derivative antihistamine

PRODUCTS

Brand-Name Products with Generic Alternatives
Antivert 12.5 mg tablet (¢¢¢)
  Generic: meclizine hydrochloride 12.5 mg tablet (¢)

---

† See page 52.   * See page 53.

Antivert 25 mg tablet (¢¢¢¢)
  Generic: meclizine hydrochloride 25 mg tablet (¢)
Antivert 50 mg tablet ($)
  Generic: meclizine hydrochloride 50 mg tablet (n/a)
Antivert 25 mg chewable tablet (n/a)
  Generic: meclizine hydrochloride 25 mg chewable tablet (n/a)

DOSING AND FOOD

Doses are taken only when needed.
This drug may be taken with or without food.
Adults and children over age 12: Up to 100 mg per day in divided doses.

ALCOHOL, DRUG, HERB, AND SUPPLEMENT INTERACTIONS

Alcohol should not be used while taking this drug.
Many OTC drugs used for appetite control, asthma, colds, cough, hay
fever, pain, or sinus problems affect the central nervous system and may
increase the risk of side effects from this drug. Check with your pharmacist for products to avoid.

**Taking this drug with any of the ones listed below may change the effect of
either drug with the possibility of causing toxicity or decreasing effectiveness:**
anesthetics, anticholinergics†, antihistamines†, anxiolytics†, barbiturates†,
narcotics†, tricyclic antidepressants†

Increased side effects are possible when this drug is taken with those listed below:
aspirin, aminoglycosides†, cisplatin, loop diuretics†, salicylates†, vancomycin

ALLERGIC REACTIONS AND SIDE EFFECTS

If you are allergic to cyclizine, you may also be allergic to this drug. You
should tell your doctor about all your allergies and any unexplained
symptoms you may have while taking this drug.
MORE COMMON SIDE EFFECTS: Drowsiness
LESS COMMON SIDE EFFECTS: Blurry vision, constipation, diarrhea, dizziness, dry mouth, excitability, hallucinations, headache, irregular heartbeat*, loss of appetite*, nausea, nervousness*, restlessness, skin rash,
ringing in the ears, sleep disorders, stomachache, urinary difficulty*,
vomiting

PRECAUTIONS

Be careful driving or handling equipment while taking this drug because
the drug may cause drowsiness.

Stopping this drug suddenly after taking it regularly for a long time may cause the original condition to return with greater severity. If you wish to stop taking this drug, ask your doctor for specific instructions.

This drug may interfere with skin tests, such as allergy tests, and should be stopped about 4 days prior to the test.

If you have an enlarged prostate, glaucoma, intestinal problems, or urinary problems, this drug may make those conditions worse.

Tell your doctor if you take large doses of aspirin on a regular basis since this drug may mask the symptoms of aspirin toxicity.

This drug may cause dry mouth, which is associated with a greater risk of cavities. Your dentist may recommend that you clean your teeth and mouth differently to avoid infection.

PREGNANCY AND BREAST-FEEDING

Safety during pregnancy has not been established although there was no evidence of harm during studies in animals.

This drug passes into breast milk, but does not appear to harm the baby. Talk to your doctor about the risks associated with breast-feeding while taking this drug.

HELPFUL COMMENTS

Tablets may be dissolved in the mouth for a more rapid effect.

Sucking on hard sugarless candy or chewing sugarless gum may help relieve dry mouth caused by this drug.

MECLOFENAMATE SODIUM

Available for over 20 years

COMMONLY USED TO TREAT

Arthritis
Menstrual pain
Mild to moderate pain

DRUG CATEGORY

analgesic
antiarthritic
antidysmenorrheal
Class: nonsteroidal antiinflammatory

---

† See page 52. * See page 53.

PRODUCTS

Brand-Name Products with Generic Alternatives
Meclomen 50 mg capsule (n/a)
  Generic: meclofenamate sodium 50 mg capsule ($$)
Meclomen 100 mg capsule (n/a)
  Generic: meclofenamate sodium 100 mg capsule ($$$)

DOSING AND FOOD

Doses are taken 4 to 6 times a day.
It is best to take this drug with food.
Adults and teens over age 14: Up to 400 mg per day in divided doses.
Forgotten doses: If you are scheduled to take the next dose within a few
   hours, do not take the forgotten dose. Otherwise take the forgotten dose
   as soon as you remember.

ALCOHOL, DRUG, HERB, AND SUPPLEMENT INTERACTIONS

Alcohol may increase the risk of serious side effects from this drug. Ask your
   doctor about the risks caused by drinking alcohol with your condition.
Do not use dong quai, feverfew, garlic, ginger, horse chestnut, red clover,
   or St. John's wort while taking this drug since they may increase the risk
   of serious side effects.

**Taking this drug with any of the ones listed below may change the effect of
either drug with the possibility of causing toxicity or decreasing effectiveness:**
ACE inhibitors†, acetaminophen, antihypertensives†, digoxin, diuretics†,
furosemide, hydrochlorothiazide, nifedipine, lithium, methotrexate,
phenytoin, probenecid, sulfonylureas†, sulindac, verapamil

Severe reactions are possible when this drug is taken with those listed below:
antibiotics†, anticoagulants†, aspirin, cefamandole, cefoperazone, cefotetan, corticosteroids†, cyclosporine, dipyridamole, gold salts†, heparin,
mezlocillin, nonsteroidal antiinflammatories†, penicillamine, piperacillin,
plicamycin, salicylates†, sulfinpyrazone, ticarcillin

ALLERGIC REACTIONS AND SIDE EFFECTS

If you are allergic to aspirin, zomepirac, salicylates†, or other nonsteroidal
   antiinflammatories†, you may also be allergic to this drug. You should
   tell your doctor about all your allergies and any unexplained symptoms
   you may have while taking this drug.
This drug promotes the effect of sunlight on the body and may cause
   severe sunburn and increased sensitivity of the eyes.

MORE COMMON SIDE EFFECTS: Abdominal pain, diarrhea, dizziness, drowsiness, headache, heartburn*, indigestion*, itching*, nausea*, ringing in ears*, skin rash*, swelling*, weight gain*

LESS COMMON SIDE EFFECTS: Bruising*, constipation, gas, high blood pressure*, sweating, vomiting

RARE SIDE EFFECTS: Back pain*, black stools*, bloody urine*, bloody vomit, blue fingernails*, blue lips*, breathing difficulty*, chest pain*, chest tightness*, chills*, confusion*, cough*, dark urine*, fainting*, fever*, hallucinations*, hearing loss*, hives*, hoarseness*, lip sores*, loss of appetite*, low blood pressure*, mood swings*, mouth sores*, muscle cramps*, nosebleeds*, pain*, pale skin*, pale stools*, puffy eyes*, rectal bleeding*, restlessness*, runny nose*, seizures*, shortness of breath*, sore throat*, stiff neck*, swollen glands*, swollen tongue*, thirst*, tiredness*, urinary changes*, vision changes*, weakness*, wheezing*, yellow eyes or skin*

PRECAUTIONS

This drug may cause serious stomach problems and possibly ulcers. Be careful to take this drug as directed with food, and let your doctor know if you develop any stomach-related symptoms.

Be careful driving or handling equipment while taking this drug because the drug may cause dizziness and drowsiness.

Do not lie down for about 30 minutes after taking this drug to help reduce the risk of heartburn and throat irritation.

If you use tobacco or have a history of alcohol abuse, stomach problems, intestinal problems, hemorrhoids, diabetes mellitus, severe fluid retention, or systemic lupus erythematosus, there is an increased risk that you will develop side effects while taking this drug.

PREGNANCY AND BREAST-FEEDING

Safety during pregnancy has not been established although the drug is known to harm animal fetuses.

Breast-feeding while taking this drug is not recommended.

HELPFUL COMMENTS

Avoid quick movements to minimize dizziness.

Several nonsteroidal antiinflammatories† are available without a prescription in lower, nonprescription strengths, including ibuprofen, ketoprofen, and naproxen.

---

†See page 52.   *See page 53.

MEDROXYPROGESTERONE ACETATE

Available for over 20 years

COMMONLY USED TO TREAT

Abnormal uterine bleeding
Menstrual dysfunction

DRUG CATEGORY

antineoplastic
progestational drug
Class: progestin

PRODUCTS

Brand-Name Products with Generic Alternatives
Provera 2.5 mg tablet (¢¢¢)
  Generic: medroxyprogesterone acetate 2.5 mg tablet (¢¢)
Provera 5 mg tablet (¢¢¢¢¢)
  Generic: medroxyprogesterone acetate 5 mg tablet (¢¢)
Provera 10 mg tablet ($)
  Generic: medroxyprogesterone acetate 10 mg tablet (¢¢)
Combination Products That Contain This Drug
PremPro tablet ($)
PremPhase tablet ($)

DOSING AND FOOD

Doses are taken once a day.
This drug may be taken with or without food.
Adults: Up to 10 mg per day.
Forgotten doses: If you are scheduled to take the next dose within a few
hours, do not take the forgotten dose. Otherwise take the forgotten dose
as soon as you remember.

ALCOHOL, DRUG, HERB, AND SUPPLEMENT INTERACTIONS

Alcohol may increase some of the side effects from this drug, depending
on the amount consumed. Ask your doctor about the risks caused by
drinking alcohol with your condition.

Taking this drug with any of the ones listed below may change the effect of
either drug with the possibility of causing toxicity or decreasing effectiveness:
aminoglutethimide, bromocriptine, carbamazepine, phenobarbital, phenytoin, rifabutin, rifampin

ALLERGIC REACTIONS AND SIDE EFFECTS

If you are allergic to any progestins†, you may also be allergic to this drug. You should tell your doctor about all your allergies and any unexplained symptoms you may have while taking this drug.

MORE COMMON SIDE EFFECTS: Abdominal pain, bloating, blood pressure increase, depression*, dizziness, dry mouth*, frequent urination*, loss of appetite*, headache*, mood swings, nervousness, swelling, thirst*, vaginal bleeding*, weight gain

LESS COMMON SIDE EFFECTS: Acne, breast-milk secretion*, breast pain, hair growth, hair loss, hot flashes, sexual dysfunction, skin rash*, skin spots, sleeping difficulty

RARE SIDE EFFECTS: Arm pain*, chest pain*, leg pain*, migraine*, numbness*, poor coordination*, shortness of breath*, speaking difficulty*, vision loss*

PRECAUTIONS

If you are diabetic, you may need a change in the dose of your antidiabetic drug† or insulin, since this drug may cause changes in blood sugar.

People with a history of blood clots, stroke, or varicose veins are at greater risk of developing blood clots when taking this drug.

If you have a history of breast cysts, depression, high cholesterol, and liver disease, this drug may make those conditions worse.

This drug may cause fluid retention, which may increase the risk of side effects in people with asthma, seizures, heart disease, kidney disease, or migraine headaches.

This drug may cause changes to your gums and mouth. Your dentist may recommend that you clean your teeth and mouth differently to avoid infection.

Be careful driving or handling equipment while taking this drug because it may cause dizziness.

PREGNANCY AND BREAST-FEEDING

This drug may cause birth defects and should not be used during pregnancy. Breast-feeding while taking this drug is not recommended.

HELPFUL COMMENTS

Sucking on hard sugarless candy or chewing sugarless gum may help relieve dry mouth caused by this drug.

---

†See page 52.   *See page 53.

This drug is usually taken in a pattern of 5 to 10 days on the drug followed by a 16- to 21-day drug-free period, unless prescribed as a contraceptive. Follow the prescription directions specific to your treatment.

This drug is not always given as a contraceptive. Birth control should be used unless this drug is specifically dosed as a contraceptive.

MEFENAMIC ACID

Available for over 20 years

COMMONLY USED TO TREAT

Menstrual pain
Mild to moderate pain

DRUG CATEGORY

analgesic
antidysmenorrheal
antiinflammatory
Class: nonsteroidal antiinflammatory

PRODUCTS

Brand-Name Products with No Generic Alternative
Ponstel 250 mg capsule ($)
No generics available.
No patents, no exclusivity.

DOSING AND FOOD

Doses are taken 4 times a day.
It is best to take this drug with food or an antacid.
Adults: Up to 1,000 mg per day in divided doses.
Forgotten doses: If you are scheduled to take the next dose within a few hours, do not take the forgotten dose. Otherwise take the forgotten dose as soon as you remember.

ALCOHOL, DRUG, HERB, AND SUPPLEMENT INTERACTIONS

Alcohol may increase the risk of serious side effects from this drug. Ask your doctor about the risks caused by drinking alcohol with your condition.

Do not use dong quai, feverfew, garlic, ginger, horse chestnut, red clover, or St. John's wort while taking this drug since they may increase the risk of serious side effects.

Taking this drug with any of the ones listed below may change the effect of either drug with the possibility of causing toxicity or decreasing effectiveness: ACE inhibitors†, acetaminophen, antihypertensives†, digoxin, diuretics†, furosemide, hydrochlorothiazide, nifedipine, lithium, methotrexate, phenytoin, probenecid, sulfonylureas†, sulindac, verapamil

Severe reactions are possible when this drug is taken with those listed below: antibiotics†, anticoagulants†, aspirin, cefamandole, cefoperazone, cefotetan, corticosteroids†, cyclosporine, dipyridamole, gold salts†, heparin, mezlocillin, nonsteroidal antiinflammatories†, penicillamine, piperacillin, plicamycin, salicylates†, sulfinpyrazone, ticarcillin

ALLERGIC REACTIONS AND SIDE EFFECTS

If you are allergic to aspirin, zomepirac, salicylates†, or other nonsteroidal antiinflammatories†, you may also be allergic to this drug. You should tell your doctor about all your allergies and any unexplained symptoms you may have while taking this drug.

This drug promotes the effect of sunlight on the body and may cause severe sunburn and increased sensitivity of the eyes.

MORE COMMON SIDE EFFECTS: Abdominal pain, diarrhea, dizziness, drowsiness, headache, heartburn*, indigestion*, itching*, mouth sores*, nausea*, skin rash*, swelling*, weight gain*

LESS COMMON SIDE EFFECTS: Bruising*, constipation, gas, high blood pressure*, sweating, vomiting

RARE SIDE EFFECTS: Back pain*, black stools*, bloody urine*, bloody vomit, blue fingernails*, blue lips*, breathing difficulty*, chest pain*, chest tightness*, chills*, confusion*, cough*, dark urine*, fainting*, fever*, hallucinations*, hearing loss*, hives*, hoarseness*, lip sores*, loss of appetite*, low blood pressure*, mood swings*, muscle cramps*, nosebleeds*, pain*, pale skin*, pale stools*, puffy eyes*, rectal bleeding*, restlessness*, ringing in ears*, runny nose*, seizures*, shortness of breath*, sore throat*, stiff neck*, swollen glands*, swollen tongue*, thirst*, tiredness*, urinary changes*, vision changes*, weakness*, wheezing*, yellow eyes or skin*

PRECAUTIONS

This drug may cause serious stomach problems and possibly ulcers. Be careful to take this drug as directed with food, and let your doctor know if you develop any stomach-related symptoms.

Be careful driving or handling equipment while taking this drug because the drug may cause dizziness and drowsiness.

†*See page 52.*   *See page 53.*

Do not lie down for about 30 minutes after taking this drug to help reduce the risk of heartburn and throat irritation.

Taking this drug for longer than 7 days increases the risk of developing serious side effects.

If you use tobacco or have a history of alcohol abuse, stomach problems, intestinal problems, hemorrhoids, diabetes mellitus, severe fluid retention, or systemic lupus erythematosus, there is an increased risk that you will develop side effects while taking this drug.

PREGNANCY AND BREAST-FEEDING

Safety during pregnancy has not been established although the drug is known to harm animal fetuses.

Breast-feeding while taking this drug is not recommended.

HELPFUL COMMENTS

Avoid quick movements to minimize dizziness.

Several nonsteroidal antiinflammatories† are available without a prescription in lower, nonprescription strengths, including ibuprofen, ketoprofen, and naproxen.

MEGESTROL ACETATE

Available for over 20 years

COMMONLY USED TO TREAT

Breast cancer
Endometrial cancer
Weight loss in people with AIDS and cancer

DRUG CATEGORY

anticachectic
antineoplastic
Class: progestin

PRODUCTS

Brand-Name Products with Generic Alternatives
Megace 20 mg tablet (¢¢¢¢)
  Generic: megestrol acetate 20 mg tablet (¢¢¢¢)
Megace 40 mg tablet ($)
  Generic: megestrol acetate 40 mg tablet (¢¢¢¢¢)

Megace 40 mg/ml oral suspension ($$$)
  Generic: megestrol acetate 40 mg/ml oral suspension ($$$)

DOSING AND FOOD

Doses are taken 1 to 4 times a day.
This drug may be taken with or without food.
Adults: Up to 800 mg per day in divided doses.
Forgotten doses: If you are scheduled to take the next dose within a few
  hours, do not take the forgotten dose. Otherwise take the forgotten dose
  as soon as you remember.

ALCOHOL, DRUG, HERB, AND SUPPLEMENT INTERACTIONS

Alcohol may increase some of the side effects from this drug, depending
  on the amount consumed. Ask your doctor about the risks caused by
  drinking alcohol with your condition.

**Taking this drug with any of the ones listed below may change the effect of
either drug with the possibility of causing toxicity or decreasing effectiveness:**
aminoglutethimide, bromocriptine, carbamazepine, phenobarbital, phenytoin, rifabutin, rifampin

ALLERGIC REACTIONS AND SIDE EFFECTS

If you are allergic to any progestins†, you may also be allergic to this drug.
  You should tell your doctor about all your allergies and any unexplained
  symptoms you may have while taking this drug.

LESS COMMON SIDE EFFECTS: Abdominal pain, acne, bloating, blood pressure increase, breast-milk secretion*, breast pain, dizziness, dry mouth*,
  frequent urination*, hair growth, hair loss, hot flashes, loss of appetite*,
  headache*, mood swings, nervousness, sexual dysfunction, skin rash*,
  skin spots, sleeping difficulty, swelling, thirst*, vaginal bleeding*, weight
  gain, wrist pain

RARE SIDE EFFECTS: Arm pain*, backache*, chest pain*, depression*, irritability*, leg pain*, migraine*, nausea*, numbness*, poor coordination*,
  round face*, shortness of breath*, speaking difficulty*, tiredness*, vision
  loss*, vomiting*, weakness*

PRECAUTIONS

If you are diabetic, you may need a change in the dose of your antidiabetic drug† or insulin, since this drug may cause changes in blood sugar.
This drug may cause fluid retention, which increases the risk of side effects

†See page 52.   *See page 53.

in people with asthma, seizures, heart disease, kidney disease, or migraine headaches.

People with a history of blood clots, stroke, or varicose veins are at greater risk of developing blood clots when taking this drug.

If you have a history of breast cysts, depression, high cholesterol, and liver disease, this drug may make those conditions worse.

This drug may cause changes to your gums and mouth. Your dentist may recommend that you clean your teeth and mouth differently to avoid infection.

PREGNANCY AND BREAST-FEEDING

This drug may cause birth defects and should not be used during pregnancy. Breast-feeding while taking this drug is not recommended.

HELPFUL COMMENTS

This drug is not always given as a contraceptive. Birth control should be used unless this drug is specifically dosed as a contraceptive.

Oral suspension should be shaken well before each dose.

Sucking on hard sugarless candy or chewing sugarless gum may help relieve dry mouth caused by this drug.

Do not measure doses of the oral suspension with anything but a measuring cup intended for use with prescription drugs. Slight inaccuracy from other measuring spoons may result in over- or under-dosing.

MELOXICAM

Available since April 2000

COMMONLY USED TO TREAT

Arthritis

DRUG CATEGORY

analgesic
antiinflammatory
Class: nonsteroidal antiinflammatory

PRODUCTS

Brand-Name Products with No Generic Alternative
Mobic 7.5 mg tablet ($$)

Mobic 15 mg tablet ($$)
No generics available.
Exclusivity until 2005.

DOSING AND FOOD

Doses are taken once a day.

It is best to take this drug on an empty stomach, but taking this drug with a little food may avoid the stomach upset that some people suffer.

Adults: Up to 15 mg per day.

Forgotten doses: If you are scheduled to take the next dose within a few hours, do not take the forgotten dose. Otherwise take the forgotten dose as soon as you remember.

ALCOHOL, DRUG, HERB, AND SUPPLEMENT INTERACTIONS

Alcohol may increase the risk of serious side effects from this drug. Ask your doctor about the risks caused by drinking alcohol with your condition.

Do not use dong quai, feverfew, garlic, ginger, horse chestnut, red clover, or St. John's wort while taking this drug since they may increase the risk of serious side effects.

Taking this drug with any of the ones listed below may change the effect of either drug with the possibility of causing toxicity or decreasing effectiveness:
ACE inhibitors†, acetaminophen, antihypertensives†, digoxin, diuretics†, furosemide, hydrochlorothiazide, nifedipine, lithium, methotrexate, probenecid, sulfonylureas†, sulindac, verapamil

Severe reactions are possible when this drug is taken with those listed below:
antibiotics†, anticoagulants†, aspirin, cefamandole, cefoperazone, cefotetan, corticosteroids†, cyclosporine, gold salts†, heparin, nonsteroidal antiinflammatories†, penicillamine, plicamycin, salicylates†, valproic acid, warfarin

ALLERGIC REACTIONS AND SIDE EFFECTS

If you are allergic to aspirin, zomepirac, salicylates†, or other nonsteroidal antiinflammatories†, you may also be allergic to this drug. You should tell your doctor about all your allergies and any unexplained symptoms you may have while taking this drug.

This drug promotes the effect of sunlight on the body and may cause severe sunburn and increased sensitivity of the eyes.

MORE COMMON SIDE EFFECTS: Diarrhea, headache, shortness of breath*, swelling*, weight gain*

---

†*See page 52.*   **See page 53.*

LESS COMMON SIDE EFFECTS: Abdominal pain, asthma, bruising*, constipation, dizziness, drowsiness, gas, heartburn*, high blood pressure*, indigestion*, itching*, mouth sores*, nausea*, skin rash*, sweating, vomiting

RARE SIDE EFFECTS: Back pain*, black stools*, bloody urine*, bloody vomit, blue fingernails*, blue lips*, breathing difficulty*, chest pain*, chest tightness*, chills*, confusion*, cough*, dark urine*, fainting*, fever*, hallucinations*, hearing loss*, hives*, hoarseness*, lip sores*, loss of appetite*, low blood pressure*, mood swings*, muscle cramps*, nosebleeds*, pain*, pale skin*, pale stools*, puffy eyes*, rectal bleeding*, restlessness*, ringing in ears*, runny nose*, seizures*, sore throat*, stiff neck*, swollen glands*, swollen tongue*, thirst*, tiredness*, urinary changes*, vision changes*, weakness*, wheezing*, yellow eyes or skin*

PRECAUTIONS

This drug may cause serious stomach problems and possibly ulcers. Be careful to take this drug as directed with food, and let your doctor know if you develop any stomach-related symptoms.

If you have a history of asthma, this drug may make that condition worse.

Do not lie down for about 30 minutes after taking this drug to help reduce the risk of heartburn and throat irritation.

If you use tobacco or have a history of alcohol abuse, stomach problems, intestinal problems, hemorrhoids, diabetes mellitus, severe fluid retention, or systemic lupus erythematosus, there is an increased risk that you will develop side effects while taking this drug.

PREGNANCY AND BREAST-FEEDING

Safety during pregnancy has not been established although the drug is known to harm animal fetuses.

Breast-feeding while taking this drug is not recommended.

HELPFUL COMMENTS

It may take several days before the effects of this drug are noticed.

Several nonsteroidal antiinflammatories† are available without a prescription in lower, nonprescription strengths, including ibuprofen, ketoprofen, and naproxen.

MEPERIDINE HYDROCHLORIDE

Available for over 20 years

COMMONLY USED TO TREAT

Pain

DRUG CATEGORY

analgesic
Class: narcotic analgesic/opioid

PRODUCTS

Brand-Name Products with Generic Alternatives
Demerol 50 mg tablet (¢¢¢¢¢)
  Generic: meperidine hydrochloride 50 mg tablet (¢¢¢¢)
Demerol 100 mg tablet ($$)
  Generic: meperidine hydrochloride 100 mg tablet ($)
Demerol 50 mg/5 ml oral syrup ($)
  Generic: meperidine hydrochloride 50 mg/5 ml oral syrup (¢¢¢¢¢)

DOSING AND FOOD

Doses are taken up to 8 times a day.
It is best to take this drug on an empty stomach, but taking this drug with
  a little food may avoid the stomach upset that some people suffer.
Adults: Up to 300 mg per day in divided doses.
Higher doses may be used in people who are under close medical supervision.
Lower doses are used in children.
Forgotten doses: If you are scheduled to take the next dose within a few
  hours, do not take the forgotten dose. Otherwise take the forgotten dose
  as soon as you remember.

ALCOHOL, DRUG, HERB, AND SUPPLEMENT INTERACTIONS

Alcohol should not be used while taking this drug.
Parsley may cause severe side effects when taken with this drug and should
  not be used.
Several OTC drugs used for asthma, colds, cough, hay fever, sleep aid, or
  sinus problems may seriously change the effects and side effects of this
  drug. Check with your pharmacist when selecting OTC products.

**Taking this drug with any of the ones listed below may change the effect of
either drug with the possibility of causing toxicity or decreasing effectiveness:**
naltrexone, rifampin

† See page 52.   * See page 53.

Severe reactions are possible when this drug is taken with those listed below: anesthetics, anticholinergics†, antihistamines†, barbiturates†, benzodiazepines†, cimetidine, isoniazid, monoamine oxidase inhibitors†, naloxone, narcotics†, phenothiazines†, sedative-hypnotics†, skeletal muscle relaxants†, tricyclic antidepressants†

ALLERGIC REACTIONS AND SIDE EFFECTS

If you are allergic to any narcotics† with the exception of morphine, you may also be allergic to this drug. You should tell your doctor about all your allergies and any unexplained symptoms you may have while taking this drug.

MORE COMMON SIDE EFFECTS: Constipation, dizziness*, drowsiness*, dry mouth, excitement*, fainting, lightheadedness, nausea, seizures*, slow breathing*, slow heartbeat*, sweating*, urinary changes*, vomiting

LESS COMMON SIDE EFFECTS: Blurry vision, breathing difficulty*, depression*, flushing*, hallucinations*, headache, hives*, irregular breathing*, irregular heartbeat*, itching*, loss of appetite, mood swings*, nervousness*, restlessness*, ringing in ears*, shortness of breath*, skin rash*, sleep disorders, spastic movements*, stomach cramps, swelling*, tiredness, trembling*, vision changes, weakness*, wheezing*

RARE SIDE EFFECTS: Body aches, clammy skin*, confusion*, diarrhea, fever, goosebumps, irritability, low blood pressure*, runny nose, shivering, small pupils*, sneezing, yawning

PRECAUTIONS

You need to wait 2 weeks after stopping a monoamine oxidase inhibitor† before starting this drug.

Be careful driving or handling equipment while taking this drug because it may cause dizziness and drowsiness.

If you have a history of head injury, brain disease, emphysema, asthma, lung disease, enlarged prostate, urinary disorders, gallbladder disease, or gallstones, you may not be able to take this drug.

People with colitis, heart disease, kidney disease, liver disease, and thyroid disease are at increased risk of developing side effects.

If you have a history of seizures, you may have an increased risk of developing a seizure while taking this drug.

This drug may cause withdrawal symptoms if stopped suddenly. If you wish to stop taking this drug, ask your doctor for specific instructions.

This drug is rarely used for more than a week because of the increased risk of developing severe side effects.

Because this drug has a high abuse potential, your prescription quantity may be limited.

This drug may cause dry mouth, which is associated with a greater risk of cavities. Your dentist may recommend that you clean your teeth and mouth differently to avoid infection.

PREGNANCY AND BREAST-FEEDING

Safety during pregnancy has not been established although the drug is known to harm animal fetuses.

Breast-feeding while taking this drug is not recommended.

HELPFUL COMMENTS

If being used for pain, this drug works best if taken before the pain gets too severe.

If the drug does not seem to be working properly, an increase in dose may not help. Talk to your doctor about other drugs and treatment options.

Sucking on hard sugarless candy or chewing sugarless gum may help relieve dry mouth caused by this drug.

Lie down for a while after taking a dose of this drug to help reduce the nausea.

Avoid quick movements to minimize dizziness. Dangling your legs over the side of the bed for a few minutes may help reduce dizziness when first waking up.

MEPHOBARBITAL

Available for over 20 years

COMMONLY USED TO TREAT

Seizures

DRUG CATEGORY

anticonvulsant
Class: barbiturate

PRODUCTS

Brand-Name Products with No Generic Alternative
Mebaral 32 mg tablet (¢¢)
Mebaral 50 mg tablet (¢¢¢)
Mebaral 100 mg tablet (¢¢¢)

---

† See page 52.   * See page 53.

No generics available.
No patents, no exclusivity.

DOSING AND FOOD

Doses are taken 3 to 4 times a day.

It is best to take this drug on an empty stomach with a full glass of water at least 1 hour before or 2 hours after meals.

Adults: Up to 600 mg per day in divided doses.

Children age 5 and older: Up to 256 mg per day in divided doses.

Children up to age 5: Up to 128 mg per day in divided doses.

Forgotten doses: If you are scheduled to take the next dose within a few hours, do not take the forgotten dose. Otherwise take the forgotten dose as soon as you remember.

ALCOHOL, DRUG, HERB, AND SUPPLEMENT INTERACTIONS

Alcohol should not be used while taking this drug.

Several OTC drugs used for appetite control, asthma, colds, cough, hay fever, pain, or sinus problems may seriously increase the side effects of this drug. Check with your pharmacist when selecting OTC products.

Taking this drug with any of the ones listed below may change the effect of either drug with the possibility of causing toxicity or decreasing effectiveness: anticoagulants†, carbamazepine, corticosteroids†, corticotropin, divalproex sodium, oral contraceptives, valproic acid

Increased side effects are possible when this drug is taken with those listed below: anesthetics, anticholinergics†, antihistamines†, anxiolytics†, barbiturates†, narcotics†, tricyclic antidepressants†

ALLERGIC REACTIONS AND SIDE EFFECTS

Allergic reactions are more likely to occur in people with a history of asthma or allergies to other drugs. You should tell your doctor about all your allergies and any unexplained symptoms you may have while taking this drug.

MORE COMMON SIDE EFFECTS: Clumsiness, dizziness, drowsiness, lightheadedness, unsteadiness

LESS COMMON SIDE EFFECTS: Anxiety, confusion*, constipation, depression*, excitement*, fainting, headache, irritability, nausea, nervousness, sleep disorders, vomiting

RARE SIDE EFFECTS: Bleeding lips*, bleeding*, bone pain*, bruising*, chest pain*, chest tightness*, fever*, hallucinations*, hives*, loss of appetite*, mouth sores*, muscle pain*, skin rash*, sore throat*, swelling*, tiredness*, weakness*, weight loss*, wheezing*, yellow eyes or skin*

PRECAUTIONS

Be careful driving or handling equipment while taking this drug because the drug may cause dizziness and drowsiness.

People over age 65 and children often get hyperactive while taking this drug.

If you have anemia, asthma, high blood sugar, hyperactivity, depression, thyroid problems, liver disease, kidney disease, or porphyria, this drug may make those conditions worse.

This drug may be habit forming when taken for a long time. It should be stopped slowly to avoid withdrawal symptoms. It may take 2 weeks for the body to adjust after the drug is stopped. If you wish to stop taking this drug, ask your doctor for specific instructions.

PREGNANCY AND BREAST-FEEDING

There is evidence that this drug may harm the fetus, but the drug may be necessary to the health of the mother.

This drug passes into breast milk, and may cause drowsiness, slow heartbeat, and breathing difficulty in the baby.

HELPFUL COMMENTS

Oral contraceptives may not work properly when taken with this drug. You need to use a barrier contraceptive, such as a condom, or other nonhormonal contraceptive to prevent pregnancy.

You may need to increase the fiber in your diet since this drug may cause constipation.

MEPROBAMATE

Available for over 20 years

COMMONLY USED TO TREAT

Anxiety
Tension

DRUG CATEGORY

anxiolytic
Class: carbamate

---

†See page 52.   * See page 53.

PRODUCTS

Brand-Name Products with Generic Alternatives
Equanil 200 mg tablet (n/a)
Miltown 200 mg tablet ($)
  Generic: meprobamate 200 mg tablet (¢¢¢)
Equanil 400 mg tablet (n/a)
Miltown 400 mg tablet ($)
  Generic: meprobamate 400 mg tablet (¢¢)
Miltown 600 mg tablet (n/a)
  Generic: meprobamate 600 mg tablet (n/a)
Other Generic Product Names
Tranmep
Combination Products That Contain This Drug
Equagesic tablet ($)
Micrainin tablet ($$)

DOSING AND FOOD

Doses are taken 3 to 4 times a day.
This drug may be taken with or without food. Do not eat raw oysters or
  other raw shellfish at any time while taking this drug.
Adults: Up to 2,400 mg per day in divided doses.
Children age 6 to 12: Up to 25 mg/kg per day in divided doses.
Forgotten doses: If more than 1 hour has passed since the forgotten dose,
  do not take the dose. Otherwise take the forgotten dose as soon as you
  remember.

ALCOHOL, DRUG, HERB, AND SUPPLEMENT INTERACTIONS

Alcohol should not be used while taking this drug.
Several OTC drugs used for appetite control, asthma, colds, cough, hay
  fever, pain, or sinus problems may seriously increase the effects of this
  drug. Check with your pharmacist when selecting OTC products.
**Taking this drug with any of the ones listed below may change the effect of
either drug with the possibility of causing toxicity or decreasing effectiveness:**
anesthetics, anticholinergics†, antihistamines†, anxiolytics†, barbiturates†,
  narcotics†, tricyclic antidepressants†

ALLERGIC REACTIONS AND SIDE EFFECTS

If you are allergic to carbromal, carisoprodol, mebutamate, or tybamate,
  you may also be allergic to this drug. You should tell your doctor about

all your allergies and any unexplained symptoms you may have while taking this drug.

MORE COMMON SIDE EFFECTS: Clumsiness, drowsiness, unsteadiness

LESS COMMON SIDE EFFECTS: Blurry vision, diarrhea, dizziness*, headache, hives*, itching*, lightheadedness*, nausea, skin rash*, tiredness, vision changes, vomiting, weakness*

RARE SIDE EFFECTS: Bleeding*, breathing difficulty*, bruising*, confusion*, excitement*, fever*, irregular heartbeat*, shortness of breath*, slurry speech*, sore throat*, staggering*, wheezing*

PRECAUTIONS

This drug may cause serious withdrawal symptoms if stopped suddenly after long-term use. If you wish to stop taking this drug, ask your doctor for specific instructions.

Be careful driving or handling equipment while taking this drug because the drug may cause drowsiness.

This drug causes changes in your blood that put you at greater risk of getting an infection. Be careful not to cut yourself or get bruised. Tell your doctor if you develop signs of infection, such as fever or sore throat. Your dentist may recommend that you clean your teeth and mouth differently to avoid infection.

This drug may be habit forming when used for long periods of time. People with a history of alcohol or drug abuse are at greater risk of developing an addiction to this drug.

If you have porphyria, this drug may make that condition worse.

People with a history of seizures are at greater risk of developing a seizure while taking this drug.

PREGNANCY AND BREAST-FEEDING

There is evidence that this drug may harm the fetus, but the drug may be necessary to the health of the mother.

Breast-feeding while taking this drug is not recommended.

HELPFUL COMMENTS

Several people have fallen out of bed or find they fall more easily after taking this drug.

Sucking on hard sugarless candy or chewing sugarless gum may help relieve dry mouth caused by this drug.

It usually takes less than 1 hour for the effects of this drug to be noticed.

† See page 52.   * See page 53.

MERCAPTOPURINE

Available for over 20 years

COMMONLY USED TO TREAT

Cancer

DRUG CATEGORY

antineoplastic
Class: antimetabolite

PRODUCTS

Brand-Name Products with No Generic Alternative
Purinethol 50 mg tablet ($$$)
No generics available.
No patents, no exclusivity.

DOSING AND FOOD

Doses are taken once a day.
This drug may be taken with or without food. Do not eat raw oysters or
other raw shellfish at any time while taking this drug.
Adults: Up to 5 mg/kg per day.
Children: Up to 2.5 mg/kg per day.
Forgotten doses: Do not take a forgotten dose. Just go back to your usual
schedule with the next dose. Let your doctor know you forgot the dose.

ALCOHOL, DRUG, HERB, AND SUPPLEMENT INTERACTIONS

Alcohol should not be used while taking this drug.

**Taking this drug with any of the ones listed below may change the effect of
either drug with the possibility of causing toxicity or decreasing effectiveness:**
allopurinol, amphotericin B, antithyroid drugs†, azathioprine, chloram-
phenicol, colchicine, corticosteroids†, co-trimoxazole, cyclosporine, flucy-
tosine, ganciclovir, interferon, muromonab-CD3, plicamycin, probenecid,
sulfinpyrazone, warfarin, zidovudine

Increased side effects are possible when this drug is taken with those listed below:
acetaminophen, amiodarone, anabolic steroids†, androgens†, antibiotics†,
carbamazepine, chloroquine, dantrolene, disulfiram, divalproex, estro-
gens†, etretinate, gold salts†, hydroxychloroquine, methyldopa, naltrex-
one, oral contraceptives, phenothiazines†, phenytoin, valproic acid

ALLERGIC REACTIONS AND SIDE EFFECTS

You should tell your doctor about all your allergies and any unexplained symptoms you may have while taking this drug.

MORE COMMON SIDE EFFECTS: Diarrhea*, loss of appetite*, nausea*, tiredness*, vomiting*, weakness*, yellow eyes or skin*

LESS COMMON SIDE EFFECTS: Back pain*, black stools*, bleeding*, bloody urine*, bruising*, chills*, cough*, fever*, hoarseness*, joint pain*, skin irritation*, swelling*, urinary difficulty*

RARE SIDE EFFECTS: Mouth sores*

PRECAUTIONS

If you vomit shortly after taking a dose, call your doctor to find out if the dose should be repeated.

You should drink a lot of water while taking this drug to reduce the risk of developing gout or kidney stones.

Avoid contact with anyone who has the chickenpox, measles, or other communicable disease since it may be easier to catch the infection while taking this drug.

Exposure to skin tests, immunizations, and people who have received immunizations may put you at a greater risk of developing the disease when you are taking this drug.

This drug causes changes in your blood that put you at greater risk of getting an infection. Be careful not to cut yourself or get bruised. Tell your doctor if you develop signs of infection, such as fever or sore throat. Your dentist may recommend that you clean your teeth and mouth differently to avoid infection.

PREGNANCY AND BREAST-FEEDING

There is evidence that this drug may harm the fetus, but the drug may be necessary to the health of the mother.

Breast-feeding while taking this drug is not recommended.

HELPFUL COMMENTS

This drug is also called by the generic name 6-MP or 6-mercaptopurine.

It may take 2 to 4 weeks before the effects of this drug are noticed.

It is very important to continue taking this drug as ordered by the doctor even if the side effects make you feel ill.

† See page 52.   * See page 53.

MESALAMINE

Available for over 20 years

COMMONLY USED TO TREAT

Inflammatory bowel disease (IBD)
Ulcerative colitis

DRUG CATEGORY

antiinflammatory
Class: salicylate

PRODUCTS

Brand-Name Products with No Generic Alternative
Asacol 400 mg delayed-release tablet (¢¢¢¢¢)
Pentasa 250 mg extended-release capsule (¢¢¢¢)
Rowasa 4 gm/60 ml rectal enema ($)
Canasa 500 mg rectal suppository ($$$)
No generics available.
No patents, no exclusivity on Canasa and Pentasa. Patents on Asacol and
   Rowasa begin to expire in 2004.

DOSING AND FOOD

Delayed-release tablets are taken 3 times a day. Extended-release capsules
   are taken 4 times a day. Rectal enemas are used once a day. Rectal sup-
   positories are used twice a day.
This drug may be taken with or without food with a full glass of water.
Adults: Up to 2,400 mg delayed-release product per day in divided doses.
Adults: Up to 2,000 mg extended-release product per day in divided doses.
Forgotten doses: If you are scheduled to take the next dose within a few
   hours, do not take the forgotten dose. Otherwise take the forgotten dose
   as soon as you remember.

ALCOHOL, DRUG, HERB, AND SUPPLEMENT INTERACTIONS

Alcohol may increase some of the side effects from this drug, depending
   on the amount consumed. Ask your doctor about the risks caused by
   drinking alcohol with your condition.

ALLERGIC REACTIONS AND SIDE EFFECTS

If you are allergic to olsalazine, sulfasalazine, aspirin, or any other salicylate†, you may also be allergic to this drug. You should tell your doctor about all your allergies and any unexplained symptoms you may have while taking this drug.

MORE COMMON SIDE EFFECTS: Abdominal pain*, diarrhea*, dizziness*, headache*, runny nose, sneezing

LESS COMMON SIDE EFFECTS: Acne, back pain, bloody diarrhea*, fever*, gas, hair loss, indigestion, itching*, joint pain, loss of appetite, skin rash*

RARE SIDE EFFECTS: Anxiety*, back pain*, bloating*, chest pain*, chills*, confusion*, drowsiness*, fast heartbeat*, hearing loss*, lightheadedness*, nausea*, pale skin*, panting*, ringing in ears*, shortness of breath*, swelling*, tiredness*, vomiting*, weakness*, yellow eyes or skin*

PRECAUTIONS

Do not open, crush, break, or chew the extended-release or delayed-release products.

If you have kidney disease, this drug may make that condition worse.

The rectal suspension product contains potassium metabisulfite, which may trigger an allergic reaction in people sensitive to sulfites.

Rectal suppositories should be retained for 1 to 3 hours.

An empty shell from the tablet and capsules products may pass in your stool without dissolving, which is not a concern.

PREGNANCY AND BREAST-FEEDING

Safety during pregnancy has not been established although there was no evidence of harm during studies in animals.

This drug passes into breast milk, but does not appear to harm the baby. Talk to your doctor about the risks associated with breast-feeding while taking this drug.

HELPFUL COMMENTS

This drug is also called by the generic name 5-aminosalicylic acid.

The effects of this drug may be noticed in 3 to 21 days. Do not stop treatment early if you start to feel better. The full cycle of therapy is typically 3 to 6 months.

If using a suppository, remove the foil and run under cold water before inserting.

---

† See page 52.   * See page 53.

MESORIDAZINE BESYLATE

Available for over 20 years

COMMONLY USED TO TREAT

Mental illness, also known as psychosis

DRUG CATEGORY

antipsychotic
Class: phenothiazine: piperidine derivative

PRODUCTS

Brand-Name Products with No Generic Alternative
Serentil 10 mg tablet (¢¢¢¢¢)
Serentil 25 mg tablet ($)
Serentil 50 mg tablet (n/a)
Serentil 100 mg tablet ($)
Serentil 25 mg/ml oral concentrate ($$$)
No generics available.
No patents, no exclusivity.

DOSING AND FOOD

Doses are taken 3 times a day.
Taking this drug with food or a full glass of milk or water may avoid the
    stomach upset that some people suffer.
Adults: Up to 400 mg per day in divided doses.
Lower doses are used in people over age 65.
Forgotten doses: If you are scheduled to take the next dose within a few
    hours, do not take the forgotten dose. Otherwise take the forgotten dose
    as soon as you remember.

ALCOHOL, DRUG, HERB, AND SUPPLEMENT INTERACTIONS

Alcohol should not be used while taking this drug.
Do not use caffeine while taking this drug since the drug effects may be
    decreased and severe reactions may occur.
Several OTC drugs used for appetite control, asthma, colds, cough, hay
    fever, pain, or sinus problems may seriously increase the effects and side
    effects of this drug. Check with your pharmacist when selecting OTC
    products.

Taking this drug with any of the ones listed below may change the effect of either drug with the possibility of causing toxicity or decreasing effectiveness: antihypertensives†, caffeine, beta blockers†, dopamine, levodopa, lithium, phenobarbital, phenytoin, warfarin

Severe reactions are possible when this drug is taken with those listed below: alcohol, amantadine, anesthetics, antiarrhythmics†, anticholinergics†, antidepressants†, antithyroid drugs†, anxiolytics†, astemizole, barbiturates†, bromocriptine, cisapride, deferoxamine, disopyramide, diuretics†, epinephrine, erythromycin, levobunolol, lithium, metipranolol, metrizamide, nabilone, narcotics†, nitrates†, pentamidine, probucol, procainamide, promethazine, propylthiouracil, quinidine, sympathomimetics†, tricyclic antidepressants†

Increased side effects are possible when this drug is taken with those listed below: antipsychotics†, metoclopramide, metyrosine, pemoline, pimozide, rauwolfia alkaloids†, trimeprazine

ALLERGIC REACTIONS AND SIDE EFFECTS

If you are allergic to any phenothiazines†, you may also be allergic to this drug. You should tell your doctor about all your allergies and any unexplained symptoms you may have while taking this drug.

This drug promotes the effect of sunlight on the body and may cause severe sunburn and increased sensitivity of the eyes.

MORE COMMON SIDE EFFECTS: Breathing difficulty*, chewing action*, congestion, constipation, decreased sweat*, dizziness, drowsiness, dry mouth, eye stare*, eyelid movement*, fainting*, lip smacking*, loss of balance*, muscle spasms*, muscle stiffness*, puffy cheeks*, restlessness*, shuffling walk*, tongue movements*, trembling*, twitching*, vision changes*

LESS COMMON SIDE EFFECTS: Breast-milk secretion, breast swelling, dark urine*, menstrual changes, rough tongue, sexual dysfunction, skin rash*, urinary difficulty*, watery mouth, weight gain

RARE SIDE EFFECTS: Abdominal pain*, aching muscles, agitation*, bleeding*, blood pressure change*, bruising*, chest pain*, chills*, clumsiness*, coma*, confusion*, diarrhea*, dreams*, drooling*, excitement*, fast heartbeat*, fever*, hair loss*, headaches*, increased sweating*, irregular heartbeat*, itching*, joint pain*, loss of bladder control*, mouth sores*, muscle stiffness*, nausea*, penile erection*, red hands*, seizures*, shivering*, skin discoloration*, sleep disorders*, sore throat*, speaking difficulty*, tiredness*, vomiting*, weakness*, yellow eyes or skin*

---

†*See page 52.*   *See page 53.*

PRECAUTIONS

If you have a history of enlarged prostate, glaucoma, ulcers, seizures, heart disease, urinary difficulty, or Parkinson's disease, this drug may make those conditions worse.

This drug may decrease the cough reflex, putting people with lung disease at greater risk of developing pneumonia.

Heavy smoking may cause this drug to be less effective.

This drug may cause false results from several diagnostic tests including pregnancy tests and should be stopped for at least 4 days before the test.

This drug should not be stopped suddenly, due to an increased risk of side effects. If you wish to stop taking this drug, ask your doctor for specific instructions.

Be careful driving or handling equipment while taking this drug because the drug may cause dizziness and drowsiness.

This drug may cause dry mouth, which is associated with a greater risk of cavities. Your dentist may recommend that you clean your teeth and mouth differently to avoid infection.

You are more likely to overheat when taking this drug and should avoid exercising in hot weather and using a sauna or hot tub.

This drug may make you more sensitive to cold temperatures.

PREGNANCY AND BREAST-FEEDING

Safety during pregnancy has not been established although the drug is known to harm animal fetuses.

Breast-feeding while taking this drug is not recommended.

HELPFUL COMMENTS

Sucking on hard sugarless candy or chewing sugarless gum may help relieve dry mouth caused by this drug.

METAPROTERENOL SULFATE

Available for over 20 years

COMMONLY USED TO TREAT

Asthma
Chronic bronchitis
Emphysema

DRUG CATEGORY

bronchodilator
Class: adrenergic

PRODUCTS

Brand-Name Products with No Generic Alternative
Alupent oral inhaler (¢¢¢¢¢)
Brand-Name Products with Generic Alternatives
Alupent 0.4% inhalation solution (n/a)
  Generic: metaproterenol sulfate 0.4% inhalation solution ($$)
Alupent 0.6% inhalation solution ($$$$)
  Generic: metaproterenol sulfate 0.6% inhalation solution ($$)
Products Only Available as Generics
metaproterenol sulfate 10 mg tablet (¢¢)
metaproterenol sulfate 20 mg tablet (¢¢¢)
metaproterenol sulfate 10 mg/5 ml oral syrup (¢¢)

DOSING AND FOOD

Oral doses are taken 3 to 4 times a day. Inhalation doses are taken up to 6
  times a day.
This drug may be taken with or without food.
Adults and children over age 9: Up to 80 mg per day in divided doses.
Children age 6 to 9: Up to 40 mg per day in divided doses.
Children under age 6: Up to 2.6 mg/kg per day in divided doses.
Forgotten doses: If more than 1 hour has passed since the forgotten dose,
  do not take the dose. Otherwise take the forgotten dose as soon as you
  remember.

ALCOHOL, DRUG, HERB, AND SUPPLEMENT INTERACTIONS

Alcohol may increase some of the side effects from this drug, depending
  on the amount consumed. Ask your doctor about the risks caused by
  drinking alcohol with your condition.
Many OTC drugs used for appetite control, asthma, colds, cough, hay
  fever, pain, or sinus problems affect the central nervous system and may
  change the severity of side effects when taken with this drug. Check with
  your pharmacist for products to avoid.

Taking this drug with any of the ones listed below may change the effect of
either drug with the possibility of causing toxicity or decreasing effectiveness:
beta blockers[†], monoamine oxidase inhibitors[†], thyroid hormones[†]

[†]*See page 52.*   [*]*See page 53.*

Severe reactions are possible when this drug is taken with those listed below: aminophylline, cocaine, digoxin, levodopa; quinidine, sympathomimetics†, theophylline, tricyclic antidepressants†

Increased side effects are possible when this drug is taken with those listed below: amphetamines†

ALLERGIC REACTIONS AND SIDE EFFECTS

If you are allergic to albuterol, ephedrine, epinephrine, isoproterenol, or terbutaline, you may also be allergic to this drug. You should tell your doctor about all your allergies and any unexplained symptoms you may have while taking this drug.

MORE COMMON SIDE EFFECTS: Dizziness, drowsiness, dry mouth, headache, heartburn, irregular heartbeat*, nausea*, nervousness, tremor, vomiting*, weakness*

LESS COMMON SIDE EFFECTS: Cough, rash*, shortness of breath*, sleeping difficulty*, sweating, throat irritation

RARE SIDE EFFECTS: Chest pain*, difficulty urinating*, hives*, mental problems*, muscle cramps*, muscle pain*, seizures*, tiredness*

PRECAUTIONS

People with cardiovascular disease, high blood pressure, hyperthyroidism, or diabetes may not be able to take this drug.

If you have a history of seizures, you may be at greater risk of developing a seizure while taking this drug.

You need to wait 2 weeks after stopping a monoamine oxidase inhibitor† before starting this drug.

If you are diabetic, you may need a change in the dose of your antidiabetic drug† or insulin, since this drug may cause changes in blood sugar.

This drug may cause dry mouth, which is associated with a greater risk of cavities. Your dentist may recommend that you clean your teeth and mouth differently to avoid infection.

PREGNANCY AND BREAST-FEEDING

Safety during pregnancy has not been established although the drug is known to harm animal fetuses.

It is not known if this drug passes into breast milk. Talk to your doctor about the risks associated with breast-feeding while taking this drug.

HELPFUL COMMENTS

The inhaler products begin to work in about 1 minute. Wait 1 to 2 minutes before taking a second dose.

If using more than one type of inhaler, you should wait at least 5 minutes between drugs.

Children may get excited and nervous when given this drug.

When used on a daily basis, this drug gradually becomes less effective.

Sucking on hard sugarless candy or chewing sugarless gum may help relieve dry mouth caused by this drug.

METAXALONE

Available for over 20 years

COMMONLY USED TO TREAT

Muscle stiffness and pain caused by injury

DRUG CATEGORY

skeletal muscle relaxant
Class: oxazolidinone derivative

PRODUCTS

Brand-Name Products with No Generic Alternative
Skelaxin 400 mg tablet (¢¢¢¢¢)
Skelaxin 800 mg tablet (n/a)
No generics available.
Patent expires in 2021.

DOSING AND FOOD

Doses are taken 3 to 4 times a day.

It is best to take this drug on an empty stomach, but taking this drug with a little food may avoid the stomach upset that some people suffer.

Adults: Up to 3,200 mg per day in divided doses.

This drug is not used in children under age 12.

Forgotten doses: If more than 1 hour has passed since the forgotten dose, do not take the dose. Just go back to your usual schedule with the next dose.

---

†*See page 52.* **See page 53.*

ALCOHOL, DRUG, HERB, AND SUPPLEMENT INTERACTIONS

Alcohol should not be used while taking this drug.

Several OTC drugs used for appetite control, asthma, colds, cough, hay fever, pain, or sinus problems may seriously increase the effects of this drug. Check with your pharmacist when selecting OTC products.

Increased side effects are possible when this drug is taken with those listed below: anesthetics, antihistamines†, anxiolytics†, barbiturates†, narcotics†, tricyclic antidepressants†

ALLERGIC REACTIONS AND SIDE EFFECTS

If you are allergic to meprobamate or other skeletal muscle relaxants†, you may also be allergic to this drug. You should tell your doctor about all your allergies and any unexplained symptoms you may have while taking this drug.

MORE COMMON SIDE EFFECTS: Blurry vision, dizziness, drowsiness, light-headedness, vision change

LESS COMMON SIDE EFFECTS: Abdominal pain, bloodshot eyes*, breathing difficulty*, burning eyes*, chest tightness*, clumsiness, confusion, constipation, depression*, diarrhea, excitement, fainting*, fever*, flushing, headache, heartburn, hiccups, hives*, irritability, itching*, nausea, nervousness, restlessness, shortness of breath*, skin rash*, sleep disorders, stomach cramps, stuffy nose*, swelling*, trembling, unsteadiness, vomiting, weakness*, wheezing*

RARE SIDE EFFECTS: Back pain*, black stools*, bleeding*, bloody urine*, bloody vomit*, bruising*, chills*, cough*, fever*, hoarseness*, irregular breathing*, mouth sores*, muscle pain*, puffy eyelids*, skin irritation*, sore throat*, swollen glands*, tiredness*, urinary difficulty*, yellow eyes or skin*

PRECAUTIONS

Be careful driving or handling equipment while taking this drug because it may cause dizziness, drowsiness, and blurry vision.

This drug may interfere with several diagnostic tests including some urine glucose tests. Diabetics should use glucose oxidase tests or glucose enzyme test strips.

Allergic reactions reported with this drug usually start with a rash or itching.

People with kidney or liver disease may not be able to take this drug.

PREGNANCY AND BREAST-FEEDING

Safety during pregnancy has not been established although there was no evidence of harm during studies in animals.

Breast-feeding while taking this drug is not recommended.

HELPFUL COMMENTS

Avoid quick movements to minimize dizziness. Dangling your legs over the side of the bed for a few minutes may help reduce dizziness when first waking up.

Tablets may be crushed and mixed with a little food or liquid for easier swallowing.

It takes about an hour for the full effects of this drug to be noticed.

METFORMIN HYDROCHLORIDE

Available since March 1995

COMMONLY USED TO TREAT

High blood sugar, specifically type 2 diabetes

DRUG CATEGORY

antidiabetic
Class: biguanide

PRODUCTS

Brand-Name Products with No Generic Alternative
Glucophage XR 500 mg extended-release tablet (¢¢¢¢)
No generic extended-release products available.
Patent expires in 2018. Exclusivity until 2003.

Brand-Name Products with Generic Alternatives
Glucophage 500 mg tablet (¢¢¢¢¢)
  Generic: metformin hydrochloride 500 mg tablet (¢¢¢¢)
Glucophage 850 mg tablet ($)
  Generic: metformin hydrochloride 850 mg tablet ($)
Glucophage 1 g tablet ($$)
  Generic: metformin hydrochloride 1 g tablet ($)

Products Only Available as Generics
metformin hydrochloride 625 mg tablet (n/a)
metformin hydrochloride 750 mg tablet (n/a)

---

† *See page 52.*   * *See page 53.*

Combination Products That Contain This Drug
Avandamet tablet (n/a)
Glucovance tablet (¢¢¢¢¢)
Metaglip tablet (n/a)

DOSING AND FOOD

Doses are taken 1 to 2 times a day. Extended-release products are taken once a day.

This drug is taken with meals, usually in the morning and evening.

Adults: Up to 2,500 mg per day in divided doses.

Lower doses are used in children.

Forgotten doses: If you are scheduled to take the next dose within a few hours, do not take the forgotten dose. Otherwise take the forgotten dose as soon as you remember.

ALCOHOL, DRUG, HERB, AND SUPPLEMENT INTERACTIONS

Alcohol may seriously increase the effects from this drug and should not be used. Ask your doctor about the risks caused by drinking alcohol with your condition.

Aloe, bilberry leaf, bitter melon, burdock, dandelion, fenugreek, garlic, ginkgo biloba, and ginseng may lower blood sugar and cause the need for a dose adjustment when taken with this drug. Tell your doctor if you are taking any of these supplements.

Several OTC drugs used for asthma, colds, cough, hay fever, sleep aid, or sinus problems may seriously change the effects of this drug. Check with your pharmacist when selecting OTC products.

Taking this drug with any of the ones listed below may change the effect of either drug with the possibility of causing toxicity or decreasing effectiveness:
alcohol, amiloride, calcium channel blockers†, cimetidine, cortico-steroids†, digoxin, diuretics†, estrogens†, furosemide, isoniazid, morphine, nicotinic acid, nifedipine, oral contraceptives, phenobarbital, phenytoin, procainamide, quinidine, quinine, ranitidine, sympatho-mimetics†, thyroid hormones†, triamterene, trimethoprim, vancomycin

ALLERGIC REACTIONS AND SIDE EFFECTS

You should tell your doctor about all your allergies and any unexplained symptoms you may have while taking this drug.

MORE COMMON SIDE EFFECTS: Gas, loss of appetite, metallic taste, stomachache, vomiting, weight loss

RARE SIDE EFFECTS: Anxiousness*, blurry vision*, cold sweats*, confusion*, diarrhea*, drowsiness*, headache*, hunger*, irregular breathing*, irregular heartbeat*, muscle pain*, nausea*, nervousness*, nightmares*, pale skin*, poor concentration*, shakiness*, sleep disorders*, sleepiness*, slurry speech*, staggering*, tiredness*, weakness*

PRECAUTIONS

People with heart disease, liver disease, or kidney disease may be at greater risk of developing serious side effects.

If you are in poor physical condition, undernourished, or have underactive adrenal or pituitary glands, the effects of this drug may be stronger than expected, requiring more frequent testing of blood sugar.

Do not crush, break, or chew the extended-release products.

If your blood sugar level is not controlled by this drug within 4 weeks, the doctor may need to increase the dose of this drug or add another drug to your treatment.

This drug is usually stopped just before surgery and restarted about 48 hours later. Blood sugar is controlled by either diet or insulin while not taking this drug.

People with fever, infections, burns, dehydration, diarrhea, hormone changes, injury, stress, intestinal disease, or vomiting may experience rapid changes in blood sugar, which increases the risk of side effects and may require emergency care.

PREGNANCY AND BREAST-FEEDING

Safety during pregnancy has not been established although there was no evidence of harm during studies in animals.

Breast-feeding while taking this drug is not recommended.

HELPFUL COMMENTS

If you do not treat high blood sugar, you may develop more serious problems such as heart failure, blood vessel disease, eye disease, or kidney disease.

If changing to another antidiabetic drug†, you may experience low blood sugar for about 2 weeks after this drug is stopped.

---

† See page 52.   * See page 53.

METHADONE HYDROCHLORIDE

Available for over 20 years

COMMONLY USED TO TREAT

Pain
Withdrawal from illegal drug addiction

DRUG CATEGORY

analgesic
antitussive
Class: narcotic analgesic/opioid

PRODUCTS

Brand-Name Products with Generic Alternatives
Dolophine 5 mg tablet (¢)
  Generic: methadone hydrochloride 5 mg tablet (¢)
Dolophine 10 mg tablet (¢¢)
  Generic: methadone hydrochloride 10 mg tablet (¢¢)
Products Only Available as Generics
methadone hydrochloride 40 mg tablet (¢¢¢)
methadone hydrochloride 5 mg/5 ml oral solution (¢¢¢)
methadone hydrochloride 10 mg/5 ml oral solution (¢¢¢¢)
methadone hydrochloride 10 mg/ml oral concentrate (¢¢¢)

DOSING AND FOOD

Doses are taken up to 8 times a day.
It is best to take this drug on an empty stomach, but taking this drug with
  a little food may avoid the stomach upset that some people suffer.
Adults: Up to 80 mg per day in divided doses.
Higher doses may be used in people who are under close medical super-
  vision.
Lower doses are used in children.
Forgotten doses: If you are scheduled to take the next dose within a few
  hours, do not take the forgotten dose. Otherwise take the forgotten dose
  as soon as you remember.

ALCOHOL, DRUG, HERB, AND SUPPLEMENT INTERACTIONS

Alcohol should not be used while taking this drug.
Several OTC drugs used for asthma, colds, cough, hay fever, sleep aid, or

sinus problems may seriously change the effects and side effects of this drug. Check with your pharmacist when selecting OTC products.

Taking this drug with any of the ones listed below may change the effect of either drug with the possibility of causing toxicity or decreasing effectiveness: natrexone, rifampin

Severe reactions are possible when this drug is taken with those listed below: anesthetics, anticholinergics†, antihistamines†, barbiturates†, benzodi-azepines†, cimetidine, monoamine oxidase inhibitors†, naloxone, narcotics†, phenothiazines†, sedative-hypnotics†, skeletal muscle relax-ants†, tricyclic antidepressants†

ALLERGIC REACTIONS AND SIDE EFFECTS

If you are allergic to any narcotics†, you may also be allergic to this drug. You should tell your doctor about all your allergies and any unexplained symptoms you may have while taking this drug.

MORE COMMON SIDE EFFECTS: Constipation, dizziness*, drowsiness*, dry mouth, excitement*, fainting, irregular breathing*, irregular heartbeat*, lightheadedness, loss of appetite, nausea, seizures*, sexual dysfunction, sweating*, urinary changes, vomiting

LESS COMMON SIDE EFFECTS: Blurry vision, breathing difficulty*, depres-sion*, flushing*, hallucinations*, headache, hives*, itching*, mood swings*, nervousness*, restlessness*, ringing in ears*, shortness of breath*, skin rash*, sleep disorders, spastic movements*, stomach cramps, swelling*, tiredness, trembling*, vision changes, weakness*, wheezing*

RARE SIDE EFFECTS: Body aches, clammy skin*, confusion*, diarrhea, fever, goosebumps, irritability, low blood pressure*, runny nose, shivering, small pupils*, sneezing, yawning

PRECAUTIONS

Be careful driving or handling equipment while taking this drug because it may cause dizziness and drowsiness.

If you have a history of head injury, brain disease, emphysema, asthma, lung disease, enlarged prostate, urinary disorders, gallbladder disease, or gallstones, you may not be able to take this drug.

People with colitis, heart disease, kidney disease, liver disease, and thyroid disease are at increased risk of developing side effects.

If you have a history of seizures, this drug may make that condition worse.

This drug may cause withdrawal symptoms if stopped suddenly. If you wish to stop taking this drug, ask your doctor for specific instructions.

---

†See page 52.   *See page 53.

Side effects may continue to develop even after the drug is stopped.

Because this drug has a high abuse potential, your prescription quantit may be limited.

This drug may cause dry mouth, which is associated with a greater risk o cavities. Your dentist may recommend that you clean your teeth and mouth differently to avoid infection.

PREGNANCY AND BREAST-FEEDING

Safety during pregnancy has not been established although the drug i known to harm animal fetuses.

Breast-feeding while taking this drug is not recommended.

HELPFUL COMMENTS

Add more fiber to your diet to help minimize the constipation that occurs with this drug. If severe, constipation may need to be treated with a stoo softener or other laxative. Ask your doctor or pharmacist for recommen- dations.

If being used for pain, this drug works best if taken before the pain gets too severe.

Sucking on hard sugarless candy or chewing sugarless gum may help re- lieve dry mouth caused by this drug.

Lie down for a while after taking a dose of this drug to help reduce the nausea.

Avoid quick movements to minimize dizziness. Dangling your legs over the side of the bed for a few minutes may help reduce dizziness when first waking up.

METHIMAZOLE

Available for over 20 years

COMMONLY USED TO TREAT

High thyroid levels, also known as hyperthyroidism

DRUG CATEGORY

antithyroid drug
Class: thyroid hormone antagonist

PRODUCTS

Brand-Name Products with No Generic Alternative
Methimazole 20 mg tablet (¢¢¢¢)

Brand-Name Products with Generic Alternatives

Tapazole 5 mg tablet (¢¢¢¢)
  Generic: methimazole 5 mg tablet (¢¢¢)
Tapazole 10 mg tablet (¢¢¢¢¢)
  Generic: methimazole 10 mg tablet (¢¢¢¢¢)

DOSING AND FOOD

Doses are taken 1 to 3 times a day.

This drug should be taken with food to reduce the stomach upset that many people suffer. Do not eat raw oysters or other raw shellfish at any time while taking this drug.

Adults: Up to 60 mg per day in divided doses.

Children: Up to 0.4 mg/kg per day in divided doses.

Forgotten doses: Take the forgotten dose as soon as you remember even if it is time for the next dose.

ALCOHOL, DRUG, HERB, AND SUPPLEMENT INTERACTIONS

Alcohol may increase the risk of liver damage from this drug. Ask your doctor about the risks caused by drinking alcohol with your condition.

OTC drugs that contain iodine should not be used while taking this drug. Ask your pharmacist for assistance when selecting OTC products.

Taking this drug with any of the ones listed below may change the effect of either drug with the possibility of causing toxicity or decreasing effectiveness: amiodarone, beta blocker†, corticosteroids†, corticotropin, digitoxin, digoxin, iodinated glycerol, lithium, potassium iodide, propylthiouracil

Severe reactions are possible when this drug is taken with those listed below: anticoagulants†

Increased side effects are possible when this drug is taken with those listed below: acetaminophen, amiodarone, anabolic steroids†, androgens†, antibiotics†, antithyroid drugs†, carbamazepine, carmustine, chloroquine, dantrolene, daunorubicin, disulfiram, divalproex, etetinate, gold salts†, hydroxy-chloroquine, isoniazid, mercaptopurine, methotrexate, naltrexone, phe-nothiazines†, phenytoin, plicamycin, valproic acid

ALLERGIC REACTIONS AND SIDE EFFECTS

If you are allergic to propylthiouracil, you may also be allergic to this drug. You should tell your doctor about all your allergies and any unexplained symptoms you may have while taking this drug.

† See page 52.   * See page 53.

MORE COMMON SIDE EFFECTS: Fever*, itching*, skin rash*

LESS COMMON SIDE EFFECTS: Chills*, cough*, dizziness, hoarseness*, joint pain*, loss of taste, mouth sores*, nausea, sore throat*, stomach pain, swelling*, vomiting, weakness*

RARE SIDE EFFECTS: Backache*, black stools*, bleeding*, bloody urine*, bruising*, coldness*, constipation*, headache*, menstrual changes*, muscle aches*, numbness*, puffy skin*, shortness of breath*, skin irritation*, sleepiness*, swollen glands*, tingling*, tiredness*, urinary changes*, weight gain*, yellow eyes or skin*

PRECAUTIONS

People with liver disease may not be able to take this drug.

This drug causes changes in your blood that put you at greater risk of getting an infection. Be careful not to cut yourself or get bruised. Tell your doctor if you develop signs of infection, such as fever or sore throat. Your dentist may recommend that you clean your teeth and mouth differently to avoid infection.

PREGNANCY AND BREAST-FEEDING

There is evidence that this drug may harm the fetus, but the drug may be necessary to the health of the mother.

Breast-feeding while taking this drug is not recommended.

HELPFUL COMMENTS

This drug is most effective when taken at equally spaced intervals. For example, if taken 3 times a day, the dose should be scheduled for every 8 hours.

It may take several months for the full effects of this drug to be noticed.

METHOCARBAMOL

Available for over 20 years

COMMONLY USED TO TREAT

Muscle stiffness and pain caused by injury

DRUG CATEGORY

skeletal muscle relaxant
Class: carbamate

PRODUCTS

Brand-Name Products with Generic Alternatives
Robaxin 500 mg tablet (¢¢¢¢)
  Generic: methocarbamol 500 mg tablet (¢)
Robaxin 750 mg tablet ($)
  Generic: methocarbamol 750 mg tablet (¢¢)
Combination Products That Contain This Drug
Robaxisal tablet (¢¢¢¢)

DOSING AND FOOD

Doses are taken 3 to 6 times a day.
It is best to take this drug on an empty stomach, but taking this drug with
  a little food may avoid the stomach upset that some people suffer.
Adults: Up to 24 g per day in divided doses.
Forgotten doses: If more than 1 hour has passed since the forgotten dose, do
  not take the dose. Just go back to your usual schedule with the next dose.

ALCOHOL, DRUG, HERB, AND SUPPLEMENT INTERACTIONS

Alcohol should not be used while taking this drug.
Several OTC drugs used for appetite control, asthma, colds, cough, hay
  fever, pain, or sinus problems may seriously increase the effects of this
  drug. Check with your pharmacist when selecting OTC products.
Increased side effects are possible when this drug is taken with those listed below:
anesthetics, antihistamines†, anxiolytics†, barbiturates†, narcotics†, tricyclic
  antidepressants†

ALLERGIC REACTIONS AND SIDE EFFECTS

If you are allergic to meprobamate or any other skeletal muscle relaxant,
  you may also be allergic to this drug. You should tell your doctor about
  all your allergies and any unexplained symptoms you may have while
  taking this drug.
MORE COMMON SIDE EFFECTS: Chest tightness*, dizziness, drowsiness,
  hives*, lightheadedness, nausea, seizures*, skin rash*, shortness of
  breath*, stomach cramps, vision changes
LESS COMMON SIDE EFFECTS: Burning eyes*, clumsiness, confusion, constipation, depression*, diarrhea, excitement, fainting*, fast heartbeat*,
  fever*, headache, heartburn, hiccups, irritability, itching*, weakness*,
  nervousness, red face, restlessness, stuffy nose*, vomiting
RARE SIDE EFFECTS: Back pain*, black stools*, bleeding*, bloody urine*,

---

†*See page 52.*   **See page 53.*

bruising*, cough*, difficulty urinating*, hoarseness*, irregular breath
ing*, mouth sores*, muscle cramps*, sore throat*, swollen eyes*, swollen
glands*, tiredness*, yellow eyes or skin*

PRECAUTIONS

Be careful driving or handling equipment while taking this drug because
the drug may cause dizziness and drowsiness.

If you have myasthenia gravis, this drug may cause severe weakness.

This drug may change the color of your urine to black, blue, brown, or
green. The color change is not associated with harm and will return to
normal once the drug is stopped.

This drug may interfere with some diagnostic urine tests. Make sure the
clinician running the test knows that you are taking this drug.

This drug may cause withdrawal symptoms if stopped suddenly after long-
term use. If you wish to stop taking this drug, ask your doctor for specific instructions.

PREGNANCY AND BREAST-FEEDING

Safety during pregnancy has not been established although there was no
evidence of harm during studies in animals.

Breast-feeding while taking this drug is not recommended.

HELPFUL COMMENTS

Avoid quick movements to minimize dizziness. Dangling your legs over the
side of the bed for a few minutes may help reduce dizziness when first
waking up.

METHOTREXATE SODIUM

Available for over 20 years

COMMONLY USED TO TREAT

Arthritis
Cancer
Psoriasis

DRUG CATEGORY

antineoplastic
antipsoriatic
antirheumatic

Class: antimetabolite

PRODUCTS

Brand-Name Products with No Generic Alternative
Trexall 5 mg tablet ($$$$)
Trexall 7.5 mg tablet ($$$$$)
Trexall 10 mg tablet ($$$$$)
Trexall 15 mg tablet ($$$$$)
Products Only Available as Generics
methotrexate sodium 2.5 mg tablet ($$$)

DOSING AND FOOD

Doses are taken 1 to 3 times a day.
It is best to take this drug on an empty stomach. Do not eat raw oysters or other raw shellfish at any time while taking this drug.
Adults: Up to 2.5 mg/kg per day in divided doses.
Children: Up to 3.3 mg/m2 per day in divided doses.
Forgotten doses: Do not take a forgotten dose. Just go back to your usual schedule with the next dose.

ALCOHOL, DRUG, HERB, AND SUPPLEMENT INTERACTIONS

Alcohol may increase the risk of liver damage from this drug. Ask your doctor about the risks caused by drinking alcohol with your condition.
Several OTC drugs used to relieve headaches and other pain may seriously increase the effects of this drug and should not be used. Ask your pharmacist for assistance when selecting OTC products.
Taking this drug with any of the ones listed below may change the effect of either drug with the possibility of causing toxicity or decreasing effectiveness: antibiotics†, aspirin, folic acid, nonsteroidal antiinflammatories†, probenecid, pyrimethamine, salicylates†, sulfonamides†, sulfonylureas†
Severe reactions are possible when this drug is taken with those listed below: phenytoin
Increased side effects are possible when this drug is taken with those listed below: acetaminophen, amiodarone, anabolic steroids†, androgens†, antithyroid drugs†, azathioprine, carbamazepine, carmustine, chloroquine, dantrolene, daunorubicin, disulfiram, divalproex, etetinate, gold salts, hydroxychloroquine, isoniazid, mercaptopurine, methotrexate, naltrexone, phenothiazines†, plicamycin, retinoids†, sulfasalazine, valproic acid

---

†See page 52.   *See page 53.

ALLERGIC REACTIONS AND SIDE EFFECTS

You should tell your doctor about all your allergies and any unexplained symptoms you may have while taking this drug.

This drug promotes the effect of sunlight on the body and may cause severe sunburn and increased sensitivity of the eyes.

MORE COMMON SIDE EFFECTS: Blisters*, flaky skin*, nausea, peeling skin* skin rash, skin redness*, urinary difficulty*, vomiting

LESS COMMON SIDE EFFECTS: Acne, boils, diarrhea*, itching, loss of appetite, mouth sores*, pale skin, stomach pain*

RARE SIDE EFFECTS: Back pain*, black stools*, bleeding*, bloody urine*, blurry vision*, bruising*, chest pain*, chills*, cough*, dark urine*, dizziness*, drowsiness*, fever*, hair loss*, headache*, hoarseness*, seizures*, shortness of breath*, skin irritation*, tiredness*, weakness*, yellow eyes or skin*

PRECAUTIONS

Avoid contact with anyone who has the chickenpox, measles, or other communicable disease since it may be easier to catch the infection while taking this drug.

Exposure to skin tests, immunizations, and people who have received immunizations may put you at a greater risk of developing the disease when you are taking this drug.

People with colitis, immune disorders, or folate deficiency are at increased risk of developing side effects.

If you have ulcers, mouth sores, or mouth swelling, this drug may make those conditions worse.

This drug causes changes in your blood that put you at greater risk of getting an infection. Be careful not to cut yourself or get bruised. Tell your doctor if you develop signs of infection, such as fever or sore throat. Your dentist may recommend that you clean your teeth and mouth differently to avoid infection.

People with a history of gout or kidney stones are at greater risk of recurrence while taking this drug.

Extremely high, toxic doses of this drug may be used in people with cancer. A second drug is given to prevent toxicity.

PREGNANCY AND BREAST-FEEDING

This drug may cause birth defects and should not be used during pregnancy. Breast-feeding while taking this drug is not recommended.

HELPFUL COMMENTS

It is very important to continue taking this drug as ordered by the doctor even if the side effects make you feel ill. Tell your doctor about any sudden or severe side effects you experience.

If you vomit shortly after taking a dose, call your doctor to find out if the dose should be repeated.

Eye irritation caused by the sun may be reduced by wearing sunglasses when outside.

Drink at least 10 to 12 glasses of water a day while taking this drug to reduce the risk of developing kidney stones or gout.

METHSUXIMIDE

Available for over 20 years

COMMONLY USED TO TREAT

Seizures

DRUG CATEGORY

anticonvulsant
Class: succinimide derivative

PRODUCTS

Brand-Name Products with No Generic Alternative
Celontin 150 mg capsule (¢¢¢¢)
Celontin 300 mg capsule (¢¢¢¢¢)
No generics available.
No patents, no exclusivity.

DOSING AND FOOD

Doses are taken once a day.

It is best to take this drug on an empty stomach, but taking this drug with a little food may avoid the stomach upset that some people suffer.

Adults and children: Up to 1,200 mg per day.

Forgotten doses: If you are scheduled to take the next dose within 4 hours, do not take the forgotten dose. Otherwise take the forgotten dose as soon as you remember.

ALCOHOL, DRUG, HERB, AND SUPPLEMENT INTERACTIONS

Alcohol should not be used while taking this drug.

† See page 52.　　* See page 53.

Several OTC drugs used for appetite control, asthma, colds, cough, hay fever, pain, or sinus problems may seriously increase the effects of this drug. Check with your pharmacist when selecting OTC products.

Taking this drug with any of the ones listed below may change the effect of either drug with the possibility of causing toxicity or decreasing effectiveness: phenytoin, valproic acid

Severe reactions are possible when this drug is taken with those listed below: haloperidol

Increased side effects are possible when this drug is taken with those listed below: anticonvulsants†, antidepressants†, antipsychotics†, anxiolytics†, narcotics†

ALLERGIC REACTIONS AND SIDE EFFECTS

If you allergic to any anticonvulsants†, you may also be allergic to this drug. You should tell your doctor about all your allergies and any unexplained symptoms you may have while taking this drug.

MORE COMMON SIDE EFFECTS: Clumsiness, dizziness, drowsiness*, fever*, headache, hiccups, itching*, loss of appetite, muscle pain*, nausea*, skin rash*, sore throat*, stomach cramps, swollen glands*, vomiting*

LESS COMMON SIDE EFFECTS: Aggressive behavior*, depression*, irritability, nightmares*, poor concentration*

RARE SIDE EFFECTS: Bleeding*, breathing difficulty*, bruising*, chest tightness*, chills*, mood swings*, mouth sores*, nosebleeds*, seizures*, shortness of breath*, tiredness*, weakness*, wheezing*

PRECAUTIONS

The contents of these capsules may melt if not stored properly. Capsules that look unusual or do not appear to be full may not be completely effective and should not be taken.

People with liver or kidney disease may not be able to take this drug.

Be careful driving or handling equipment while taking this drug because the drug may cause dizziness and drowsiness.

Stopping this drug suddenly may cause you to have a seizure. If you wish to stop taking this drug, ask your doctor for specific instructions.

This drug may cause the urine to turn pink or reddish in color.

PREGNANCY AND BREAST-FEEDING

Safety during pregnancy has not been established although the drug is known to harm animal fetuses.

Breast-feeding while taking this drug is not recommended.

HELPFUL COMMENTS

Avoid quick movements to minimize dizziness. Dangling your legs over the side of the bed for a few minutes may help reduce dizziness when first waking up.

METHYCLOTHIAZIDE

Available for over 20 years

COMMONLY USED TO TREAT

Fluid retention, also known as edema
Frequent urination in people with diabetes
High blood pressure, also known as hypertension

DRUG CATEGORY

antihypertensive
Class: thiazide diuretic

PRODUCTS

Brand-Name Products with Generic Alternatives
Enduron 2.5 mg tablet (¢¢¢¢)
  Generic: methyclothiazide 2.5 mg tablet (n/a)
Enduron 5 mg tablet (¢¢¢¢¢)
  Generic: methyclothiazide 5 mg tablet (¢¢¢¢)

Other Generic Product Names
Aquatensen

Combination Products That Contain This Drug
Enduronyl tablet ($$)

DOSING AND FOOD

Doses are taken once a day but may be taken as little as 3 times a week.
Adults: Up to 10 mg per day.
Lower doses may be used in children.
It is best to take this drug on an empty stomach, but taking this drug with a little food may avoid the stomach upset that some people suffer. Avoid food with excess salt.
Forgotten doses: If you are scheduled to take the next dose within a few hours, do not take the forgotten dose. Otherwise take the forgotten dose as soon as you remember.

---

† See page 52.   * See page 53.

ALCOHOL, DRUG, HERB, AND SUPPLEMENT INTERACTIONS

Alcohol may cause your blood pressure to rise, making this drug less effective. Ask your doctor about the risks caused by drinking alcohol with your condition.

Licorice root may increase potassium loss and should not be used while taking this drug.

Several OTC drugs used for appetite control, asthma, colds, cough, hay fever, or sinus problems may cause an increase in blood pressure when taken with this drug. Check with your pharmacist when selecting OTC products.

Taking this drug with any of the ones listed below may change the effect of either drug with the possibility of causing toxicity or decreasing effectiveness: antidiabetics†, cholestyramine, colestipol, digoxin, insulin, lithium

ALLERGIC REACTIONS AND SIDE EFFECTS

If you are allergic to acetazolamide, bumetanide, dichlorphenamide, furosemide, methazolamide, sulfonamides†, or thiazide diuretics†, you may also be allergic to this drug. You should tell your doctor about all your allergies and any unexplained symptoms you may have while taking this drug.

This drug promotes the effect of sunlight on the body and may cause severe sunburn and increased sensitivity of the eyes.

LESS COMMON SIDE EFFECTS: Diarrhea*, dizziness, lightheadedness, loss of appetite, sexual dysfunction, stomach upset

RARE SIDE EFFECTS: Back pain*, black stools*, bleeding*, bloody urine*, breathing difficulty*, bruising*, burning sensation*, chest pain*, chills*, confusion*, cough*, fatigue*, fever*, hives*, headache*, hoarseness*, irregular heartbeat*, joint pain*, leg pain*, muscle cramps*, nausea*, numbness*, painful urination*, shortness of breath*, skin rash*, stomach pain*, swelling*, vomiting*, weakness*, yellow eyes or skin*

PRECAUTIONS

This drug may cause your blood sugar level to rise and lead to type 2 diabetes.

Your body may lose potassium while taking this drug, which may cause severe side effects. Potassium levels should be monitored periodically and may need to be supplemented while taking this drug. Eat food rich in potassium, such as apricots, bananas, citrus fruit, dates, and tomatoes, if you are not taking a potassium supplement or potassium-sparing diuretic†.

People with kidney disease may not be able to take this drug.

This drug may increase the level of uric acid in the body that may lead to gout or kidney stones.

If you have lupus erythematosus or pancreatitis, this drug may make those conditions worse.

Nicotine in cigarettes may increase blood pressure, making this drug less effective.

This drug may cause an increase in the levels of cholesterol or triglyceride in the blood.

PREGNANCY AND BREAST-FEEDING

Safety during pregnancy has not been established although the drug is known to harm animal fetuses.

Breast-feeding while taking this drug is not recommended.

HELPFUL COMMENTS

Take your last dose of the day no later than 6 P.M. to avoid urination during the night.

Avoid quick movements to minimize dizziness. Dangling your legs over the side of the bed for a few minutes may help reduce dizziness when first waking up.

Record your weight twice a day, when first getting up in the morning and after the drug causes urination. A weight gain or loss of more than 2 pounds per day should be reported to your doctor.

The antihypertensive effects of this drug may last about 1 week after it is stopped.

METHYLDOPA

Available for over 20 years

COMMONLY USED TO TREAT

High blood pressure, also known as hypertension

DRUG CATEGORY

antihypertensive
Class: centrally acting antiadrenergic

PRODUCTS

Brand-Name Products with Generic Alternatives
Aldomet 125 mg tablet (n/a)
  Generic: methyldopa 125 mg tablet (¢)

---

† See page 52.   * See page 53.

Aldomet 250 mg tablet (¢¢¢)
  Generic: methyldopa 250 mg tablet (¢¢)
Aldomet 500 mg tablet (n/a)
  Generic: methyldopa 500 mg tablet (¢¢)
Combination Products That Contain This Drug
Aldoril 15 tablet (¢¢¢¢)
Aldoril 25 tablet (¢¢¢¢)
Aldoril D30 tablet ($)
Aldoril D50 tablet (n/a)

DOSING AND FOOD

Doses are taken 2 to 4 times a day.

This drug may be taken with or without food. Do not eat raw oysters or other raw shellfish at any time while taking this drug.

Adults: Up to 3,000 mg per day in divided doses.

Children: Up to 65 mg/kg (maximum 3 grams) per day in divided doses.

Lower doses may be needed in people with kidney disease.

Forgotten doses: If you are scheduled to take the next dose within a few hours, do not take the forgotten dose. Otherwise take the forgotten dose as soon as you remember.

ALCOHOL, DRUG, HERB, AND SUPPLEMENT INTERACTIONS

Alcohol may cause your blood pressure to rise, making this drug less effective. Ask your doctor about the risks caused by drinking alcohol with your condition.

Capsaicin and other foods or supplements derived from the capsicum family of plants, including hot peppers, sweet peppers, paprika, and chili powder, may interfere with the effects of this drug and should not be consumed.

Several OTC drugs used for appetite control, asthma, colds, cough, hay fever, or sinus problems may cause an increase in blood pressure when taken with this drug. Check with your pharmacist when selecting OTC products.

Taking this drug with any of the ones listed below may change the effect of either drug with the possibility of causing toxicity or decreasing effectiveness: anesthetics, antihypertensives†, diuretics†, iron supplements, lithium, phenothiazines†, sympathomimetics†, tolbutamide, tricyclic antidepressants†

Severe reactions are possible when this drug is taken with those listed below: haloperidol, phenoxybenzamide

ALLERGIC REACTIONS AND SIDE EFFECTS

You should tell your doctor about all your allergies and any unexplained symptoms you may have while taking this drug.

MORE COMMON SIDE EFFECTS: Drowsiness, dry mouth, headache, swelling*

LESS COMMON SIDE EFFECTS: Anxiety*, breast-milk secretion, breast swelling, depression*, diarrhea*, dizziness, fever*, irregular heartbeat*, lightheadedness, nausea*, numbness, sexual dysfunction, stuffy nose, tingling, vivid dreams*, vomiting*, weakness*

RARE SIDE EFFECTS: Breathing difficulty*, chills*, dark urine*, itching*, joint pain*, pale stools*, skin rash*, stomach pain*, tiredness*, yellow eyes or skin*

PRECAUTIONS

You need to wait 2 weeks after stopping a monoamine oxidase inhibitor† before starting this drug.

This drug causes changes in your blood that put you at greater risk of getting an infection. Be careful not to cut yourself or get bruised. Tell your doctor if you develop signs of infection, such as fever or sore throat. Your dentist may recommend that you clean your teeth and mouth differently to avoid infection.

If you have chest pain or Parkinson's disease, this drug may make those conditions worse.

People with a history of depression are at greater risk of relapse while taking this drug.

This drug may cause dry mouth, which is associated with a greater risk of cavities. Your dentist may recommend that you clean your teeth and mouth differently to avoid infection.

Be careful driving or handling equipment while taking this drug because the drug may cause drowsiness.

This drug is drawn out of the blood during kidney dialysis, which may result in an increase in blood pressure after dialysis. Make sure the dialysis center knows that you are taking this drug.

Record your weight each day while taking this drug. A weight gain or loss of more than 5 pounds per week should be reported to your doctor.

This drug loses its effect in some people after 2 to 3 weeks, and a change in therapy may be required.

PREGNANCY AND BREAST-FEEDING

Safety during pregnancy has not been established although there was no evidence of harm during studies in animals.

---

†See page 52.   * See page 53.

This drug passes into breast milk, but does not appear to harm the baby. The American Academy of Pediatrics considers this drug acceptable for use while breast-feeding.

HELPFUL COMMENTS

Sucking on hard sugarless candy or chewing sugarless gum may help relieve dry mouth caused by this drug.

Avoid quick movements to minimize dizziness. Dangling your legs over the side of the bed for a few minutes may help reduce dizziness when first waking up.

If you do not treat high blood pressure, you may develop more serious problems such as heart failure, blood vessel disease, stroke, or kidney disease. Losing weight, exercising, eating more fruits and vegetables, and avoiding salty foods, such as lunchmeat and pickles, may help make drug treatment more successful.

It takes about 2 days for the full effects of this drug to be noticed although blood pressure will begin to lower with the first dose.

METHYLERGONOVINE MALEATE

Available for over 20 years

COMMONLY USED TO TREAT

Uterine bleeding after childbirth

DRUG CATEGORY

oxytocic
Class: ergot alkaloid

PRODUCTS

Brand-Name Products with No Generic Alternative
Metherine 0.2 mg tablet (¢¢¢¢)
No generics available.
No patents, no exclusivity.

DOSING AND FOOD

Doses are taken 2 to 4 times a day.
This drug may be taken with or without food.
Women: Up to 1.6 mg per day in divided doses.

Forgotten doses: Do not take a forgotten dose. Just go back to your usual schedule with the next dose.

ALCOHOL, DRUG, HERB, AND SUPPLEMENT INTERACTIONS

Alcohol may increase some of the side effects from this drug, depending on the amount consumed. Ask your doctor about the risks caused by drinking alcohol with your condition.

Taking this drug with any of the ones listed below may change the effect of either drug with the possibility of causing toxicity or decreasing effectiveness: nitrates†

Severe reactions are possible when this drug is taken with those listed below: bromocriptine, epinephrine, ergoloid, ergonovine, ergotamine, methylergonovine, methysergide, sympathomimetics†

ALLERGIC REACTIONS AND SIDE EFFECTS

If you are allergic to any other ergot alkaloid†, you may also be allergic to this drug. You should tell your doctor about all your allergies and any unexplained symptoms you may have while taking this drug.

MORE COMMON SIDE EFFECTS: Diarrhea*, nausea*, seizures*, uterine cramps, vomiting*

LESS COMMON SIDE EFFECTS: Anxiety*, blisters*, chest pain*, coldness*, confusion*, congestion, dizziness*, drowsiness*, dry mouth, excitement*, headaches*, increased blood pressure*, irregular heartbeat*, itching*, muscle pain*, nervousness, numbness*, pale skin*, restlessness, ringing in ears, shortness of breath*, stomach pain*, swelling*, taste changes, tingling*, thirst*, vision changes*, weakness*

PRECAUTIONS

Smoking may increase the side effects of this drug. You should stop smoking while taking this drug, or wait several hours after taking your dose before smoking.

PREGNANCY AND BREAST-FEEDING

Safety during pregnancy has not been established although the drug is known to harm animal fetuses.

Breast-feeding while taking this drug is not recommended.

HELPFUL COMMENTS

This drug is used for a maximum of 7 days.

---

†See page 52. *See page 53.

METHYLPHENIDATE HYDROCHLORIDE

Available for over 20 years

COMMONLY USED TO TREAT

Attention deficit hyperactivity disorder (ADHD)
Sudden sleeping attacks, also known as narcolepsy

DRUG CATEGORY

analeptic
behavioral agent
Class: CNS stimulant: piperidine

PRODUCTS

Brand-Name Products with No Generic Alternative
Concerta 18 mg extended-release tablet ($$)
Concerta 27 mg extended-release tablet (n/a)
Concerta 36 mg extended-release tablet ($$)
Concerta 54 mg extended-release tablet ($$$)
Methylin 5 mg/5 ml oral solution (n/a)
Methylin 10 mg/5 ml oral solution (n/a)
Mendate CD 20 mg extended-release capsule (n/a)
Ritalin LA 20 mg extended-release capsule (n/a)
Ritalin LA 40 mg extended-release capsule (n/a)
Ritalin LA 30 mg extended-release capsule (n/a)

Brand-Name Products with Generic Alternatives
Ritalin 5 mg tablet (¢¢¢)
  Generic: methylphenidate hydrochloride 5 mg tablet (¢¢¢)
Ritalin 10 mg tablet (¢¢¢¢)
  Generic: methylphenidate hydrochloride 10 mg tablet (¢¢¢)
Ritalin 20 mg tablet (¢¢¢¢)
  Generic: methylphenidate hydrochloride 20 mg tablet (¢¢¢¢)
Ritalin-SR 20 mg extended-release tablet ($)
  Generic: methylphenidate hydrochloride 20 mg extended-release
tablet ($)

Other Generic Product Names
Methylin ER, Metadate ER

DOSING AND FOOD

Doses are taken 1 to 3 times a day.

It is best to take this drug with a meal or snack.

Adults and children age 6 and older: Up to 60 mg per day in divided doses.

Forgotten doses: Take the forgotten dose as soon as you remember even if it is time for the next dose. Then adjust the schedule to space doses evenly for the remainder of the day.

ALCOHOL, DRUG, HERB, AND SUPPLEMENT INTERACTIONS

Alcohol should not be used while taking this drug.

Do not use caffeine while taking this drug since the drug effects may be decreased.

Many OTC drugs used for appetite control, asthma, colds, cough, hay fever, pain, or sinus problems affect the central nervous system and may cause severe side effects when taken with this drug. Check with your pharmacist for products to avoid.

Taking this drug with any of the ones listed below may change the effect of either drug with the possibility of causing toxicity or decreasing effectiveness: anticonvulsants†, bretylium, guanethidine, phenobarbital, phenylbutazone, phenytoin, primidone, tricyclic antidepressants†, warfarin

Severe reactions are possible when this drug is taken with those listed below: monoamine oxidase inhibitors†

Increased side effects are possible when this drug is taken with those listed below: amantadine, amphetamines, bupropion, caffeine, chlorphedianol, cocaine, nabilone, pemoline

ALLERGIC REACTIONS AND SIDE EFFECTS

You should tell your doctor about all your allergies and any unexplained symptoms you may have while taking this drug.

More Common Side Effects: Fast heartbeat*, increased blood pressure*, loss of appetite, nervousness, sleep disorders

Less Common Side Effects: Chest pain*, dizziness, drowsiness, fever*, headache*, hives*, joint pain*, nausea, skin rash*, spastic movements*, stomach pain

Rare Side Effects: Agitation*, black stools*, bleeding*, bloody urine*, blurry vision*, bruising*, confusion*, delusions*, depersonalization*, dilated pupils*, dry mouth*, hallucinations*, irregular heartbeat*, mood swings*, muscle cramps*, seizures*, shaking*, skin irritation*, sweating*, trembling*, twitching*, vision changes*, vocal outbursts*, vomiting*, weight loss*

---

†See page 52.   * See page 53.

PRECAUTIONS

Because this drug has a high abuse potential, your prescription quantity may be limited.

People with a history of seizures are at greater risk of developing a seizure while taking this drug.

If you have glaucoma, high blood pressure, anxiety, depression, agitation, muscle tics, or Tourette's syndrome, this drug may make those conditions worse.

Do not open, crush, break, or chew the extended-release products.

An empty shell from the Concerta extended-release products may pass in your stool without dissolving, which is not a concern.

Be careful driving or handling equipment while taking this drug because it may cause dizziness, drowsiness, and blurry vision.

This drug may become habit forming over time. Withdrawal symptoms may occur if the drug is stopped suddenly. If you wish to stop taking this drug, ask your doctor for specific instructions.

People with a history of alcohol or drug abuse have a greater risk of addiction to this drug.

You need to wait 2 weeks after stopping a monoamine oxidase inhibitor† before starting this drug.

PREGNANCY AND BREAST-FEEDING

Safety during pregnancy has not been established although the drug is known to harm animal fetuses.

It is not known if this drug passes into breast milk. Talk to your doctor about the risks associated with breast-feeding while taking this drug.

HELPFUL COMMENTS

Take the last dose of the day before 6 P.M. to reduce the chance of sleep disorders.

Contact your doctor if your symptoms do not improve after about a week.

It is very important to get enough sleep while taking this drug to prevent exhaustion between doses.

METHYLPREDNISOLONE

Available for over 20 years

COMMONLY USED TO TREAT

Allergic reactions
Multiple sclerosis
Severe inflammation

DRUG CATEGORY

antiinflammatory
immunosuppressant
Class: corticosteroid

PRODUCTS

Brand-Name Products with No Generic Alternative
Medrol 2 mg tablet (¢¢¢)
Medrol Acetate 0.25% topical ointment (n/a)

Brand-Name Products with Generic Alternatives
Medrol 4 mg tablet (¢¢¢¢¢)
  Generic: methylprednisolone 4 mg tablet (¢¢¢¢)
Medrol 8 mg tablet ($)
  Generic: methylprednisolone 8 mg tablet (n/a)
Medrol 16 mg tablet ($$)
  Generic: methylprednisolone 16 mg tablet (n/a)
Medrol 24 mg tablet ($$)
  Generic: methylprednisolone 24 mg tablet (n/a)
Medrol 32 mg tablet ($$$)
  Generic: methylprednisolone 32 mg tablet (n/a)

DOSING AND FOOD

Doses are taken 1 to 4 times a day.
The oral form of this drug should be taken with food.
Adults: Up to 60 mg per day in divided doses.
Children: Up to 1.66 mg/kg per day in divided doses.
Topical preparations should be applied in a thin layer.
Forgotten doses: Determining when to take a forgotten dose will depend on your prescription schedule. If you remember the forgotten dose within a few hours of when it was due, you may take the dose immediately and continue with your regular schedule. If you are tapering the drug to

avoid withdrawal symptoms, you may need to evaluate the time since the last dose and the interval between the next doses. A complete change in schedule may be needed. Talk to your doctor or pharmacist for more help.

ALCOHOL, DRUG, HERB, AND SUPPLEMENT INTERACTIONS

Alcohol may increase the risk of side effects from this drug, especially stomach problems. Ask your doctor about the risks caused by drinking alcohol with your condition.

Taking this drug with any of the ones listed below may change the effect of either drug with the possibility of causing toxicity or decreasing effectiveness: aminoglutethimide, antacids, anticoagulants†, antidiabetics†, barbiturates†, carbamazepine, cholestyramine, colestipol, diuretics†, estrogens†, griseofulvin, insulin, isoniazid, mitotane, phenylbutazone, phenytoin, primidone, rifampin, salicylates†, somatrem, somatropin

Severe reactions are possible when this drug is taken with those listed below: aspirin, amphotericin B, cardiac glycosides†, immunizations, nonsteroidal antiinflammatories†, ritodrine

ALLERGIC REACTIONS AND SIDE EFFECTS

If you are allergic to any corticosteroids†, you may also be allergic to this drug. You should tell your doctor about all your allergies and any unexplained symptoms you may have while taking this drug.

This drug may cause your eyes to be more sensitive to sunlight, but there are no special risks associated with sunburn while taking this drug.

MORE COMMON SIDE EFFECTS: Excitement*, indigestion, irregular heartbeat*, leg pain*, nervousness, restlessness, seizures*, sleep disorders, stomach pain*, swelling*

LESS COMMON SIDE EFFECTS: Acne*, bloody stools*, bruising*, dizziness, eye pain*, flushing, frequent urination*, headache*, hiccups, increased appetite, hair growth*, thirst*, lightheadedness, menstrual problems*, muscle cramps*, nausea*, pain*, red eyes*, rounding of the face*, skin discoloration, skin irritation*, spinning sensation, stunted growth*, sweating, tearing of eyes*, tiredness*, vision changes*, vomiting*, weakness*, weight gain*

RARE SIDE EFFECTS: Confusion*, depression*, hallucinations*, hives*, mood swings*, restlessness*, skin rash*

PRECAUTIONS

This drug may cause severe and possibly fatal withdrawal symptoms if stopped abruptly. The drug must be stopped over 7 to 10 days by gradually decreasing the dose or time between doses. If you wish to stop taking this drug, ask your doctor for specific instructions.

The topical form of this drug is absorbed through the skin and may carry the same warnings as the oral product if it is used for a long time, covers a large area, or is used on broken or irritated skin.

This drug may cause an increase in blood sugar or cholesterol level, calcium loss, and/or retention of fluid.

Avoid contact with anyone who has the chickenpox, measles, or other communicable disease since it may be easier to catch the infection while taking this drug.

Exposure to skin tests, immunizations, and people who have received immunizations may put you at a greater risk of developing the disease when you are taking this drug.

PREGNANCY AND BREAST-FEEDING

Safety during pregnancy has not been established although the drug is known to harm animal fetuses.

This drug passes into breast milk and may cause growth problems in the baby. The risk is related to the dose and route of the drug. Small amounts of the drug are absorbed into the body from topical products. Talk to your doctor about the risks associated with breast-feeding while taking this drug.

HELPFUL COMMENTS

If you need to take an antacid, take it either 2 hours before or after taking this drug.

METHYLTESTOSTERONE

Available for over 20 years

COMMONLY USED TO TREAT

Delayed puberty
Testosterone deficiency

DRUG CATEGORY

antineoplastic
male hormone replacement
Class: androgen

---

† See page 52.   * See page 53.

PRODUCTS

Brand-Name Products with Generic Alternatives

Android 10 mg tablet ($$)
  Generic: methyltestosterone 10 mg tablet ($)
Android 25 mg tablet (n/a)
  Generic: methyltestosterone 25 mg tablet (n/a)

Other Generic Product Names

Testred, Virilon

DOSING AND FOOD

Doses are taken 1 to 4 times a day.
It is best to take this drug at mealtime.

Men: Up to 50 mg per day in divided doses.

Women: Up to 200 mg per day in divided doses.

Boys: Up to 25 mg per day in divided doses.

Forgotten doses: If more than half the time between doses has passed, do not take the forgotten dose. Just return to your normal schedule with the next dose. If less than half the time between doses has passed, take the forgotten dose as soon as you remember.

ALCOHOL, DRUG, HERB, AND SUPPLEMENT INTERACTIONS

Alcohol may increase the risk of liver damage from this drug. Ask your doctor about the risks caused by drinking alcohol with your condition.

Taking this drug with any of the ones listed below may change the effect of either drug with the possibility of causing toxicity or decreasing effectiveness: anticoagulants†, oxyphenbutazone

Increased side effects are possible when this drug is taken with those listed below: acetaminophen, amiodarone, anabolic steroids†, antibiotics†, antithyroid drugs†, carmustine, chloroquine, dantrolene, daunorubicin, disulfiram, divalproex, estrogens†, etretinate, gold salts†, hydroxychloroquine, mercaptopurine, methotrexate, methyldopa, naltrexone, oral contraceptives, phenothiazines†, phenytoin, plicamycin, valproic acid

ALLERGIC REACTIONS AND SIDE EFFECTS

If you are allergic to any androgens† or anabolic steroids†, you may also be allergic to this drug. You should tell your doctor about all your allergies and any unexplained symptoms you may have while taking this drug.

MORE COMMON SIDE EFFECTS: Acne*, breast size change*, masculine characteristics in women*, menstrual irregularities*, penile erection*, urinary changes*

LESS COMMON SIDE EFFECTS: Black stools*, bleeding*, bloody vomit*, chills*, confusion*, constipation*, decreased testicle size, depression*, diarrhea, dizziness*, flushing*, hair loss, headache*, itching*, mood swings*, nausea*, nervousness, paranoia*, pubic-hair growth, sexual dysfunction, skin irritation*, sleep disorders, stomach pain, swelling*, thirst*, tiredness*, vomiting*, weakness*, weight gain*, yellow eyes or skin*

RARE SIDE EFFECTS: Abdominal tenderness*, abdominal pain*, bad breath*, dark urine*, fever*, hives*, loss of appetite*, mouth sores*, pain*, sore throat*

PRECAUTIONS

If you are a diabetic, you may need a change in the dose of your antidiabetic drug† or insulin, since this drug may cause changes in blood sugar.

Men have a small risk of developing painful, prolonged erection of the penis, which requires treatment by a doctor. If this happens, go to your doctor or the nearest emergency room immediately.

This drug may cause the body to retain water. If you have a history of headaches, seizures, heart disease, liver disease, or kidney disease, make sure your doctor knows about these conditions before this drug is prescribed. Report any swelling of your face, feet, hands, or legs right away.

If you have an enlarged prostate, this drug may make the condition worse.

High-dose treatment in men may temporarily decrease sperm production. Talk to your doctor if you are planning to have children.

PREGNANCY AND BREAST-FEEDING

This drug may cause birth defects and should not be used during pregnancy. Breast-feeding while taking this drug is not recommended.

HELPFUL COMMENTS

Treatment with this drug should be re-evaluated at least every 6 months.

This drug has been used to increase athletic performance without adequate safety information and is classified by the FDA as a controlled substance. The International Olympic Committee and World Anti-Doping Agency have banned this drug from use in competitive sports.

† See page 52.   * See page 53.

METHYSERGIDE MALEATE

Available for over 20 years

COMMONLY USED TO TREAT

People at risk of developing migraine headaches

DRUG CATEGORY

antimigraine
Class: ergot alkaloid

PRODUCTS

Brand-Name Products with No Generic Alternative
Sansert 2 mg tablet ($$$)
No generics available.
No patents, no exclusivity.

DOSING AND FOOD

Doses are taken 2 to 4 times a day.
This drug may be taken with or without food.

Adults: Up to 8 mg per day in divided doses.

Forgotten doses: Do not take a forgotten dose. Just go back to your usual
  schedule with the next dose.

ALCOHOL, DRUG, HERB, AND SUPPLEMENT INTERACTIONS

Alcohol may make your headache worse. You should ask your doctor about
  the risks caused by drinking alcohol with your condition.

**Taking this drug with any of the ones listed below may change the effect of
either drug with the possibility of causing toxicity or decreasing effectiveness:**
narcotics†

Severe reactions are possible when this drug is taken with those listed below:
cocaine, epinephrine, ergoloid, ergonovine, methylergonovine

ALLERGIC REACTIONS AND SIDE EFFECTS

If you are allergic to any other ergot alkaloid†, you may also be allergic to
  this drug. You should tell your doctor about all your allergies and any un-
  explained symptoms you may have while taking this drug.

MORE COMMON SIDE EFFECTS: Abdominal pain*, coldness*, diarrhea, dizziness*, drowsiness, itching*, lightheadedness, muscle pain*, nausea, numbness*, tingling*, vomiting

LESS COMMON SIDE EFFECTS: Breathing difficulty*, chest pain*, chest tightness*, chills*, clumsiness*, constipation, cough*, depression*, excitement*, fever*, flushing*, hair loss, hallucinations*, heartburn, hoarseness*, irregular heartbeat*, leg cramps*, loss of appetite*, nightmares*, pale skin*, seizures*, shortness of breath*, skin rash*, sleep disorders, swelling*, unsteadiness*, urinary changes*, vision changes*, weight changes*

PRECAUTIONS

This drug works to prevent headaches but is not effective for relieving headache pain. If you get a headache while taking this drug, call your doctor for the recommended treatment.

This drug is usually taken for no more than 6 months at a time followed by a drug-free interval of at least 2 months to prevent serious side effects.

Be careful driving or handling equipment while taking this drug because it may cause dizziness and drowsiness.

Smoking may increase the side effects of this drug. You should stop smoking while taking this drug, or wait several hours after taking your dose before smoking.

If you have high blood pressure or stomach ulcers, this drug may make those conditions worse.

Stopping this drug suddenly may trigger a headache. If you wish to stop taking this drug, ask your doctor for specific instructions.

PREGNANCY AND BREAST-FEEDING

This drug may cause birth defects and should not be used during pregnancy. Breast-feeding while taking this drug is not recommended.

HELPFUL COMMENTS

Avoid quick movements to minimize dizziness. Dangling your legs over the side of the bed for a few minutes may help reduce dizziness when first waking up.

It takes about 3 weeks for the effects of this drug to be noticed.

Dress warmly while taking this drug since it may cause you to be more sensitive to cold temperatures.

† See page 52.   * See page 53.

METOCLOPRAMIDE HYDROCHLORIDE

Available for over 20 years

COMMONLY USED TO TREAT

Heartburn, specifically gastroesophageal reflux disease (GERD)
Stomach problems, specifically delayed gastric emptying

DRUG CATEGORY

antiemetic
gastrointestinal stimulant
Class: para-aminobenzoic acid derivative

PRODUCTS

Brand-Name Products with No Generic Alternative
Metoclopramide Intensol 10 mg/ml oral concentrate ($$$)
Brand-Name Products with Generic Alternatives
Reglan 5 mg tablet (¢¢¢¢)
  Generic: metoclopramide hydrochloride 5 mg tablet (¢¢¢)
Reglan 10 mg tablet (¢¢¢¢¢)
  Generic: metoclopramide hydrochloride 10 mg tablet (¢¢)
Products Only Available as Generics
metoclopramide hydrochloride 5 mg/5 ml oral solution (¢¢)

DOSING AND FOOD

Doses are taken 1 to 4 times a day.
Always take your dose 30 minutes before a meal.
Adults: Up to 60 mg per day in divided doses.
Lower doses are used in children, people over age 65, and people with
  kidney disease.
Forgotten doses: If you are scheduled to take the next dose within a few
  hours, do not take the forgotten dose. Otherwise take the forgotten dose
  as soon as you remember.

ALCOHOL, DRUG, HERB, AND SUPPLEMENT INTERACTIONS

Alcohol should not be used while taking this drug.
Several OTC drugs used for appetite control, asthma, colds, cough, hay
  fever, pain, or sinus problems may seriously increase the side effects of
  this drug. Check with your pharmacist when selecting OTC products.

Taking this drug with any of the ones listed below may change the effect of either drug with the possibility of causing toxicity or decreasing effectiveness: acetaminophen, anticholinergics†, aspirin, cyclosporine, diazepam, digoxin, levodopa, lithium, narcotics†, tetracycline

Severe reactions are possible when this drug is taken with those listed below: anesthetics, antihistamines†, antihypertensives†, antipsychotics†, anxiolytics†, barbiturates†, monoamine oxidase inhibitors†, phenothiazines†, tricyclic antidepressants†

ALLERGIC REACTIONS AND SIDE EFFECTS

If you are allergic to procaine or procainamide, you may also be allergic to this drug. You should tell your doctor about all your allergies and any unexplained symptoms you may have while taking this drug.

MORE COMMON SIDE EFFECTS: Depression, diarrhea, drowsiness*, panic attack*, restlessness, sleeping difficulty

LESS COMMON SIDE EFFECTS: Breast-milk secretion, breast swelling, breast tenderness, constipation, depression, dry mouth, irritability*, menstrual changes, nausea, skin rash

RARE SIDE EFFECTS: Blood pressure increase*, chewing motion*, chills*, confusion*, dizziness*, expressionless face*, fainting*, fever*, headache*, irregular heartbeat*, leg pain*, lip smacking*, muscle spasms*, nervousness*, poor balance*, puckering*, puffy cheeks*, restlessness*, seizures*, shaking*, shuffling walk*, sore throat*, spastic movements*, speaking difficulty*, stiffness*, still eyes*, suicidal thoughts*, tiredness*, tongue movements*, trembling*, twitching*, weakness*

PRECAUTIONS

If you have stomach bleeding, asthma, high blood pressure, intestinal problems, depression, or Parkinson's disease, this drug may make those conditions worse.

People with a history of seizures are at greater risk of developing a seizure while taking this drug.

Be careful driving or handling equipment while taking this drug because the drug may cause drowsiness.

This drug is not taken for longer than 12 weeks.

Involuntary body movement and twitches may be a sign of toxicity and should be reported to your doctor right away.

This drug may cause dry mouth, which is associated with a greater risk of cavities. Your dentist may recommend that you clean your teeth and mouth differently to avoid infection.

† See page 52.   * See page 53.

PREGNANCY AND BREAST-FEEDING

Safety during pregnancy has not been established although there was no evidence of harm during studies in animals.

Breast-feeding while taking this drug is not recommended.

HELPFUL COMMENTS

The oral concentrate may be mixed with water, juice, soda, or soft food such as applesauce or pudding to make swallowing easier.

Do not measure doses of the oral solution with anything but a measuring cup intended for use with prescription drugs. Slight inaccuracy from other measuring spoons may result in over- or under-dosing.

Sucking on hard sugarless candy or chewing sugarless gum may help relieve dry mouth caused by this drug.

METOLAZONE

Available for over 20 years

COMMONLY USED TO TREAT

Fluid retention, also known as edema

Frequent urination in people with diabetes

High blood pressure, also known as hypertension

DRUG CATEGORY

antihypertensive

Class: thiazidelike diuretic

PRODUCTS

Brand-Name Products with No Generic Alternative

Mykrox 0.5 mg tablet ($)

Zaroxolyn 2.5 mg tablet (¢¢¢¢¢)

Zaroxolyn 5 mg tablet ($)

Zaroxolyn 10 mg tablet ($)

No generics available.

No patents, no exclusivity.

DOSING AND FOOD

Doses are taken once a day.

Adults: Up to 20 mg per day.

This drug is not used in children.

Taking this drug with food may avoid the stomach upset that some people suffer. Avoid food with excess salt.

Forgotten doses: If you are scheduled to take the next dose within a few hours, do not take the forgotten dose. Otherwise take the forgotten dose as soon as you remember.

ALCOHOL, DRUG, HERB, AND SUPPLEMENT INTERACTIONS

Alcohol may cause your blood pressure to rise, making this drug less effective. Ask your doctor about the risks caused by drinking alcohol with your condition.

Licorice root may increase potassium loss and should not be used while taking this drug.

Several OTC drugs used for appetite control, asthma, colds, cough, hay fever, or sinus problems may cause an increase in blood pressure when taken with this drug. Check with your pharmacist when selecting OTC products.

Taking this drug with any of the ones listed below may change the effect of either drug with the possibility of causing toxicity or decreasing effectiveness: amphetamines, antidiabetics†, antihypertensive†, cholestyramine, colestipol, digoxin, insulin, lithium, methenamine, quinidine

Severe reactions are possible when this drug is taken with those listed below: diazoxide

ALLERGIC REACTIONS AND SIDE EFFECTS

If you are allergic to acetazolamide, bumetanide, dichlorphenamide, furosemide, methazolamide, sulfonamides†, or thiazide diuretics†, you may also be allergic to this drug. You should tell your doctor about all your allergies and any unexplained symptoms you may have while taking this drug.

This drug promotes the effect of sunlight on the body and may cause severe sunburn and increased sensitivity of the eyes.

LESS COMMON SIDE EFFECTS: Diarrhea*, dizziness, lightheadedness, loss of appetite, sexual dysfunction, stomach upset

RARE SIDE EFFECTS: Back pain*, black stools*, bleeding*, bloody urine*, breathing difficulty*, bruising*, burning sensation*, chest pain*, chills*, confusion*, cough*, fatigue*, fever*, hives*, headache*, hoarseness*, irregular heartbeat*, joint pain*, leg pain*, muscle cramps*, nausea*,

---

†See page 52.   * See page 53.

numbness*, painful urination*, shortness of breath*, skin rash*, stomach pain*, swelling*, vomiting*, weakness*, yellow eyes or skin*

PRECAUTIONS

This drug may cause your blood sugar level to rise and may lead to type 2 diabetes.

Your body may lose potassium while taking this drug, which may cause severe side effects. Potassium levels should be monitored periodically and may need to be supplemented while taking this drug. Eat food rich in potassium, such as apricots, bananas, citrus fruit, dates, and tomatoes, if you are not taking a potassium supplement or potassium-sparing diuretic†.

This drug may increase the level of uric acid in the body, which may lead to gout or kidney stones.

If you have lupus erythematosus or pancreatitis, this drug may make those conditions worse.

Nicotine in cigarettes may increase blood pressure, making this drug less effective.

This drug may cause an increase in the levels of cholesterol or triglyceride in the blood.

PREGNANCY AND BREAST-FEEDING

Safety during pregnancy has not been established although the drug is known to harm animal fetuses.

Breast-feeding while taking this drug is not recommended.

HELPFUL COMMENTS

Take your last dose of the day no later than 6 P.M. to avoid urination during the night.

Avoid quick movements to minimize dizziness. Dangling your legs over the side of the bed for a few minutes may help reduce dizziness when first waking up.

Record your weight twice a day, when first getting up in the morning and after the drug causes urination. A weight gain or loss of more than 2 pounds per day should be reported to your doctor.

The antihypertensive effects of this drug will last about 1 week after it is stopped.

METOPROLOL TARTRATE

Available for over 20 years

COMMONLY USED TO TREAT

Chest pain, also known as angina
High blood pressure, also known as hypertension
Irregular heart rhythm, also known as arrhythmia
People at risk of complications after a heart attack

DRUG CATEGORY

antianginal
antiarrhythmic
antihypertensive
Class: beta blocker

PRODUCTS

Brand-Name Products with No Generic Alternative
Toprol-XL 25 mg extended-release tablet (¢¢¢¢)
Toprol-XL 50 mg extended-release tablet (¢¢¢¢)
Toprol-XL 100 mg extended-release tablet (¢¢¢¢¢)
Toprol-XL 200 mg extended-release tablet ($$)
No generic extended-release products.
Multiple patents that begin to expire in 2007.
Brand-Name Products with Generic Alternatives
Lopressor 50 mg tablet (¢¢¢¢¢)
  Generic: metoprolol tartrate 50 mg tablet (¢¢)
Lopressor 100 mg tablet ($)
  Generic: metoprolol tartrate 100 mg tablet (¢¢¢)
Combination Products That Contain This Drug
Lopressor HCT tablet (¢¢¢¢¢) to ($$)

DOSING AND FOOD

Doses are taken 1 to 2 times a day.
It is best to take this drug with food.
Adults: Up to 400 mg per day in divided doses.
Lower doses are used in people with liver disease and heart failure.
This drug is rarely used in children.
Forgotten doses: If you are taking the extended-release tablets and are
  scheduled to take the next dose within 8 hours, do not take the forgotten

---

† See page 52.   * See page 53.

dose. Otherwise take the forgotten dose as soon as you remember. If you are taking the regular tablets and are scheduled to take the next dose within 4 hours, do not take the forgotten dose. Otherwise take the forgotten dose as soon as you remember.

ALCOHOL, DRUG, HERB, AND SUPPLEMENT INTERACTIONS

Alcohol may increase some of the side effects from this drug, depending on the amount consumed. Ask your doctor about the risks caused by drinking alcohol with your condition.

Several OTC drugs used for appetite control, asthma, colds, cough, hay fever, or sinus problems may cause an increase in blood pressure when taken with this drug. Check with your pharmacist when selecting OTC products.

Taking this drug with any of the ones listed below may change the effect of either drug with the possibility of causing toxicity or decreasing effectiveness:
aminophylline, anesthetics†, antidiabetics†, caffeine, calcium channel blockers†, carbonic anhydrase inhibitors†, clonidine, digoxin, dyphylline, epinephrine, guanabenz, lidocaine, nonsteroidal antiinflammatories†, oxtriphylline, pilocarpine, reserpine, sympathomimetics†, theophylline, verapamil

Severe reactions are possible when this drug is taken with those listed below:
allergy shots, beta blockers†, cocaine, monoamine oxidase inhibitors†

Increased effects or side effects are possible when this drug is taken with those listed below:
antihypertensives†

ALLERGIC REACTIONS AND SIDE EFFECTS

If you are allergic to any other beta blockers†, you may also be allergic to this drug. This drug may exaggerate the reaction from your current allergies. Inform your doctor of any allergies that you have as well as the severity of the allergic reaction before starting this drug.

MORE COMMON SIDE EFFECTS: Dizziness*, drowsiness, lightheadedness*, sexual dysfunction, sleep disorders, tiredness, weakness

LESS COMMON SIDE EFFECTS: Anxiety, breathing difficulty*, cold hands or feet*, constipation, depression*, diarrhea, itching, nausea, nervousness, numbness, shortness of breath*, slow heartbeat*, sore eyes, stomachache, stuffy nose, swollen legs or feet, tingling, vivid dreams, vomiting, wheezing

RARE SIDE EFFECTS: Back pain*, bleeding*, bruising*, chest pain*, confusion*, fever*, hallucinations*, irregular heartbeat*, joint pain*, rash*, scaly skin*, sore throat*

PRECAUTIONS

People with asthma, heart disease, or a heart rate that is routinely less than 45 beats per minute (bradycardia) may not be able to take this drug.

Stopping this drug suddenly may cause chest pain or heart attack. If you wish to stop taking this drug, ask your doctor for specific instructions.

Be careful driving or handling equipment while taking this drug because the drug may cause drowsiness.

You need to wait 2 weeks after stopping a monoamine oxidase inhibitor† before starting this drug.

If you are diabetic, this drug may increase blood sugar levels or make the symptoms of low blood sugar less noticeable.

This drug may cause nondiabetics to develop type 2 diabetes.

If you have psoriasis or myasthenia gravis, this drug may make those conditions worse.

PREGNANCY AND BREAST-FEEDING

Safety during pregnancy has not been established although the drug is known to harm animal fetuses.

It is not known if this drug passes into breast milk. Talk to your doctor about the risks associated with breast-feeding while taking this drug.

HELPFUL COMMENTS

This drug may make you more sensitive to cold temperatures.

If you do not treat high blood pressure, you may develop more serious problems such as heart failure, blood vessel disease, stroke, or kidney disease. Losing weight, exercising, eating more fruits and vegetables, and avoiding salty foods, such as lunchmeat and pickles, may help make drug treatment more successful.

METRONIDAZOLE

Available for over 20 years

COMMONLY USED TO TREAT

Bedsores, also known as decubitus pressure ulcers

Crohn's disease

Infection

Pelvic inflammatory disease

Rosacea, also known as "adult acne"

---

† See page 52.   * See page 53.

DRUG CATEGORY

amebicide
antibiotic
antiprotozoal
Class: nitroimidazole

PRODUCTS

Brand-Name Products with No Generic Alternative
Flagyl 375 mg capsule ($$$)
Nortate 1% topical cream (¢¢¢¢)
Metrocream 0.75% topical cream (¢¢¢)
Metrogel 0.75% topical gel (¢¢¢)
Metrogel-Vaginal 0.75% vaginal gel (¢¢)
Metrolotion 0.75% topical lotion (¢¢)
Flagyl ER 750 mg extended-release tablet ($$$$)
Brand-Name Products with Generic Alternatives
Flagyl 250 mg tablet ($$)
  Generic: metronidazole 250 mg tablet (¢¢)
Flagyl 500 mg tablet ($$$)
  Generic: metronidazole 500 mg tablet (¢¢¢)
Other Generic Product Names
Metromidol
Combination Products That Contain This Drug
Helidac chewable tablets ($$)

DOSING AND FOOD

Oral doses are taken 1 to 3 times a day. Topical and vaginal products are
  used 2 to 3 times a day.
This drug may be taken with or without food, but taking this drug with
  food may avoid the stomach upset that some people suffer.
Adults: Up to 4,000 mg per day in divided doses.
Lower doses are used in children.
Forgotten doses: If you are scheduled to take the next dose within a few
  hours, do not take the forgotten dose. Otherwise take the forgotten dose
  as soon as you remember.

ALCOHOL, DRUG, HERB, AND SUPPLEMENT INTERACTIONS

Alcohol should not be used while taking this drug and for 3 days after the
  drug is stopped.

Taking this drug with any of the ones listed below may change the effect of either drug with the possibility of causing toxicity or decreasing effectiveness: anticoagulants†, barbiturates†, cimetidine, lithium, phenytoin

Severe reactions are possible when this drug is taken with those listed below: disulfiram

ALLERGIC REACTIONS AND SIDE EFFECTS

If you are allergic to clotrimazole or tioconazole, you may also be allergic to this drug. You should tell your doctor about all your allergies and any unexplained symptoms you may have while taking this drug.

MORE COMMON SIDE EFFECTS: Diarrhea, dizziness, headache, lightheadedness, loss of appetite, nausea*, stomach cramps, vomiting*

LESS COMMON SIDE EFFECTS: Back pain*, black stools*, bleeding*, bloody urine*, bruising*, clumsiness*, dry mouth, fever*, hives*, itching*, metallic taste, mood swings*, numbness*, pain*, redness*, skin irritation*, skin rash*, sore throat*, taste changes, tingling*, unsteadiness*, urinary changes*, vaginal discharge*, vaginal dryness*, vaginal irritation*, weakness*

RARE SIDE EFFECTS: Seizures*

PRECAUTIONS

Do not crush, break, or chew the extended-release products.

People with a history of seizures are at greater risk of developing a seizure while taking this drug.

If you have a history of blood disease, vaginal yeast infection, or oral thrush, this drug may make those conditions worse.

Be careful driving or handling equipment while taking this drug because it may cause dizziness.

Vaginal gel is absorbed into the body and carries the same warning and precautions as the oral products. When applied topically, only a small amount of drug is absorbed into the body. Most of the warnings and precautions in the summary do not apply to topical products.

When used to treat vaginal infections, this drug does not prevent transmission of the disease. A barrier contraceptive should be used to avoid spread of the infection.

PREGNANCY AND BREAST-FEEDING

Safety during pregnancy has not been established although there was no evidence of harm during studies in animals.

Breast-feeding while taking this drug is not recommended.

---

† See page 52.   * See page 53.

HELPFUL COMMENTS

Contact your doctor if your symptoms do not improve after a couple of days.

Do not stop treatment early if you start to feel better. It takes the full prescription for this drug to work completely.

Sucking on hard sugarless candy or chewing sugarless gum may help relieve dry mouth caused by this drug.

Avoid quick movements to minimize dizziness. Dangling your legs over the side of the bed for a few minutes may help reduce dizziness when first waking up.

MEXILETINE

Available since December 1985

COMMONLY USED TO TREAT

Irregular heartbeat, also known as arrhythmias

DRUG CATEGORY

antiarrhythmic
Class: sodium channel blocker

PRODUCTS

Brand-Name Products with Generic Alternatives
Mexitil 150 mg capsule ($)
  Generic: mexiletine 150 mg capsule (¢¢¢)
Mexitil 200 mg capsule ($)
  Generic: mexiletine 200 mg capsule (¢¢¢¢¢)
Mexitil 250 mg capsule ($$)
  Generic: mexiletine 250 mg capsule (¢¢¢¢¢)

DOSING AND FOOD

Doses are taken 2 to 4 times a day.

This drug may be taken with or without food but is best taken with food to reduce the stomach upset that some people suffer.

Adults: Up to 1,200 mg per day in divided doses.

Lower doses are used in children.

Forgotten doses: If more than 4 hours have passed since the forgotten dose, do not take the dose. Otherwise take the forgotten dose as soon as you remember.

ALCOHOL, DRUG, HERB, AND SUPPLEMENT INTERACTIONS

Alcohol may increase some of the side effects from this drug, depending on the amount consumed. Ask your doctor about the risks caused by drinking alcohol with your condition.

Several OTC drugs used for appetite control, asthma, colds, cough, hay fever, pain, or sinus problems may seriously increase the side effects of this drug. Check with your pharmacist when selecting OTC products.

Taking this drug with any of the ones listed below may change the effect of either drug with the possibility of causing toxicity or decreasing effectiveness:
ammonium chloride, antacids, atropine, carbonic anhydrase inhibitors†, cimetidine, metoclopramide, narcotics†, phenobarbital, phenytoin, rifampin, theophylline

ALLERGIC REACTIONS AND SIDE EFFECTS

If you are allergic to lidocaine or tocainide, you may also be allergic to this drug. You should tell your doctor about all your allergies and any unexplained symptoms you may have while taking this drug.

MORE COMMON SIDE EFFECTS: Dizziness, heartburn, lightheadedness, nausea, nervousness, shaky hands*, trembling, unsteadiness*, vomiting

LESS COMMON SIDE EFFECTS: Blurry vision, chest pain*, confusion, constipation, diarrhea, headache, irregular heartbeat*, numbness, ringing in ears, shortness of breath*, skin rash, sleep disorders, slurry speech, tingling, tiredness, weakness

RARE SIDE EFFECTS: Bleeding*, bruising*, chills*, fever*, seizures*

PRECAUTIONS

People with a history of seizures are at greater risk of developing a seizure while taking this drug.

If you have low blood pressure or congestive heart failure, this drug may make those conditions worse.

Be careful driving or handling equipment while taking this drug because it may cause dizziness.

PREGNANCY AND BREAST-FEEDING

Safety during pregnancy has not been established although the drug is known to harm animal fetuses.

Breast-feeding while taking this drug is not recommended.

---

† See page 52.   * See page 53.

HELPFUL COMMENTS

If you need to take an antacid, take it either 1 hour before or after taking this drug.

Avoid quick movements to minimize dizziness. Dangling your legs over the side of the bed for a few minutes may help reduce dizziness when first waking up.

It takes 2 to 3 days for the full effect of this drug to be noticed.

If your condition is stable and you are taking this drug 3 times a day, talk to your doctor about changing the schedule to every 12 hours.

MIDODRINE HYDROCHLORIDE

Available since September 1996

COMMONLY USED TO TREAT

Low blood pressure, also known as hypotension

DRUG CATEGORY

antihypotensive
Class: vasopressor

PRODUCTS

Brand-Name Products with No Generic Alternative
Proamatine 2.5 mg tablet ($)
Proamatine 5 mg tablet ($$)
Proamatine 10 mg tablet (n/a)
No generics available.
Exclusivity until 2003.

DOSING AND FOOD

Doses are taken 3 times a day, usually when first waking, mid-morning, and mid-afternoon.

This drug may be taken with or without food.

Adults: Up to 30 mg per day in divided doses.

Forgotten doses: If you are scheduled to take the next dose within a few hours, do not take the forgotten dose. Otherwise take the forgotten dose as soon as you remember.

ALCOHOL, DRUG, HERB, AND SUPPLEMENT INTERACTIONS

Alcohol may cause your blood pressure to rise, increasing the risk of side effects from this drug. Ask your doctor about the risks caused by drinking alcohol with your condition.

Several OTC drugs used for asthma, colds, cough, hay fever, sleep aid, or sinus problems may seriously change the effects of this drug. Check with your pharmacist when selecting OTC products.

Taking this drug with any of the ones listed below may change the effect of either drug with the possibility of causing toxicity or decreasing effectiveness: alpha adrenergic blockers†, digitoxin, digoxin, dihydroergotamine, ephedrine, fludrocortisone, phenylephrine, pheylpropanolamine, pseudoephedrine

ALLERGIC REACTIONS AND SIDE EFFECTS

You should tell your doctor about all your allergies and any unexplained symptoms you may have while taking this drug.

MORE COMMON SIDE EFFECTS: Blurry vision*, burning, chills, goosebumps, headache*, itching, pounding in ears*, urinary changes

LESS COMMON SIDE EFFECTS: Anxiety, confusion, dry mouth, flushing, headache, nervousness, skin rash

RARE SIDE EFFECTS: Backache, dizziness*, drowsiness, dry skin, fainting*, gas, heartburn, leg cramps, lip sores, nausea, sensitivity to touch, sleep disorders, slow pulse*, vision changes, weakness

PRECAUTIONS

Do not lie down for 3 to 4 hours after taking a dose of this drug since it may cause extreme elevation in blood pressure.

If you have heart disease, high blood pressure, bladder problems, high thyroid levels, or vision problems, this drug may make those conditions worse.

This drug may cause dry mouth, which is associated with a greater risk of cavities. Your dentist may recommend that you clean your teeth and mouth differently to avoid infection.

Be careful driving or handling equipment while taking this drug because it may cause blurry vision.

PREGNANCY AND BREAST-FEEDING

Safety during pregnancy has not been established although the drug is known to harm animal fetuses.

It is not known if this drug passes into breast milk. Talk to your doctor about the risks associated with breast-feeding while taking this drug.

---

† *See page 52.*   * *See page 53.*

HELPFUL COMMENTS

The last dose of the day should be taken before 6 P.M. to avoid side effects associated with laying down too soon after a dose.

You may need to sleep with extra pillows under your head to avoid side effects such as pounding in the ears.

Sucking on hard sugarless candy or chewing sugarless gum may help relieve dry mouth caused by this drug.

MIGLITOL

Available since December 1996

COMMONLY USED TO TREAT

High blood sugar, specifically type 2 diabetes

DRUG CATEGORY

antidiabetic
Class: alphaglucosidase Inhibitor

PRODUCTS

Brand-Name Products with No Generic Alternative
Glyset 25 mg tablet (¢¢¢¢)
Glyset 50 mg tablet (¢¢¢¢)
Glyset 100 mg tablet (¢¢¢¢¢)
No generics available.
Patent expires in 2009.

DOSING AND FOOD

Doses are taken 3 times a day.
Always take your dose with the first bite of each meal.
Adults: Up to 300 mg per day in divided doses.
Lower doses may be needed in people with kidney disease.
Forgotten doses: If you have finished eating your meal, do not take a forgotten dose. Just go back to your usual schedule with the next dose.

ALCOHOL, DRUG, HERB, AND SUPPLEMENT INTERACTIONS

Alcohol may cause a change in your blood sugar, altering the effects of this drug. Ask your doctor about the risks caused by drinking alcohol with your condition.

Aloe, bilberry leaf, bitter melon, burdock, dandelion, fenugreek, garlic, ginkgo biloba, and ginseng may lower blood sugar and cause the need for a dose adjustment when taken with this drug. Tell your doctor if you are taking any of these supplements.

Taking this drug with any of the ones listed below may change the effect of either drug with the possibility of causing toxicity or decreasing effectiveness: amylase, charcoal, digoxin, pancreatin, propranolol, ranitidine

ALLERGIC REACTIONS AND SIDE EFFECTS

You should tell your doctor about all your allergies and any unexplained symptoms you may have while taking this drug.

MORE COMMON SIDE EFFECTS: Abdominal pain, bloating, gas, loose stools, soft stools

LESS COMMON SIDE EFFECTS: Skin rash

PRECAUTIONS

People with inflammatory bowel disease, intestinal problems, or digestive problems may not be able to take this drug.

If you are anemic, this drug may make that condition worse.

Blood glucose levels may be measured 1 hour after eating to evaluate the effectiveness of this drug.

Burns, diarrhea, fever, hormonal changes, infection, malnourishment, severe stress, uncontrolled thyroid disease, and vomiting may cause changes in blood sugar that may make this drug less effective.

PREGNANCY AND BREAST-FEEDING

Safety during pregnancy has not been established although there was no evidence of harm during studies in animals.

Breast-feeding while taking this drug is not recommended.

HELPFUL COMMENTS

The side effects of this drug are usually noticed for 1 to 2 weeks after starting the drug, but may then start to go away.

If you do not treat high blood sugar, you may develop more serious problems such as heart failure, blood vessel disease, eye disease, or kidney disease.

---

† See page 52. * See page 53.

MINOCYCLINE HYDROCHLORIDE

Available for over 20 years

COMMONLY USED TO TREAT

Infection

DRUG CATEGORY

antibiotic
Class: tetracycline

PRODUCTS

Brand-Name Products with No Generic Alternative
Arestin 1 mg extended-release dental powder (n/a)
Brand-Name Products with Generic Alternatives
Minocin 50 mg capsule ($$)
  Generic: minocycline hydrochloride 50 mg capsule (¢¢¢¢)
Minocin 75 mg capsule (n/a)
  Generic: minocycline hydrochloride 75 mg capsule ($$)
Minocin 100 mg capsule ($$$)
  Generic: minocycline hydrochloride 100 mg capsule (¢¢¢¢¢)
Other Generic Product Names
Vectrin

DOSING AND FOOD

Doses are taken 2 to 4 times a day.
This drug may be taken with or without food although dairy products may
  decrease the drug absorption and should not be taken at the same time.
Adults: Up to 200 mg per day in divided doses.
Children over age 8: Up to 4 mg/kg per day in divided doses.
This drug is not used in children under age 8 because of potential damage
  to developing teeth and bones.
Forgotten doses: If you are scheduled to take the next dose within a few
  hours, do not take the forgotten dose. Otherwise take the forgotten dose
  as soon as you remember.

ALCOHOL, DRUG, HERB, AND SUPPLEMENT INTERACTIONS

Alcohol may increase some of the side effects from this drug, depending
  on the amount consumed. Ask your doctor about the risks caused by
  drinking alcohol with your condition.

Many OTC drugs, including antacids, laxatives, and mineral supplements such as calcium, magnesium or iron, may decrease the effects of this drug when taken at the same time as the drug. If you need to take an OTC drug take it either 2 hours before or after taking this drug.

Taking this drug with any of the ones listed below may change the effect of either drug with the possibility of causing toxicity or decreasing effectiveness: antacids, anticoagulants†, calcium supplements, cholestyramine, cimetidine, colestipol, digoxin, iron supplements, mineral supplements, oral contraceptives, penicillins, sodium bicarbonate, zinc

Severe reactions are possible when this drug is taken with those listed below: methoxyflurane, tetracycline

ALLERGIC REACTIONS AND SIDE EFFECTS

If you are allergic to any tetracyclines†, you may also be allergic to this drug. You should tell your doctor about all your allergies and any unexplained symptoms you may have while taking this drug.

This drug promotes the effect of sunlight on the body and may cause severe sunburn and increased sensitivity of the eyes. This effect may last as long as 2 to 4 weeks after the drug is stopped.

MORE COMMON SIDE EFFECTS: Diarrhea, dizziness, lightheadedness, stomach cramps, sun sensitivity*, unsteadiness

LESS COMMON SIDE EFFECTS: Genital itching, rectal itch, skin discoloration*, sore mouth

RARE SIDE EFFECTS: Abdominal pain*, headache*, loss of appetite*, nausea*, vomiting*, visual changes*, yellow eyes or skin*

PRECAUTIONS

Be careful driving or handling equipment while taking this drug because the drug may cause dizziness.

People with kidney disease have a greater risk of developing side effects.

This drug decomposes after the expiration date and may be harmful if taken. Make sure you destroy any leftover capsules as soon as you are done with the prescription.

Some people get a discolored tongue when taking this drug, but the coloring will return to normal when the drug is stopped.

Do not crush, open, or break the capsules.

PREGNANCY AND BREAST-FEEDING

This drug may cause toxic effects to the fetus and should not be used during pregnancy.

---

† See page 52.   * See page 53.

Breast-feeding while taking this drug is not recommended.

HELPFUL COMMENTS

Oral contraceptives may not work properly when taken with this drug. You need to use a barrier contraceptive, such as a condom, or other nonhormonal contraceptive to prevent pregnancy.

Contact your doctor if your symptoms do not improve after a couple of days. Do not stop treatment early if you start to feel better. It takes the full prescription for this drug to work completely.

MINOXIDIL

Available for over 20 years

COMMONLY USED TO TREAT

High blood pressure, also known as hypertension

DRUG CATEGORY

antihypertensive
Class: peripheral vasodilator

PRODUCTS

Brand-Name Products with Generic Alternatives
Loniten 2.5 mg tablet (¢¢¢¢¢)
  Generic: minoxidil 2.5 mg tablet (¢¢¢)
Loniten 10 mg tablet ($$)
  Generic: minoxidil 10 mg tablet (¢¢¢)

DOSING AND FOOD

Doses are taken once a day.
This drug may be taken with or without food.
Adults and children over age 12: Up to 100 mg per day.
Children under age 12: Up to 1 mg/kg (maximum 50 mg) per day.
Forgotten doses: If you are scheduled to take the next dose within 3 to 4 hours, do not take the forgotten dose. Otherwise take the forgotten dose as soon as you remember.

ALCOHOL, DRUG, HERB, AND SUPPLEMENT INTERACTIONS

Alcohol may cause your blood pressure to rise, making this drug less effective. Ask your doctor about the risks caused by drinking alcohol with your condition.

Several OTC drugs used for appetite control, asthma, colds, cough, hay fever, or sinus problems may cause an increase in blood pressure when taken with this drug. Check with your pharmacist when selecting OTC products.

Taking this drug with any of the ones listed below may change the effect of either drug with the possibility of causing toxicity or decreasing effectiveness: diuretics†, guanethidine, nitrates†

ALLERGIC REACTIONS AND SIDE EFFECTS

You should tell your doctor about all your allergies and any unexplained symptoms you may have while taking this drug.

MORE COMMON SIDE EFFECTS: Bloating*, flushing*, hair growth increase, irregular heartbeat*, skin redness*, swelling*, weight gain*

LESS COMMON SIDE EFFECTS: Breast tenderness, chest pain*, headache, numbness*, shortness of breath*, tingling*

RARE SIDE EFFECTS: Itching*, skin rash*

PRECAUTIONS

Record your weight each day while taking this drug. A weight gain or loss of more than 5 pounds per day (2 pounds per day in children) should be reported to your doctor.

If you have a history of chest pains, this drug may make that condition worse.

This drug may cause fluid retention, which may be harmful in people with heart disease or blood vessel disease.

Learn how to measure your heart rate when resting and track it on a daily basis. Call your doctor if it rises 20 beats per minute above the usual.

PREGNANCY AND BREAST-FEEDING

Safety during pregnancy has not been established although the drug is known to harm animal fetuses.

Breast-feeding while taking this drug is not recommended.

HELPFUL COMMENTS

This drug may cause an increase in hair growth, but growth will return to normal within 6 months of stopping the drug.

If you do not treat high blood pressure, you may develop more serious problems such as heart failure, blood vessel disease, stroke, or kidney disease. Losing weight, exercising, eating more fruits and vegetables, and avoiding salty foods, such as lunchmeat and pickles, may help make drug treatment more successful.

† See page 52.   * See page 53.

MIRTAZAPINE

Available since June 1996

COMMONLY USED TO TREAT

Depression

DRUG CATEGORY

antidepressant
Class: tetracyclic antidepressant

PRODUCTS

Brand-Name Products with No Generic Alternative
Remeron 45 mg tablet ($$$)
Remeron Soltab 15 mg disintegrating tablet ($$$)
Remeron Soltab 30 mg disintegrating tablet ($$$)
Remeron Soltab 45 mg disintegrating tablet ($$$)

Brand-Name Products with Generic Alternatives
Remeron 15 mg tablet ($$$)
  Generic: mirtazapine 15 mg tablet (n/a)
Remeron 30 mg tablet ($$$)
  Generic: mirtazapine 30 mg tablet (n/a)

DOSING AND FOOD

Doses are taken once a day just before bedtime.

This drug may be taken with or without food. Do not eat raw oysters or other raw shellfish at any time while taking this drug.

Adults: Up to 45 mg per day.

Forgotten doses: If more than 8 hours have passed since the forgotten dose, do not take the forgotten dose. Otherwise take the forgotten dose as soon as you remember.

ALCOHOL, DRUG, HERB, AND SUPPLEMENT INTERACTIONS

Alcohol should not be used while taking this drug.

Many OTC drugs used for appetite control, asthma, colds, cough, hay fever, pain, or sinus problems affect the central nervous system and may cause serious side effects when taken with this drug. Check with your pharmacist for products to avoid.

Taking this drug with any of the ones listed below may change the effect of either drug with the possibility of causing toxicity or decreasing effectiveness: alcohol, analgesics, anesthetics, antihistamines†, anxiolytics†, barbiturates†, narcotics†

Severe reactions are possible when this drug is taken with those listed below: monoamine oxidase inhibitors†

ALLERGIC REACTIONS AND SIDE EFFECTS

You should tell your doctor about all your allergies and any unexplained symptoms you may have while taking this drug.

MORE COMMON SIDE EFFECTS: Constipation, dizziness, drowsiness, dry mouth, increased appetite, weight gain

LESS COMMON SIDE EFFECTS: Abdominal pain, abnormal thinking*, agitation*, anxiety*, back pain, confusion*, fainting, low blood pressure, mood swings*, motionlessness*, muscle pain, nausea, nightmares, shaking, shortness of breath*, skin rash*, swelling*, thirst, trembling, urinary changes, vomiting, weakness

RARE SIDE EFFECTS: Anger*, chills*, excitement*, fever*, hallucinations*, menstrual pain*, missed periods*, mouth sores*, seizures*, sexual dysfunction*, sore throat*

PRECAUTIONS

You need to wait 2 weeks after stopping a monoamine oxidase inhibitor† before starting this drug.

People with a history of seizures have a greater risk of developing a seizure while taking this drug.

Liver function should be tested periodically while taking this drug.

The oral disintegrating tablets may contain aspartame, which should not be taken by people with phenylketonuria (PKU).

Disintegrating tablets should be placed on top of the tongue for a few seconds, then swallowed with saliva.

This drug causes changes in your blood that put you at greater risk of getting an infection. Be careful not to cut yourself or get bruised. Tell your doctor if you develop signs of infection, such as fever or sore throat. Your dentist may recommend that you clean your teeth and mouth differently to avoid infection.

Be careful driving or handling equipment while taking this drug because the drug may cause dizziness and drowsiness.

---

†See page 52. *See page 53.

This drug may cause dry mouth, which is associated with a greater risk of cavities. Your dentist may recommend that you clean your teeth and mouth differently to avoid infection.

PREGNANCY AND BREAST-FEEDING

Safety during pregnancy has not been established although the drug is known to harm animal fetuses.

It is not known if this drug passes into breast milk. Talk to your doctor about the risks associated with breast-feeding while taking this drug.

HELPFUL COMMENTS

Disintegrating tablets may fall apart if pushed through the foil when removing from the packaging. Instead, the foil should be peeled back to open.

Sucking on hard sugarless candy or chewing sugarless gum may help relieve dry mouth caused by this drug.

Avoid quick movements to minimize dizziness. Dangling your legs over the side of the bed for a few minutes may help reduce dizziness when first waking up.

MISOPROSTOL

Available since December 1988

COMMONLY USED TO TREAT

People at risk of developing stomach ulcers from taking nonsteroidal anti-inflammatories†

DRUG CATEGORY

antiulcer
gastric mucosal protectant
Class: prostaglandin E1 analogue

PRODUCTS

Brand-Name Products with Generic Alternatives
Cytotec 0.1 mg tablet (¢¢¢¢¢)
  Generic: misoprostol 0.1 mg tablet (n/a)
Cytotec 0.2 mg tablet ($)
  Generic: misoprostol 0.2 mg tablet (n/a)
Combination Products That Contain This Drug
Arthrotec delayed-release tablet ($$)

DOSING AND FOOD

Doses are taken 4 times a day.

It is best to take this drug with meals and at bedtime.

Adults: Up to 0.8 mg per day in divided doses.

Forgotten doses: If you are scheduled to take the next dose within a few hours, do not take the forgotten dose. Otherwise take the forgotten dose as soon as you remember.

ALCOHOL, DRUG, HERB, AND SUPPLEMENT INTERACTIONS

Alcohol may increase some of the side effects from this drug, depending on the amount consumed. Ask your doctor about the risks caused by drinking alcohol with your condition.

Antacids and other OTC products containing magnesium may increase the risk of side effects from this drug and should not be used.

ALLERGIC REACTIONS AND SIDE EFFECTS

You should tell your doctor about all your allergies and any unexplained symptoms you may have while taking this drug.

MORE COMMON SIDE EFFECTS: Abdominal pain*, diarrhea*

LESS COMMON SIDE EFFECTS: Constipation*, gas*, headache*, heartburn*, indigestion*, nausea*, stomach cramps*, vaginal bleeding*, vomiting*

RARE SIDE EFFECTS: Breathing difficulty*, drowsiness*, fever*, irregular heartbeat*, low blood pressure*, seizures*, slow heartbeat*, tremor*

PRECAUTIONS

People with a history of seizures are at greater risk of developing a seizure while taking this drug.

If you have blood vessel disease, this drug may make that condition worse.

PREGNANCY AND BREAST-FEEDING

This drug may cause miscarriage in pregnant women.

This drug may cause birth defects and should not be used during pregnancy.

Breast-feeding while taking this drug is not recommended.

HELPFUL COMMENTS

Many of the intestinal side effects begin to go away after this drug has been taken for a few days. Call your doctor if diarrhea continues for over a week.

---

† See page 52.   * See page 53.

MODAFINIL

Available since December 1988

COMMONLY USED TO TREAT

Sudden sleeping attacks, also known as narcolepsy

DRUG CATEGORY

analeptic
Class: CNS stimulant: nonamphetamine

PRODUCTS

Brand-Name Products with No Generic Alternative
Provigil 100 mg tablet ($$$)
Provigil 200 mg tablet ($$$$)
No generics available.
Multiple patents that begin to expire in 2007. Exclusivity until 2005.

DOSING AND FOOD

Doses are taken once a day in the morning.
This drug may be taken with or without food.
Adults: Up to 200 mg per day.
Lower doses are used in people with liver disease.
Forgotten doses: If more than 4 hours have passed since the forgotten
dose, do not take the dose. Otherwise take the forgotten dose as soon as
you remember.

ALCOHOL, DRUG, HERB, AND SUPPLEMENT INTERACTIONS

Alcohol should not be used while taking this drug.
Several OTC drugs used for asthma, colds, cough, hay fever, sleep aid, or
sinus problems may seriously increase the side effects of this drug. Check
with your pharmacist when selecting OTC products.

Taking this drug with any of the ones listed below may change the effect of
either drug with the possibility of causing toxicity or decreasing effectiveness:
carbamazepine, cyclosporine, diazepam, itraconazole, ketoconazole,
methylphenidate, oral contraceptives, phenobarbital, propranolol,
rifampin, theophylline, tricyclic antidepressants†, warfarin

Increased side effects are possible when this drug is taken with those listed below:
amantadine, amphetamines†, bupropion, caffeine, chlophedianol, co-
caine, nabilone, pemoline

ALLERGIC REACTIONS AND SIDE EFFECTS

If you are allergic to methylphenidate or dextroamphetamine, you may also be allergic to this drug. You should tell your doctor about all your allergies and any unexplained symptoms you may have while taking this drug.

MORE COMMON SIDE EFFECTS: Anxiety, headache, nausea, nervousness, runny nose, sleep disorders*

LESS COMMON SIDE EFFECTS: Diarrhea, dry mouth, dry skin, loss of appetite, shaking, skin irritation, stiffness, tingling, trembling, vomiting

RARE SIDE EFFECTS: Agitation*, blurry vision*, chills*, clumsiness*, confusion*, depression*, dizziness*, excitement*, fainting*, fever*, increased blood pressure*, irregular heartbeat*, memory loss*, mood swings*, mouth movements*, shortness of breath*, sore throat*, thirst*, tongue movement*, unsteadiness*, urinary difficulty*, vision changes*

PRECAUTIONS

If you have a history of mental illness, this drug may make that condition worse.

Be careful driving or handling equipment while taking this drug because it may cause dizziness.

People with heart disease may not be able to take this drug.

Call your doctor right away if you develop hives or a rash while taking this drug, since they may be signs of allergy.

PREGNANCY AND BREAST-FEEDING

Safety during pregnancy has not been established although the drug is known to harm animal fetuses.

It is not known if this drug passes into breast milk. Talk to your doctor about the risks associated with breast-feeding while taking this drug.

HELPFUL COMMENTS

Oral contraceptives may not work properly when taken with this drug. You need to use a barrier contraceptive, such as a condom, or other nonhormonal contraceptive to prevent pregnancy while taking this drug and for 1 month after the drug is stopped.

The effects of this drug are noticed quicker if taken on an empty stomach.

† See page 52.   * See page 53.

MOEXIPRIL HYDROCHLORIDE

Available since April 1995

COMMONLY USED TO TREAT

High blood pressure, also known as hypertension

DRUG CATEGORY

antihypertensive
Class: ACE inhibitor

PRODUCTS

Brand-Name Products with No Generic Alternative
Univasc 7.5 mg tablet (¢¢¢¢¢)
Univasc 15 mg tablet (¢¢¢¢¢)
No generics available.
Patent expires in 2007.

Combination Products That Contain This Drug
Uniretic tablet (¢¢¢¢¢)

DOSING AND FOOD

Doses are taken 1 to 2 times a day.
It is best to take this drug on an empty stomach at least 1 hour before
meals.
Adults: Up to 30 mg per day in divided doses.
Lower doses are used in people with kidney disease.
This drug is rarely used in children.
Forgotten doses: If you are scheduled to take the next dose within a few
hours, do not take the forgotten dose. Otherwise take the forgotten dose
as soon as you remember.

ALCOHOL, DRUG, HERB, AND SUPPLEMENT INTERACTIONS

Alcohol may cause your blood pressure to rise, making this drug less effective. Ask your doctor about the risks caused by drinking alcohol with
your condition.
Black catechu should not be used with this drug because there is an
increased risk of lowering the blood pressure too much.
Licorice may interfere with the effects of this drug.
Capsaicin and other foods or supplements, including hot peppers, sweet
peppers, paprika, and chili powder, derived from the capsicum family of

plants may increase the risk of developing a cough and should not be
taken with this drug.

Several OTC drugs used for appetite control, asthma, colds, cough, hay
fever, or sinus problems may cause an increase in blood pressure when
taken with this drug. Check with your pharmacist when selecting OTC
products.

**Taking this drug with any of the ones listed below may change the effect of
either drug with the possibility of causing toxicity or decreasing effectiveness:**
antacids, antidiabetics†, antihypertensives†, digoxin, diuretics†, insulin,
lithium, nonsteroidal antiinflammatories†, potassium supplements

ALLERGIC REACTIONS AND SIDE EFFECTS

If you are allergic to any ACE inhibitors†, you may also be allergic to this
drug. You should tell your doctor about all your allergies and any unexplained symptoms you may have while taking this drug.

More Common Side Effects: Dry cough, headache

Less Common Side Effects: Diarrhea, dizziness*, fainting*, fever*, joint
pain*, lightheadedness*, loss of taste, nausea, skin rash*, tiredness

Rare Side Effects: Abdominal pain*, breathing difficulty*, chest pain*,
chills*, confusion*, hoarseness*, irregular heartbeat*, itching*, nausea*,
nervousness*, numbness*, stomach pain*, swallowing difficulty*, swelling*, vomiting*, weakness*, yellow eyes or skin*

PRECAUTIONS

Be careful driving or handling equipment while taking this drug because
the drug may cause dizziness.

People with systemic lupus erythematosus may be at greater risk of developing blood problems while taking this drug.

Do not use potassium-containing products, including salt substitutes, while
taking this drug.

Diuretics† should be stopped 2 to 3 days prior to starting this drug. If it is
not possible to stop the diuretic, the dose of this drug should be lowered.

Drink plenty of fluids to avoid dehydration when sweating, such as in hot
weather and during exercise.

PREGNANCY AND BREAST-FEEDING

Safety during pregnancy has not been established although the drug is
known to harm animal fetuses.

Breast-feeding while taking this drug is not recommended.

---

† See page 52.   * See page 53.

HELPFUL COMMENTS

It may take several weeks before the full effects of this drug are noticed.

A persistent dry cough may appear while taking this drug, but it will go away when the drug is stopped.

If you need to take an antacid, take it either 2 hours before or after taking this drug.

Avoid quick movements to minimize dizziness. Dangling your legs over the side of the bed for a few minutes may help reduce dizziness when first waking up.

MOLINDONE HYDROCHLORIDE

Available for over 20 years

COMMONLY USED TO TREAT

Mental retardation
Psychosis

DRUG CATEGORY

antipsychotic
Class: dihydroindolone

PRODUCTS

Brand-Name Products with No Generic Alternative
Moban 5 mg tablet ($)
Moban 10 mg tablet ($$)
Moban 25 mg tablet ($$$)
Moban 50 mg tablet ($$$)
Moban 100 mg tablet ($$$)
Moban 20 mg/ml oral concentrate ($$$$$)
No generics available.
No patents, no exclusivity.

DOSING AND FOOD

Doses are taken 3 to 4 times a day.

This drug may be taken with or without food but is best taken with a full glass of water or milk to reduce the stomach upset that some people suffer.

Adults: Up to 225 mg per day in divided doses.

Lower doses are used in children and adults over age 65.

Forgotten doses: If you are scheduled to take the next dose within 2 hours, do not take the forgotten dose. Otherwise take the forgotten dose as soon as you remember.

ALCOHOL, DRUG, HERB, AND SUPPLEMENT INTERACTIONS

Alcohol should not be used while taking this drug.

Several OTC drugs used for asthma, colds, cough, hay fever, sleep aid, or sinus problems may seriously change the side effects of this drug. Check with your pharmacist when selecting OTC products.

Taking this drug with any of the ones listed below may change the effect of either drug with the possibility of causing toxicity or decreasing effectiveness:

amoxapine, antipsychotics†, beta blockers†, bromocriptine, clonidine, dopamine, guanabenz, guanadrel, guanethidine, levodopa, methyldopa, metoclopramide, metyrosine, pemoline, phenytoin, pimozide, promethazine, rauwolfia alkaloids†, reserpine, tetracycline, trimeprazine

Severe reactions are possible when this drug is taken with those listed below:

analgesics, anesthetics, antiarrhythmics†, anticholinergics†, antidepressants†, antidyskinetics†, antihistamines†, anxiolytics†, barbiturates†, disopyramide, lithium, magnesium sulfate, meperidine, metrizamide, monoamine oxidase inhibitors†, narcotics†, phenothiazines†, procainamide, quinidine

Increased side effects are possible when this drug is taken with those listed below:

nitrates†, propylthiouracil, sympathomimetics†

ALLERGIC REACTIONS AND SIDE EFFECTS

If you are allergic to any phenothiazines†, thioxanthenes†, haloperidol, or loxapine, you may also be allergic to this drug. You should tell your doctor about all your allergies and any unexplained symptoms you may have while taking this drug.

This drug promotes the effect of sunlight on the body and may cause severe sunburn and increased sensitivity of the eyes.

MORE COMMON SIDE EFFECTS: Blurry vision, chewing motion*, constipation, dizziness, drowsiness, dry mouth, emotionless face*, eye stillness*, headache, lack of sweat, lightheadedness, lip smacking*, muscle spasms*, nausea, puffy cheeks*, restlessness*, shaky hands*, shuffling walk*, spastic movements*, speech dysfunction*, stiffness*, stuffy nose, swallowing difficulty*, tongue movements*, trembling*, urinary difficulty

---

† See page 52.   * See page 53.

LESS COMMON SIDE EFFECTS: Breast-milk secretion, breast swelling, depression*, menstrual changes, sexual dysfunction

RARE SIDE EFFECTS: Blood pressure change*, confusion*, dry skin*, fever*, irregular heartbeat*, pale skin*, poor bladder control*, rapid breathing*, seizures*, skin rash*, stiffness*, sweating*, tiredness*, weakness*, yellow eyes or skin*

PRECAUTIONS

This drug makes you sweat less, putting you at greater risk of developing heatstroke. Avoid exercising in hot weather and using hot tubs or saunas.

If you have urinary problems, enlarged prostate, glaucoma, liver disease, or Parkinson's disease, this drug may make those conditions worse.

The oral concentrate product contains sodium metabisulfite, which may cause an allergic reaction in sulfite-sensitive people.

Be careful driving or handling equipment while taking this drug because it may cause dizziness, drowsiness, and blurry vision.

Your urine may turn pink or brown in color while taking this drug.

This drug may cause false positive results in urine pregnancy tests.

Touching the oral concentrate solution may cause skin irritation. You should wash your hands immediately after taking the dose.

This drug may cause dry mouth, which is associated with a greater risk of cavities. Your dentist may recommend that you clean your teeth and mouth differently to avoid infection.

PREGNANCY AND BREAST-FEEDING

Safety during pregnancy has not been established although the drug is known to harm animal fetuses.

It is not known if this drug passes into breast milk. Talk to your doctor about the risks associated with breast-feeding while taking this drug.

HELPFUL COMMENTS

The oral concentrate product should be mixed with about 1/4 to 1/2 cup of fruit juice, soup, milk, pudding, water, or soda just before taking a dose.

It may take several weeks before the full effects of this drug are noticed.

If you need to take an antacid or diarrhea drug, take it either 2 hours before or after taking this drug.

Sucking on hard sugarless candy or chewing sugarless gum may help relieve dry mouth caused by this drug.

Avoid quick movements to minimize dizziness. Dangling your legs over the side of the bed for a few minutes may help reduce dizziness when first waking up.

Eye irritation caused by the sun may be reduced by wearing sunglasses when outside.

MONTELUKAST SODIUM

Available since February 1998

COMMONLY USED TO TREAT

People with asthma to prevent an attack

DRUG CATEGORY

antiasthmatic
Class: leukotriene receptor antagonist

PRODUCTS

Brand-Name Products with No Generic Alternative
Singulair 10 mg tablet ($$$)
Singulair 4 mg chewable tablet ($$$)
Singulair 5 mg chewable tablet ($$$)
Singulair 4 mg granule packet (n/a)
No generics available.
Patents expire in 2012. Exclusivity begins to expire in 2003.

DOSING AND FOOD

Doses are taken once a day in the evening.
This drug may be taken with or without food.
Adults and children over age 15: Up to 10 mg per day.
Children age 6 to 14: Up to 5 mg per day.
Children age 2 to 5: Up to 4 mg per day.
Forgotten doses: If you are scheduled to take the next dose within a few hours, do not take the forgotten dose. Otherwise take the forgotten dose as soon as you remember.

ALCOHOL, DRUG, HERB, AND SUPPLEMENT INTERACTIONS

Alcohol may increase some of the side effects from this drug, depending on the amount consumed. Ask your doctor about the risks caused by drinking alcohol with your condition.

---

† See page 52.   * See page 53.

Taking this drug with any of the ones listed below may change the effect of either drug with the possibility of causing toxicity or decreasing effectiveness: phenobarbital, rifampin

ALLERGIC REACTIONS AND SIDE EFFECTS

You should tell your doctor about all your allergies and any unexplained symptoms you may have while taking this drug.

MORE COMMON SIDE EFFECTS: Headache

LESS COMMON SIDE EFFECTS: Abdominal pain, cough, dental pain, dizziness, fever, heartburn, skin rash, congestion, tiredness, weakness

PRECAUTIONS

This drug is used to prevent asthma attacks but is NOT effective in treating an attack that has already started.

Chewable tablets contain aspartame and should not be used in people with phenylketonuria.

Tell your dentist that you are taking this drug and talk about the risk and treatment of dental pain that may occur while taking this drug.

Granules may be either placed directly in the mouth and swallowed, or mixed with cold or room-temperature food. Doses mixed with food must be taken within 15 minutes or they will begin to go bad.

PREGNANCY AND BREAST-FEEDING

Safety during pregnancy has not been established although there was no evidence of harm during studies in animals.

It is not known if this drug passes into breast milk. Talk to your doctor about the risks associated with breast-feeding while taking this drug.

HELPFUL COMMENTS

Contact your doctor if your symptoms do not improve or get worse after a couple of days. Aspirin or nonsteroidal antiinflammatories† may be taken to treat headache, which is commonly caused by this drug.

Do not stop treatment early if you start to feel better.

MORICIZINE HYDROCHLORIDE

Available since June 1990

COMMONLY USED TO TREAT

Irregular heartbeat, also known as arrhythmias

DRUG CATEGORY

antiarrhythmic
Class: sodium channel blocker

PRODUCTS

Brand-Name Products with No Generic Alternative
Ethmozine 200 mg tablet ($)
Ethmozine 250 mg tablet ($)
Ethmozine 300 mg tablet ($$)
No generics available.
No patents, no exclusivity.

DOSING AND FOOD

Doses are taken 2 to 3 times a day.
It is better to take this drug on an empty stomach, but taking this drug
with a little food may avoid the stomach upset that some people suffer.
Adults: Up to 900 mg per day in divided doses.
Lower doses are used in people with kidney disease or liver disease.
Forgotten doses: If more than 4 hours have passed since the forgotten
dose, do not take the dose. Otherwise take the forgotten dose as soon as
you remember.

ALCOHOL, DRUG, HERB, AND SUPPLEMENT INTERACTIONS

Alcohol may increase some of the side effects from this drug, depending
on the amount consumed. Ask your doctor about the risks caused by
drinking alcohol with your condition.

**Taking this drug with any of the ones listed below may change the effect of
either drug with the possibility of causing toxicity or decreasing effectiveness:**
cimetidine, digoxin, propranolol, theophylline

ALLERGIC REACTIONS AND SIDE EFFECTS

You should tell your doctor about all your allergies and any unexplained
symptoms you may have while taking this drug.
MORE COMMON SIDE EFFECTS: Abdominal pain, diarrhea, dizziness, dry
mouth, headache, indigestion, nausea, tiredness, vomiting
LESS COMMON SIDE EFFECTS: Blurry vision, chest pain*, irregular heart-
beat*, leg pain, nervousness, numbness, shortness of breath*, sleep dis-
orders, stomach pain, swelling*, tingling, urinary changes, weakness
RARE SIDE EFFECTS: Fever*

†See page 52.   * See page 53.

PRECAUTIONS

People with a pacemaker, or who have recently had a heart attack, may be at greater risk of developing irregular heartbeats while taking this drug.

Be careful driving or handling equipment while taking this drug because it may cause dizziness.

If switching from a different antiarrhythmic† to this drug, there is a 6- to 24-hour waiting period that is recommended depending on the drug. Ask your doctor or pharmacist for more information.

This drug may cause dry mouth, which is associated with a greater risk of cavities. Your dentist may recommend that you clean your teeth and mouth differently to avoid infection.

PREGNANCY AND BREAST-FEEDING

Safety during pregnancy has not been established although there was no evidence of harm during studies in animals.

This drug passes into breast milk, but does not appear to harm the baby. Talk to your doctor about the risks associated with breast-feeding while taking this drug.

HELPFUL COMMENTS

Sucking on hard sugarless candy or chewing sugarless gum may help relieve dry mouth caused by this drug.

MORPHINE SULFATE

Available for over 20 years

COMMONLY USED TO TREAT

Pain

DRUG CATEGORY

analgesic
antidiarrheal
antitussive
Class: narcotic analgesic/opioid

PRODUCTS

Brand-Name Products with No Generic Alternative
Avinza 30 mg extended-release capsule (n/a)
Avinza 60 mg extended-release capsule (n/a)

Avinza 120 mg extended-release capsule (n/a)
Kadian 20 mg extended-release capsule ($$)
Kadian 30 mg extended-release capsule ($$)
Kadian 50 mg extended-release capsule ($$$)
Kadian 60 mg extended-release capsule ($$$)
Kadian 100 mg extended-release capsule ($$$$)

Brand-Name Products with Generic Alternatives
MS Contin 15 mg extended-release tablet (¢¢¢¢¢)
  Generic: morphine sulfate 15 mg extended-release tablet (¢¢¢¢¢)
MS Contin 30 mg extended-release tablet ($$)
  Generic: morphine sulfate 30 mg extended-release tablet ($$)
MS Contin 60 mg extended-release tablet ($$$)
  Generic: morphine sulfate 60 mg extended-release tablet ($$$)
MS Contin 100 mg extended-release tablet ($$$$)
  Generic: morphine sulfate 100 mg extended-release tablet ($$$)
MS Contin 200 mg extended-release tablet ($$$$$)
  Generic: morphine sulfate 200 mg extended-release tablet ($$$$)

Products Only Available as Generics
morphine sulfate 10 mg tablet (¢¢¢)
morphine sulfate 15 mg tablet (¢¢)
morphine sulfate 30 mg tablet (¢¢¢)
morphine sulfate 10 mg/5 ml oral solution (¢¢¢)
morphine sulfate 20 mg/5 ml oral solution (¢¢¢¢)
morphine sulfate 20 mg/ml oral solution ($$$)
morphine sulfate 5 mg rectal suppository ($)
morphine sulfate 10 mg rectal suppository ($)
morphine sulfate 20 mg rectal suppository ($$)
morphine sulfate 30 mg rectal suppository ($$)

Other Generic Product Names
MSIR, Oramorph SR, RMS, Roxanol

DOSING AND FOOD

Regular oral doses are taken up to 6 times a day. Extended-release products are taken twice a day. Rectal doses are used up to 6 times a day.
It is best to take this drug on an empty stomach, but taking this drug with a little food may avoid the stomach upset that some people suffer.
Adults: Up to 180 mg per day in divided doses.
Higher doses may be used in people who are under close medical supervision.

---

† See page 52.   * See page 53.

Lower doses are used in children.

Forgotten doses: If you are scheduled to take the next dose within a few hours, do not take the forgotten dose. Otherwise take the forgotten dose as soon as you remember.

ALCOHOL, DRUG, HERB, AND SUPPLEMENT INTERACTIONS

Alcohol should not be used while taking this drug.

Several OTC drugs used for asthma, colds, cough, hay fever, sleep aid, or sinus problems may seriously change the effects and side effects of this drug. Check with your pharmacist when selecting OTC products.

Taking this drug with any of the ones listed below may change the effect of either drug with the possibility of causing toxicity or decreasing effectiveness: natrexone, rifampin

Severe reactions are possible when this drug is taken with those listed below: anesthetics, anticholinergicst, antihistaminest, barbituratest, benzodiazepinest, cimetidine, monoamine oxidase inhibitorst, naloxone, narcoticst, phenothiazinest, sedative-hypnoticst, skeletal muscle relaxantst, tricyclic antidepressantst

ALLERGIC REACTIONS AND SIDE EFFECTS

If you are allergic to any narcoticst, you may also be allergic to this drug. You should tell your doctor about all your allergies and any unexplained symptoms you may have while taking this drug.

MORE COMMON SIDE EFFECTS: Constipation, dizziness*, drowsiness*, dry mouth, excitement*, fainting, irregular breathing*, irregular heartbeat*, lightheadedness, nausea, sweating*, urinary changes*, vomiting

LESS COMMON SIDE EFFECTS: Blurry vision, breathing difficulty*, depression*, flushing*, hallucinations*, headache, hives*, itching*, loss of appetite, mood swings*, nervousness*, restlessness*, ringing in ears*, shortness of breath*, skin rash*, sleep disorders, spastic movements*, stomach cramps, swelling*, tiredness, trembling*, vision changes, weakness*, wheezing*

RARE SIDE EFFECTS: Body aches, clammy skin*, confusion*, diarrhea, fever, goosebumps, irritability, low blood pressure*, runny nose, seizures*, shivering, small pupils*, sneezing, yawning

PRECAUTIONS

Do not open, crush, break, or chew the extended-release products.

Be careful driving or handling equipment while taking this drug because it may cause dizziness and drowsiness.

If you have a history of head injury, brain disease, emphysema, asthma, lung disease, enlarged prostate, urinary disorders, gallbladder disease, or gallstones, you may not be able to take this drug.

People with colitis, heart disease, kidney disease, liver disease, and thyroid disease are at increased risk of developing side effects.

If you have a history of seizures, you may be at greater risk of developing a seizure while taking this drug.

This drug may cause withdrawal symptoms if stopped suddenly. If you wish to stop taking this drug, ask your doctor for specific instructions.

Side effects may continue to develop even after this drug is stopped.

Pain relief from the extended-release products many not be as dependable as the regular-release products.

This drug may cause dry mouth, which is associated with a greater risk of cavities. Your dentist may recommend that you clean your teeth and mouth differently to avoid infection.

Because this drug has a high abuse potential, your prescription quantity may be limited.

PREGNANCY AND BREAST-FEEDING

Safety during pregnancy has not been established although the drug is known to harm animal fetuses.

Breast-feeding while taking this drug is not recommended.

HELPFUL COMMENTS

If the drug does not seem to be working properly, an increase in dose may not help. Talk to your doctor about other drugs and treatment options.

Sucking on hard sugarless candy or chewing sugarless gum may help relieve dry mouth caused by this drug.

Lie down for a while after taking a dose of this drug to help reduce the nausea.

Avoid quick movements to minimize dizziness. Dangling your legs over the side of the bed for a few minutes may help reduce dizziness when first waking up.

If being used for pain, this drug works best when taken before the pain gets too severe.

Add more fiber to your diet to help minimize the constipation that occurs with this drug. If severe, constipation may need to be treated with a stool softener. Ask your doctor or pharmacist for recommendations.

If using a suppository, remove the foil and run under cold water before inserting.

---

† See page 52.   * See page 53.

MOXIFLOXACIN HYDROCHLORIDE

Available since December 1999

COMMONLY USED TO TREAT

Infection

DRUG CATEGORY

antibiotic
Class: fluoroquinolone

PRODUCTS

Brand-Name Products with No Generic Alternative
Avelox 400 mg tablet ($$$$)
No generics available.
Multiple patents that begin to expire in 2009.

DOSING AND FOOD

Doses are taken once a day.
It is best to take this drug on an empty stomach, 2 hours after a meal.
Adults: Up to 400 mg per day.
Lower doses are used in people with kidney disease.
This drug is rarely used by mouth in children under age 18 because it may
   interfere with bone development.
Forgotten doses: If you are scheduled to take the next dose within a few
   hours, do not take the forgotten dose. Otherwise take the forgotten dose
   as soon as you remember.

ALCOHOL, DRUG, HERB, AND SUPPLEMENT INTERACTIONS

Alcohol may increase some of the side effects from this drug, depending
   on the amount consumed. Ask your doctor about the risks caused by
   drinking alcohol with your condition.

Taking this drug with any of the ones listed below may change the effect of
either drug with the possibility of causing toxicity or decreasing effectiveness:
antacids, antidiabetics†, digoxin, iron supplements, mineral supplements,
   probenecid, sucralfate, theophylline, warfarin

Severe reactions are possible when this drug is taken with those listed below:
amiodarone, antipsychotics†, astemizole, bepridil, cisapride, erythromycin,
   nonsteroidal antiinflammatories†, phenothiazines†, procainamide, quinidine, sotalol, tricyclic antidepressants†

ALLERGIC REACTIONS AND SIDE EFFECTS

If you are allergic to any fluoroquinolones†, you may also be allergic to this drug. You should tell your doctor about all your allergies and any unexplained symptoms you may have while taking this drug.

This drug promotes the effect of sunlight on the body and may cause severe sunburn and increased sensitivity of the eyes.

MORE COMMON SIDE EFFECTS: Diarrhea*, nausea, nervousness, rash, seizures*, skin irritation*, vomiting

LESS COMMON SIDE EFFECTS: Back pain, blisters*, difficulty urinating, dreams, dizziness, drowsiness, headache, lightheadedness, muscle pain, sleep disorders, sore mouth, stomachache, vaginal discharge, vaginal pain, taste changes, vision changes

RARE SIDE EFFECTS: Abdominal pain*, agitation*, bloody urine*, confusion*, dark urine*, fever*, flushing*, hallucinations*, irregular heartbeat*, joint pain*, leg pain*, loss of appetite*, pale stools*, shakiness*, shortness of breath*, sweating*, swelling*, tiredness*, tremors*, weakness*, yellow eyes or skin*

PRECAUTIONS

Be careful driving or handling equipment while taking this drug because the drug may cause dizziness and drowsiness.

If you have a history of tendinitis, this drug may make that condition worse.

PREGNANCY AND BREAST-FEEDING

Safety during pregnancy has not been established although the drug is known to harm animal fetuses.

Breast-feeding while taking this drug is not recommended.

HELPFUL COMMENTS

Contact your doctor if your symptoms do not improve after a couple of days.

Do not stop treatment early if you start to feel better. It takes the full prescription for this drug to work completely.

If you need to take an antacid, minerals, or iron supplements, take them either 4 hours before or 2 hours after taking this drug.

Drink a lot of water while taking this drug.

---

†See page 52.   *See page 53.

MYCOPHENOLATE MOFETIL

Available since May 1995

COMMONLY USED TO TREAT

Organ transplant recipients to reduce the risk of rejection

DRUG CATEGORY

immunosuppressant
Class: mycophenolic acid derivative

PRODUCTS

Brand-Name Products with No Generic Alternative
Cellcept 250 mg capsule ($$$)
Cellcept 500 mg tablet ($$$$)
Cellcept 200 mg/ml oral suspension ($$$$$)
No generics available.
No patents, no exclusivity.

DOSING AND FOOD

Doses are taken twice a day.
It is best to take this drug on an empty stomach with a full glass of water.
  Do not eat raw oysters or other raw shellfish at any time while taking this
  drug.
Adults: Up to 3,000 mg per day in divided doses.
Forgotten doses: If you are scheduled to take the next dose within 12
  hours, do not take the forgotten dose. Otherwise take the forgotten dose
  as soon as you remember.

ALCOHOL, DRUG, HERB, AND SUPPLEMENT INTERACTIONS

Alcohol may increase some of the side effects from this drug, depending
  on the amount consumed. Ask your doctor about the risks caused by
  drinking alcohol with your condition.

Taking this drug with any of the ones listed below may change the effect of
either drug with the possibility of causing toxicity or decreasing effectiveness:
acyclovir, antacids, cholestyramine, ganciclovir, oral contraceptives

Increased side effects are possible when this drug is taken with those listed below:
antithymocyte globulin, azathioprine, chlorambucil, corticosteroids†, cyclo-
  phosphamide, cyclosporine, mercaptopurine, muromonab-CD3, tacrolimus

ALLERGIC REACTIONS AND SIDE EFFECTS

You should tell your doctor about all your allergies and any unexplained symptoms you may have while taking this drug.

MORE COMMON SIDE EFFECTS: Back pain*, bloody urine*, chest pain*, chills*, constipation, cough*, diarrhea, fever*, headache, heartburn, hoarseness*, nausea, shortness of breath*, stomach pain, swelling*, urinary difficulty*, vomiting, weakness

LESS COMMON SIDE EFFECTS: Abdominal pain*, acne, black stools*, bleeding gums*, bleeding*, bloody vomit*, bruising*, dizziness, irregular heartbeat*, joint pain*, mouth sores*, muscle pain*, shaky hands*, skin irritation*, sleep disorders, swollen gums*, trembling*

PRECAUTIONS

Do not open, crush, break, or chew the capsules.

This drug may cause changes to your gums and mouth. Your dentist may recommend that you clean your teeth and mouth differently to avoid infection.

Avoid contact with anyone who has the chickenpox, measles, or other communicable disease since it may be easier to catch the infection while taking this drug.

Exposure to skin tests, immunizations, and people who have received immunizations may put you at a greater risk of developing the disease when you are taking this drug.

This drug causes changes in your blood that put you at greater risk of getting an infection. Be careful not to cut yourself or get bruised. Tell your doctor if you develop signs of infection, such as fever or sore throat. Your dentist may recommend that you clean your teeth and mouth differently to avoid infection.

Touching these tablets may cause skin irritation. You should wash your hands immediately after taking the dose.

PREGNANCY AND BREAST-FEEDING

Safety during pregnancy has not been established although the drug is known to harm animal fetuses.

Breast-feeding while taking this drug is not recommended.

HELPFUL COMMENTS

Oral contraceptives may not work properly when taken with this drug. You need to use two other forms of contraceptive, such as a condom and

---

†See page 52.　*See page 53.

foam, to prevent pregnancy. Start taking precautions at least 1 week before taking this drug and for 6 weeks after the drug is stopped.

If you need to take an antacid, take it either 2 hours before or after taking this drug.

NABUMETONE

Available since December 1991

COMMONLY USED TO TREAT

Arthritis

DRUG CATEGORY

antiarthritic
Class: nonsteroidal antiinflammatory

PRODUCTS

Brand-Name Products with Generic Alternatives
Relafen 500 mg tablet ($)
  Generic: nabumetone 500 mg tablet ($)
Relafen 750 mg tablet ($$)
  Generic: nabumetone 750 mg tablet ($$)

DOSING AND FOOD

Doses are taken 1 to 2 times a day.
It is best to take this drug with food.
Adults: Up to 2,000 mg per day in divided doses.
Forgotten doses: If you are scheduled to take the next dose within a few hours, do not take the forgotten dose. Otherwise take the forgotten dose as soon as you remember.

ALCOHOL, DRUG, HERB, AND SUPPLEMENT INTERACTIONS

Alcohol may increase the risk of serious side effects from this drug. Ask your doctor about the risks caused by drinking alcohol with your condition.

Do not use dong quai, feverfew, garlic, ginger, horse chestnut, red clover, or St. John's wort while taking this drug since they may increase the risk of serious side effects.

Taking this drug with any of the ones listed below may change the effect of either drug with the possibility of causing toxicity or decreasing effectiveness: acetaminophen, antihypertensives†, digoxin, diuretics†, furosemide, hydrochlorothiazide, nifedipine, lithium, methotrexate, probenecid, sulfonylureas†, sulindac, verapamil

Severe reactions are possible when this drug is taken with those listed below: antibiotics†, anticoagulants†, aspirin, cefamandole, cefoperazone, cefotetan, corticosteroids†, cyclosporine, gold salts, heparin, nonsteroidal antiinflammatories†, penicillamine, plicamycin, salicylates†, valproic acid, warfarin

ALLERGIC REACTIONS AND SIDE EFFECTS

If you are allergic to aspirin, zomepirac, salicylates†, or other nonsteroidal antiinflammatories†, you may also be allergic to this drug. You should tell your doctor about all your allergies and any unexplained symptoms you may have while taking this drug.

This drug promotes the effect of sunlight on the body and may cause severe sunburn and increased sensitivity of the eyes.

MORE COMMON SIDE EFFECTS: Abdominal pain, diarrhea, dizziness, drowsiness, headache, heartburn*, indigestion*, itching*, mouth sores*, nausea*, skin rash*, swelling*, weight gain*

LESS COMMON SIDE EFFECTS: Bruising*, constipation, gas, high blood pressure*, sweating, vomiting

RARE SIDE EFFECTS: Back pain*, black stools*, bloody urine*, bloody vomit, blue fingernails*, blue lips*, breathing difficulty*, chest pain*, chest tightness*, chills*, confusion*, cough*, dark urine*, fainting*, fever*, hallucinations*, hearing loss*, hives*, hoarseness*, lip sores*, loss of appetite*, low blood pressure*, mood swings*, muscle cramps*, nosebleeds*, pain*, pale skin*, pale stools*, puffy eyes*, rectal bleeding*, restlessness*, ringing in ears*, runny nose*, seizures*, shortness of breath*, sore throat*, stiff neck*, swollen glands*, swollen tongue*, thirst*, tiredness*, urinary changes*, vision changes*, weakness*, wheezing*, yellow eyes or skin*

PRECAUTIONS

This drug may cause serious stomach problems and possibly ulcers. Be careful to take this drug as directed with food, and let your doctor know if you develop any stomach-related symptoms.

Be careful driving or handling equipment while taking this drug because the drug may cause dizziness and drowsiness.

Do not lie down for about 30 minutes after taking this drug to help reduce the risk of heartburn and throat irritation.

† See page 52.   * See page 53.

If you use tobacco or have a history of alcohol abuse, stomach problems, intestinal problems, hemorrhoids, diabetes mellitus, severe fluid retention, or systemic lupus erythematosus, there is an increased risk that you will develop side effects while taking this drug.

PREGNANCY AND BREAST-FEEDING

Safety during pregnancy has not been established although the drug is known to harm animal fetuses.

Breast-feeding while taking this drug is not recommended.

HELPFUL COMMENTS

Avoid quick movements to minimize dizziness.

Several nonsteroidal antiinflammatories† are available without a prescription in lower, nonprescription strengths, including ibuprofen, ketoprofen, and naproxen.

NADOLOL

Available for over 20 years

COMMONLY USED TO TREAT

Chest pain, also known as angina
High blood pressure, also known as hypertension
Irregular heart rhythm, also known as arrhythmia
People at risk of complications after a heart attack
People at risk of developing vascular headaches, also known as migraines

DRUG CATEGORY

antianginal
antiarrhythmic
antihypertensive
Class: beta blocker

PRODUCTS

Brand-Name Products with Generic Alternatives
Corgard 20 mg tablet ($$)
   Generic: nadolol 20 mg tablet (¢¢¢¢¢)
Corgard 40 mg tablet ($$)
   Generic: nadolol 40 mg tablet ($)

Corgard 80 mg tablet ($$$)
  Generic: nadolol 80 mg tablet ($)
Corgard 120 mg tablet ($$$)
  Generic: nadolol 120 mg tablet ($$)
Corgard 160 mg tablet ($$$)
  Generic: nadolol 160 mg tablet ($$)
Combination Products That Contain This Drug
Corzide tablet ($$)

DOSING AND FOOD

Doses are taken once a day.
This drug may be taken with or without food.
Adults: Up to 320 mg per day.
Doses are taken less frequently in people with renal disease.
This drug is rarely used in children.
Forgotten doses: If you are scheduled to take the next dose within 8 hours, do not take the forgotten dose. Otherwise take the forgotten dose as soon as you remember.

ALCOHOL, DRUG, HERB, AND SUPPLEMENT INTERACTIONS

Alcohol may increase some of the side effects from this drug, depending on the amount consumed. Ask your doctor about the risks caused by drinking alcohol with your condition.

Several OTC drugs used for appetite control, asthma, colds, cough, hay fever, or sinus problems may cause an increase in blood pressure when taken with this drug. Check with your pharmacist when selecting OTC products.

Taking this drug with any of the ones listed below may change the effect of either drug with the possibility of causing toxicity or decreasing effectiveness:
aminophylline, anesthetics[†], antidiabetics[†], caffeine, calcium channel blockers[†], carbonic anhydrase inhibitors[†], clonidine, dyphylline, epinephrine, guanabenz, isoproterenol, lidocaine, nonsteroidal anti inflammatories[†], oxtriphylline, pilocarpine, reserpine, theophylline

Severe reactions are possible when this drug is taken with those listed below:
allergy shots, antiarrhythmics[†], atropine, beta blockers[†], cocaine, monoamine oxidase inhibitors[†]

Increased effects or side effects are possible when this drug is taken with those listed below:
antihypertensives[†]

[†] *See page 52.*   [*] *See page 53.*

ALLERGIC REACTIONS AND SIDE EFFECTS

If you are allergic to any other beta blockers†, you may also be allergic to this drug. This drug may exaggerate the reaction from your current allergies. Inform your doctor of any allergies that you have as well as the severity of the allergic reaction before starting this drug.

More Common Side Effects: Dizziness, drowsiness, lightheadedness*, sexual dysfunction, sleeping difficulty*, tiredness, sleeping difficulty, weakness

Less Common Side Effects: Anxiety, breathing difficulty*, cold hands and feet*, constipation, depression*, diarrhea, itching, nausea, nervousness, numbness, shortness of breath*, slow heartbeat*, sore eyes, stomachache, stuffy nose, swollen legs or feet, tingling, vivid dreams, vomiting, wheezing

Rare Side Effects: Back pain*, bleeding*, bruising*, chest pain*, confusion*, dizziness*, fever*, hallucinations*, irregular heartbeat*, joint pain*, rash*, scaly skin*, sore throat*

PRECAUTIONS

People with asthma, heart disease, or a heart rate that is routinely less than 60 beats per minute (bradycardia) may not be able to take this drug.

Stopping this drug suddenly may cause chest pain or heart attack. If you wish to stop taking this drug, ask your doctor for specific instructions.

Be careful driving or handling equipment while taking this drug because the drug may cause dizziness and drowsiness.

You need to wait 2 weeks after stopping a monoamine oxidase inhibitor† before starting this drug.

If you are diabetic, this drug may increase blood sugar levels or make the symptoms of low blood sugar less noticeable.

This drug may cause nondiabetics to develop type 2 diabetes.

If you have psoriasis or myasthenia gravis, this drug may make those conditions worse.

PREGNANCY AND BREAST-FEEDING

Safety during pregnancy has not been established although the drug is known to harm animal fetuses.

Breast-feeding while taking this drug is not recommended.

HELPFUL COMMENTS

This drug may make you more sensitive to cold temperatures.

If you do not treat high blood pressure, you may develop more serious problems such as heart failure, blood vessel disease, stroke, or kidney disease. Losing weight, exercising, eating more fruits and vegetables, and avoiding salty foods, such as lunchmeat and pickles, may help make drug treatment more successful.

NAPROXEN

Available for over 20 years

COMMONLY USED TO TREAT

Arthritis in children
Gout
Mild to moderate pain

DRUG CATEGORY

antiarthritic
antidysmenorrheal
antigout
antiinflammatory
antipyretic
Class: nonsteroidal antiinflammatory

PRODUCTS

Brand-Name Products with Generic Alternatives
Anaprox 275 mg tablet (¢¢¢¢¢)
  Generic: naproxen sodium 275 mg tablet (¢¢)
Anaprox DS 550 mg tablet ($$)
  Generic: naproxen sodium 550 mg tablet (¢¢¢)
Naprosyn 250 mg tablet ($)
  Generic: naproxen 250 mg tablet (¢¢)
Naprosyn 375 mg tablet ($)
  Generic: naproxen 375 mg tablet (¢¢)
Naprosyn 500 mg tablet ($$)
  Generic: naproxen 500 mg tablet (¢¢¢)
Naprosyn EC 375 mg delayed-release tablet ($)
Naprelan 375 mg delayed-release tablet ($)
  Generic: naproxen 375 mg delayed-release tablet ($)
Naprosyn EC 500 mg delayed-release tablet ($$)
Naprelan 500 mg delayed-release tablet ($$)
  Generic: naproxen 500 mg delayed-release tablet ($)

---

† See page 52.   * See page 53.

Naprosyn 25 mg/ml oral suspension (¢¢¢¢)
   Generic: naproxen 25 mg/ml oral suspension (¢¢¢)

DOSING AND FOOD

Doses are taken 2 to 4 times a day. Extended-release products are taken once a day.

It is best to take this drug with food or milk.

Adults: Up to 1,000 mg per day in divided doses.

Children: Up to 10 mg/kg per day in divided doses.

Forgotten doses: If you are scheduled to take the next dose within a few hours, do not take the forgotten dose. Otherwise take the forgotten dose as soon as you remember.

ALCOHOL, DRUG, HERB, AND SUPPLEMENT INTERACTIONS

Alcohol may increase the risk of serious side effects from this drug. Ask your doctor about the risks caused by drinking alcohol with your condition.

Do not use dong quai, feverfew, garlic, ginger, horse chestnut, red clover, or St. John's wort while taking this drug since they may increase the risk of serious side effects.

Taking this drug with any of the ones listed below may change the effect of either drug with the possibility of causing toxicity or decreasing effectiveness: ACE inhibitors†, acetaminophen, antihypertensives†, digoxin, diuretics†, furosemide, hydrochlorothiazide, nifedipine, lithium, methotrexate, phenytoin, probenecid, sulfonylureas†, sulindac, verapamil

Severe reactions are possible when this drug is taken with those listed below: antibiotics†, anticoagulants†, aspirin, cefamandole, cefoperazone, cefotetan, corticosteroids†, cyclosporine, dipyridamole, gold salts†, heparin, mezlocillin, nonsteroidal antiinflammatories†, penicillamine, piperacillin, plicamycin, salicylates†, sulfinpyrazone, ticarcillin

ALLERGIC REACTIONS AND SIDE EFFECTS

If you are allergic to aspirin, zomepirac, salicylates†, or other nonsteroidal antiinflammatories†, you may also be allergic to this drug. You should tell your doctor about all your allergies and any unexplained symptoms you may have while taking this drug.

This drug promotes the effect of sunlight on the body and may cause severe sunburn and increased sensitivity of the eyes.

MORE COMMON SIDE EFFECTS: Abdominal pain, black stools*, dizziness, drowsiness, headache, heartburn*, indigestion*, itching*, nausea*, ringing in ears*, skin rash*, swelling*, weight gain*

LESS COMMON SIDE EFFECTS: Bruising*, constipation, diarrhea, gas, high blood pressure*, mouth sores*, sweating, vomiting

RARE SIDE EFFECTS: Back pain*, bloody urine*, bloody vomit, blue fingernails*, blue lips*, breathing difficulty*, chest pain*, chest tightness*, chills*, confusion*, cough*, dark urine*, fainting*, fever*, hallucinations*, hearing loss*, hives*, hoarseness*, lip sores*, loss of appetite*, low blood pressure*, mood swings*, muscle cramps*, nosebleeds*, pain*, pale skin*, pale stools*, puffy eyes*, rectal bleeding*, restlessness*, runny nose*, seizures*, shortness of breath*, sore throat*, stiff neck*, swollen glands*, swollen tongue*, thirst*, tiredness*, urinary changes*, vision changes*, weakness*, wheezing*, yellow eyes or skin*

PRECAUTIONS

This drug may cause serious stomach problems and possibly ulcers. Be careful to take this drug as directed with food, and let your doctor know if you develop any stomach-related symptoms.

Do not crush, break, or chew the extended-release products.

Be careful driving or handling equipment while taking this drug because the drug may cause dizziness and drowsiness.

Do not lie down for about 30 minutes after taking this drug to help reduce the risk of heartburn and throat irritation.

If you use tobacco or have a history of alcohol abuse, stomach problems, intestinal problems, hemorrhoids, diabetes mellitus, severe fluid retention, or systemic lupus erythematosus, there is an increased risk that you will develop side effects while taking this drug.

People over age 60 are at greater risk of developing fluid retention and swelling when taking this drug.

Measure your weight every 2 to 3 days. Weight gain of more than 3 pounds in a week may be a sign of a serious reaction and should be reported to your doctor.

PREGNANCY AND BREAST-FEEDING

Safety during pregnancy has not been established although the drug is known to harm animal fetuses.

Breast-feeding while taking this drug is not recommended.

HELPFUL COMMENTS

Do not mix the oral suspension product with anything before taking the dose.

It takes about 2 weeks before the full effects of this drug are noticed.

Avoid quick movements to minimize dizziness.

---

† See page 52.   * See page 53.

Several nonsteroidal antiinflammatories† are available without a prescription in lower, nonprescription strengths, including ibuprofen, ketoprofen, and naproxen.

If you are taking the OTC form of this drug for more than 14 days, you should talk to your doctor to verify your diagnosis and consider higher doses or another drug.

NARATRIPTAN HYDROCHLORIDE

Available since February 1998

COMMONLY USED TO TREAT

Migraine headache

DRUG CATEGORY

antimigraine
Class: triptan

PRODUCTS

Brand-Name Products with No Generic Alternative
Amerge 1 mg tablet ($$$$$)
Amerge 2.5 mg tablet ($$$$$)
No generics available.
Patent expires in 2010.

DOSING AND FOOD

Doses are taken as a single dose repeated after 4 hours if needed.
This drug may be taken with or without food.
Adults: Up to 5 mg per day.
Lower doses are used in people with kidney disease or liver disease.

ALCOHOL, DRUG, HERB, AND SUPPLEMENT INTERACTIONS

Alcohol may increase some of the side effects from this drug, depending on the amount consumed. Ask your doctor about the risks caused by drinking alcohol with your condition.

Taking this drug with any of the ones listed below may change the effect of either drug with the possibility of causing toxicity or decreasing effectiveness:
oral contraceptives

Severe reactions are possible when this drug is taken with those listed below:
ergot alkaloids†, SSRIs†, triptans†

ALLERGIC REACTIONS AND SIDE EFFECTS

You should tell your doctor about all your allergies and any unexplained symptoms you may have while taking this drug.

This drug may cause your eyes to be more sensitive to sunlight, but there are no special risks associated with sunburn while taking this drug.

MORE COMMON SIDE EFFECTS: Chest pain*, dizziness, drowsiness, nausea, numbness*, throat tightness*, tingling*, tiredness, vomiting

LESS COMMON SIDE EFFECTS: Acne, anxiety, blurry vision, bone pain, chills, confusion, constipation, diarrhea, fainting, fever, irregular heartbeat*, itching, joint pain, mood swings, muscle spasms, restlessness, rigidity, seizures*, shaky hands, skin rash, sleep disorders, slow heartbeat*, stiffness, stomachache, taste changes, thirst, trembling, urinary changes, weakness

PRECAUTIONS

This drug does not prevent a migraine headache and is not useful if taken on a regular basis.

Heavy smoking may cause this drug to be less effective.

People with a history of stroke, chest pain, high blood pressure, kidney disease, liver disease, or heart disease may be at greater risk of developing side effects while taking this drug.

This drug is NOT a pain reliever and should not be used for non-migraine headaches.

Be careful driving or handling equipment while taking this drug because it may cause drowsiness and dizziness.

Talk to your doctor before you get a headache to plan what to do if this drug is not effective.

PREGNANCY AND BREAST-FEEDING

Safety during pregnancy has not been established although the drug is known to harm animal fetuses.

Breast-feeding while taking this drug is not recommended.

HELPFUL COMMENTS

This drug works best if taken as soon as the headache starts, not earlier when visual auras or warnings appear.

Eye irritation caused by the sun may be reduced by wearing sunglasses when outside.

---

†See page 52.   * See page 53.

NATEGLINIDE

Available since December 2000

COMMONLY USED TO TREAT

High blood sugar, specifically type 2 diabetes

DRUG CATEGORY

antidiabetic
Class: biguanide: meglitinide

PRODUCTS

Brand-Name Products with No Generic Alternative
Starlix 60 mg tablet (¢¢¢¢¢)
Starlix 120 mg tablet (¢¢¢¢¢)
No generics available.
Multiple patents that begin to expire in 2006. Exclusivity until 2005.

DOSING AND FOOD

Doses are taken 3 times a day.
Always take your dose 30 minutes or less before each meal.
Adults: Up to 360 mg per day in divided doses.
Forgotten doses: Do not take a forgotten dose. Just go back to your usual
schedule with the next dose.

ALCOHOL, DRUG, HERB, AND SUPPLEMENT INTERACTIONS

Alcohol may cause a change in your blood sugar, altering the effects of this
drug. Ask your doctor about the risks caused by drinking alcohol with
your condition.

Aloe, bilberry leaf, bitter melon, burdock, dandelion, fenugreek, garlic,
ginkgo biloba, and ginseng may lower blood sugar and cause the need
for a dose adjustment when taken with this drug. Tell your doctor if you
are taking any of these supplements.

Several OTC drugs used for headache or pain may seriously increase the
effects of this drug, while drugs used for cold and allergies may decrease
the effects of this drug. Check with your pharmacist when selecting OTC
products.

Taking this drug with any of the ones listed below may change the effect of
either drug with the possibility of causing toxicity or decreasing effectiveness:
aspirin, beta blockers†, corticosteroids†, monoamine oxidase inhibitors†,

nonsteroidal antiinflammatories†, sympathomimetics†, thiazide diuretics†, thyroid hormones†

ALLERGIC REACTIONS AND SIDE EFFECTS

You should tell your doctor about all your allergies and any unexplained symptoms you may have while taking this drug.

MORE COMMON SIDE EFFECTS: Cough, runny nose, sore throat

LESS COMMON SIDE EFFECTS: Abdominal pain, anxiety*, back pain, blurry vision*, chills, cold sweats*, confusion*, dizziness, drowsiness*, fast heartbeat*, headache*, hunger*, joint pain, nausea*, nervousness*, nightmares*, pale skin*, poor concentration*, seizures*, shakiness*, slurry speech*, sneezing, swelling, tiredness*, unconsciousness*, weakness*

PRECAUTIONS

This drug is not effective in people with type 1 diabetes or people with ketoacidosis.

If you skip a meal, you should also skip the dose of this drug.

This drug may be combined with metformin or insulin for control of blood sugar levels, but should not be used with other antidiabetic drugs†.

This drug may become less effective when taken for a long period of time.

Burns, diarrhea, fever, hormonal changes, infection, malnourishment, severe stress, uncontrolled thyroid disease, and vomiting may cause changes in blood sugar, which may make this drug less effective.

This drug may cause your blood sugar level to drop below normal. Make sure your doctor explains what symptoms to watch for and the action you should take.

PREGNANCY AND BREAST-FEEDING

Safety during pregnancy has not been established although the drug is known to harm animal fetuses.

Breast-feeding while taking this drug is not recommended.

HELPFUL COMMENTS

If you do not treat high blood sugar, you may develop more serious problems such as heart failure, blood vessel disease, eye disease, or kidney disease.

---

†See page 52.   *See page 53.

NEFAZODONE HYDROCHLORIDE

Available since December 1994

COMMONLY USED TO TREAT

Depression

DRUG CATEGORY

antidepressant
Class: phenylpiperazine

PRODUCTS

Brand-Name Products with No Generic Alternative
Serzone 50 mg tablet ($)
Serzone 100 mg tablet ($)
Serzone 150 mg tablet ($)
Serzone 200 mg tablet ($$)
Serzone 250 mg tablet ($$)
No generics available.
Multiple patents that begin to expire in 2003.

DOSING AND FOOD

Doses are taken twice a day.
This drug may be taken with or without food.
Adults: Up to 600 mg per day in divided doses.
Lower doses are used in people over age 65 and people with liver disease.
Forgotten doses: If you are scheduled to take the next dose within a few
hours, do not take the forgotten dose. Otherwise take the forgotten dose
as soon as you remember.

ALCOHOL, DRUG, HERB, AND SUPPLEMENT INTERACTIONS

Alcohol should not be used while taking this drug.
Many OTC drugs used for appetite control, asthma, colds, cough, hay
fever, pain, or sinus problems affect the central nervous system and may
increase the effects or side effects when taken with this drug. Check with
your pharmacist for products to avoid.

**Taking this drug with any of the ones listed below may change the effect of
either drug with the possibility of causing toxicity or decreasing effectiveness:**
alprazolam, aspirin, digoxin, triazolam, warfarin

Severe reactions are possible when this drug is taken with those listed below: astemizole, cisapride, monoamine oxidase inhibitors†, terfenadine

ALLERGIC REACTIONS AND SIDE EFFECTS

If you are allergic to trazodone, you may also be allergic to this drug. You should tell your doctor about all your allergies and any unexplained symptoms you may have while taking this drug.

This drug promotes the effect of sunlight on the body and may cause severe sunburn and increased sensitivity of the eyes.

MORE COMMON SIDE EFFECTS: Agitation, blurry vision*, clumsiness*, confusion, constipation, cough, diarrhea*, dizziness, dreams, drowsiness, dry mouth, fainting*, flushing, headache, heartburn, increased appetite, itching*, lightheadedness*, memory loss, nausea, ringing in ears*, skin rash*, sleep disorders, swelling*, tingling, tremor, unsteadiness*, vision changes*, vomiting*

LESS COMMON SIDE EFFECTS: Breast tenderness, breathing difficulty*, chest tightness*, eye pain*, lack of energy, nausea*, shortness of breath*, stomach pain*, thirst*, weakness*, wheezing*, yellow eyes or skin*

RARE SIDE EFFECTS: Asthma*, back pain*, black stools*, bleeding*, bloody vomit*, breast enlargement, breast-milk secretion, bruising*, chest pain*, chills*, confusion*, dark urine*, double vision*, dry eyes*, ear pain*, excitability*, eye irritation*, fainting*, fast heartbeat*, fever*, hallucinations*, hives*, joint pain*, kidney stones*, lack of appetite*, large pupils*, loss of consciousness*, menstrual changes*, mood swings*, mouth irritation*, muscle pain*, nerve pain*, pale stools*, pelvic pain*, penile erection*, rectal bleeding*, sexual dysfunction*, skin irritation*, sore throat*, stiffness*, sweating*, swollen glands*, tiredness*, twitching*, urinary changes*

PRECAUTIONS

People with a history of seizures are at greater risk of developing a seizure while taking this drug.

Be careful driving or handling equipment while taking this drug because it may cause drowsiness, dizziness, and vision changes.

You need to wait 2 weeks after stopping a monoamine oxidase inhibitor† before starting this drug.

Drink plenty of fluids to avoid dehydration when sweating, such as in hot weather and during exercise.

This drug may cause serious harm to your liver and requires regular testing and follow-up with the doctor. Call your doctor right away if you begin to

---

† See page 52.   * See page 53.

feel poorly, lose your appetite, have stomach pains, or notice a yellowing of the skin or eyes.

If you have a history of mania, this drug may make that condition worse.

Men have a very small risk of developing painful, prolonged erection of the penis, which requires treatment by a doctor. If this happens, go to your doctor or the nearest emergency room immediately.

This drug may cause dry mouth, which is associated with a greater risk of cavities. Your dentist may recommend that you clean your teeth and mouth differently to avoid infection.

Tell your doctor if you take large doses of aspirin on a regular basis since this drug may mask the symptoms of aspirin toxicity.

PREGNANCY AND BREAST-FEEDING

Safety during pregnancy has not been established although the drug is known to harm animal fetuses.

It is not known if this drug passes into breast milk. Talk to your doctor about the risks associated with breast-feeding while taking this drug.

HELPFUL COMMENTS

It may take several weeks before you begin to notice the effects of this drug.

Your prescription quantity may be limited because of the need for frequent doctor visits while taking this drug.

Sucking on hard sugarless candy or chewing sugarless gum may help relieve dry mouth caused by this drug.

Avoid quick movements to minimize dizziness. Dangling your legs over the side of the bed for a few minutes may help reduce dizziness when first waking up.

Eye irritation caused by the sun may be reduced by wearing sunglasses when outside.

NELFINAVIR MESYLATE

Available since March 1997

COMMONLY USED TO TREAT

HIV infection

DRUG CATEGORY

antiretroviral
Class: protease inhibitor (PI)

PRODUCTS

Brand-Name Products with No Generic Alternative
Viracept 250 mg tablet ($$$)
Viracept 50 mg/scoop oral powder (¢)
No generics available.
Multiple patents that begin to expire in 2013.

DOSING AND FOOD

Doses are taken 2 to 3 times a day.
It is best to take this drug with a meal or light snack.

Adults and children over age 13: Up to 2,500 mg per day in divided doses.

Children age 2 to 13: Up to 90 mg/kg (maximum 2,250 mg) per day in divided doses.

Forgotten doses: If you are scheduled to take the next dose within a few hours, do not take the forgotten dose. Otherwise take the forgotten dose as soon as you remember.

ALCOHOL, DRUG, HERB, AND SUPPLEMENT INTERACTIONS

Alcohol may increase some of the side effects from this drug, depending on the amount consumed. Ask your doctor about the risks caused by drinking alcohol with your condition.

St. John's wort may noticeably interfere with the effects of this drug and should not be used at any time during treatment.

Taking this drug with any of the ones listed below may change the effect of either drug with the possibility of causing toxicity or decreasing effectiveness:
amiodarone, astemizole, calcium channel blockers†, carbamazepine, cisapride, dihydropyridine, ergot alkaloids†, lovastatin, midazolam, oral contraceptives, phenobarbital, phenytoin, protease inhibitors†, quinidine, rifabutin, rifampin, ritonavir, sildenafil, simvastatin, terfenadine, triazolam

ALLERGIC REACTIONS AND SIDE EFFECTS

You should tell your doctor about all your allergies and any unexplained symptoms you may have while taking this drug.

MORE COMMON SIDE EFFECTS: Diarrhea

LESS COMMON SIDE EFFECTS: Abdominal pain, anxiety, breath odor*, confusion*, dehydration*, depression, dizziness, drowsiness, dry skin*, ex-

---

†*See page 52.*   **See page 53.*

citement, eye irritation, fatigue*, gas, headache, hunger*, itching*, loss of appetite, mouth sores, nausea*, runny nose, seizures*, skin rash, sleep disorders, suicidal thoughts*, sweating, thirst*, urinary changes*, vomiting*, weight loss*

RARE SIDE EFFECTS: Back pain, breathing difficulty*, fever*, increased blood sugar, muscle pain, sexual dysfunction, shortness of breath*, yellow eyes or skin*

PRECAUTIONS

The oral powder product contains phenylalanine and should not be used in people with phenylketonuria. Oral powder should be mixed with water, milk, soy liquids, or formula and taken within 6 hours of mixing. Mixing with fruit juice will give the drug a bitter taste. Put the powder into the glass before adding fluids for better mixing.

If also taking didanosine, you need to wait 1 hour before taking this drug. Otherwise take this drug first and didanosine 2 hours later.

This drug does not prevent transmission of the infection.

Drink plenty of fluids to avoid dehydration when sweating, such as in hot weather and during exercise.

This drug may cause you to build up fat on your body.

PREGNANCY AND BREAST-FEEDING

Safety during pregnancy has not been established although there was no evidence of harm during studies in animals.

Breast-feeding while taking this drug is not recommended.

HELPFUL COMMENTS

Oral contraceptives may not work properly when taken with this drug. You need to use a barrier contraceptive, such as a condom, or other nonhormonal contraceptive to prevent pregnancy.

Contact your doctor if your symptoms do not improve after a couple of days.

Do not stop treatment early if you start to feel better. It takes the full prescription for this drug to work completely.

Tablets may be crushed and mixed with water for easier swallowing.

Diarrhea caused by this drug is often treated with loperamide, the active drug found in the OTC product Imodium.

NEOMYCIN SULFATE

Available for over 20 years

COMMONLY USED TO TREAT

High cholesterol levels, also known as hypercholesterolemia
Intestinal infection

DRUG CATEGORY

antibiotic
Class: aminoglycoside

PRODUCTS

Brand-Name Products with No Generic Alternative
Neomycin sulfate 350 mg tablet (n/a)
Neo-Fradin 87.5 mg/5 ml oral solution (¢¢¢)
No generics available.
No patent, no exclusivity.

Combination Products That Contain This Drug
Coly-Mycin S ear suspension ($$$$$)
Cortisporin ear solution ($$$$$)
Cortisporin ear suspension ($$$$$)
Cortisporin ophthalmic ointment ($$$$$)
Cortisporin ophthalmic suspension ($$$$$)
Cortisporin topical cream ($$$$)
Cortisporin topical ointment ($$)
Dexacidin ophthalmic suspension ($$$$$)
Dexasporin ophthalmic suspension ($$$$$)
Maxitrol ophthalmic ointment ($$$$$)
Maxitrol ophthalmic suspension ($$$$$)
Neo-Cort-Dome ear suspension (n/a)
Neo-Cort-Dome topical cream (n/a)
Neosporin ophthalmic ointment ($$$$$)
Oticair ear suspension (n/a)
Pediotic ear suspension ($$$$$)
Poly-Pred ophthalmic suspension ($$$$$)

DOSING AND FOOD

Doses are taken 2 to 6 times a day.
This drug may be taken with or without food.

---

† See page 52.   * See page 53.

Adults: Up to 1,200 mg per day in divided doses.

Children: Up to 100 mg/kg per day in divided doses.

Lower doses are used in people with kidney disease.

Forgotten doses: If you are scheduled to take the next dose within a few hours, do not take the forgotten dose. Otherwise take the forgotten dose as soon as you remember.

ALCOHOL, DRUG, HERB, AND SUPPLEMENT INTERACTIONS

Alcohol may increase some of the side effects from this drug, depending on the amount consumed. Ask your doctor about the risks caused by drinking alcohol with your condition.

Taking this drug with any of the ones listed below may change the effect of either drug with the possibility of causing toxicity or decreasing effectiveness: anticoagulants†

ALLERGIC REACTIONS AND SIDE EFFECTS

If you are allergic to amikacin, gentamicin, kanamycin, netilmicin, streptomycin, or tobramycin, you may also be allergic to this drug. You should tell your doctor about all your allergies and any unexplained symptoms you may have while taking this drug.

MORE COMMON SIDE EFFECTS: Diarrhea*, hearing loss*, mouth irritation, nausea, poor balance*, rectal sores, skin rash*, vomiting

RARE SIDE EFFECTS: Breathing difficulty*, clumsiness*, dizziness*, drowsiness*, fatty stools*, gas*, itching, pale stools*, ringing in ears*, thirst*, unsteadiness*, urinary changes*, weakness*

PRECAUTIONS

The topical form of this drug is not absorbed into the body unless it is applied to open cuts, wounds, or burns.

This drug is found in topical OTC products and should be used with caution in people with kidney disease.

People with kidney disease or intestinal problems may be at greater risk of developing side effects.

If you have myasthenia gravis or Parkinson's disease, this drug may make those conditions worse.

PREGNANCY AND BREAST-FEEDING

Safety during pregnancy has not been established although the drug is known to harm animal fetuses.

It is not known if this drug passes into breast milk. Talk to your doctor about the risks associated with breast-feeding while taking this drug.

HELPFUL COMMENTS

You should drink a lot of water while taking this drug.

Do not measure doses of the oral solution with anything but a measuring cup that is intended for use with prescription drugs. Slight inaccuracy from other measuring spoons may result in over- or under-dosing.

Contact your doctor if your symptoms do not improve after a couple of days.

Do not stop treatment early if you start to feel better. It takes the full prescription for this drug to work completely.

NEVIRAPINE

Available since June 1996

COMMONLY USED TO TREAT

HIV infection

DRUG CATEGORY

antiretroviral
Class: nonnucleoside reverse transcriptase inhibitor (NNRTI)

PRODUCTS

Brand-Name Products with No Generic Alternative
Viramune 200 mg tablet ($$$$)
Viramune 50 mg/5 ml oral suspension ($$)
No generics available.
Patent expires in 2011.

DOSING AND FOOD

Doses are taken 1 to 2 times a day.
This drug may be taken with or without food.
Adults and teens: Up to 400 mg per day in divided doses.
Children over age 8: Up to 8 mg/kg (maximum 400 mg) per day in divided doses.
Children age 2 months to 8 years: Up to 14 mg/kg (maximum 400 mg) per day in divided doses.
Infants: Up to 200 mg/m^2 per day in divided doses.
Lower doses are used for the first 2 weeks of treatment.

---

†*See page 52.*   **See page 53.*

Forgotten doses: If you are scheduled to take the next dose within a few hours, do not take the forgotten dose. Otherwise take the forgotten dose as soon as you remember.

ALCOHOL, DRUG, HERB, AND SUPPLEMENT INTERACTIONS

Alcohol may increase the risk of liver damage from this drug. Ask your doctor about the risks caused by drinking alcohol with your condition.

St. John's wort may noticeably interfere with the effects of this drug and should not be used at any time during treatment.

Taking this drug with any of the ones listed below may change the effect of either drug with the possibility of causing toxicity or decreasing effectiveness: ketoconazole, methadone, oral contraceptives, rifabutin, rifampin

Increased side effects are possible when this drug is taken with those listed below: prednisone

ALLERGIC REACTIONS AND SIDE EFFECTS

You should tell your doctor about all your allergies and any unexplained symptoms you may have while taking this drug.

MORE COMMON SIDE EFFECTS: Abdominal pain*, blisters*, chills*, cough*, dark urine*, diarrhea*, eye irritation*, fever*, headache, itching*, joint pain*, mouth sores*, muscle pain*, nausea*, pale stools*, skin irritation*, skin rash*, sore throat*, tiredness*, vomiting*, weakness*, yellow eyes or skin*

LESS COMMON SIDE EFFECTS: Hives*, loss of appetite*

RARE SIDE EFFECTS: Drowsiness*, numbness*, tingling*

PRECAUTIONS

This drug is usually prescribed in combination with another antiretroviral drug†. Ask your pharmacist about the type of drug interaction that may occur between antiretroviral drugs† to coordinate the administration times of multiple drugs.

A rash may be the first sign of a serious side effect when taking this drug and should be reported to your doctor right away. Most rashes appear in the first 6 weeks of treatment. Lower doses are used for the first 2 weeks to reduce the chance of developing a rash.

This drug may cause changes to the liver and requires regular testing to ensure safety.

If this drug is stopped for more than 7 days and then restarted, a low dose should be used initially to avoid side effects.

This drug does not prevent transmission of the HIV virus.

PREGNANCY AND BREAST-FEEDING

Safety during pregnancy has not been established although the drug is known to harm animal fetuses.

Breast-feeding while taking this drug is not recommended.

HELPFUL COMMENTS

Contact your doctor if your symptoms do not improve after a couple of days.

Do not stop treatment early if you start to feel better. It takes the full prescription for this drug to work completely.

Oral contraceptives may not work properly when taken with this drug. You need to use a barrier contraceptive, such as a condom, or other nonhormonal contraceptive to prevent pregnancy.

NICARDIPINE HYDROCHLORIDE

Available since December 1988

COMMONLY USED TO TREAT

Chest pain, also known as angina

High blood pressure, also known as hypertension

DRUG CATEGORY

antianginal

antihypertensive

Class: calcium channel blocker

PRODUCTS

Brand-Name Products with No Generic Alternative

Cardene SR 30 mg extended-release capsule (¢¢¢¢¢)

Cardene SR 45 mg extended-release capsule ($)

Cardene SR 60 mg extended-release capsule ($$)

No generic extended-release product.

Patent expires in 2010.

Brand-Name Products with Generic Alternatives

Cardene 20 mg capsule (¢¢¢¢)

  Generic: nicardipine hydrochloride 20 mg capsule (¢¢¢)

Cardene 30 mg capsule (¢¢¢¢¢)

  Generic: nicardipine hydrochloride 30 mg capsule (¢¢¢¢)

---

† See page 52.   * See page 53.

DOSING AND FOOD

Doses are taken 3 times a day. Extended-release products are taken twice a day.

It is best to take this drug on an empty stomach. Do not drink grapefruit juice while taking this drug.

Adults: Up to 120 mg per day in divided doses.

Forgotten doses: If you are scheduled to take the next dose within a few hours, do not take the forgotten dose. Otherwise take the forgotten dose as soon as you remember.

ALCOHOL, DRUG, HERB, AND SUPPLEMENT INTERACTIONS

Alcohol may increase some of the side effects from this drug, depending on the amount consumed. Ask your doctor about the risks caused by drinking alcohol with your condition.

Several OTC drugs used for appetite control, asthma, colds, cough, hay fever, or sinus problems may cause an increase in blood pressure when taken with this drug. Check with your pharmacist when selecting OTC products.

Taking this drug with any of the ones listed below may change the effect of either drug with the possibility of causing toxicity or decreasing effectiveness: anesthetics, carbamazepine, cimetidine, cyclosporine, digoxin, procainamide, quinidine

Severe reactions are possible when this drug is taken with those listed below: beta blockers†

ALLERGIC REACTIONS AND SIDE EFFECTS

If you are allergic to any other calcium channel blocker†, you may also be allergic to this drug. You should tell your doctor about all your allergies and any unexplained symptoms you may have while taking this drug.

MORE COMMON SIDE EFFECTS: Flushing, fluid retention, irregular heartbeat*, swelling*

LESS COMMON SIDE EFFECTS: Abdominal pain, breathing difficulty*, cough*, dizziness, dry mouth, headache, nausea, shortness of breath*, skin rash*, tiredness, weakness, wheezing*

RARE SIDE EFFECTS: Chest pain*, fainting*, tender gums*

PRECAUTIONS

Do not open, crush, break, or chew the extended-release products.

This drug may cause changes to your gums and mouth. Your dentist may recommend that you clean your teeth and mouth differently to avoid infection.

People with heart failure or liver disease may not be able to use this drug.

PREGNANCY AND BREAST-FEEDING

Safety during pregnancy has not been established although the drug is known to harm animal fetuses.

Breast-feeding while taking this drug is not recommended.

HELPFUL COMMENTS

Sucking on hard sugarless candy or chewing sugarless gum may help relieve dry mouth caused by this drug.

NIFEDIPINE

Available for over 20 years

COMMONLY USED TO TREAT

Chest pain, also known as angina
High blood pressure, also known as hypertension

DRUG CATEGORY

antianginal
antihypertensive
Class: calcium channel blocker

PRODUCTS

Brand-Name Products with Generic Alternatives
Procardia 10 mg capsule (¢¢¢¢)
  Generic: nifedipine 10 mg capsule (¢¢)
Procardia 20 mg capsule ($)
  Generic: nifedipine 20 mg capsule (¢¢)
Adalat CC 30 mg extended-release tablet§ ($)
Procardia XL 30 mg extended-release tablet§ ($$)
  Generic: nifedipine 30 mg extended-release tablet§ ($)
Adalat CC 60 mg extended-release tablet§ ($$)
Procardia XL 60 mg extended-release tablet§ ($$$)
  Generic: nifedipine 60 mg extended-release tablet§ ($$)
Adalat CC 90 mg extended-release tablet§ ($$$)
Procardia XL 90 mg extended-release tablet§ ($$$)
  Generic: nifedipine 90 mg extended-release tablet§ ($$$)

---

† See page 52.   * See page 53.   § See "Precautions" in this entry.

Other Generic Product Names
Adalat, Nifedical XL

DOSING AND FOOD

Doses are taken 3 to 4 times a day. Extended-release products are taken once a day.

It is best to take this drug on an empty stomach, but taking this drug with a little food may avoid the stomach upset that some people suffer. Do NOT drink grapefruit juice while taking this drug.

Adults: Up to 120 mg per day in divided doses.

Forgotten doses: If you are scheduled to take the next dose within a few hours, do not take the forgotten dose. Otherwise take the forgotten dose as soon as you remember.

ALCOHOL, DRUG, HERB, AND SUPPLEMENT INTERACTIONS

Alcohol may increase some of the side effects from this drug, depending on the amount consumed. Ask your doctor about the risks caused by drinking alcohol with your condition.

Several OTC drugs used for appetite control, asthma, colds, cough, hay fever, or sinus problems may cause an increase in blood pressure when taken with this drug. Check with your pharmacist when selecting OTC products.

Taking this drug with any of the ones listed below may change the effect of either drug with the possibility of causing toxicity or decreasing effectiveness: benzodiazepines†, carbamazepine, cimetidine, cyclosporine, dalfopristin, digoxin, fentanyl, procainamide, quinidine, quinupristin

Severe reactions are possible when this drug is taken with those listed below: beta blockers†

ALLERGIC REACTIONS AND SIDE EFFECTS

If you are allergic to any other calcium channel blocker†, you may also be allergic to this drug. You should tell your doctor about all your allergies and any unexplained symptoms you may have while taking this drug.

MORE COMMON SIDE EFFECTS: Dizziness, fluid retention, flushing, headache, lightheadedness, nausea, swelling*, weakness

LESS COMMON SIDE EFFECTS: Abdominal pain, breathing difficulty*, congestion, constipation, cough*, diarrhea, fainting*, fever*, irregular heartbeat*, muscle cramps, nervousness, shortness of breath*, skin rash*, tiredness, wheezing*

RARE SIDE EFFECTS: Chest pain*, tender gums*

PRECAUTIONS

§The manufacturing process for the extended-release products may make a difference in the effect of this drug. Some products cause a greater effect than others. Talk to your pharmacist to make sure that you continue taking product from the same manufacturer.

Do not crush, break, or chew the extended-release products.

Be careful driving or handling equipment while taking this drug because it may cause dizziness and lightheadedness.

This drug may cause changes to your gums and mouth. Your dentist may recommend that you clean your teeth and mouth differently to avoid infection.

People with heart failure or liver disease may not be able to use this drug.

PREGNANCY AND BREAST-FEEDING

Safety during pregnancy has not been established although the drug is known to harm animal fetuses.

Breast-feeding while taking this drug is not recommended.

HELPFUL COMMENTS

Avoid quick movements to minimize dizziness. Dangling your legs over the side of the bed for a few minutes may help reduce dizziness when first waking up.

NILUTAMIDE

Available since April 1999

COMMONLY USED TO TREAT

Prostate cancer

DRUG CATEGORY

antineoplastic
Class: nonsteroidal antiandrogen

PRODUCTS

Brand-Name Products with No Generic Alternative
Niladron 150 mg tablet ($$$$$)
No generics available.
No patents, no exclusivity.

---

†See page 52.   *See page 53.

DOSING AND FOOD

Doses are taken once a day.

This drug may be taken with or without food.

Men: Up to 300 mg per day.

Forgotten doses: If you are scheduled to take the next dose in less than 8 hours, do not take the forgotten dose. Otherwise take the forgotten dose as soon as you remember. If you vomit shortly after taking a dose, call your doctor to find out if the dose should be repeated.

ALCOHOL, DRUG, HERB, AND SUPPLEMENT INTERACTIONS

Alcohol may increase some of the side effects from this drug, depending on the amount consumed. Ask your doctor about the risks caused by drinking alcohol with your condition.

Taking this drug with any of the ones listed below may change the effect of either drug with the possibility of causing toxicity or decreasing effectiveness: anticoagulants†, phenytoin, theophylline

ALLERGIC REACTIONS AND SIDE EFFECTS

If you are allergic to bicalutamide or flutamide, you may also be allergic to this drug. You should tell your doctor about all your allergies and any unexplained symptoms you may have while taking this drug.

This drug may cause your eyes to be more sensitive to sunlight, but there are no special risks associated with sunburn while taking this drug.

MORE COMMON SIDE EFFECTS: Breast tenderness, breast swelling, chest tightness*, constipation, cough*, diarrhea, dizziness*, fever*, headache, hoarseness*, loss of appetite, loss of color vision, nausea, runny nose*, sexual dysfunction, sleep disorders, sneezing*, sore throat*, urinary difficulty, wheezing*

LESS COMMON SIDE EFFECTS: Bloating, bloody stools*, breathing difficulty*, chest pain*, confusion, depression*, drowsiness, dry mouth, gas, indigestion, itching*, nervousness, numbness*, pain*, shortness of breath*, skin rash*, swelling*, tingling*, tiredness*, vomiting, weakness*

RARE SIDE EFFECTS: Abdominal pain*, bleeding*, bruising*, dark urine*, skin irritation*, yellow eyes or skin*

PRECAUTIONS

If you have liver disease, you may not be able to take this drug.

Be careful driving or handling equipment while taking this drug because it may cause dizziness.

This drug may change the way your eyes react to light, making it more difficult to see when going from a light to a dark place. Be especially careful when stepping outdoors, turning on lights, driving out of tunnels, and driving at night.

If you have lung disease or a history of breathing problems, this drug may make your condition worse.

People of Asian descent are at greater risk of developing serious lung problems. Make sure to tell your doctor right away if you develop shortness of breath.

PREGNANCY AND BREAST-FEEDING

This drug should not be used in women, but if necessary, it should not be used during pregnancy. This drug may interfere with the normal development of a male fetus.

Breast-feeding while taking this drug is not recommended.

HELPFUL COMMENTS

For best results, this drug should be started the day of or the day after surgery.

It is very important to continue taking this drug as ordered by the doctor even if the side effects make you feel ill.

Avoid quick movements to minimize dizziness. Dangling your legs over the side of the bed for a few minutes may help reduce dizziness when first waking up.

Eye irritation caused by the sun may be reduced by wearing sunglasses when outside.

NIMODIPINE

Available since December 1988

COMMONLY USED TO TREAT

People with bleeding inside the head who are at risk of brain damage

DRUG CATEGORY

subarachnoid hemorrhage therapy
Class: calcium channel blocker

PRODUCTS

Brand-Name Products with No Generic Alternative
Nimotop 30 mg capsule ($$$$)

---

†See page 52.　　*See page 53.

No generics available.
No patents, no exclusivity.

DOSING AND FOOD

Doses are taken 6 times a day.

It is best to take this drug on an empty stomach at least 1 hour before or 2 hours after a meal.

Adults: Up to 360 mg per day in divided doses.

Lower doses are used in people with liver disease.

Forgotten doses: If you are scheduled to take the next dose within a few hours, do not take the forgotten dose. Otherwise take the forgotten dose as soon as you remember.

ALCOHOL, DRUG, HERB, AND SUPPLEMENT INTERACTIONS

Alcohol may increase some of the side effects from this drug, depending on the amount consumed. Ask your doctor about the risks caused by drinking alcohol with your condition.

Taking this drug with any of the ones listed below may change the effect of either drug with the possibility of causing toxicity or decreasing effectiveness: antihypertensives†, cimetidine

ALLERGIC REACTIONS AND SIDE EFFECTS

If you are allergic to any other calcium channel blocker†, you may also be allergic to this drug. You should tell your doctor about all your allergies and any unexplained symptoms you may have while taking this drug.

MORE COMMON SIDE EFFECTS: Diarrhea, fainting*, irregular heartbeat*, lightheadedness*, low blood pressure, nausea, skin rash*, swelling*

LESS COMMON SIDE EFFECTS: Breathing difficulty*, constipation, cough*, dizziness, fluid retention, flushing, headache, muscle cramps, shortness of breath*, tiredness, weakness, wheezing*

RARE SIDE EFFECTS: Chest pain*

PRECAUTIONS

Blood pressure should be checked regularly while taking this drug.
People with heart failure or liver disease may not be able to use this drug.

PREGNANCY AND BREAST-FEEDING

Safety during pregnancy has not been established although the drug is known to harm animal fetuses.
Breast-feeding while taking this drug is not recommended.

HELPFUL COMMENTS

This drug is only taken for 21 days.

NISOLDIPINE

Available since February 1995

COMMONLY USED TO TREAT

High blood pressure, also known as hypertension

DRUG CATEGORY

antihypertensive
Class: calcium channel blocker

PRODUCTS

Brand-Name Products with No Generic Alternative
Sular 10 mg extended-release tablet ($)
Sular 20 mg extended-release tablet ($)
Sular 30 mg extended-release tablet ($)
Sular 40 mg extended-release tablet ($)
No generics available.
Multiple patents that begin to expire in 2005.

DOSING AND FOOD

Doses are taken once a day.
It is best to take this drug on an empty stomach. Do not drink grapefruit
juice or eat high-fat foods or grapefruit while taking this drug.
Adults: Up to 60 mg per day.
Lower doses are used in people over age 65 and people with liver disease.
Forgotten doses: If you are scheduled to take the next dose within a few
hours, do not take the forgotten dose. Otherwise take the forgotten dose
as soon as you remember.

ALCOHOL, DRUG, HERB, AND SUPPLEMENT INTERACTIONS

Alcohol may increase some of the side effects from this drug, depending
on the amount consumed. Ask your doctor about the risks caused by
drinking alcohol with your condition.
Several OTC drugs used for appetite control, asthma, colds, cough, hay fever,
or sinus problems may cause an increase in blood pressure when taken
with this drug. Check with your pharmacist when selecting OTC products.

†See page 52.   *See page 53.

Taking this drug with any of the ones listed below may change the effect of either drug with the possibility of causing toxicity or decreasing effectiveness: cimetidine, quinidine

ALLERGIC REACTIONS AND SIDE EFFECTS

If you are allergic to any other calcium channel blocker†, you may also be allergic to this drug. You should tell your doctor about all your allergies and any unexplained symptoms you may have while taking this drug.

MORE COMMON SIDE EFFECTS: Headache, swelling*

LESS COMMON SIDE EFFECTS: Chest pain*, dizziness, fainting*, hoarseness, irregular heartbeat, lightheadedness*, skin rash*, sore throat, stuffy nose

RARE SIDE EFFECTS: Shortness of breath*

PRECAUTIONS

Do not crush, break, or chew the extended-release products.

Learn how to measure your heart rate and call your doctor if it falls below 60 beats per minute.

If you have congestive heart failure, this drug may make that condition worse.

PREGNANCY AND BREAST-FEEDING

Safety during pregnancy has not been established although the drug is known to harm animal fetuses.

Breast-feeding while taking this drug is not recommended.

HELPFUL COMMENTS

Avoid quick movements to minimize dizziness.

NITAZOXANIDE

Available since November 2002

COMMONLY USED TO TREAT

Diarrhea caused by protozoa infections
Infection caused by *Cryptosporidium* or *Giargia*

DRUG CATEGORY

antiprotozoal
Class: benzamide derivative

PRODUCTS

Brand-Name Products with No Generic Alternative
Alinia 100 mg/5 ml oral suspension (n/a)
No generics available.
No patents. Exclusivity begins to expire in 2007.

DOSING AND FOOD

Doses are taken twice a day.
It is best to take this drug with food.
Children age 4 to 11: Up to 30 ml per day in divided doses.
Children age 12 months to 4 years: Up to 15 ml per day in divided doses.
Forgotten doses: If more than 4 hours have passed since the forgotten dose, you should call your doctor to talk about a change in your prescription. Otherwise take the forgotten dose right away.

ALCOHOL, DRUG, HERB, AND SUPPLEMENT INTERACTIONS

Taking this drug with any of the ones listed below may change the effect of either drug with the possibility of causing toxicity or decreasing effectiveness: aspirin, warfarin

ALLERGIC REACTIONS AND SIDE EFFECTS

You should tell your doctor about all your allergies and any unexplained symptoms you may have while taking this drug.
MORE COMMON SIDE EFFECTS: Abdominal pain
LESS COMMON SIDE EFFECTS: Diarrhea, headache, vomiting
RARE SIDE EFFECTS: Anorexia, discolored urine, dizziness, fever, gas, itching, loss of appetite, nausea, runny nose, sweating, swollen glands, tiredness

PRECAUTIONS

Diabetics need to know that the oral suspension products contain 1.48 grams of sucrose per 5 ml.
This product loses effectiveness 7 days after mixing and should then be thrown out.

PREGNANCY AND BREAST-FEEDING

Safety during pregnancy has not been established although the drug is known to harm animal fetuses.

---

† See page 52.   * See page 53.

It is not known if this drug passes into breast milk. Talk to your doctor about the risks associated with breast-feeding while taking this drug.

HELPFUL COMMENTS

Contact your doctor if your symptoms do not improve after a couple of days. Do not stop treatment early if you start to feel better. It takes the full prescription for this drug to work completely.

The oral suspension product contains natural strawberry flavoring.

NITISINONE

Available since January 2002

COMMONLY USED TO TREAT

Hereditary tyrosinemia, type 1

DRUG CATEGORY

tyrosine degredation inhibitor
Class: cyclohexane dione

PRODUCTS

Brand-Name Products with No Generic Alternative
Orfadin 2 mg capsule ($$$$$)
Orfadin 5 mg capsule ($$$$$)
Orfadin 10 mg capsule ($$$$$)
No generics available.
No patents. Exclusivity begins to expire in 2007.

DOSING AND FOOD

Doses are taken twice a day.
It is best to take this drug on an empty stomach about 1 hour before meals.
Adults and children: Up to 2 mg/kg per day in divided doses.
Forgotten doses: If you are scheduled to take the next dose within a few hours, do not take the forgotten dose. Otherwise take the forgotten dose as soon as you remember.

ALCOHOL, DRUG, HERB, AND SUPPLEMENT INTERACTIONS

Alcohol may increase the risk of liver damage from this drug. Ask your doctor about the risks caused by drinking alcohol with your condition.

This drug is still relatively new and there are no known interactions. Check with your pharmacist for more-current information.

ALLERGIC REACTIONS AND SIDE EFFECTS

You should tell your doctor about all your allergies and any unexplained symptoms you may have while taking this drug.

This drug promotes the effect of sunlight on the body and may cause severe sunburn and increased sensitivity of the eyes.

MORE COMMON SIDE EFFECTS: Abdominal pain*, bloating*, dark urine*, headache*, loss of appetite*, pale stools*, tiredness*, vomiting*, weakness*, weight loss*, yellow eyes or skin*

LESS COMMON SIDE EFFECTS: Black stools*, bleeding*, blindness*, blisters*, bloody nose*, bloody urine*, blurry vision*, bruising*, chest pain*, chills*, cough*, dry eyes*, dry skin*, eye irritation*, fever*, hair loss, heartburn, indigestion, itching*, menstrual changes, mouth sores*, shortness of breath*, skin irritation*, sleepiness, sore throat*, swollen eyelids*, swollen glands*, tooth discoloration*, urinary changes*, vision changes*

RARE SIDE EFFECTS: Agitation*, anxiety*, back pain*, behavior change*, bloody vomit*, blue fingers*, blue lips*, breathing difficulty*, chest tightness*, coma*, confusion*, constipation*, diarrhea*, dizziness*, drowsiness*, dry mouth*, earache*, fainting*, hallucinations*, hunger*, infection*, irregular breathing*, irregular heartbeat*, lightheadedness*, mood swings*, nausea*, nervousness*, pale skin*, shakiness*, skin rash*, spastic movements*, stiff neck*, sunken eyes*, sweating*, swelling*, thirst*, wheezing*, wrinkles*

PRECAUTIONS

It is necessary to follow strict diet recommendations if you want this drug to work effectively. Your doctor will provide details.

Because this drug may be harmful to the eyes, frequent eye exams are needed. Tell your doctor about any changes in your vision right away.

People with a history of liver disease may be at greater risk of developing serious side effects from this drug.

PREGNANCY AND BREAST-FEEDING

Safety during pregnancy has not been established although the drug is known to harm animal fetuses.

Breast-feeding while taking this drug is not recommended.

---

† See page 52.   * See page 53.

HELPFUL COMMENTS

The capsules may be opened and the contents mixed with water, formula, or applesauce for easier swallowing.

Eye irritation caused by the sun may be reduced by wearing sunglasses when outside.

NITROGLYCERIN

Available for over 20 years

COMMONLY USED TO TREAT

Chest pain, also known as angina
People at risk of developing chest pain

DRUG CATEGORY

antianginal
Class: nitrate

PRODUCTS

Brand-Name Products with No Generic Alternative
Nitrogard 2 mg controlled-release buccal tablet (¢¢¢)
Nitrogard 3 mg controlled-release buccal tablet (¢¢¢¢)
NitroQuick 0.3 mg sublingual tablet (¢)
NitroQuick 0.4 mg sublingual tablet (¢)
NitroQuick 0.6 mg sublingual tablet (¢)
Nitrolingual 0.4 mg sublingual spray ($)
Nitro-Dur 0.3 mg/hr extended-release topical patch ($$)
Nitro-Dur 0.8 mg/hr extended-release topical patch ($$)
Transderm-Nitro 0.8 mg/hr extended-release topical patch (n/a)
Brand-Name Products with Generic Alternatives
Nitrostat 0.3 mg sublingual tablet (¢)
  Generic: nitroglycerin 0.3 mg sublingual tablet (¢)
Nitrostat 0.4 mg sublingual tablet (¢)
  Generic: nitroglycerin 0.4 mg sublingual tablet (¢)
Nitrostat 0.6 mg sublingual tablet (¢)
  Generic: nitroglycerin 0.6 mg sublingual tablet (¢)
Nitrong 2.6 mg extended-release tablet (n/a)
  Generic: nitroglycerin 2.6 mg extended-release tablet (¢)
Nitrong 6.5 mg extended-release tablet (n/a)
  Generic: nitroglycerin 6.5 mg extended-release tablet (¢)

Nitrong 9 mg extended-release tablet (n/a)
  Generic: nitroglycerin 9 mg extended-release tablet (¢)
Nitro-Dur 0.1 mg/hr extended-release topical patch ($$)
Transderm-Nitro 0.1 mg/hr extended-release topical patch (n/a)
  Generic: nitroglycerin 0.1 mg/hr extended-release topical patch ($$)
Nitro-Dur 0.2 mg/hr extended-release topical patch ($$)
Transderm-Nitro 0.2 mg/hr extended-release topical patch (n/a)
  Generic: nitroglycerin 0.2 mg/hr extended-release topical patch ($)
Nitro-Dur 0.4 mg/hr extended-release topical patch ($$)
Transderm-Nitro 0.4 mg/hr extended-release topical patch (n/a)
  Generic: nitroglycerin 0.4 mg/hr extended-release topical patch ($$)
Nitro-Dur 0.6 mg/hr extended-release topical patch ($$)
Transderm-Nitro 0.6 mg/hr extended-release topical patch (n/a)
  Generic: nitroglycerin 0.6 mg/hr extended-release topical patch ($$)
Nitro-Bid 2% topical ointment (¢)
  Generic: nitroglycerin 2% topical ointment (¢)

Products Only Available as Generics
nitroglyn 13 mg extended-release tablet (n/a)

Other Generic Product Names
Minitran, Nitrol, Nitroglyn, Nitro-Time, Nitro-Dur, Nitrek, Nitrodisk,
  Deponit

DOSING AND FOOD

Doses are taken 2 to 8 times a day depending on the product.
It is best to take this drug on an empty stomach, about 1 hour before or
  2 hours after meals.
Adult doses are individualized based on the product.
Forgotten doses: Have your doctor or pharmacist explain what to do
  about forgotten doses when you get your prescription.

ALCOHOL, DRUG, HERB, AND SUPPLEMENT INTERACTIONS

Alcohol should not be used while taking this drug.

Taking this drug with any of the ones listed below may change the effect of
either drug with the possibility of causing toxicity or decreasing effectiveness:
antihypertensives†, calcium channel blockers†, phenothiazines†, vaso-
  dilators†

Severe reactions are possible when this drug is taken with those listed below:
ergot alkaloids†, silfenafil

---

†*See page 52.*   **See page 53.*

ALLERGIC REACTIONS AND SIDE EFFECTS

You should tell your doctor about all your allergies and any unexplained symptoms you may have while taking this drug.

MORE COMMON SIDE EFFECTS: Dizziness*, fast pulse, flushing, headache*, lightheadedness, restlessness, swelling*

RARE SIDE EFFECTS: Blue hands*, blue lips*, blurry vision*, dry mouth*, fainting*, fever*, head pressure*, irregular heartbeat*, nausea, seizures*, shortness of breath*, skin rash*, tiredness*, vomiting, weakness*

PRECAUTIONS

Most products are used to prevent chest pain from occurring, but only sublingual tablets and translingual sprays are used to stop the pain once it starts.

The effect of sublingual, or translingual, products should be noticed within about 2 to 4 minutes. If chest pain continues, go to the hospital.

Do not apply ointment to the forearm or lower leg. Apply instead to a hairless part of the trunk, upper arm, or upper leg. Do not rub the ointment into the skin, but cover it with plastic wrap.

This drug should not be stopped suddenly once it has been taken for more than a few weeks since severe chest pains may occur. If you wish to stop taking this drug, ask your doctor for specific instructions.

Be careful driving or handling equipment while taking this drug because it may cause dizziness and blurry vision.

Do not crush, break, or chew the extended-release products.

If taken too often, it is possible that this drug will become less effective over time. Make sure you follow the prescription exactly as written, and tell your doctor how often you have chest pain.

Your cholesterol level may appear lower while taking this drug, but the drug interferes with the test, causing a false result.

Sublingual tablets should be moistened with saliva when placed under the tongue and allowed to dissolve without chewing, sucking, or swallowing.

You should not swallow for at least 10 seconds after using the translingual spray under the tongue.

Buccal tablets and sublingual tablets are placed in different areas of the mouth and will not work properly if placed in the wrong area. If you are taking a buccal or sublingual tablet, make sure your doctor or pharmacist has explained the difference.

Transdermal patches have an aluminum back that may burn the skin if you are standing too close to a microwave that is leaking radiation.

If you have a history of head injury, stroke, anemia, or glaucoma, this drug may make those conditions worse.

PREGNANCY AND BREAST-FEEDING

Safety during pregnancy has not been established although the drug is known to harm animal fetuses.

Breast-feeding while taking this drug is not recommended.

HELPFUL COMMENTS

Aspirin or acetaminophen may be used to relieve the headache pain that many people suffer while taking this drug.

Avoid quick movements to minimize dizziness. Dangling your legs over the side of the bed for a few minutes may help reduce dizziness when first waking up.

People should always be sitting down when taking a sublingual, translingual, or chewable dose of this drug.

This drug is also called by the generic name glyceryl trinitrate.

Sucking on hard sugarless candy or chewing sugarless gum may help relieve dry mouth caused by this drug.

Keep sublingual or translingual products with you at all times.

NIZATIDINE

Available since April 1988

COMMONLY USED TO TREAT

Stomach ulcers, specifically duodenal ulcers and gastric ulcers

DRUG CATEGORY

antiulcer
Class: H2 receptor antagonist

PRODUCTS

Brand-Name Products with Generic Alternatives
Axid 150 mg capsule ($$$)
  Generic: nizatidine 150 mg capsule (n/a)
Axid 300 mg capsule ($$$$)
  Generic: nizatidine 300 mg capsule (n/a)

DOSING AND FOOD

Doses are taken 1 to 2 times a day.

It is best to take this drug with food or milk, or within 1 hour before meals.
Vegetable-based tomato juice may decrease the effect of this drug.

Adults: Up to 300 mg per day in divided doses.

Children over age 12: Up to 150 mg per day in divided doses.

Lower doses are used in people with kidney disease.

Forgotten doses: If you are scheduled to take the next dose within a few
hours, do not take the forgotten dose. Otherwise take the forgotten dose
as soon as you remember.

ALCOHOL, DRUG, HERB, AND SUPPLEMENT INTERACTIONS

Alcohol may increase some of the side effects from this drug, depending
on the amount consumed. Ask your doctor about the risks caused by
drinking alcohol with your condition.

Taking this drug with any of the ones listed below may change the effect of
either drug with the possibility of causing toxicity or decreasing effectiveness:
aspirin

ALLERGIC REACTIONS AND SIDE EFFECTS

If you are allergic to any H2 receptor antagonists†, you may also be allergic
to this drug. You should tell your doctor about all your allergies and any
unexplained symptoms you may have while taking this drug.

MORE COMMON SIDE EFFECTS: Irregular heartbeat*, sweating

LESS COMMON SIDE EFFECTS: Drowsiness

RARE SIDE EFFECTS: Abdominal pain*, back pain*, bleeding*, blisters*,
bloody stool*, breathing difficulty*, bruising*, chest tightness*, chills*,
dark urine*, fainting*, fever*, hives*, itching*, pale stools*, shallow
breathing*, shortness of breath*, skin irritation*, swelling*, tiredness*,
vomiting*, weakness*, wheezing*, yellow eyes or skin*

PRECAUTIONS

Smoking may increase stomach acids, making your condition worse.

The OTC product Axid AR should not be taken for longer than 2 weeks unless recommended by your doctor.

PREGNANCY AND BREAST-FEEDING

Safety during pregnancy has not been established although there was no
evidence of harm during studies in animals.

Breast-feeding while taking this drug is not recommended.

HELPFUL COMMENTS

Once-a-day doses should be taken at bedtime.
This drug is available without a prescription in 75 mg tablets under the
brand name Axid AR. No generic OTC product is available.

NORETHINDRONE

Available for over 20 years

COMMONLY USED TO TREAT

Abnormal uterine bleeding
Endometriosis
Women of childbearing age to prevent pregnancy

DRUG CATEGORY

progestational drug
Class: progestin

PRODUCTS

Brand-Name Products with Generic Alternatives
Aygestin 5 mg tablet ($$)
  Generic: norethindrone acetate 5 mg tablet§ ($)
Micronor 0.35 mg tablet ($)
  Generic: norethindrone 0.35 mg tablet ($)

Other Generic Product Names
Camila, Errin, Nor-QD

Combination Products That Contain This Drug

Activella tablet (¢¢¢¢¢)	Modicon tablet ($)
Brevicon tablet (¢¢¢¢¢)	Norcept tablet (n/a)
CombiPatch 24-hour patch ($$$)	Norethin tablet (n/a)
Estrostep FE tablet ($)	Norinyl tablet ($)
Femhrt tablet (¢¢¢¢¢)	Nortrel tablet ($)
Gencept tablet (n/a)	Ortho-Novum tablet ($)
Loestrin tablet ($$)	Ovcon tablet ($)
Microgestin tablet ($)	Tri-Norinyl tablet ($)

DOSING AND FOOD

Doses are taken once a day.
This drug may be taken with or without food.
Adults: Up to 15 mg per day.

---

† See page 52.   * See page 53.   § See "Precautions" in this entry.

Forgotten doses: If you are scheduled to take the next dose within a few hours, do not take the forgotten dose. Otherwise take the forgotten dose as soon as you remember.

ALCOHOL, DRUG, HERB, AND SUPPLEMENT INTERACTIONS

Alcohol may increase some of the side effects from this drug, depending on the amount consumed. Ask your doctor about the risks caused by drinking alcohol with your condition.

Taking this drug with any of the ones listed below may change the effect of either drug with the possibility of causing toxicity or decreasing effectiveness: aminoglutethimide, bromocriptine, carbamazepine, phenobarbital, phenytoin, rifabutin, rifampin

ALLERGIC REACTIONS AND SIDE EFFECTS

If you are allergic to any progestins†, you may also be allergic to this drug. You should tell your doctor about all your allergies and any unexplained symptoms you may have while taking this drug.

MORE COMMON SIDE EFFECTS: Abdominal pain, bloating, blood pressure increase, depression*, dizziness, dry mouth*, frequent urination*, loss of appetite*, headache*, mood swings, nervousness, swelling, thirst*, vaginal bleeding*, weight gain

LESS COMMON SIDE EFFECTS: Acne, breast-milk secretion*, breast pain, hair growth, hair loss, hot flashes, sexual dysfunction, skin rash*, skin spots, sleeping difficulty

RARE SIDE EFFECTS: Arm pain*, chest pain*, leg pain*, migraine*, numbness*, poor coordination*, shortness of breath*, speaking difficulty*, vision loss*

PRECAUTIONS

§Norethindrone acetate is twice as strong as regular norethindrone and cannot be used as a substitute for the other without a new prescription.

If you are diabetic, you may need a change in the dose of your antidiabetic drug† or insulin, since this drug may cause changes in blood sugar.

People with a history of blood clots, stroke, or varicose veins are at greater risk of developing blood clots when taking this drug.

If you have a history of breast cysts, depression, high cholesterol, or liver disease, this drug may make those conditions worse.

This drug may cause fluid retention, which may increase the risk of side effects in people with asthma, seizures, heart disease, kidney disease, or migraine headaches.

Be careful driving or handling equipment while taking this drug because it may cause dizziness.

This drug may cause dry mouth, which is associated with a greater risk of cavities. Your dentist may recommend that you clean your teeth and mouth differently to avoid infection.

PREGNANCY AND BREAST-FEEDING

This drug may cause birth defects and should not be used during pregnancy. Breast-feeding while taking this drug is not recommended.

HELPFUL COMMENTS

There is a special patient instruction sheet that the FDA requires people to read before taking the first dose of this drug. Talk to your pharmacist if that information is not supplied with your prescription.

Sucking on hard sugarless candy or chewing sugarless gum may help relieve dry mouth caused by this drug.

This drug is usually taken in a pattern of 5 to 14 days taking the drug followed by a 14- to 21-day drug-free period unless prescribed as a contraceptive. Follow the prescription directions specific to your treatment.

This drug is not always given as a contraceptive. Birth control should be used unless this drug is specifically dosed as a contraceptive.

NORFLOXACIN

Available since October 1986

COMMONLY USED TO TREAT

Infection

DRUG CATEGORY

antibiotic
Class: fluoroquinolone

PRODUCTS

Brand-Name Products with No Generic Alternative
Noroxin 400 mg tablet ($$$)
Chibroxin 0.3% ophthalmic solution (n/a)
No generics available.
Patent expires in 2005.

---

† See page 52.   * See page 53.

DOSING AND FOOD

Doses are taken twice a day.

This drug should be taken on an empty stomach.

Adults: Up to 800 mg per day in divided doses.

Lower doses are used in people with kidney disease.

This drug is rarely used in children under age 18 because it may interfere with bone development.

Forgotten doses: If you are scheduled to take the next dose within a few hours, do not take the forgotten dose. Otherwise take the forgotten dose as soon as you remember.

ALCOHOL, DRUG, HERB, AND SUPPLEMENT INTERACTIONS

Alcohol may increase some of the side effects from this drug, depending on the amount consumed. Ask your doctor about the risks caused by drinking alcohol with your condition.

Taking this drug with any of the ones listed below may change the effect of either drug with the possibility of causing toxicity or decreasing effectiveness: aminophylline, antacids, didanosine, iron and mineral supplements, nitrofurantoin, oxtriphylline, probenecid, sucralfate, theophylline, warfarin

ALLERGIC REACTIONS AND SIDE EFFECTS

If you are allergic to any fluoroquinolones†, you may also be allergic to this drug. You should tell your doctor about all your allergies and any unexplained symptoms you may have while taking this drug.

This drug promotes the effect of sunlight on the body and may cause severe sunburn and increased sensitivity of the eyes.

MORE COMMON SIDE EFFECTS: Diarrhea*, nausea, nervousness, rash*, seizures*, shortness of breath*, skin irritation*, swelling*, vomiting

LESS COMMON SIDE EFFECTS: Back pain*, blisters*, difficulty urinating, dreams, dizziness, drowsiness, headache, lightheadedness, muscle pain, sleep disorders, sore mouth, stomachache, vaginal discharge, vaginal pain, taste changes, vision changes

RARE SIDE EFFECTS: Abdominal pain*, agitation*, bloody urine*, confusion*, dark urine*, fever*, flushing*, hallucinations*, irregular heartbeat*, joint pain*, leg pain*, loss of appetite*, pale stools*, shakiness*, sweating*, tiredness*, tremors*, weakness*, yellow eyes or skin*

PRECAUTIONS

Be careful driving or handling equipment while taking this drug because the drug may cause dizziness and drowsiness.

If you have a history of tendinitis, this drug may make that condition worse.
This drug may interfere with the results of urine opiate tests. If you have a
pre-employment drug-screening test, make sure the laboratory knows
that you are taking this drug.

PREGNANCY AND BREAST-FEEDING

Safety during pregnancy has not been established although the drug is
known to harm animal fetuses.
Breast-feeding while taking this drug is not recommended.

HELPFUL COMMENTS

Contact your doctor if your symptoms do not improve after a couple of days.
Do not stop treatment early if you start to feel better. It takes the full pre-
scription for this drug to work completely.
If you need to take an antacid, minerals, or iron supplements, take them
either 1 hour before or 2 hours after taking this drug.
Drink a lot of water while taking this drug.

NORGESTREL

Available for over 20 years

COMMONLY USED TO TREAT

Women of childbearing age to prevent pregnancy

DRUG CATEGORY

progestational drug
Class: progestin

PRODUCTS

Brand-Name Products with No Generic Alternative
Ovrette 0.075 mg tablet (¢¢¢)
No generics available.
No patents, no exclusivity.
Combination Products That Contain This Drug
Cryselle tablet (n/a)
Lo/Ovral tablet ($$)
Low-Ogestrel tablet (n/a)
Ogestrol tablet ($$)
Ovral tablet ($$)

---

† See page 52.   * See page 53.

DOSING AND FOOD

Doses are taken once a day starting on the first day of menstruation. This drug may be taken with or without food.

Adult women: Up to 0.075 mg per day.

Forgotten doses: If more than 3 hours have passed since the forgotten dose, call your doctor to determine if the dose should be taken. Otherwise take the forgotten dose as soon as you remember. Use another form of birth control for the next 2 days.

ALCOHOL, DRUG, HERB, AND SUPPLEMENT INTERACTIONS

Alcohol may increase some of the side effects from this drug, depending on the amount consumed. Ask your doctor about the risks caused by drinking alcohol with your condition.

Taking this drug with any of the ones listed below may change the effect of either drug with the possibility of causing toxicity or decreasing effectiveness: aminoglutethimide, carbamazepine, phenobarbital, phenytoin, rifabutin, rifampin

Severe reactions are possible when this drug is taken with those listed below: bromocriptine

ALLERGIC REACTIONS AND SIDE EFFECTS

If you are allergic to any progestins†, you may also be allergic to this drug. You should tell your doctor about all your allergies and any unexplained symptoms you may have while taking this drug.

The Ovrette product contains tartrazine, which may cause an allergic reaction in people sensitive to aspirin.

MORE COMMON SIDE EFFECTS: Abdominal pain, diarrhea, dizziness, fatigue, headache, menstrual dysfunction*, mood swings, nausea, nervousness, swelling, tiredness, uterine bleeding*, vomiting, weakness, weight gain

LESS COMMON SIDE EFFECTS: Acne, breast-milk secretion*, breast tenderness, depression*, hair gain, hair loss, hot flashes, sexual dysfunction, skin rash*, skin spots, sleep disorders

PRECAUTIONS

People with high cholesterol may not be able to take this drug since it may cause elevation in blood cholesterol levels.

If you have asthma, seizures, breast disease, heart disease, kidney disease, or migraine headaches, this drug may make those conditions worse.

If you are diabetic, you may need a change in the dose of your antidiabetic drug† or insulin, since this drug may cause changes in blood sugar.

This drug does not protect women from sexually transmitted diseases.

Be careful driving or handling equipment while taking this drug because it may cause dizziness.

This drug, when given alone, is about one-third less effective in preventing pregnancy when compared to combination products.

Heavy smoking may increase the risk of stroke when taking this drug.

PREGNANCY AND BREAST-FEEDING

This drug may cause birth defects and should not be used during pregnancy. Breast-feeding while taking this drug is not recommended.

HELPFUL COMMENTS

This drug is also called the "mini pill."

NORTRIPTYLINE HYDROCHLORIDE

Available for over 20 years

COMMONLY USED TO TREAT

Depression
Panic attacks
People trying to stop smoking

DRUG CATEGORY

antidepressant
antineuralgic
antipanic
Class: tricyclic antidepressant

PRODUCTS

Brand-Name Products with Generic Alternatives
Pamelor 10 mg capsule (¢¢¢¢¢)
  Generic: nortriptyline hydrochloride 10 mg capsule (¢¢)
Pamelor 25 mg capsule ($$)
  Generic: nortriptyline hydrochloride 25 mg capsule (¢¢)
Pamelor 50 mg capsule ($$$)
  Generic: nortriptyline hydrochloride 50 mg capsule (¢¢)

---

† *See page 52.*   * *See page 53.*

Pamelor 75 mg capsule ($$$)
   Generic: nortriptyline hydrochloride 75 mg capsule ($$)
Pamelor 10 mg/5 ml oral solution ($)
   Generic: nortriptyline hydrochloride 10 mg/5 ml oral solution (¢¢¢)
Other Generic Product Names
Aventyl

DOSING AND FOOD

Doses are taken 1 to 4 times a day. Once-daily doses are usually taken at
  bedtime.
Taking this drug with food or milk may avoid the stomach upset that some
  people suffer.
Adults: Up to 150 mg per day.
Lower doses are used in teens and adults over age 65.
Forgotten doses: If you have forgotten a bedtime dose, do not take the
  forgotten dose. Just go back to your usual schedule with the next dose. If
  you have forgotten a daytime dose and are scheduled to take the next
  dose within a few hours, do not take the forgotten dose. Otherwise take
  the forgotten dose as soon as you remember.

ALCOHOL, DRUG, HERB, AND SUPPLEMENT INTERACTIONS

Alcohol should not be used while taking this drug.
Evening primrose oil, SAMe, St. John's wort, and yohimbe may cause serious reactions when taken with this drug. Tell your doctor if you are taking
  any of these supplements.
Several OTC drugs used for asthma, colds, cough, hay fever, sleep aid, or
  sinus problems may seriously change the effects and side effects of this
  drug. Check with your pharmacist when selecting OTC products.
**Taking this drug with any of the ones listed below may change the effect of
either drug with the possibility of causing toxicity or decreasing effectiveness:**
anesthetics, antipsychotics†, anxiolytics†, barbiturates†, beta blockers†,
cimetidine, clonidine, fluoxetine, guanabenz, guanadrel, guanethidine,
haloperidol, methyldopa, methylphenidate, narcotics†, oral contraceptives, phenothiazines†, propoxyphene, reserpine

Severe reactions are possible when this drug is taken with those listed below:
amphetamines†, anesthetics, anticholinergics†, antidyskinetics†, antihista-
mines†, antithyroid drugs†, anxiolytics†, appetite suppressants, barbitu-
rates†, disopyramide, disulfiram, ephedrine, epinephrine, ethchlorvynol,
isoproterenol, meperidine, metrizamide, monoamine oxidase inhibitors†,

phenylephrine, pimozide, procainamide, quinidine, tricyclic antidepressants†, warfarin

Increased side effects are possible when this drug is taken with those listed below:
alseroxylon, deserpidine, metoclopramide, metyrosine, pemoline, pimozide, promethazine, rauwolfia serpentine, reserpine, trimeprazine

ALLERGIC REACTIONS AND SIDE EFFECTS

If you are allergic to carbamazepine, maprotiline, trazodone, or any tricyclic antidepressants†, you may also be allergic to this drug. You should tell your doctor about all your allergies and any unexplained symptoms you may have while taking this drug.

This drug promotes the effect of sunlight on the body and may cause severe sunburn and increased sensitivity of the eyes.

MORE COMMON SIDE EFFECTS: Blurry vision*, constipation*, dizziness, drowsiness, fever*, irregular heartbeat*, seizures*, sweating, tiredness, urinary changes*

LESS COMMON SIDE EFFECTS: Confusion*, diarrhea, dry mouth, expressionless face*, eye pain*, fainting*, hallucinations*, headache, heartburn, loss of balance*, nausea, nervousness*, restlessness*, shakiness*, shuffling walk*, sleeping difficulty, slowed movements*, stiffness*, swallowing difficulty*, trembling*, vomiting, weakness*

RARE SIDE EFFECTS: Anxiety*, breast enlargement*, hair loss, irritability*, muscle twitching*, ringing in ears*, skin rash*, sore throat*, swelling*, taste changes, teeth or gum problems*, yellow eyes or skin*

PRECAUTIONS

You need to wait 2 weeks after stopping a monoamine oxidase inhibitor† before starting this drug.

Be careful driving or handling equipment while taking this drug because it may cause drowsiness, dizziness, and blurry vision.

Stopping this drug abruptly may result in withdrawal symptoms that include nausea, headache, and general discomfort. If you wish to stop taking this drug, ask your doctor for specific instructions.

This drug may cause dry mouth, which is associated with a greater risk of cavities. Your dentist may recommend that you clean your teeth and mouth frequently to avoid infection.

If you have a history of asthma, blood disorders, seizures, enlarged prostate, glaucoma, heart disease, high blood pressure, urinary difficulty, schizophrenia, or manic depression, this drug may make those conditions worse.

---

†See page 52.　　*See page 53.

PREGNANCY AND BREAST-FEEDING

Safety during pregnancy has not been established although the drug is known to harm animal fetuses.

Breast-feeding while taking this drug is not recommended.

HELPFUL COMMENTS

When first starting this drug, you may need to lie down for about 30 minutes after each dose due to extreme dizziness.

Heavy smoking may decrease the effectiveness of this drug.

It may take 4 weeks before the effects of this drug are noticed.

Sucking on hard sugarless candy or chewing sugarless gum may help relieve dry mouth caused by this drug.

NYSTATIN

Available for over 20 years

COMMONLY USED TO TREAT

Fungal infections, specifically candida
Thrush

DRUG CATEGORY

antifungal
Class: polyene macrolide

PRODUCTS

Brand-Name Products with No Generic Alternative
Mycostatin Pastilles 200,000 units lozenge ($)

Brand-Name Products with Generic Alternatives
Mycostatin 500,000 units tablet (¢¢¢¢¢)
  Generic: nystatin 500,000 units tablet (¢¢)
Mycostatin 100,000 units/g topical cream (¢¢)
  Generic: nystatin 100,000 units/g topical cream (¢)
Mycostatin 100,000 units/g topical powder (¢¢¢¢)
  Generic: Nystop 100,000 units/g topical powder (¢¢¢¢)
Mycostatin 100,000 units/ml oral suspension ($$)
  Generic: nystatin 100,000 units/ml oral suspension (¢¢¢)

Products Only Available as Generics
nystatin 100,000 units/g topical ointment (¢)

nystatin oral powder (¢¢¢¢)
nystatin 100,000 units vaginal tablet (¢¢¢¢)

Other Generic Product Names
Nilstat, Nilstatin, Nystex

Combination Products That Contain This Drug
Mycolog-II 0.1% topical cream (¢¢)
Mycolog-II 0.1% topical ointment (¢¢)

DOSING AND FOOD

Oral doses are taken 3 to 5 times a day. Topical products are used 2 to 3 times a day. Vaginal tablets are used twice a day.

This drug may be taken with or without food.

Adults: Up to 5,000,000 units orally per day in divided doses.

Children: Up to 2,400,000 units orally per day in divided doses.

Infants: Up to 800,000 units per day in divided doses.

Forgotten doses: If you are scheduled to take the next dose within a few hours, do not take the forgotten dose. Otherwise take the forgotten dose as soon as you remember.

ALCOHOL, DRUG, HERB, AND SUPPLEMENT INTERACTIONS

This drug works directly on the site of contact and is not absorbed into the body. There are no known interactions.

ALLERGIC REACTIONS AND SIDE EFFECTS

You should tell your doctor about all your allergies and any unexplained symptoms you may have while taking this drug.

LESS COMMON SIDE EFFECTS: Diarrhea, nausea, stomach pain, vomiting

PRECAUTIONS

Touching these tablets or powder may cause skin irritation. You should wash your hands immediately after taking the dose.

Your mouth should be rinsed with water before using the lozenges or oral suspension. Skin should be washed before applying topical products.

Do not cover the skin with bandages or other type of tight wrap since it may lead to the development of secondary yeast infections.

Vaginal products should be continued even if the menstrual period starts.

PREGNANCY AND BREAST-FEEDING

Safety during pregnancy has not been established although there was no evidence of harm during studies in animals.

† See page 52.   * See page 53.

This drug passes into breast milk, but does not appear to harm the baby. Talk to your doctor about the risks associated with breast-feeding while taking this drug.

HELPFUL COMMENTS

Contact your doctor if your symptoms do not improve after a couple of days.

Do not stop treatment early if you start to feel better. Treatment should be continued for at least 2 days after symptoms are completely gone to prevent recurrence of the condition.

Washing and changing clothes that come in contact with the affected area may help prevent reinfection.

OFLOXACIN

Available since December 1990

COMMONLY USED TO TREAT

Infection

DRUG CATEGORY

antibiotic
Class: fluoroquinolone

PRODUCTS

Brand-Name Products with No Generic Alternative
Floxin 200 mg tablet ($$$)
Floxin 300 mg tablet ($$$$)
Floxin 400 mg tablet ($$$$)
Floxin 0.3% ophthalmic solution ($$$$$)
Ocuflox 0.3% ophthalmic solution ($$$$$)
No generics available.
Patent expires in 2003.

DOSING AND FOOD

Doses are taken 1 to 2 times a day.
This drug may be taken with or without food.
Adults: Up to 800 mg per day in divided doses.
Lower doses are used in people with kidney disease.
This drug is rarely used by mouth in children under age 18 because it

may interfere with bone development. Eyedrops are used in children over age 1.

Eyedrops: 1 to 2 drops per dose, 1 to 10 times per day.

Forgotten doses: If you are scheduled to take the next dose within a few hours, do not take the forgotten dose. Otherwise take the forgotten dose as soon as you remember.

ALCOHOL, DRUG, HERB, AND SUPPLEMENT INTERACTIONS

Alcohol may increase some of the side effects from this drug, depending on the amount consumed. Ask your doctor about the risks caused by drinking alcohol with your condition.

Taking this drug with any of the ones listed below may change the effect of either drug with the possibility of causing toxicity or decreasing effectiveness: aminophylline, antacids, antidiabetics†, didanosine, oxtriphylline, sucralfate, theophylline, warfarin

ALLERGIC REACTIONS AND SIDE EFFECTS

If you are allergic to any fluoroquinolones†, you may also be allergic to this drug. You should tell your doctor about all your allergies and any unexplained symptoms you may have while taking this drug.

This drug promotes the effect of sunlight on the body and may cause severe sunburn and increased sensitivity of the eyes.

MORE COMMON SIDE EFFECTS: Nausea, nervousness, rash*, seizures*, skin irritation*, severe diarrhea*, shortness of breath*, vomiting

LESS COMMON SIDE EFFECTS: Back pain, blisters*, difficulty urinating, dreams, dizziness, drowsiness, headache, lightheadedness, muscle pain, sleep disorders, sore mouth, stomachache, vaginal discharge, vaginal pain, taste changes, vision changes

RARE SIDE EFFECTS: Abdominal pain*, agitation*, bloody urine*, confusion*, dark urine*, fever*, flushing*, hallucinations*, irregular heartbeat*, joint pain*, leg pain*, loss of appetite*, pale stools*, shakiness*, sweating*, swelling*, tiredness*, tremors*, weakness*, yellow eyes or skin*

PRECAUTIONS

Be careful driving or handling equipment while taking this drug because the drug may cause dizziness and drowsiness.

If you have a history of tendinitis, this drug may make that condition worse.

A rash may be the first symptom of an allergic reaction and should be reported to your doctor immediately.

---

†*See page 52.*   **See page 53.*

If you are using eyedrops, many of the side effects and warnings, do not apply. Watch for burning and irritation when the drops are used and report any rash, itching, swelling, or redness around the eye.

PREGNANCY AND BREAST-FEEDING

Safety during pregnancy has not been established although the drug is known to harm animal fetuses.

Breast-feeding while taking this drug is not recommended.

HELPFUL COMMENTS

Drink a lot of water while taking this drug.

Contact your doctor if your symptoms do not improve after a couple of days.

Do not stop treatment early if you start to feel better. It takes the full prescription for this drug to work completely.

If you need to take an antacid, vitamins, minerals, or iron supplements, take them either 2 hours before or after taking this drug.

OLANZAPINE

Available since September 1996

COMMONLY USED TO TREAT

Mental disturbances

DRUG CATEGORY

antipsychotic
Class: thienobenzodiazepine derivative

PRODUCTS

Brand-Name Products with No Generic Alternative
Zyprexa 2.5 mg tablet ($$$$)
Zyprexa 5 mg tablet ($$$$)
Zyprexa 7.5 mg tablet ($$$$)
Zyprexa 10 mg tablet ($$$$)
Zyprexa 15 mg tablet ($$$$$)
Zyprexa 20 mg tablet ($$$$$)
Zyprexa Zydis 5 mg disintegrating tablet ($$$$)
Zyprexa Zydis 10 mg disintegrating tablet ($$$$$)
Zyprexa Zydis 15 mg disintegrating tablet ($$$$$)
Zyprexa Zydis 20 mg disintegrating tablet ($$$$$)

No generics available.
Patent expires in 2011.

DOSING AND FOOD

Doses are taken once a day.
This drug may be taken with or without food.
Adults: Up to 20 mg per day.
Forgotten doses: If you are scheduled to take the next dose within a few hours, do not take the forgotten dose. Otherwise take the forgotten dose as soon as you remember.

ALCOHOL, DRUG, HERB, AND SUPPLEMENT INTERACTIONS

Alcohol should not be used while taking this drug.
Nutmeg may decrease the effects of this drug and should not be used.
Many OTC drugs used for appetite control, asthma, colds, cough, hay fever, pain, or sinus problems affect the central nervous system and may cause a change in the effects or side effects of this drug. Check with your pharmacist for products to avoid.

Taking this drug with any of the ones listed below may change the effect of either drug with the possibility of causing toxicity or decreasing effectiveness: carbamazepine, fluvoxamine, levodopa, omeprazole, rifampin

Severe reactions are possible when this drug is taken with those listed below: antihypertensives†, diazepam

ALLERGIC REACTIONS AND SIDE EFFECTS

You should tell your doctor about all your allergies and any unexplained symptoms you may have while taking this drug.
This drug promotes the effect of sunlight on the body and may cause severe sunburn and increased sensitivity of the eyes.

MORE COMMON SIDE EFFECTS: Agitation*, behavior changes*, constipation, dizziness, drowsiness, dry mouth, fainting, headache, restlessness*, runny nose, shaking*, speech dysfunction*, stiffness*, swallowing difficulty*, trembling*, vision changes, weakness, weight gain

LESS COMMON SIDE EFFECTS: Abdominal pain, anger*, anxiety*, chest pain*, chewing motion*, cough, double vision, eye stillness*, fever*, giddiness*, increased appetite, irregular heartbeat*, joint pain, lip smacking*, low blood pressure, memory loss*, mood swings*, muscle spasms*, nausea, nervousness*, puckering*, puffy cheeks*, sexual dysfunction, sleeping difficulty, sore throat, spastic movements*, stuttering, swelling*,

---

†*See page 52.* **See page 53.*

thirst, tongue movements*, twitching*, urinary changes, vomiting, watery mouth, weight loss

RARE SIDE EFFECTS: Breathing difficulty*, confusion*, menstrual changes*, skin rash*, sluggishness*

PRECAUTIONS

People with a history of seizures or Alzheimer's disease may be at greater risk of developing a seizure while taking this drug.

Drink plenty of fluids to avoid dehydration when sweating, such as in hot weather and during exercise.

If you have a history of breast cancer, enlarged prostate, intestinal disorders, heart disease, or glaucoma, this drug may make those conditions worse.

Be careful driving or handling equipment while taking this drug because it may cause drowsiness and dizziness.

This drug may cause dry mouth, which is associated with a greater risk of cavities. Your dentist may recommend that you clean your teeth and mouth differently to avoid infection.

PREGNANCY AND BREAST-FEEDING

Safety during pregnancy has not been established although the drug is known to harm animal fetuses.

Breast-feeding while taking this drug is not recommended.

HELPFUL COMMENTS

Avoid quick movements to minimize dizziness. Dangling your legs over the side of the bed for a few minutes may help reduce dizziness when first waking up.

Sucking on hard sugarless candy or chewing sugarless gum may help relieve dry mouth caused by this drug.

OLMESARTAN MEDOXOMIL

Available since April 2002

COMMONLY USED TO TREAT

High blood pressure, also known as hypertension

DRUG CATEGORY

antihypertensive

Class: angiotensin II receptor antagonist

PRODUCTS

Brand-Name Products with No Generic Alternative
Benicar 5 mg tablet (n/a)
Benicar 20 mg tablet (n/a)
Benicar 40 mg tablet (n/a)
No generics available.
Exclusivity until 2007.

DOSING AND FOOD

Doses are taken once a day.
This drug may be taken with or without food.

Adults: Up to 40 mg per day.

Forgotten doses: If you are scheduled to take the next dose within a few
hours, do not take the forgotten dose. Otherwise take the forgotten dose
as soon as you remember.

ALCOHOL, DRUG, HERB, AND SUPPLEMENT INTERACTIONS

Alcohol may increase some of the side effects from this drug, depending
on the amount consumed. Ask your doctor about the risks caused by
drinking alcohol with your condition.

Several OTC drugs used for appetite control, asthma, colds, cough, hay
fever, or sinus problems may cause an increase in blood pressure when
taken with this drug. Check with your pharmacist when selecting OTC
products.

**Taking this drug with any of the ones listed below may change the effect of
either drug with the possibility of causing toxicity or decreasing effectiveness:**
diuretics†

ALLERGIC REACTIONS AND SIDE EFFECTS

You should tell your doctor about all your allergies and any unexplained
symptoms you may have while taking this drug.

LESS COMMON SIDE EFFECTS: Abdominal pain, back pain*, bloody urine*,
blurry vision*, body aches*, breath odor*, breathing difficulty*, chills*,
cough*, diarrhea, dizziness*, dry mouth*, dry skin*, ear congestion*, fatigue*, fever*, headache*, hunger, loss of appetite, nasal congestion*,
nausea, runny nose*, shivering, shortness of breath*, sleep disorders,
sneezing*, sore throat*, swallowing difficulty*, sweating*, swollen glands,
thirst, tiredness*, urinary changes*, vomiting, weakness*, weight loss,
wheezing*

---

† See page 52.   * See page 53.

RARE SIDE EFFECTS: Belching, bloating, bone pain, chest pain*, confusion*, faintness*, heartburn, indigestion, irregular heartbeat*, joint pain*, light-headedness*, muscle pains, puffy face, rash, sour stomach, stiffness*, stomach pain, swelling*, tingling, weight gain

PRECAUTIONS

If you are dehydrated, the blood-pressure-lowering effect of this drug may be increased. Drink plenty of fluids to avoid dehydration when sweating, such as in hot weather and during exercise.

Be careful driving or handling equipment while taking this drug because the drug may cause dizziness.

If you have congestive heart failure, this drug may make that condition worse.

PREGNANCY AND BREAST-FEEDING

There is evidence that this drug may harm the fetus. The drug should be discontinued immediately if pregnancy is diagnosed.

Breast-feeding while taking this drug is not recommended.

HELPFUL COMMENTS

The full effects of this drug should be noticed within a week.

If you do not treat high blood pressure, you may develop more serious problems such as heart failure, blood vessel disease, stroke, or kidney disease. Losing weight, exercising, eating more fruits and vegetables, and avoiding salty foods, such as lunchmeat and pickles, may help make drug treatment more successful.

OLSALAZINE SODIUM

Available since July 1990

COMMONLY USED TO TREAT

Intestinal inflammation, also known as irritable bowel syndrome (IBS)
Ulcerative colitis

DRUG CATEGORY

antiinflammatory
Class: salicylate

PRODUCTS

Brand-Name Products with No Generic Alternative
Dipentum 250 mg capsule ($)
No generics available.
Patent expires in 2004.

DOSING AND FOOD

Doses are taken twice a day.
It is best to take this drug with food.
Adults: Up to 1 mg per day in divided doses.
Forgotten doses: If you are scheduled to take the next dose within a few hours, do not take the forgotten dose. Otherwise take the forgotten dose as soon as you remember.

ALCOHOL, DRUG, HERB, AND SUPPLEMENT INTERACTIONS

Alcohol may increase some of the side effects from this drug, depending on the amount consumed. Ask your doctor about the risks caused by drinking alcohol with your condition.

Taking this drug with any of the ones listed below may change the effect of either drug with the possibility of causing toxicity or decreasing effectiveness:
warfarin

ALLERGIC REACTIONS AND SIDE EFFECTS

If you are allergic to aspirin, mesalamine, sulfasalazine, or any salicylates†, you may also be allergic to this drug. You should tell your doctor about all your allergies and any unexplained symptoms you may have while taking this drug.

MORE COMMON SIDE EFFECTS: Abdominal pain, diarrhea*, loss of appetite, stomach upset

LESS COMMON SIDE EFFECTS: Acne, anxiety, depression, dizziness, drowsiness, headache, joint pain, muscle pain, sleeping difficulty

RARE SIDE EFFECTS: Back pain*, bloating*, bloody diarrhea*, fever*, irregular heartbeat*, nausea*, skin rash*, stomach pain*, vomiting*, yellow eyes or skin*

PRECAUTIONS

If you have kidney disease, this drug may make that condition worse.
It is difficult to determine if diarrhea is caused by the drug or by the illness.

---

† See page 52.　　* See page 53.

Call your doctor if you get diarrhea that was not present before taking the drug or if your diarrhea gets worse.

PREGNANCY AND BREAST-FEEDING

Safety during pregnancy has not been established although the drug is known to harm animal fetuses.

Breast-feeding while taking this drug is not recommended.

HELPFUL COMMENTS

Do not stop treatment early if you start to feel better.

OMEPRAZOLE

Available since September 1989

COMMONLY USED TO TREAT

Excess stomach acid
Heartburn, specifically gastroesophageal reflux disease (GERD)
Ulcers

DRUG CATEGORY

antiulcer
Class: proton pump inhibitor

PRODUCTS

Brand-Name Products with Generic Alternatives
Prilosec 10 mg delayed-release capsule ($$$)
  Generic: omeprazole 10 mg delayed-release capsule (n/a)
Prilosec 20 mg delayed-release capsule ($$$)
  Generic: omeprazole 20 mg delayed-release capsule (n/a)
Prilosec 40 mg delayed-release capsule ($$$$)
  Generic: omeprazole 40 mg delayed-release capsule (n/a)

DOSING AND FOOD

Doses are taken 1 to 2 times a day.
It is best to take this drug on an empty stomach about 30 minutes before a meal.
Adults: Up to 360 mg per day in divided doses.
Lower doses are used in people with kidney disease.
Forgotten doses: If you are scheduled to take the next dose within a few

hours, do not take the forgotten dose. Otherwise take the forgotten dose as soon as you remember.

ALCOHOL, DRUG, HERB, AND SUPPLEMENT INTERACTIONS

Alcohol may increase some of the side effects from this drug, depending on the amount consumed. Ask your doctor about the risks caused by drinking alcohol with your condition.

The herb male fern may not be effective when taken with this drug.

The toxic effects of pennyroyal may be enhanced when taken with this drug.

Taking this drug with any of the ones listed below may change the effect of either drug with the possibility of causing toxicity or decreasing effectiveness: ampicillin, diazepam, iron, itraconazole, ketoconazole, phenytoin, propranolol, theophylline, warfarin

ALLERGIC REACTIONS AND SIDE EFFECTS

You should tell your doctor about all your allergies and any unexplained symptoms you may have while taking this drug.

MORE COMMON SIDE EFFECTS: Abdominal pain

LESS COMMON SIDE EFFECTS: Back pain*, chest pain, constipation, diarrhea, dizziness, drowsiness*, gas, headache*, heartburn, itching*, muscle pain, nausea*, skin rash*, tiredness*, vomiting

RARE SIDE EFFECTS: Bleeding*, blisters*, bloody urine*, blurry vision*, bruising*, chills*, confusion*, dry mouth*, eye irritation*, fever*, flushing*, irregular heartbeat*, joint pain*, leg pain*, lip sores*, loss of appetite*, mouth sores*, muscle cramps*, skin irritation*, sore throat*, stomach pain*, sweating*, urinary changes*, weakness*

PRECAUTIONS

Do not crush, break, or chew the delayed-release products.

Liver function should be monitored regularly while taking this drug.

PREGNANCY AND BREAST-FEEDING

Safety during pregnancy has not been established although the drug is known to harm animal fetuses.

Breast-feeding while taking this drug is not recommended.

HELPFUL COMMENTS

It may take several days before the effects of this drug are noticed. Antacids may be taken if needed while on this drug.

Contact your doctor if your symptoms do not improve after a couple of days.

---

†See page 52.   *See page 53.

ONDANSETRON HYDROCHLORIDE

Available since January 1991

COMMONLY USED TO TREAT

Nausea and vomiting after chemotherapy or radiation

DRUG CATEGORY

antiemetic
Class: selective 5-HT3 receptor antagonist

PRODUCTS

Brand-Name Products with No Generic Alternative
Zofran 4 mg tablet ($$$$$)
Zofran 8 mg tablet ($$$$$)
Zofran 24 mg tablet ($$$$$)
Zofran 4 mg/5 ml oral solution ($$$$$)
Zofran 4 mg disintegrating tablet ($$$$$)
Zofran 8 mg disintegrating tablet ($$$$$)
No generics available.
Multiple patents that begin to expire in 2005.

DOSING AND FOOD

Doses are taken 2 to 3 times a day.
This drug may be taken with or without food.
Adults and children over age 12: Up to 32 mg per day in divided doses.
Children age 4 to 11: Up to 12 mg per day in divided doses.
Lower doses are used in people with liver disease.
Forgotten doses: If feeling nauseated, take the forgotten dose as soon as you remember. Otherwise just return to your usual schedule with the next dose. If you vomit within 30 minutes of a dose, the dose should be repeated. If you vomit after 2 doses, call your doctor for further instructions.

ALCOHOL, DRUG, HERB, AND SUPPLEMENT INTERACTIONS

Alcohol may increase some of the side effects from this drug, depending on the amount consumed. Ask your doctor about the risks caused by drinking alcohol with your condition.
The herb horehound may interfere with the effects of this drug and should not be used.

ALLERGIC REACTIONS AND SIDE EFFECTS

If you are allergic to granisetron or dolasetron, you may also be allergic to this drug. You should tell your doctor about all your allergies and any unexplained symptoms you may have while taking this drug.

MORE COMMON SIDE EFFECTS: Constipation, diarrhea, fever, headache

LESS COMMON SIDE EFFECTS: Abdominal pain, burning, cold, dizziness, drowsiness, dry mouth, itching, lightheadedness, tingling, tiredness, weakness

RARE SIDE EFFECTS: Breathing difficulty*, chest pain*, chest tightness*, hives*, itching*, shortness of breath*, skin rash*, wheezing*

PRECAUTIONS

The oral disintegrating tablets may contain aspartame, which should not be taken by people with phenylketonuria (PKU).

Liver function should be tested periodically while taking this drug.

Disintegrating tablets should be placed on top of the tongue for a few seconds, then swallowed with saliva.

PREGNANCY AND BREAST-FEEDING

Safety during pregnancy has not been established although there was no evidence of harm during studies in animals.

It is not known if this drug passes into breast milk. Talk to your doctor about the risks associated with breast-feeding while taking this drug.

HELPFUL COMMENTS

Disintegrating tablets may fall apart if pushed through the foil when removing from the packaging. Instead, the foil should be peeled back to open.

ORLISTAT

Available since April 1999

COMMONLY USED TO TREAT

Obesity

DRUG CATEGORY

antiobesity
Class: lipase inhibitor

---

† See page 52.   * See page 53.

PRODUCTS

Brand-Name Products with No Generic Alternative
Xenical 120 mg capsule ($)
No generics available.
Multiple patents that begin to expire in 2009.

DOSING AND FOOD

Doses are taken 3 times a day.
This drug should be taken with a meal or within 1 hour after the meal.
Adults: Up to 360 mg per day in divided doses.
Forgotten doses: If it is less than 1 hour since the end of the meal, take the forgotten dose as soon as you remember. Otherwise do not take the forgotten dose.

ALCOHOL, DRUG, HERB, AND SUPPLEMENT INTERACTIONS

Taking this drug with any of the ones listed below may change the effect of either drug with the possibility of causing toxicity or decreasing effectiveness: pravastatin, vitamin A, vitamin D, vitamin E, vitamin K, warfarin

ALLERGIC REACTIONS AND SIDE EFFECTS

You should tell your doctor about all your allergies and any unexplained symptoms you may have while taking this drug.

MORE COMMON SIDE EFFECTS: Back pain, body aches, bowel movement changes, chills, cough, diarrhea*, fever, gas*, headache, nasal congestion, runny nose, sneezing, sore throat

LESS COMMON SIDE EFFECTS: Anxiety, breathing difficulty*, chest tightness*, gum and tooth problems*, menstrual changes, rectal pain, wheezing*

RARE SIDE EFFECTS: Bloody urine*, ear pain*, hearing changes*, urinary changes*

PRECAUTIONS

This drug interferes with the absorption of fat-soluble vitamins. You should take a daily multivitamin supplement at least 2 hours before or after taking this drug.
If you have kidney stones or gallbladder problems, this drug may make those conditions worse.
Diabetics who lose weight when taking this drug may need a change in their dose of antidiabetic drug† or insulin.

If your diet is high in fat, you are more likely to have side effects from this drug.

This drug may cause changes to your gums and mouth. Your dentist may recommend that you clean your teeth and mouth differently to avoid infection.

PREGNANCY AND BREAST-FEEDING

Safety during pregnancy has not been established although there was no evidence of harm during studies in animals.

It is not known if this drug passes into breast milk. Talk to your doctor about the risks associated with breast-feeding while taking this drug.

HELPFUL COMMENTS

Side effects may continue for 2 to 3 days after this drug is stopped.

This drug does nothing when you eat a fat-free meal, and the dose may be omitted.

This drug may cause oily spots and stains on undergarments.

ORPHENADRINE CITRATE

Available for over 20 years

COMMONLY USED TO TREAT

Muscle pain caused by injury

DRUG CATEGORY

skeletal muscle relaxant
Class: diphenhydramine analogue

PRODUCTS

Brand-Name Products with Generic Alternatives
Norflex 100 mg extended-release tablet ($$)
  Generic: orphenadrine citrate 100 mg extended-release tablet ($$)
Combination Products That Contain This Drug
Norgesic tablet ($)
Norgesic Forte tablet ($)

DOSING AND FOOD

Doses are taken 1 to 4 times a day.
This drug may be taken with or without food.

---

† See page 52.　　* See page 53.

Adults: Up to 200 mg per day in divided doses.

Forgotten doses: If more than 1 hour has passed since the forgotten dose, do not take the dose. Otherwise take the forgotten dose as soon as you remember.

ALCOHOL, DRUG, HERB, AND SUPPLEMENT INTERACTIONS

Alcohol should not be used while taking this drug.

Many OTC drugs used for appetite control, asthma, colds, cough, hay fever, pain, or sinus problems affect the central nervous system and may change the effects or side effects of this drug. Check with your pharmacist for products to avoid.

Severe reactions are possible when this drug is taken with those listed below: anesthetics, anticholinergics†, antipsychotics†, anxiolytics†, barbiturates†, monoamine oxidase inhibitors†, narcotics†, tricyclic antidepressants†

ALLERGIC REACTIONS AND SIDE EFFECTS

You should tell your doctor about all your allergies and any unexplained symptoms you may have while taking this drug.

MORE COMMON SIDE EFFECTS: Dry mouth

LESS COMMON SIDE EFFECTS: Abdominal pain, blurry vision, confusion, constipation, dizziness, drowsiness, excitement, eye pain*, fainting*, headache, irregular heartbeat*, irritability, large pupils, lightheadedness, nausea, nervousness, restlessness, trembling, urinary changes*, vision changes, vomiting

RARE SIDE EFFECTS: Bleeding*, breathing difficulty*, bruising*, chest tightness*, hallucinations*, hives*, itching*, mouth sores*, shortness of breath*, skin rash*, swollen glands*, tiredness*, weakness*, wheezing*

PRECAUTIONS

Some products contain sodium bisulfite, which may cause allergic reactions in sensitive people. Make sure your pharmacist knows if you have this condition.

If you have an enlarged prostate, glaucoma, stomach problems, intestinal disorders, myasthenia gravis, urinary problems, or irregular heartbeat, this drug may make those conditions worse.

Do not crush, break, or chew the extended-release products.

Be careful driving or handling equipment while taking this drug because it may cause dizziness, drowsiness, and vision changes.

This drug may cause dry mouth, which is associated with a greater risk of cavities. Your dentist may recommend that you clean your teeth and mouth differently to avoid infection.

PREGNANCY AND BREAST-FEEDING

Safety during pregnancy has not been established although the drug is known to harm animal fetuses.

It is not known if this drug passes into breast milk. Talk to your doctor about the risks associated with breast-feeding while taking this drug.

HELPFUL COMMENTS

Sucking on hard sugarless candy or chewing sugarless gum may help relieve dry mouth caused by this drug.

Avoid quick movements to minimize dizziness. Dangling your legs over the side of the bed for a few minutes may help reduce dizziness when first waking up.

OSELTAMIVIR PHOSPHATE

Available since October 1999

COMMONLY USED TO TREAT

Flu virus

DRUG CATEGORY

antiviral
Class: influenza virus neuraminidase inhibitor

PRODUCTS

Brand-Name Products with No Generic Alternative
Tamiflu 75 mg capsule ($$$$)
Tamiflu 12 mg/ml oral suspension ($$$$)
No generics available.
Patents expire in 2016. Exclusivity until 2004.

DOSING AND FOOD

Doses are taken 1 to 2 times a day.
This drug may be taken with or without food but is best taken with food to reduce the stomach upset that some people suffer.
Adults: Up to 150 mg per day in divided doses.

---

† See page 52.   * See page 53.

Lower doses are used in children.

Forgotten doses: If you are scheduled to take the next dose within a few hours, do not take the forgotten dose. Otherwise take the forgotten dose as soon as you remember.

ALCOHOL, DRUG, HERB, AND SUPPLEMENT INTERACTIONS

Alcohol may increase some of the side effects from this drug, depending on the amount consumed. Ask your doctor about the risks caused by drinking alcohol with your condition.

Taking this drug with any of the ones listed below may change the effect of either drug with the possibility of causing toxicity or decreasing effectiveness: probenecid

ALLERGIC REACTIONS AND SIDE EFFECTS

You should tell your doctor about all your allergies and any unexplained symptoms you may have while taking this drug.

MORE COMMON SIDE EFFECTS: Diarrhea*, nausea*, vomiting*

LESS COMMON SIDE EFFECTS: Abdominal pain, bloody nose, congestion*, cough*, dizziness, ear disorders, eye irritation, fatigue, headache, sleep disorders, swollen eyelids, tear production, wheezing*

PRECAUTIONS

If treating the flu virus, this drug should be started within 2 days of the first symptoms. When taken to prevent the flu after exposure, the drug should be started within 2 days of exposure.

This drug does not provide long-term protection against getting the flu. Talk to your doctor about getting a flu shot each fall.

PREGNANCY AND BREAST-FEEDING

Safety during pregnancy has not been established although the drug is known to harm animal fetuses.

It is not known if this drug passes into breast milk. Talk to your doctor about the risks associated with breast-feeding while taking this drug.

HELPFUL COMMENTS

Contact your doctor if your symptoms do not improve after a couple of days.

Do not stop treatment early if you start to feel better. It takes the full prescription for this drug to work completely.

Do not measure doses of the oral suspension with anything but a measuring cup intended for use with prescription drugs. Slight inaccuracy from other measuring spoons may result in over- or under-dosing.

OXACILLIN SODIUM

Available for over 20 years

COMMONLY USED TO TREAT

Infection

DRUG CATEGORY

antibiotic
Class: penicillinase-resistant penicillin

PRODUCTS

Brand-Name Products with Generic Alternatives
Bactocill 250 mg capsule (n/a)
  Generic: oxacillin 250 mg capsule (n/a)
Bactocill 500 mg capsule (n/a)
  Generic: oxacillin 500 mg capsule (n/a)
Bactocill 250 mg/5 ml oral solution (n/a)
  Generic: oxacillin 250 mg/5 ml oral solution (n/a)

DOSING AND FOOD

Doses are taken 4 to 6 times a day.
This drug works best if taken on an empty stomach with a full glass of water, but taking it with food may avoid the stomach upset that some people suffer.
Adults: Up to 6 g per day in divided doses.
Children more than 40 kg: Up to 100 mg/kg per day in divided doses.
Forgotten doses: If you are scheduled to take the next dose within a few hours, do not take the forgotten dose. Otherwise take the forgotten dose as soon as you remember.

ALCOHOL, DRUG, HERB, AND SUPPLEMENT INTERACTIONS

Alcohol may increase some of the side effects from this drug, depending on the amount consumed. Ask your doctor about the risks caused by drinking alcohol with your condition.

†*See page 52.*   **See page 53.*

Taking this drug with any of the ones listed below may change the effect of either drug with the possibility of causing toxicity or decreasing effectiveness: chloramphenicol, erythromycins†, methotrexate, probenecid, sulfonamides†, tetracyclines†

Increased side effects are possible when this drug is taken with those listed below: acetaminophen, amiodarone, androgens†, antithyroid drugs†, carmustine, chloroquine, dantrolene, daunorubicin, disulfiram, divalproex, estrogens†, etretinate, gold salts†, hydroxychloroquine, mercaptopurine, methotrexate, methyldopa, naltrexone, nandrolone, oral contraceptives, oxandrolone, oxymetholone, phenothiazines†, plicamycin, stanozolol, valproic acid

ALLERGIC REACTIONS AND SIDE EFFECTS

If you are allergic to any penicillins† or cephalosporins†, you may also be allergic to this drug. You should tell your doctor about all your allergies and any unexplained symptoms you may have while taking this drug.

MORE COMMON SIDE EFFECTS: Headache, diarrhea*, mouth sores*, vaginal discharge, vaginal itching

LESS COMMON SIDE EFFECTS: Fainting*, fever*, hives*, irregular breathing*, itching*, joint pain*, lightheadedness*, scaly skin*, shortness of breath*, skin rash*, swelling*

RARE SIDE EFFECTS: Abdominal pain*, bleeding*, bruising*, decreased urine output, depression*, nausea*, seizures*, sore throat*, stomach cramps*, vomiting*, yellow eyes or skin*

PRECAUTIONS

If you have a history of stomach or intestinal disease, you may be at greater risk of developing colitis while taking this drug. Tell your doctor if you get severe or watery diarrhea.

PREGNANCY AND BREAST-FEEDING

Safety during pregnancy has not been established although there was no evidence of harm during studies in animals.

This drug passes into breast milk. Allergic reactions, diarrhea, fungal infections, and skin rash have been reported in babies.

HELPFUL COMMENTS

Contact your doctor if your symptoms do not improve after a couple of days. Do not stop treatment early if you start to feel better. It takes full prescription for this drug to work completely.

OXAPROZIN

Available since October 1992

COMMONLY USED TO TREAT

Arthritis

DRUG CATEGORY

antiarthritic
Class: nonsteroidal antiinflammatory

PRODUCTS

Brand-Name Products with No Generic Alternative
Daypro Alta 600 mg tablet (n/a)
Brand-Name Products with Generic Alternatives
Daypro 600 mg tablet ($$)
  Generic: oxaprozin 600 mg tablet ($)

DOSING AND FOOD

Doses are taken 1 to 2 times a day.
It is best to take this drug on an empty stomach, but taking this drug with a little food may avoid the stomach upset that some people suffer.

Adults: Up to 26 mg/kg (maximum 1,800 mg) per day in divided doses.

Forgotten doses: If you are scheduled to take the next dose within a few hours, do not take the forgotten dose. Otherwise take the forgotten dose as soon as you remember.

ALCOHOL, DRUG, HERB, AND SUPPLEMENT INTERACTIONS

Alcohol may increase the risk of serious side effects from this drug. Ask your doctor about the risks caused by drinking alcohol with your condition.

Do not use dong quai, feverfew, garlic, ginger, horse chestnut, red clover, or St. John's wort while taking this drug since they may increase the risk of serious side effects.

Taking this drug with any of the ones listed below may change the effect of either drug with the possibility of causing toxicity or decreasing effectiveness:
acetaminophen, antihypertensives†, beta blockers†, digoxin, diuretics†, furosemide, hydrochlorothiazide, nifedipine, lithium, methotrexate, probenecid, sulfonylureas†, sulindac, verapamil

---

†See page 52.   *See page 53.

Severe reactions are possible when this drug is taken with those listed below: antibiotics†, anticoagulants†, aspirin, cefamandole, cefoperazone, cefotetan, corticosteroids†, cyclosporine, gold salts†, heparin, nonsteroidal antiinflammatories†, penicillamine, plicamycin, salicylates†, valproic acid, warfarin

ALLERGIC REACTIONS AND SIDE EFFECTS

If you are allergic to aspirin, zomepirac, salicylates†, or other nonsteroidal antiinflammatories†, you may also be allergic to this drug. You should tell your doctor about all your allergies and any unexplained symptoms you may have while taking this drug.

This drug promotes the effect of sunlight on the body and may cause severe sunburn and increased sensitivity of the eyes.

MORE COMMON SIDE EFFECTS: Diarrhea, constipation, heartburn*, indigestion*, itching*, nausea*, skin rash*

LESS COMMON SIDE EFFECTS: Abdominal pain, bruising*, gas, high blood pressure*, sweating, vomiting

RARE SIDE EFFECTS: Back pain*, black stools*, bloody urine*, bloody vomit*, blue fingernails*, blue lips*, breathing difficulty*, chest pain*, chest tightness*, chills*, confusion*, cough*, dark urine*, dizziness, drowsiness, fainting*, fever*, hallucinations*, headache, hearing loss*, hoarseness*, lip sores*, loss of appetite*, low blood pressure*, mood swings*, mouth sores*, muscle cramps*, nosebleeds*, pain*, pale skin*, pale stools*, puffy eyes*, rectal bleeding*, restlessness*, ringing in ears*, runny nose*, seizures*, shortness of breath*, sore throat*, stiff neck*, swelling*, swollen glands*, swollen tongue*, thirst*, tiredness*, urinary changes*, vision changes*, weakness*, weight gain*, wheezing*, yellow eyes or skin*

PRECAUTIONS

This drug may cause serious stomach problems and possibly ulcers. Be careful to take this drug as directed with food, and let your doctor know if you develop any stomach-related symptoms.

Do not lie down for about 30 minutes after taking this drug to help reduce the risk of heartburn and throat irritation.

If you use tobacco or have a history of alcohol abuse, stomach problems, intestinal problems, hemorrhoids, diabetes mellitus, severe fluid retention, or systemic lupus erythematosus, there may be an increased risk that you will develop side effects while taking this drug.

PREGNANCY AND BREAST-FEEDING

Safety during pregnancy has not been established although the drug is
known to harm animal fetuses.

Breast-feeding while taking this drug is not recommended.

HELPFUL COMMENTS

Several nonsteroidal antiinflammatories† are available without a prescription in lower, nonprescription strengths, including ibuprofen, ketoprofen, and naproxen.

OXAZEPAM

Available for over 20 years

COMMONLY USED TO TREAT

Anxiety

DRUG CATEGORY

anxiolytic
sedative-hypnotic
Class: benzodiazepine

PRODUCTS

Brand-Name Products with No Generic Alternative
Serax 15 mg tablet ($)
Brand-Name Products with Generic Alternatives
Serax 10 mg capsule (¢¢¢¢¢)
  Generic: oxazepam 10 mg capsule (¢¢)
Serax 15 mg capsule ($)
  Generic: oxazepam 15 mg capsule (¢¢¢)
Serax 30 mg capsule ($$)
  Generic: oxazepam 30 mg capsule (¢¢¢)

DOSING AND FOOD

Doses are taken 3 to 4 times a day.
This drug may be taken with or without food.
Adults: Up to 120 mg per day in divided doses.
Lower doses are used in people over age 65.
Forgotten doses: If you are scheduled to take the next dose within a few

† See page 52.   * See page 53.

hours, do not take the forgotten dose. Otherwise take the forgotten dose as soon as you remember.

ALCOHOL, DRUG, HERB, AND SUPPLEMENT INTERACTIONS

Alcohol should not be used while taking this drug.

Catnip, kava, lady's slipper, lemon balm, passion flower, sassafras, skullcap, and valerian should not be used while taking this drug due to an increased sedative effect.

Taking this drug with any of the ones listed below may change the effect of either drug with the possibility of causing toxicity or decreasing effectiveness: antacids, cimetidine, disulfiram, fluvoxamine, itraconazole, ketoconazole, levodopa, nefazodone

Severe reactions are possible when this drug is taken with those listed below: anesthetics, antidepressants†, antihistamines†, barbiturates†, monoamine oxidase inhibitors†, narcotics†, phenothiazines†

Increased side effects are possible when this drug is taken with those listed below: aminophylline, theophylline

ALLERGIC REACTIONS AND SIDE EFFECTS

If you are allergic to any benzodiazepines†, you may also be allergic to this drug. You should tell your doctor about all your allergies and any unexplained symptoms you may have while taking this drug.

MORE COMMON SIDE EFFECTS: Clumsiness, drowsiness, fever*, lightheadedness, yellow eyes or skin*

LESS COMMON SIDE EFFECTS: Anxiety*, confusion*, constipation, depression*, diarrhea, difficulty urinating, dizziness, dry mouth, headache, irregular heartbeat*, memory loss*, muscle spasm, nausea, sexual dysfunction, slurry speech, stomach cramps, thirst, trembling, vision changes, vomiting, watery mouth

RARE SIDE EFFECTS: Agitation*, behavior changes*, bleeding*, bruising*, chills*, delusions*, disorientation*, excitement*, eye movement*, hallucinations*, irritability*, low blood pressure*, mouth sores*, nervousness*, seizures*, skin irritation*, sore throat*, spastic movements*, tiredness*, weakness*

PRECAUTIONS

This drug may be habit forming and will cause severe withdrawal symptoms if stopped abruptly. If you wish to stop taking this drug, ask your doctor for specific instructions.

You need to wait 2 weeks after stopping a monoamine oxidase inhibitor†
before starting this drug.

If you have difficulty swallowing, emphysema, asthma, bronchitis, glaucoma, hyperactivity, mental depression, mental illness, myasthenia gravis,
porphyria, or sleep apnea, this drug may make those conditions worse.

Heavy smoking may cause this drug to be less effective.

Be careful driving or handling equipment while taking this drug because
the drug may cause dizziness and drowsiness.

PREGNANCY AND BREAST-FEEDING

There is evidence that this drug may harm the fetus, but the drug may be
necessary to the health of the mother.

Breast-feeding while taking this drug is not recommended.

HELPFUL COMMENTS

If you need to take an antacid, take it either 2 hours before or after taking
this drug.

Dangling your legs over the side of the bed for a few minutes may help reduce dizziness when first waking up.

It may take up to 2 hours for this drug to cause drowsiness.

OXCARBAZEPINE

Available since January 2000

COMMONLY USED TO TREAT

Seizures

DRUG CATEGORY

anticonvulsant
Class: carboxamide derivative

PRODUCTS

Brand-Name Products with No Generic Alternative
Trileptal 150 mg tablet (¢¢¢¢¢)
Trileptal 300 mg tablet ($$)
Trileptal 600 mg tablet ($$$)
Trileptal 300 mg/5 ml oral suspension ($$)
No generics available.
Exclusivity until 2005.

---

† See page 52.   * See page 53.

DOSING AND FOOD

Doses are taken twice a day.

This drug may be taken with or without food.

Adults: Up to 2,400 mg per day in divided doses.

Lower doses are used in children.

Forgotten doses: If you are scheduled to take the next dose within a few hours, do not take the forgotten dose. Otherwise take the forgotten dose as soon as you remember.

ALCOHOL, DRUG, HERB, AND SUPPLEMENT INTERACTIONS

Alcohol should not be used while taking this drug.

Many OTC drugs used for appetite control, asthma, colds, cough, hay fever, pain, or sinus problems affect the central nervous system and may change the effects or side effects of this drug. Check with your pharmacist for products to avoid.

Taking this drug with any of the ones listed below may change the effect of either drug with the possibility of causing toxicity or decreasing effectiveness: carbamazepine, felodipine, oral contraceptives, phenobarbital, phenytoin, valproic acid, verapamil

ALLERGIC REACTIONS AND SIDE EFFECTS

If you are allergic to carbamazepine, you may also be allergic to this drug. You should tell your doctor about all your allergies and any unexplained symptoms you may have while taking this drug.

MORE COMMON SIDE EFFECTS: Abdominal pain, clumsiness*, cough*, crying*, depression*, dizziness*, drowsiness, eye movements*, fever*, nausea, poor balance*, sneezing*, sore throat*, stuffy nose*, unsteadiness*, vision changes*, vomiting.

LESS COMMON SIDE EFFECTS: Acne, agitation*, awkwardness*, back pain, belching, bloody nose, bloody urine*, blurry vision*, breathing difficulty*, bruising*, chest tightness*, confusion*, congestion*, constipation, convulsions*, diarrhea, disorientation*, dry mouth, faintness*, headache*, heartburn, hoarseness*, irregular heartbeat*, lightheadedness*, memory loss*, muscle cramps*, nervousness*, shaking*, shortness of breath*, skin rash*, sleep disorders, sour stomach*, speech disturbances, sweating, taste changes, thirst*, tiredness*, trembling*, unconsciousness*, urinary changes*, vaginal itch*, weakness*, wheezing*

RARE SIDE EFFECTS: Anxiety*, chest pain*, chills*, hives*, irritability*, itching*, joint pain*, lip sores*, mouth sores*, rectal bleeding*, restlessness*, skin irritation*, swelling*, swollen glands*

PRECAUTIONS

Stopping this drug suddenly may cause a severe reaction including seizure. If you wish to stop taking this drug, ask your doctor for specific instructions.

Be careful driving or handling equipment while taking this drug because it may cause dizziness, drowsiness, and vision changes.

Make sure to include salt in your diet since this drug may cause your body to lose sodium.

PREGNANCY AND BREAST-FEEDING

Safety during pregnancy has not been established although the drug is known to harm animal fetuses.

Breast-feeding while taking this drug is not recommended.

HELPFUL COMMENTS

This drug is also called by the generic name GP 47680.

Oral contraceptives may not work properly when taken with this drug. You need to use a barrier contraceptive, such as a condom, or other nonhormonal contraceptive to prevent pregnancy.

Avoid quick movements to minimize dizziness. Dangling your legs over the side of the bed for a few minutes may help reduce dizziness when first waking up.

The oral suspension product may be mixed with water for easier swallowing.

OXYBUTYNIN CHLORIDE

Available for over 20 years

COMMONLY USED TO TREAT

Frequent urination
Overactive bladder (OAB)

DRUG CATEGORY

antispasmodic
Class: tertiary amine

PRODUCTS

Brand-Name Products with No Generic Alternative
Ditropan XL 5 mg extended-release tablet ($$$)
Ditropan XL 10 mg extended-release tablet ($$$)

---

† See page 52.   * See page 53.

Ditropan XL 15 mg extended-release tablet ($$$)
Oxytrol 3.9 mg/24 hour topical patch (n/a)

Brand-Name Products with Generic Alternatives
Ditropan 5 mg tablet (¢¢¢¢¢)
  Generic: oxybutynin chloride 5 mg tablet (¢¢)
Ditropan 5 mg/5 ml oral syrup (¢¢¢¢¢)
  Generic: oxybutynin chloride 5 mg/5 ml oral syrup (¢¢¢)

DOSING AND FOOD

Doses are taken 2 to 4 times a day.
This drug may be taken with or without food.
Adults: Up to 20 mg per day in divided doses.
Children age 5 and older: Up to 15 mg per day in divided doses.
Forgotten doses: If you are scheduled to take the next dose within a few
  hours, do not take the forgotten dose. Otherwise take the forgotten dose
  as soon as you remember.

ALCOHOL, DRUG, HERB, AND SUPPLEMENT INTERACTIONS

Alcohol may increase some of the side effects from this drug, depending
  on the amount consumed. Ask your doctor about the risks caused by
  drinking alcohol with your condition.
Many OTC drugs used for appetite control, asthma, colds, cough, hay
  fever, pain, or sinus problems affect the central nervous system and may
  change the effects or side effects of this drug. Check with your pharma-
  cist for products to avoid.

**Taking this drug with any of the ones listed below may change the effect of
either drug with the possibility of causing toxicity or decreasing effectiveness:**
amantadine, anticholinergics†, antidepressants†, antidyskinetics†, antihista-
mines†, antipsychotics†, buclizine, carbamazepine, cyclizine, cyclobenza-
prine, digoxin, disopyramide, flavoxate, ipratropium, meclizine, methylphen-
idate, orphenadrine, procainamide, promethazine, quinidine, trimeprazine

Severe reactions are possible when this drug is taken with those listed below:
haloperidol

Increased side effects are possible when this drug is taken with those listed below:
phenothiazines†

ALLERGIC REACTIONS AND SIDE EFFECTS

You should tell your doctor about all your allergies and any unexplained
  symptoms you may have while taking this drug.

This drug may cause your eyes to be more sensitive to sunlight, but there are no special risks associated with sunburn while taking this drug.

MORE COMMON SIDE EFFECTS: Constipation, drowsiness*, dry mouth, lack of sweat

LESS COMMON SIDE EFFECTS: Blurry vision, headache, lack of breast milk, nausea, sexual dysfunction, sleep disorders, swallowing disorder, tiredness, urinary changes, vomiting, weakness

RARE SIDE EFFECTS: Breathing difficulty*, clumsiness*, confusion*, dizziness*, excitement*, eye pain*, fast heartbeat*, fever*, flushing*, hallucinations*, hives*, irritability*, nervousness*, restlessness*, shortness of breath*, skin rash*, unsteadiness*

PRECAUTIONS

Do not crush, break, or chew the extended-release products.

If you have colitis, dry mouth, enlarged prostate, glaucoma, heart disease, hiatal hernia, high blood pressure, intestinal problems, myasthenia gravis, urinary problems, or toxemia of pregnancy, this drug may make those conditions worse.

Be careful driving or handling equipment while taking this drug because it may cause drowsiness and blurry vision.

This drug may cause dry mouth, which is associated with a greater risk of cavities. Your dentist may recommend that you clean your teeth and mouth differently to avoid infection.

Drink plenty of fluids to avoid dehydration when sweating, such as in hot weather and during exercise.

PREGNANCY AND BREAST-FEEDING

Safety during pregnancy has not been established although there was no evidence of harm during studies in animals.

It is not known if this drug passes into breast milk. Talk to your doctor about the risks associated with breast-feeding while taking this drug.

HELPFUL COMMENTS

Eye irritation caused by the sun may be reduced by wearing sunglasses when outside.

Sucking on hard sugarless candy or chewing sugarless gum may help relieve dry mouth caused by this drug.

† *See page 52.*   * *See page 53.*

OXYCODONE HYDROCHLORIDE

Available for over 20 years

COMMONLY USED TO TREAT

Pain

DRUG CATEGORY

analgesic
Class: narcotic analgesic/opioid

PRODUCTS

Brand-Name Products with No Generic Alternative
Oxycontin 10 mg extended-release tablet (n/a)
Oxycontin 20 mg extended-release tablet (n/a)
Oxycontin 40 mg extended-release tablet (n/a)
Oxycontin 80 mg extended-release tablet (n/a)
Roxicodone 5 mg tablet (¢¢¢)
Roxicodone 15 mg tablet ($)
Roxicodone 30 mg tablet ($)
Roxicodone 5 mg/5 ml oral solution (¢¢¢)
Roxicodone 20 mg/ml oral solution ($$$$)
No generic available.
Multiple patents on extended-release products that begin to expire
 in 2006. No patents or exclusivity on regular tablets.

Combination Products That Contain This Drug
Percodan tablet ($)
Percocet tablet (¢¢¢¢) to ($$)
Roxicet oral solution (¢¢¢)
Roxicet tablet (¢¢¢) to (¢¢¢¢)
Tylox capsule (¢¢¢¢¢)

DOSING AND FOOD

Doses are taken 4 to 6 times a day. Extended-release products are taken
 twice a day.
It is best to take this drug on an empty stomach, but taking this drug with
 a little food may avoid the stomach upset that some people suffer.
Adults: Up to 90 mg per day in divided doses.
Higher doses may be used in people who are under close medical super-
 vision.

Forgotten doses: If you are scheduled to take the next dose within a few hours, do not take the forgotten dose. Otherwise take the forgotten dose as soon as you remember.

ALCOHOL, DRUG, HERB, AND SUPPLEMENT INTERACTIONS

Alcohol should not be used while taking this drug.

Several OTC drugs used for asthma, colds, cough, hay fever, sleep aid, or sinus problems may seriously change the effects and side effects of this drug. Check with your pharmacist when selecting OTC products.

Many combination products that contain this drug also contain aspirin, which may interfere with anticoagulants†.

Taking this drug with any of the ones listed below may change the effect of either drug with the possibility of causing toxicity or decreasing effectiveness: natrexone, rifampin

Severe reactions are possible when this drug is taken with those listed below: anesthetics, anticholinergics†, antihistamines†, barbiturates†, benzodiazepines†, cimetidine, monoamine oxidase inhibitors†, naloxone, narcotics†, phenothiazines†, sedative-hypnotics†, skeletal muscle relaxants†, tricyclic antidepressants†

ALLERGIC REACTIONS AND SIDE EFFECTS

If you are allergic to any narcotics†, you may also be allergic to this drug. You should tell your doctor about all your allergies and any unexplained symptoms you may have while taking this drug.

MORE COMMON SIDE EFFECTS: Constipation, dizziness*, drowsiness*, dry mouth, excitement*, fainting, irregular breathing*, irregular heartbeat*, lightheadedness, nausea, sweating*, urinary changes*, vomiting

LESS COMMON SIDE EFFECTS: Blurry vision, breathing difficulty*, depression*, flushing*, hallucinations*, headache, hives*, itching*, loss of appetite, mood swings*, nervousness*, restlessness*, ringing in ears*, shortness of breath*, skin rash*, sleep disorders, spastic movements*, stomach cramps, swelling*, tiredness, trembling*, vision changes, weakness*, wheezing*

RARE SIDE EFFECTS: Body aches, clammy skin*, confusion*, diarrhea, fever, goosebumps, irritability, low blood pressure*, runny nose, seizures*, shivering, small pupils*, sneezing, yawning

PRECAUTIONS

Do not crush, break, or chew the extended-release products.

---

†See page 52.   *See page 53.

Be careful driving or handling equipment while taking this drug because it may cause dizziness and drowsiness.

If you have a history of head injury, brain disease, emphysema, asthma, lung disease, enlarged prostate, urinary disorders, gallbladder disease, or gallstones, you may not be able to take this drug.

This drug may cause dry mouth, which is associated with a greater risk of cavities. Your dentist may recommend that you clean your teeth and mouth differently to avoid infection.

People with colitis, heart disease, kidney disease, liver disease, and thyroid disease are at increased risk of developing side effects.

People with a history of seizures are at greater risk of developing a seizure while taking this drug.

This drug may cause withdrawal symptoms if stopped suddenly. If you wish to stop taking this drug, ask your doctor for specific instructions.

Side effects may continue to develop even after the drug is stopped.

Because this drug has a high abuse potential, your prescription quantity may be limited.

PREGNANCY AND BREAST-FEEDING

Safety during pregnancy has not been established although the drug is known to harm animal fetuses.

Breast-feeding while taking this drug is not recommended.

HELPFUL COMMENTS

If the drug does not seem to be working properly, an increase in dose may not help. Talk to your doctor about other drugs and treatment options.

Sucking on hard sugarless candy or chewing sugarless gum may help relieve dry mouth caused by this drug.

Lie down for a while after taking a dose of this drug to help reduce the nausea.

Avoid quick movements to minimize dizziness. Dangling your legs over the side of the bed for a few minutes may help reduce dizziness when first waking up.

If being used for pain, this drug works best when taken before the pain gets too severe.

Add more fiber to your diet to help minimize the constipation that occurs with this drug. If severe, constipation may need to be treated with a stool softener. Ask your doctor or pharmacist for recommendations.

OXYTETRACYCLINE

Available for over 20 years

COMMONLY USED TO TREAT

Infection

DRUG CATEGORY

antibiotic
Class: tetracycline

PRODUCTS

Brand-Name Products with No Generic Alternative
Terramycin 250 mg capsule (n/a)
No generics available.
No patents, no exclusivity.
Combination Products That Contain This Drug
Terra-Cortril ophthalmic suspension (n/a)
Terramycin with Polymyxin B Sulfate ophthalmic ointment ($)

DOSING AND FOOD

Doses are taken 4 times a day.
It is better to take this drug on an empty stomach with a full glass of water,
  but taking this drug with a little food may avoid the stomach upset that
  some people suffer. Do not drink milk or eat dairy products within 2
  hours of taking this drug.
Adults: Up to 2,000 mg per day in divided doses.
Children over age 8: Up to 50 mg/kg per day in divided doses.
This drug is not used in children under age 8 because of potential damage
  to developing teeth and bones.
Forgotten doses: If you are scheduled to take the next dose within a few
  hours, do not take the forgotten dose. Otherwise take the forgotten dose
  as soon as you remember.

ALCOHOL, DRUG, HERB, AND SUPPLEMENT INTERACTIONS

Alcohol may increase some of the side effects from this drug, depending
  on the amount consumed. Ask your doctor about the risks caused by
  drinking alcohol with your condition.
Many OTC drugs, including antacids, laxatives, and mineral supplements
  such as calcium, magnesium, or iron, may decrease the effects of this

---

†See page 52.   *See page 53.

drug when taken at the same time. If you need an OTC drug, take it either 2 hours before or after taking this drug.

Taking this drug with any of the ones listed below may change the effect of either drug with the possibility of causing toxicity or decreasing effectiveness: antacids, calcium supplements, cholestyramine, colestipol, iron supplements, mineral supplements, oral contraceptives, penicillins†

ALLERGIC REACTIONS AND SIDE EFFECTS

If you are allergic to any tetracyclines†, you may also be allergic to this drug. You should tell your doctor about all your allergies and any unexplained symptoms you may have while taking this drug.

This drug promotes the effect of sunlight on the body and may cause severe sunburn and increased sensitivity of the eyes. This effect may last as long as 2 to 4 weeks after the drug is stopped.

MORE COMMON SIDE EFFECTS: Diarrhea, stomach cramps, sun sensitivity*

LESS COMMON SIDE EFFECTS: Genital itch, rectal itch, sore mouth

RARE SIDE EFFECTS: Abdominal pain*, headache*, loss of appetite*, nausea*, vomiting*, visual changes*, yellow eyes or skin*

PRECAUTIONS

People with kidney disease have a greater risk of developing side effects.

This drug decomposes after the expiration date and may be harmful if taken. Make sure you destroy any leftover tablets as soon as you are done with the prescription.

Some people get a discolored tongue when taking this drug, but the coloring will return to normal when the drug is stopped.

PREGNANCY AND BREAST-FEEDING

This drug may cause toxic effects to the fetus and should not be used during pregnancy.

Breast-feeding while taking this drug is not recommended.

HELPFUL COMMENTS

Oral contraceptives may not work properly when taken with this drug. You need to use a barrier contraceptive, such as a condom, or other nonhormonal contraceptive to prevent pregnancy.

Contact your doctor if your symptoms do not improve after a couple of days.

Do not stop treatment early if you start to feel better. It takes the full prescription for this drug to work completely.

PANTOPRAZOLE SODIUM

Available since February 2000

COMMONLY USED TO TREAT

Heartburn, specifically gastroesophageal reflux disease (GERD)
Too much acid in the stomach
Ulcers

DRUG CATEGORY

antiulcer
Class: proton pump inhibitor

PRODUCTS

Brand-Name Products with No Generic Alternative
Protonix 20 mg delayed-release tablet ($$$)
Protonix 40 mg delayed-release tablet ($$$)
No generics available.
Multiple patents that begin to expire in 2005.

DOSING AND FOOD

Doses are taken once a day.
This drug may be taken with or without food.
Adults: Up to 40 mg per day.
Forgotten doses: If you are scheduled to take the next dose within a few
hours, do not take the forgotten dose. Otherwise take the forgotten dose
as soon as you remember.

ALCOHOL, DRUG, HERB, AND SUPPLEMENT INTERACTIONS

Alcohol may increase some of the side effects from this drug, depending
on the amount consumed. Ask your doctor about the risks caused by
drinking alcohol with your condition.
If you are taking St. John's wort when taking this drug, you may be at
greater risk of developing a sunburn when outdoors.

**Taking this drug with any of the ones listed below may change the effect of
either drug with the possibility of causing toxicity or decreasing effectiveness:**
ampicillin, iron, ketoconazole

ALLERGIC REACTIONS AND SIDE EFFECTS

You should tell your doctor about all your allergies and any unexplained
symptoms you may have while taking this drug.

†See page 52.　　*See page 53.

MORE COMMON SIDE EFFECTS: Headache

LESS COMMON SIDE EFFECTS: Abdominal pain*, anxiety, back pain, belching, blisters*, blurry vision, breathing difficulty*, chest pain*, chest tightness*, chills, confusion, constipation, cough, diarrhea*, dizziness, drooling, gas, hives*, hoarseness, indigestion, infection*, irregular breathing, itching*, joint pain*, loss of appetite*, loss of energy, muscle pain*, nausea*, neck pain, rectal irritation, ringing in ears, runny nose, shortness of breath*, sinus trouble, skin discoloration*, skin irritation*, skin rash*, sleep disorders, sneezing, sore throat, speech disorders*, stiffness*, swollen eyelids*, swollen tongue*, thirst*, tiredness*, urinary changes*, vision changes*, vomiting*, weakness*, wheezing*, yellow eyes or skin*

PRECAUTIONS

Do not crush, break, or chew the delayed release products.

This drug is usually prescribed for only 8 weeks and should not be used longer than 16 weeks.

If you get a headache from this drug, take acetaminophen for relief. Aspirin and other nonsteroidal antiinflammatories† may cause your condition to get worse.

PREGNANCY AND BREAST-FEEDING

Safety during pregnancy has not been established although there was no evidence of harm during studies in animals.

Breast-feeding while taking this drug is not recommended.

HELPFUL COMMENTS

It may take several days before the effects of this drug are noticed.

Do not stop treatment early if you start to feel better. It takes the full prescription for this drug to work completely.

PAPAVERINE HYDROCHLORIDE

Available for over 20 years

COMMONLY USED TO TREAT

Poor circulation

DRUG CATEGORY

antispasmotic
Class: peripheral vasodilator

PRODUCTS

Products Only Available as Generics
papaverine hydrochloride 150 mg extended-release capsule (¢)

Other Generic Product Names
Papacon, Para-Time SR, Pavacot

DOSING AND FOOD

Doses are taken 2 to 3 times a day.

This drug may be taken with or without food but is best taken with food, milk, or antacids to reduce the stomach upset that some people suffer.

Adults: Up to 600 mg per day in divided doses.

Forgotten doses: If you are scheduled to take the next dose within a few hours, do not take the forgotten dose. Otherwise take the forgotten dose as soon as you remember.

ALCOHOL, DRUG, HERB, AND SUPPLEMENT INTERACTIONS

Alcohol may increase some of the side effects from this drug, depending on the amount consumed. Ask your doctor about the risks caused by drinking alcohol with your condition.

Several OTC drugs used for appetite control, asthma, colds, cough, hay fever, pain, or sinus problems may seriously increase the side effects of this drug. Check with your pharmacist when selecting OTC products.

Taking this drug with any of the ones listed below may change the effect of either drug with the possibility of causing toxicity or decreasing effectiveness: levodopa

Severe reactions are possible when this drug is taken with those listed below: anesthetics, antihistamines†, anxiolytics†, barbiturates†, narcotics†

ALLERGIC REACTIONS AND SIDE EFFECTS

You should tell your doctor about all your allergies and any unexplained symptoms you may have while taking this drug.

MORE COMMON SIDE EFFECTS: Flushing, headache, irregular heartbeat*, nausea*, sweating*

LESS COMMON SIDE EFFECTS: Breathing changes, dizziness

RARE SIDE EFFECTS: Abdominal pain*, blurry vision*, constipation*, diarrhea*, drowsiness*, loss of appetite*, rash*, tiredness*, weakness*, yellow eyes or skin*

---

†*See page 52.*   *See page 53.*

PRECAUTIONS

People with glaucoma, heart disease, chest pain, or who have had a recent heart attack or stroke are at increased risk of developing side effects.

Do not crush, break, or chew the extended-release products. Capsules may be opened and the contents mixed with jam or jelly for easier swallowing. Do not chew the pellets inside the capsule.

Heavy smoking may cause this drug to be less effective.

Drink plenty of fluids to avoid dehydration when sweating, such as in hot weather and during exercise.

PREGNANCY AND BREAST-FEEDING

Safety during pregnancy has not been established although the drug is known to harm animal fetuses.

It is not known if this drug passes into breast milk. Talk to your doctor about the risks associated with breast-feeding while taking this drug.

HELPFUL COMMENTS

Avoid quick movements to minimize dizziness. Dangling your legs over the side of the bed for a few minutes may help reduce dizziness when first waking up.

It may take several days to weeks for the full effects of this drug to be noticed.

PAROXETINE HYDROCHLORIDE

Available since December 1992

COMMONLY USED TO TREAT

Headache
Obsessive compulsive disorder
Panic attack
Phobia
Post-traumatic stress disorder
Premature ejaculation

DRUG CATEGORY

antidepressant
antipanic
anxiolytic
Class: selective serotonin reuptake inhibitor (SSRI)

PRODUCTS

Brand-Name Products with No Generic Alternative
Paxil 10 mg tablet ($$$)
Paxil 20 mg tablet ($$$)
Paxil 30 mg tablet ($$$)
Paxil 40 mg tablet ($$$)
Paxil 10 mg/5 ml oral suspension ($$$)
Paxil 12.5 mg extended-release tablet (n/a)
Paxil 25 mg extended-release tablet (n/a)
Paxil 37.5 mg extended-release tablet (n/a)
No generics available.
Multiple patents that begin to expire in 2006.

DOSING AND FOOD

Doses are taken once a day.
This drug may be taken with or without food.

Adults: Up to 60 mg per day.

Lower doses are used in children, people over age 65, and people with kidney or liver disease.

Forgotten doses: If you are scheduled to take the next dose within a few hours, do not take the forgotten dose. Otherwise take the forgotten dose as soon as you remember.

ALCOHOL, DRUG, HERB, AND SUPPLEMENT INTERACTIONS

Alcohol should not be used while taking this drug.
Use of SAMe or St. John's wort may cause serious side effects while taking this drug.

Taking this drug with any of the ones listed below may change the effect of either drug with the possibility of causing toxicity or decreasing effectiveness: cimetidine, digoxin, phenobarbital, phenytoin, procyclidine, theophylline, warfarin

Severe reactions are possible when this drug is taken with those listed below: monoamine oxidase inhibitors†, moclobemide, tryptophan

Increased side effects are possible when this drug is taken with those listed below: astemizole, bromocriptine, buspirone, dextromethorphan, levodopa, lithium, LSD, marijuana, MDMA (ecstasy), meperidine, nefazodone, pentazocine, SSRI†, sumatriptan, tramadol, trazodone, tricyclic antidepressants†, venlafaxine

---

†*See page 52.*   *See page 53.*

ALLERGIC REACTIONS AND SIDE EFFECTS

You should tell your doctor about all your allergies and any unexplained symptoms you may have while taking this drug.

MORE COMMON SIDE EFFECTS: Constipation, diarrhea*, dizziness*, drowsiness*, dry mouth*, headache, nausea*, sexual dysfunction, shaking*, sleep disorders, sweating*, tiredness, trembling*, urinary difficulty, vomiting, weakness*

LESS COMMON SIDE EFFECTS: Agitation*, anxiety, appetite changes, blurry vision, burning, irregular heartbeat*, muscle pain*, nervousness, skin rash*, taste changes, tingling, weight gain, weight loss

RARE SIDE EFFECTS: Body stillness*, confusion*, excitability*, eye stillness*, facial movements*, fever*, flushing*, irregular heartbeat*, irritability*, lack of energy*, large pupils*, poor coordination*, restlessness*, seizures*, shivering*, skin irritation*, spastic movements*, speech difficulty*, thirst*, twitching*, vomiting*

PRECAUTIONS

People with a history of brain disease, mental retardation, or seizures are at greater risk of developing a seizure while taking this drug.

If you have a manic disorder, this drug may make that condition worse.

Do not crush, break, or chew the extended-release products.

Stopping this drug suddenly may cause severe reactions. If you wish to stop taking this drug, ask your doctor for specific instructions.

You need to wait 2 weeks after stopping a monoamine oxidase inhibitor† before starting this drug.

This drug may cause dry mouth, which is associated with a greater risk of cavities. Your dentist may recommend that you clean your teeth and mouth differently to avoid infection.

Be careful driving or handling equipment while taking this drug because the drug may cause dizziness and drowsiness.

PREGNANCY AND BREAST-FEEDING

Safety during pregnancy has not been established although the drug is known to harm animal fetuses.

Breast-feeding while taking this drug is not recommended.

HELPFUL COMMENTS

It may take several weeks for the effects of this drug to be noticed.

PEMOLINE

Available for over 20 years

COMMONLY USED TO TREAT

Children with attention deficit hyperactivity disorder (ADHD)

DRUG CATEGORY

behavioral agent
Class: CNS stimulant

PRODUCTS

Brand-Name Products with Generic Alternatives
Cylert 18.75 mg tablet ($)
  Generic: pemoline 18.75 mg tablet (¢¢¢¢¢)
Cylert 37.5 mg tablet ($$)
  Generic: pemoline 37.5 mg tablet ($)
Cylert 75 mg tablet ($$$)
  Generic: pemoline 75 mg tablet ($$)
Cylert 37.5 mg chewable tablet ($$)
  Generic: pemoline 37.5 mg chewable tablet ($$)

DOSING AND FOOD

Doses are taken once a day in the morning.
This drug may be taken with or without food.
Children over age 6: Up to 112.5 mg per day in divided doses.
Forgotten doses: If you are scheduled to take the next dose within a few
  hours, do not take the forgotten dose. Otherwise take the forgotten dose
  as soon as you remember.

ALCOHOL, DRUG, HERB, AND SUPPLEMENT INTERACTIONS

Alcohol should not be used while taking this drug.
Many OTC drugs used for appetite control, asthma, colds, cough, hay
  fever, pain, or sinus problems affect the central nervous system and may
  change the effects or side effects of this drug. Check with your pharma-
  cist for products to avoid.
**Taking this drug with any of the ones listed below may change the effect of
either drug with the possibility of causing toxicity or decreasing effectiveness:**
anticonvulsants†
Severe reactions are possible when this drug is taken with those listed below:
monoamine oxidase inhibitors†

---

† See page 52.   * See page 53.

Increased side effects are possible when this drug is taken with those listed below:
amantadine, amphetamines†, antiasthmatics†, appetite suppressants†, caffeine, cocaine, methylphenidate, nabilone

ALLERGIC REACTIONS AND SIDE EFFECTS

You should tell your doctor about all your allergies and any unexplained symptoms you may have while taking this drug.

MORE COMMON SIDE EFFECTS: Loss of appetite, sleep disorders, weight loss

LESS COMMON SIDE EFFECTS: Depression, dizziness, drowsiness, headache*, irritability, stomachache

RARE SIDE EFFECTS: Agitation*, bleeding*, breathing difficulty*, bruising*, chest tightness*, dark urine*, delayed growth*, dilated pupils*, fever*, hallucinations*, high blood pressure*, irregular heartbeat*, mouth sores*, nausea*, restlessness*, seizures*, shortness of breath*, skin rash*, spastic movements*, sweating*, swollen glands*, tiredness*, trembling*, vocalization*, vomiting*, wheezing*, yellow eyes or skin*

PRECAUTIONS

This drug is only used when other treatment has failed, because of the risk of developing severe liver disease.

You must have your blood tested every other week while taking this drug to ensure safe use.

You need to wait 2 weeks after stopping a monoamine oxidase inhibitor† before starting this drug.

This drug may become habit forming if taken for a long time. Suddenly stopping the drug may cause withdrawal symptoms. If you wish to stop taking this drug, ask your doctor for specific instructions.

Chewable tablets must be completely chewed before swallowing.

Be careful driving or handling equipment while taking this drug because it may cause dizziness and drowsiness.

PREGNANCY AND BREAST-FEEDING

Safety during pregnancy has not been established although there was no evidence of harm during studies in animals.

It is not known if this drug passes into breast milk. Talk to your doctor about the risks associated with breast-feeding while taking this drug.

HELPFUL COMMENTS

It may take 3 to 4 weeks for the effects of this drug to be noticed.

PENBUTOLOL SULFATE

Available since January 1985

COMMONLY USED TO TREAT

Chest pain, also known as angina
High blood pressure, also known as hypertension

DRUG CATEGORY

antianginal
antihypertensive
Class: beta blocker

PRODUCTS

Brand-Name Products with No Generic Alternative
Levatol 20 mg tablet ($$)
No generics available.
No patents, no exclusivity.

DOSING AND FOOD

Doses are taken once a day.
This drug may be taken with or without food.

Adults: Up to 20 mg per day.

Lower doses are used in people with renal disease, liver disease or heart failure.

This drug is rarely used in children.

Forgotten doses: If you are scheduled to take the next dose within 8 hours, do not take the forgotten dose. Otherwise take the forgotten dose as soon as you remember.

ALCOHOL, DRUG, HERB, AND SUPPLEMENT INTERACTIONS

Alcohol may increase some of the side effects from this drug, depending on the amount consumed. Ask your doctor about the risks caused by drinking alcohol with your condition.

Several OTC drugs used for appetite control, asthma, colds, cough, hay fever, or sinus problems may cause an increase in blood pressure when taken with this drug. Check with your pharmacist when selecting OTC products.

---

† See page 52. * See page 53.

Taking this drug with any of the ones listed below may change the effect of either drug with the possibility of causing toxicity or decreasing effectiveness: aminophylline, anesthetics†, antidiabetics†, caffeine, calcium channel blockers†, carbonic anhydrase inhibitors†, clonidine, dyphylline, epinephrine, guanabenz, lidocaine, nonsteroidal antiinflammatories†, oxtriphylline, pilocarpine, reserpine, theophylline

Severe reactions are possible when this drug is taken with those listed below: allergy shots, beta blockers†, cocaine, monoamine oxidase inhibitors†

Increased effects or side effects are possible when this drug is taken with those listed below:
antihypertensives†

ALLERGIC REACTIONS AND SIDE EFFECTS

If you are allergic to any other beta blockers†, you may also be allergic to this drug.

This drug may exaggerate the reaction you get from your current allergies. Inform your doctor of any allergies that you have as well as the severity of the allergic reaction before starting this drug.

MORE COMMON SIDE EFFECTS: Dizziness, drowsiness, lightheadedness*, sexual dysfunction, sleeping difficulty, tiredness, weakness

LESS COMMON SIDE EFFECTS: Anxiety, breathing difficulty*, cold hands and feet*, constipation, depression*, diarrhea, itching, nausea, nervousness, numbness, shortness of breath*, slow heartbeat*, sore eyes, stomachache, stuffy nose, swollen legs or feet, tingling, vivid dreams, vomiting, wheezing

RARE SIDE EFFECTS: Back pain*, bleeding*, bruising*, chest pain*, confusion*, dizziness*, fever*, hallucinations*, irregular heartbeat*, joint pain*, rash*, scaly skin*, sore throat*

PRECAUTIONS

This drug should not be used in people with a heart rate that is routinely less than 60 beats per minute (bradycardia), or in people with heart block, heart failure, or cardiogenic shock.

People with asthma may not be able to take this drug.

Stopping this drug suddenly may cause chest pain or heart attack. If you wish to stop taking this drug, ask your doctor for specific instructions.

Be careful driving or handling equipment while taking this drug because the drug may cause dizziness and drowsiness.

You need to wait 2 weeks after stopping a monoamine oxidase inhibitor† before starting this drug.

If you are diabetic, this drug may increase blood sugar levels or make the symptoms of low blood sugar less noticeable.

This drug may cause nondiabetics to develop type 2 diabetes.

If you have psoriasis or myasthenia gravis, this drug may make those conditions worse.

PREGNANCY AND BREAST-FEEDING

Safety during pregnancy has not been established although the drug is known to harm animal fetuses.

Breast-feeding while taking this drug is not recommended.

HELPFUL COMMENTS

This drug may make you more sensitive to cold temperatures.

If you do not treat high blood pressure, you may develop more serious problems such as heart failure, blood vessel disease, stroke, or kidney disease. Losing weight, exercising, eating more fruits and vegetables, and avoiding salty foods, such as lunchmeat and pickles, may help make drug treatment more successful.

PENICILLAMINE

Available for over 20 years

COMMONLY USED TO TREAT

Arthritis

People at risk of developing kidney stones

Too much copper in the body, also known as Wilson's disease

DRUG CATEGORY

antirheumatic

chelating drug

Class: heavy metal antagonist

PRODUCTS

Brand-Name Products with No Generic Alternative

Cuprimine 125 mg capsule (¢¢¢¢¢)

Cuprimine 250 mg capsule ($)

Depen 250 mg tablet ($$$)

No generics available.

No patents, no exclusivity.

---

† See page 52.   * See page 53.

DOSING AND FOOD

Doses are taken 1 to 4 times a day.

It is best to take this drug on an empty stomach at least 1 hour before or 2 hours after a meal.

Adults: Up to 2,000 mg per day in divided doses.

Lower doses are used in children.

Forgotten doses: If more than 3 hours have passed since the forgotten dose, do not take the dose. Otherwise, take the forgotten dose as soon as you remember.

ALCOHOL, DRUG, HERB, AND SUPPLEMENT INTERACTIONS

Alcohol may increase some of the side effects from this drug, depending on the amount consumed. Ask your doctor about the risks caused by drinking alcohol with your condition.

Taking this drug with any of the ones listed below may change the effect of either drug with the possibility of causing toxicity or decreasing effectiveness: antacids, digoxin, iron supplements

Severe reactions are possible when this drug is taken with those listed below: antimalarials†, antineoplastics†, gold salts, oxyphenbutazone, phenylbutazone

ALLERGIC REACTIONS AND SIDE EFFECTS

About 30% of the people who take this drug have an allergic reaction. Call your doctor right away if you notice a rash, joint pain, bruises, or other signs of allergy. If you are allergic to penicillin, you may also be allergic to this drug. You should tell your doctor about all your allergies and any unexplained symptoms you may have while taking this drug.

MORE COMMON SIDE EFFECTS: Diarrhea, fever*, hives*, itching*, joint pain*, loss of appetite, loss of taste, mouth sores*, nausea, skin rash*, skin sores*, stomach pain, swollen glands*, vomiting

LESS COMMON SIDE EFFECTS: Bleeding*, bloody urine*, breathing difficulty*, bruising*, chest tightness*, chills*, fever*, shortness of breath*, sore throat*, swelling*, tiredness*, weakness*, weight gain*, wheezing*

RARE SIDE EFFECTS: Abdominal pain*, back pain*, black stools*, blisters*, blurry vision*, chest pain*, chewing*, cough*, dark urine*, excessive talking*, eye irritation*, eye pain*, hoarseness*, itching*, pale stools*, ringing in ears*, skin irritation*, spitting blood*, swallowing difficulty*, urinary changes*, vision change*, weakness*, yellow eyes or skin*

PRECAUTIONS

This drug may cause changes to your gums and mouth. Your dentist may recommend that you clean your teeth and mouth differently to avoid infection.

People with a history of kidney disease or blood disease may be at greater risk of developing side effects while taking this drug.

Periodic testing of liver function and kidney function is needed to ensure the safe use of this drug.

PREGNANCY AND BREAST-FEEDING

Safety during pregnancy has not been established although the drug is known to harm animal fetuses.

Breast-feeding while taking this drug is not recommended.

HELPFUL COMMENTS

You should drink 8 to 10 glasses of water a day while taking this drug.

If you need to take an antacid or iron supplement, take it either 2 hours before or after taking this drug.

It may take several months before the effects of this drug are noticed.

PENICILLIN V POTASSIUM

Available for over 20 years

COMMONLY USED TO TREAT

Infection

DRUG CATEGORY

Antibiotic
Class: Natural Penicillin

PRODUCTS

Products Only Available as Generics
penicillin V potassium 250 mg tablet (¢)
penicillin V potassium 500 mg tablet (¢¢)
penicillin V potassium 125 mg/5 ml oral solution (¢)
penicillin V potassium 250 mg/5 ml oral solution (¢¢)

Other Generic Product Names
Beepen-VK, Ledercillin-VK, Pen-Vee K, Penicillin VK, Veetids, Uticillin VK

---

†See page 52.   *See page 53.

DOSING AND FOOD

Doses are taken 3 to 4 times a day.

This drug works best if taken on an empty stomach with a full glass of water, but taking it with food may avoid the stomach upset that some people suffer.

Adults: Up to 2 g per day in divided doses.

Children: Up to 70 mg/kg per day in divided doses.

Forgotten doses: If you are scheduled to take the next dose within a few hours, do not take the forgotten dose. Otherwise take the forgotten dose as soon as you remember.

ALCOHOL, DRUG, HERB, AND SUPPLEMENT INTERACTIONS

Alcohol may increase some of the side effects from this drug, depending on the amount consumed. Ask your doctor about the risks caused by drinking alcohol with your condition.

Taking this drug with any of the ones listed below may change the effect of either drug with the possibility of causing toxicity or decreasing effectiveness: chloramphenicol, erythromycins†, methotrexate, probenecid, sulfonamides†, tetracyclines†

ALLERGIC REACTIONS AND SIDE EFFECTS

If you are allergic to any penicillins† or cephalosporins†, you may also be allergic to this drug. You should tell your doctor about all your allergies and any unexplained symptoms you may have while taking this drug.

MORE COMMON SIDE EFFECTS: Headache, diarrhea*, mouth sore*, vaginal discharge, vaginal itching

LESS COMMON SIDE EFFECTS: Fainting*, fever*, hives*, irregular breathing*, itching*, joint pain*, lightheadedness*, scaly skin*, shortness of breath*, skin rash*, swelling*

RARE SIDE EFFECTS: Abdominal pain*, bleeding*, bruising*, decreased urine output, depression*, nausea*, seizures*, sore throat*, stomach cramps*, vomiting*, yellow eyes or skin*

PRECAUTIONS

If you have a history of stomach or intestinal disease, you may be at greater risk of developing colitis while taking this drug. Tell your doctor if you get severe or watery diarrhea.

There are several injectable forms of penicillin that are different from the oral form. This drug cannot be used in place of injectable penicillin.

PREGNANCY AND BREAST-FEEDING

Safety during pregnancy has not been established although there was no evidence of harm during studies in animals.

This drug passes into breast milk. Allergic reactions, diarrhea, fungal infections, and skin rash have been reported in babies.

HELPFUL COMMENTS

Contact your doctor if your symptoms do not improve after a couple of days.

Do not stop treatment early if you start to feel better. It takes full prescription for this drug to work completely.

PENTOBARBITAL SODIUM

Available for over 20 years

COMMONLY USED TO TREAT

Sleeping difficulty, also known as insomnia

DRUG CATEGORY

sedative-hypnotic
Class: barbiturate

PRODUCTS

Brand-Name Products with No Generic Alternative
Nembutal Sodium 30 mg capsule (n/a)
Brand-Name Products with Generic Alternatives
Nembutal Sodium 100 mg capsule (n/a)
  Generic: pentobarbital sodium 100 mg capsules (n/a)

DOSING AND FOOD

Doses are taken 1 to 4 times a day.

It is best to take this drug on an empty stomach with a full glass of water at least 1 hour before or 2 hours after meals.

Adults: Up to 100 mg per day.

Children: Up to 6 mg/kg (maximum 100 mg) per day in divided doses.

Forgotten doses: Do not take a forgotten dose. Just go back to your usual schedule with the next dose.

ALCOHOL, DRUG, HERB, AND SUPPLEMENT INTERACTIONS

Alcohol should not be used while taking this drug.

†See page 52.   *See page 53.

Several OTC drugs used for appetite control, asthma, colds, cough, hay fever, pain, or sinus problems may seriously increase the side effects of this drug. Check with your pharmacist when selecting OTC products.

Taking this drug with any of the ones listed below may change the effect of either drug with the possibility of causing toxicity or decreasing effectiveness: anticoagulants†, carbamazepine, corticosteroids†, corticotropin, divalproex sodium, oral contraceptives†, valproic acid

Increased side effects are possible when this drug is taken with those listed below: anesthetics, antihistamines†, anxiolytics†, barbiturates†, narcotics†, tricyclic antidepressants†

ALLERGIC REACTIONS AND SIDE EFFECTS

Allergic reactions are more likely to occur in people with a history of asthma or allergies to other drugs. You should tell your doctor about all your allergies and any unexplained symptoms you may have while taking this drug.

MORE COMMON SIDE EFFECTS: Clumsiness, dizziness, drowsiness, lightheadedness, unsteadiness

LESS COMMON SIDE EFFECTS: Anxiety, confusion*, constipation, depression*, excitement*, fainting, headache, irritability, nausea, nervousness, sleep disorders, vomiting

RARE SIDE EFFECTS: Bleeding lips*, bleeding*, bone pain*, bruising*, chest pain*, chest tightness*, fever*, hallucinations*, hives*, loss of appetite*, mouth sores*, muscle pain*, skin rash*, sore throat*, swelling*, tiredness*, weakness*, weight loss*, wheezing*, yellow eyes or skin*

PRECAUTIONS

Be careful driving or handling equipment while taking this drug because the drug may cause dizziness and drowsiness.

Children and people over age 65 often get hyperactive when taking this drug.

If you have anemia, asthma, high blood sugar, hyperactivity, depression, thyroid problems, liver disease, kidney disease, or porphyria, this drug may make those conditions worse.

This drug may be habit forming when taken for a long time. It should be stopped slowly to avoid withdrawal symptoms. It may take 2 weeks for the body to adjust after the drug is stopped. If you wish to stop taking this drug, ask your doctor for specific instructions.

PREGNANCY AND BREAST-FEEDING

There is evidence that this drug may harm the fetus, but the drug may be necessary to the health of the mother.

This drug passes into breast milk, and may cause drowsiness, slow heart-beat, and breathing difficulty in the baby.

HELPFUL COMMENTS

If used regularly for more than 2 weeks, this drug may lose the ability to make you sleep.

Oral contraceptives may not work properly when taken with this drug. You need to use a barrier contraceptive, such as a condom, or other nonhormonal contraceptive to prevent pregnancy.

This drug has a calming effect and is also used to treat anxiety.

You may need to increase the fiber in your diet since this drug may cause constipation.

PENTOSAN POLYSULFATE SODIUM

Available since September 1996

COMMONLY USED TO TREAT

Bladder pain caused by interstitial cystitis

DRUG CATEGORY

urinary analgesic
Class: carbohydrate derivative

PRODUCTS

Brand-Name Products with No Generic Alternative
Elmiron 100 mg capsule ($$)
No generics available.
Patent expires in 2010.

DOSING AND FOOD

Doses are taken 3 times a day.

It is best to take this drug on an empty stomach with a full glass of water at least 1 hour before or 2 hours after meals.

Adults: Up to 300 mg per day in divided doses.

Forgotten doses: If you are scheduled to take the next dose within a few

---

†*See page 52.*   ** See page 53.*

hours, do not take the forgotten dose. Otherwise take the forgotten dose as soon as you remember.

ALCOHOL, DRUG, HERB, AND SUPPLEMENT INTERACTIONS

Alcohol may increase some of the side effects from this drug, depending on the amount consumed. Ask your doctor about the risks caused by drinking alcohol with your condition.

Increased side effects are possible when this drug is taken with those listed below: alteplase, anticoagulants†, aspirin, heparin, streptokinase

ALLERGIC REACTIONS AND SIDE EFFECTS

You should tell your doctor about any allergies and any unexplained symptoms you may have while taking this drug.

This drug promotes the effect of sunlight on the body and may cause severe sunburn and increased sensitivity of the eyes.

LESS COMMON SIDE EFFECTS: Abdominal pain, bleeding gums, constipation, diarrhea, dizziness, dry throat, eye irritation, gas, hair loss, headache, heartburn, itching, loss of appetite, mouth sores, nausea, nosebleeds, ringing in ears, runny nose, stomachache, swallowing difficulty, vomiting

RARE SIDE EFFECTS: Bleeding*, breathing difficulty*, bruising*, chills*, fever*, hives*, skin rash*, sore throat*, tiredness*, vision changes*, weakness*

PRECAUTIONS

People with blood disease, blood vessel problems, polyps, ulcers, or liver disease may not be able to take this drug.

If you are planning any medical or dental procedures, make sure your surgeon or dentist knows that you are taking this drug since it may thin the blood, making you bleed more easily.

This drug may put you at greater risk of developing problems in the mouth, such as bleeding gums. Your dentist may recommend that you clean your teeth and mouth differently to avoid infection.

PREGNANCY AND BREAST-FEEDING

Safety during pregnancy has not been established although there was no evidence of harm during studies in animals.

It is not known if this drug passes into breast milk. Talk to your doctor about the risks associated with breast-feeding while taking this drug.

HELPFUL COMMENTS

This drug is usually used for less than 3 months, but may be continued longer if pain continues and there are no major side effects. If you have not responded to this drug after 6 months, it is not likely that you will notice any improvement by staying on the drug longer.

Hair loss that may occur while taking this drug is usually limited to a single area on the scalp and will be noticed within 4 weeks of starting the drug.

Oral contraceptives may not work properly when taken with this drug. You need to use a barrier contraceptive, such as a condom, or other non-hormonal contraceptive to prevent pregnancy.

PENTOXIFYLLINE

Available for over 20 years

COMMONLY USED TO TREAT

Leg cramps caused by lack of blood, specifically known as intermittent claudication

DRUG CATEGORY

hemorrheologic
Class: xanthine derivative

PRODUCTS

Brand-Name Products with Generic Alternatives
Trental 400 mg extended-release tablet (¢¢¢¢)
  Generic: pentoxifylline 400 mg extended-release tablet (¢¢¢)

Other Generic Product Names
pentoxil

DOSING AND FOOD

Doses are taken 3 times a day.
It is best to take this drug with meals.
Adults: Up to 1,200 mg per day in divided doses.
Forgotten doses: If you are scheduled to take the next dose within a few hours, do not take the forgotten dose. Otherwise take the forgotten dose as soon as you remember.

---

† See page 52.   * See page 53.

ALCOHOL, DRUG, HERB, AND SUPPLEMENT INTERACTIONS

Alcohol may increase some of the side effects from this drug, depending on the amount consumed. Ask your doctor about the risks caused by drinking alcohol with your condition.

Taking this drug with any of the ones listed below may change the effect of either drug with the possibility of causing toxicity or decreasing effectiveness: anticoagulants†, antihypertensives†, theophylline

ALLERGIC REACTIONS AND SIDE EFFECTS

If you are allergic to aminophylline, caffeine, dyphylline, ethylenediamine, oxtriphylline, theobromine, or theophylline you may also be allergic to this drug. You should tell your doctor about all your allergies and any unexplained symptoms you may have while taking this drug.

LESS COMMON SIDE EFFECTS: Bloating, dizziness, gas, headache, nausea, upset stomach, vomiting,

RARE SIDE EFFECTS: Chest pain*, drowsiness*, excitement*, faintness*, flushing*, irregular heartbeat*, seizures*

PRECAUTIONS

Do not crush, break, or chew the extended-release products.
Heavy smoking may cause this drug to be less effective.

PREGNANCY AND BREAST-FEEDING

Safety during pregnancy has not been established although the drug is known to harm animal fetuses.
Breast-feeding while taking this drug is not recommended.

HELPFUL COMMENTS

Take this drug with an antacid if you get an upset stomach after a dose.
It may take several weeks for the effects of this drug to be noticed.
Do not stop treatment early if you start to feel better. It takes the full 8-week prescription for this drug to work completely.

PERGOLIDE MESYLATE

Available since December 1988

COMMONLY USED TO TREAT

Parkinson's disease

DRUG CATEGORY

antidyskinetic
Class: dopaminergic agonist

PRODUCTS

Brand-Name Products with Generic Alternatives
Permax 0.05 mg tablet ($)
  Generic: pergolide mesylate 0.05 mg tablet (n/a)
Permax 0.25 mg tablet ($$)
  Generic: pergolide mesylate 0.25 mg tablet (n/a)
Permax 1 mg tablet ($$$)
  Generic: pergolide mesylate 1 mg tablet (n/a)

DOSING AND FOOD

Doses are taken 1 to 3 times a day.
This drug may be taken with or without food but is best taken with food to
  reduce the stomach upset that some people suffer.
Adults: Up to 3 mg per day in divided doses.
Forgotten doses: If you are scheduled to take the next dose within a few
  hours, do not take the forgotten dose. Otherwise take the forgotten dose
  as soon as you remember.

ALCOHOL, DRUG, HERB, AND SUPPLEMENT INTERACTIONS

Alcohol may increase some of the side effects from this drug, depending
  on the amount consumed. Ask your doctor about the risks caused by
  drinking alcohol with your condition.

Taking this drug with any of the ones listed below may change the effect of
either drug with the possibility of causing toxicity or decreasing effectiveness:
aspirin, haloperidol, metoclopramide, phenothiazines†, thioxanthenes†,
warfarin

ALLERGIC REACTIONS AND SIDE EFFECTS

If you are allergic to ergotamine or any ergot alkaloids†, you may also be
  allergic to this drug. You should tell your doctor about all your allergies
  and any unexplained symptoms you may have while taking this drug.
MORE COMMON SIDE EFFECTS: Anxiety*, back pain*, congestion, bloody
  urine*, confusion*, constipation, dizziness, drowsiness, hallucinations*,
  heartburn, lightheadedness, muscle pain, nausea*, runny nose, sleep disorders, spastic movements*, urinary changes*, weakness*

---

†See page 52.   * See page 53.

LESS COMMON SIDE EFFECTS: Diarrhea, dizziness*, dry mouth, headache*, loss of appetite, swelling*, vomiting*

RARE SIDE EFFECTS: Abdominal pain*, blurry vision*, breathing problems*, chest pain*, chills*, cough*, fainting*, fever*, irregular blood pressure*, irregular heartbeat*, nervousness*, pale skin*, poor bladder control*, seizures*, shortness of breath*, stiffness*, sweating*, tiredness*, vision changes*

PRECAUTIONS

If you have a history of mental disorders or heart disease, this drug may make those conditions worse.

Be careful driving or handling equipment while taking this drug because it may cause drowsiness and dizziness.

If you have high blood pressure, the dose of your antihypertensive† drug may need to be adjusted while taking this drug.

PREGNANCY AND BREAST-FEEDING

Safety during pregnancy has not been established although there was no evidence of harm during studies in animals.

Breast-feeding while taking this drug is not recommended.

HELPFUL COMMENTS

Avoid quick movements to minimize dizziness. Dangling your legs over the side of the bed for a few minutes may help reduce dizziness when first waking up.

Sucking on hard sugarless candy or chewing sugarless gum may help relieve dry mouth caused by this drug.

It may take several weeks before the effects of this drug are noticed.

PERINDOPRIL ERBUMINE

Available since December 1993

COMMONLY USED TO TREAT

High blood pressure, also known as hypertension

DRUG CATEGORY

antihypertensive
Class: ACE inhibitor

PRODUCTS

Brand-Name Products with No Generic Alternative
Aceon 2 mg tablet ($)
Aceon 4 mg tablet ($)
Aceon 8 mg tablet ($$)
No generics available.
Patent expires in 2006.

DOSING AND FOOD

Doses are taken 1 to 2 times a day.
This drug may be taken with or without food.
Adults: Up to 16 mg per day in divided doses.
Lower doses are used in people with kidney disease.
This drug is rarely used in children.
Forgotten doses: If you are scheduled to take the next dose within a few hours, do not take the forgotten dose. Otherwise take the forgotten dose as soon as you remember.

ALCOHOL, DRUG, HERB, AND SUPPLEMENT INTERACTIONS

Alcohol may cause your blood pressure to rise, making this drug less effective. Ask your doctor about the risks caused by drinking alcohol with your condition.
Licorice may interfere with the effects of this drug.
Capsaicin and other foods or supplements, including hot peppers, sweet peppers, paprika, and chili powder, derived from the capsicum family of plants may increase the risk of developing a cough and should not be taken with this drug.
Several OTC drugs used for appetite control, asthma, colds, cough, hay fever, or sinus problems may cause an increase in blood pressure when taken with this drug. Check with your pharmacist when selecting OTC products.
Taking this drug with any of the ones listed below may change the effect of either drug with the possibility of causing toxicity or decreasing effectiveness: antidiabetics[†], antihypertensives[†], diuretics[†], insulin, lithium, potassium supplements

ALLERGIC REACTIONS AND SIDE EFFECTS

If you are allergic to any ACE inhibitors[†], you may also be allergic to this drug. You should tell your doctor about all your allergies and any unexplained symptoms you may have while taking this drug.

[†] *See page 52.*   [*] *See page 53.*

MORE COMMON SIDE EFFECTS: Breathing difficulty*, cough, headache, swallowing difficulty*, swelling*

LESS COMMON SIDE EFFECTS: Diarrhea, dizziness*, fainting*, fever*, joint pain*, lightheadedness*, loss of taste, nausea, skin rash*, tiredness

RARE SIDE EFFECTS: Abdominal pain*, chest pain*, chills*, confusion*, hoarseness*, irregular heartbeat*, itching*, nausea*, nervousness*, numbness*, vomiting*, weakness*, yellow eyes or skin*

PRECAUTIONS

Be careful driving or handling equipment while taking this drug because the drug may cause dizziness.

People with systemic lupus erythematosus may be at greater risk of developing blood problems while taking this drug.

Do not use potassium-containing products, including salt substitutes, while taking this drug.

Diuretics† should be stopped 2 to 3 days prior to starting this drug. If it is not possible to stop the diuretic, the dose of this drug should be lowered.

Drink plenty of fluids to avoid dehydration when sweating, such as in hot weather and during exercise.

PREGNANCY AND BREAST-FEEDING

Safety during pregnancy has not been established although the drug is known to harm animal fetuses.

Breast-feeding while taking this drug is not recommended.

HELPFUL COMMENTS

A persistent dry cough may appear while taking this drug, but it will go away when the drug is stopped.

Avoid quick movements to minimize dizziness. Dangling your legs over the side of the bed for a few minutes may help reduce dizziness when first waking up.

PERPHENAZINE

Available for over 20 years

COMMONLY USED TO TREAT

Mental illness, also known as psychosis
Nausea and vomiting

DRUG CATEGORY

antiemetic
antipsychotic
Class: phenothiazine: piperazine derivative

PRODUCTS

Brand-Name Products with Generic Alternatives
Trilafon 2 mg tablet (¢¢¢¢¢)
  Generic: perphenazine 2 mg tablet (¢¢¢)
Trilafon 4 mg tablet ($)
  Generic: perphenazine 4 mg tablet (¢¢¢)
Trilafon 8 mg tablet ($)
  Generic: perphenazine 8 mg tablet (¢¢¢)
Trilafon 16 mg tablet ($$)
  Generic: perphenazine 16 mg tablet ($)
Products Only Available as Generics
perphenazine 16 mg/5 ml oral concentrate ($$)

DOSING AND FOOD

Doses are taken 2 to 4 times a day.
Taking this drug with food or a full glass of milk or water may avoid the
  stomach upset that some people suffer.
Adults: Up to 64 mg per day in divided doses.
Lower doses are used in people over age 65.
Forgotten doses: If you are scheduled to take the next dose within a few
  hours, do not take the forgotten dose. Otherwise take the forgotten dose
  as soon as you remember.

ALCOHOL, DRUG, HERB, AND SUPPLEMENT INTERACTIONS

Alcohol should not be used while taking this drug.
Do not use caffeine, kava, or yohimbe while taking this drug since the drug
  effects may be decreased and severe reactions may occur.
Several OTC drugs used for appetite control, asthma, colds, cough, hay fever,
  pain, or sinus problems may seriously increase the effects and side effects
  of this drug. Check with your pharmacist when selecting OTC products.

**Taking this drug with any of the ones listed below may change the effect of
either drug with the possibility of causing toxicity or decreasing effectiveness:**
antacids, antihypertensives[†], beta blockers[†], bromocriptine, caffeine,
dopamine, levodopa, lithium, phenobarbital, phenytoin, warfarin

---

† See page 52.   * See page 53.

Severe reactions are possible when this drug is taken with those listed below:
alcohol, amantadine, anesthetics, antiarrhythmics†, anticholinergics†, antidepressants†, antihistamines†, antithyroid drugs†, anxiolytics†, astemizole, barbiturates†, bromocriptine, cisapride, deferoxamine, disopyramide, diuretics†, epinephrine, erythromycin, levobunolol, lithium, metipranolol, metrizamide, nabilone, narcotics†, nitrates, pentamidine, probucol, procainamide, promethazine, propylthiouracil, quinidine, sympathomimetics†, tricyclic antidepressants†

Increased side effects are possible when this drug is taken with those listed below:
antipsychotics†, metoclopramide, metyrosine, pemoline, pimozide, rauwolfia alkaloids†, trimeprazine

ALLERGIC REACTIONS AND SIDE EFFECTS

If you are allergic to any phenothiazines†, you may also be allergic to this drug. You should tell your doctor about all your allergies and any unexplained symptoms you may have while taking this drug.

This drug promotes the effect of sunlight on the body and may cause severe sunburn and increased sensitivity of the eyes.

MORE COMMON SIDE EFFECTS: Breathing difficulty*, chewing action*, congestion, constipation, decreased sweating, difficulty breathing*, dizziness, drowsiness, dry mouth, eye stare*, eyelid movement*, fainting*, lip smacking*, loss of balance*, muscle spasms*, muscle stiffness*, puffy cheeks*, restlessness*, shuffling walk*, tongue movements*, trembling*, twitching*, urinary difficulty*, vision changes*

LESS COMMON SIDE EFFECTS: Breast-milk secretion, breast swelling, dark urine*, fever*, menstrual changes, rough tongue, sexual dysfunction, skin rash*, watery mouth, weight gain

RARE SIDE EFFECTS: Abdominal pain*, agitation*, bleeding*, blood pressure change*, bruising*, chest pain*, chills*, clumsiness*, coma*, confusion*, diarrhea*, dreams*, drooling*, excitement*, fast heartbeat*, hair loss*, headaches*, irregular heartbeat*, itching*, joint pain*, lack of sweat*, loss of bladder control*, mouth sores*, muscle stiffness*, muscle weakness*, nausea*, penile erection*, red hands*, seizures*, shivering*, skin discoloration*, sleep disorders*, sore throat*, speaking difficulty*, sweating*, tiredness*, vomiting*, weakness*, yellow eyes or skin*

PRECAUTIONS

If you have a history of enlarged prostate, glaucoma, ulcers, seizures, heart disease, urinary difficulty, or Parkinson's disease, this drug may make those conditions worse.

This drug may decrease the cough reflex, putting people with lung disease at greater risk of developing pneumonia.

Heavy smoking may cause this drug to be less effective.

This drug may cause false results from several diagnostic tests, including pregnancy tests, and should be stopped for at least 4 days before the test.

This drug should not be stopped suddenly, due to an increased risk of side effects. If you wish to stop taking this drug, ask your doctor for specific instructions.

Be careful driving or handling equipment while taking this drug because the drug may cause dizziness and drowsiness.

You are more likely to overheat when taking this drug and should avoid exercising in hot weather and using a sauna or hot tub.

This drug may make you more sensitive to cold temperatures.

Touching the liquid form of this drug may cause skin irritation. Make sure you do not spill the liquid, and wash your hands immediately after taking the dose.

This drug may cause dry mouth, which is associated with a greater risk of cavities. Your dentist may recommend that you clean your teeth and mouth differently to avoid infection.

PREGNANCY AND BREAST-FEEDING

Safety during pregnancy has not been established although the drug is known to harm animal fetuses.

Breast-feeding while taking this drug is not recommended.

HELPFUL COMMENTS

If you need to take an antacid, take it either 2 hours before or after taking this drug.

Sucking on hard sugarless candy or chewing sugarless gum may help relieve dry mouth caused by this drug.

The liquid form of this drug should be mixed in $1/4$ to $1/2$ cup of a caffeine-free carbonated beverage, fruit juice (not apple), milk, pudding, soup, tomato juice, or water just before taking the dose.

---

† See page 52.   * See page 53.

PHENOBARBITAL

Available for over 20 years

COMMONLY USED TO TREAT

Seizures

DRUG CATEGORY

anticonvulsant
sedative-hypnotic
Class: barbiturate

PRODUCTS

Products Only Available as Generics
phenobarbital 15 mg tablet (¢)
phenobarbital 30 mg tablet (¢)
phenobarbital 32.4 mg tablet (¢)
phenobarbital 60 mg tablet (¢)
phenobarbital 64.8 mg tablet (¢)
phenobarbital 97.2 mg tablet (¢)
phenobarbital 100 mg tablet (¢)
phenobarbital 20 mg/5 ml elixir (¢)

DOSING AND FOOD

Doses are taken 1 to 4 times a day.

It is best to take this drug on an empty stomach with a full glass of water at least 1 hour before or 2 hours after meals.

Adults: Up to 320 mg per day in divided doses.

Children: Up to 6 mg/kg per day in divided doses.

Forgotten doses: If you are scheduled to take the next dose within a few hours, do not take the forgotten dose. Otherwise take the forgotten dose as soon as you remember.

ALCOHOL, DRUG, HERB, AND SUPPLEMENT INTERACTIONS

Alcohol should not be used while taking this drug.

Several OTC drugs used for appetite control, asthma, colds, cough, hay fever, pain, or sinus problems may seriously increase the side effects of this drug. Check with your pharmacist when selecting OTC products.

Taking this drug with any of the ones listed below may change the effect of either drug with the possibility of causing toxicity or decreasing effectiveness: anticoagulants†, carbamazepine, corticosteroids†, corticotropin, divalproex sodium, oral contraceptives†, valproic acid

Increased side effects are possible when this drug is taken with those listed below: anesthetics, antihistamines†, anxiolytics†, barbiturates†, narcotics†, tricyclic antidepressants†

ALLERGIC REACTIONS AND SIDE EFFECTS

Allergic reactions are more likely to occur in people with a history of asthma or allergies to other drugs. You should tell your doctor about all your allergies and any unexplained symptoms you may have while taking this drug.

MORE COMMON SIDE EFFECTS: Clumsiness, dizziness, drowsiness, lightheadedness, unsteadiness

LESS COMMON SIDE EFFECTS: Anxiety, confusion*, constipation, depression*, excitement*, fainting, headache, irritability, nausea, nervousness, sleep disorders, vomiting

RARE SIDE EFFECTS: Bleeding lips*, bleeding*, bone pain*, bruising*, chest pain*, chest tightness*, fever*, hallucinations*, hives*, loss of appetite*, mouth sores*, muscle pain*, skin rash*, sore throat*, swelling*, tiredness*, weakness*, weight loss*, wheezing*, yellow eyes or skin*

PRECAUTIONS

Be careful driving or handling equipment while taking this drug because the drug may cause dizziness and drowsiness.

Children and people over age 65 may get hyperactive while taking this drug.

If you have anemia, asthma, high blood sugar, hyperactivity, depression, thyroid problems, liver disease, kidney disease, or porphyria, this drug may make those conditions worse.

This drug may be habit forming when taken for a long time. It should be stopped slowly to avoid withdrawal symptoms. It may take 2 weeks for the body to adjust after the drug is stopped. If you wish to stop taking this drug, ask your doctor for specific instructions.

PREGNANCY AND BREAST-FEEDING

There is evidence that this drug may harm the fetus, but the drug may be necessary to the health of the mother.

---

†*See page 52.* ** See page 53.*

This drug passes into breast milk, and may cause drowsiness, slow heart-beat, and breathing difficulty in the baby.

HELPFUL COMMENTS

Oral contraceptives may not work properly when taken with this drug. You need to use a barrier contraceptive, such as a condom, or other nonhormonal contraceptive to prevent pregnancy.

You may need to increase the fiber in your diet since this drug may cause constipation.

PHENTERMINE

Available for over 20 years

COMMONLY USED TO TREAT

Overeating

DRUG CATEGORY

appetite suppressant
Class: sympathomimetic

PRODUCTS

Brand-Name Products with No Generic Alternative
Ionamin 15 mg extended-release capsule§ ($$)
Ionamin 30 mg extended-release capsule§ ($$$)

Brand-Name Products with Generic Alternatives
Adipex-P 37.5 mg capsule ($$)
  Generic: phentermine hydrochloride 37.5 mg capsule (¢¢¢)
Adipex-P 37.5 mg tablet ($$)
  Generic: phentermine hydrochloride 37.5 mg tablet (¢¢¢)

Products Only Available as Generics
phentermine hydrochloride 8 mg tablet (¢¢)
phentermine hydrochloride 15 mg capsule (¢¢)
phentermine hydrochloride 18.75 mg capsule (¢)
phentermine hydrochloride 30 mg capsule (¢)

Other Generic Product Names
Ona-Mast, Phentercot, Phentride

DOSING AND FOOD

Doses are taken 1 to 3 times a day.

§ *See "Precautions" in this entry.*

This drug should be taken 1 hour before meals.

Adults: Up to 37.5 mg per day in divided doses.

Forgotten doses: Do not take a forgotten dose. Just go back to your usual schedule with the next dose.

ALCOHOL, DRUG, HERB, AND SUPPLEMENT INTERACTIONS

Alcohol may increase some of the side effects from this drug, depending on the amount consumed. Ask your doctor about the risks caused by drinking alcohol with your condition.

Do not use caffeine while taking this drug since the drug effects may be increased and severe reactions may occur.

Several OTC drugs used for appetite control, asthma, colds, cough, hay fever, pain, or sinus problems may seriously increase the effects of this drug. Check with your pharmacist when selecting OTC products.

Taking this drug with any of the ones listed below may change the effect of either drug with the possibility of causing toxicity or decreasing effectiveness: acetazolamide, antacids, antidiabetics†, antihypertensives†, haloperidol, insulin, phenothiazines†, sodium bicarbonate

Severe reactions are possible when this drug is taken with those listed below: amantadine, amphetamines†, caffeine, cocaine, methylphenidate, monoamine oxidase inhibitors†, nabilone, pemoline, tricyclic antidepressants†

Increased side effects are possible when this drug is taken with those listed below: anesthetics, SSRI†

ALLERGIC REACTIONS AND SIDE EFFECTS

If you are allergic to amphetamine, dextroamphetamine, ephedrine, epinephrine, isoproterenol, metaproterenol, methamphetamine, norepinephrine, phenylephrine, phenylpropanolamine, pseudoephedrine, terbutaline, or other appetite suppressants, you may also be allergic to this drug. You should tell your doctor about all your allergies and any unexplained symptoms you may have while taking this drug.

MORE COMMON SIDE EFFECTS: Constipation, dizziness*, dry mouth, blood pressure changes*, irregular heartbeat*, irritability*, lightheadedness*, nausea*, nervousness, restlessness, shaking*, sleep disorders*, stomach cramps, trembling*, vomiting*

LESS COMMON SIDE EFFECTS: Abdominal cramps*, behavior changes*, blurry vision, coma*, confusion*, depression*, diarrhea*, drowsiness, excitability*, fainting*, fever*, hallucinations*, hives*, hostility*, irregular breathing*, numbness*, panic attack*, restlessness*, seizures*, sexual

---

† See page 52.   * See page 53.

dysfunction, skin disease*, skin rash*, sweating, taste changes, tiredness*, urinary changes*, weakness*

RARE SIDE EFFECTS: Breathing difficulty*, Chest pain*, fainting*, swelling

PRECAUTIONS

§The strength of Ionamin capsules is not the same as the strength of other products and may not be substituted without a new prescription.

This drug is habit forming and may cause severe withdrawal symptoms if stopped suddenly. If you wish to stop taking this drug, ask your doctor for specific instructions. People with a history of alcohol or substance abuse have a greater risk of becoming dependent on this drug.

If you are diabetic, you may need a change in the dose of your antidiabetic drug† or insulin, since this drug may cause changes in blood sugar.

Be careful driving or handling equipment while taking this drug because it may cause dizziness.

Do not open, crush, break, or chew the extended-release products.

You need to wait 2 weeks after stopping a monoamine oxidase inhibitor† before starting this drug.

This drug may cause positive results for amphetamine when performing urine screening. If you have a pre-employment drug-screening test, make sure the laboratory knows that you are taking this drug.

If you have glaucoma, heart disease, blood vessel disease, high blood pressure, mental problems, or thyroid problems, this drug may make those conditions worse.

If you notice a decrease in your ability to exercise, it may be a sign of serious side effects and you should call your doctor right away.

PREGNANCY AND BREAST-FEEDING

This drug may cause birth defects and should not be used during pregnancy. Breast-feeding while taking this drug is not recommended.

HELPFUL COMMENTS

Sucking on hard sugarless candy or chewing sugarless gum may help relieve dry mouth caused by this drug.

Increasing the dose of this drug may not increase the effectiveness. If the drug does not appear to be working within a few weeks, call your doctor.

Take the last dose of the day at least 6 hours before bedtime to reduce insomnia.

PHENYTOIN

Available for over 20 years

COMMONLY USED TO TREAT

Nerve pain
Seizures

DRUG CATEGORY

anticonvulsant
Class: hydantoin derivative

PRODUCTS

Brand-Name Products with No Generic Alternative
Dilantin 50 mg chewable tablet (¢¢¢)
Dilantin 30 mg extended-release capsule (¢¢¢)
Dilantin 200 mg extended-release capsule (n/a)
Phenytek 200 mg extended-release capsule (¢¢¢¢)
Phenytek 300 mg extended-release capsule (¢¢¢¢¢)
Phenytoin 100 mg prompt-release capsule (¢¢)
Brand-Name Products with Generic Alternatives
Dilantin 100 mg extended-release capsule§ (¢¢¢)
  Generic: phenytoin 100 mg extended-release capsule§ (¢¢¢)
Dilantin 125 mg/5 ml oral suspension§ (¢¢¢¢¢)
  Generic: phenytoin 125 mg/5 ml oral suspension§ (¢¢¢¢)

DOSING AND FOOD

Doses are taken 1 to 3 times a day.
This drug may be taken with or without food but is best taken with food to reduce the stomach upset that some people suffer.
Adults: Up to 600 mg per day in divided doses.
Children: Up to 8 mg/kg per day in divided doses.
Forgotten doses: If it is 4 hours or less before the next scheduled dose, do not take the forgotten dose. Otherwise take the forgotten dose as soon as you remember.

ALCOHOL, DRUG, HERB, AND SUPPLEMENT INTERACTIONS

Alcohol should not be used while taking this drug.
Several OTC drugs used for appetite control, asthma, colds, cough, hay

---

† See page 52.   * See page 53.   § See "Precautions" in this entry.

fever, pain, or sinus problems may seriously increase the effects of this drug. Check with your pharmacist when selecting OTC products.

Taking this drug with any of the ones listed below may change the effect of either drug with the possibility of causing toxicity or decreasing effectiveness: acetaminophen, allopurinol, amiodarone, antacids, anticoagulants†, antineoplastics†, antipsychotics†, aspirin, barbiturates†, benzodiazepines†, calcium supplements, carbamazepine, charcoal, chloramphenicol, chlorpheniramine, cimetidine, corticosteroids†, cyclosporine, diazepam, diazoxide, dicumerol, digitoxin, disopyramide, disulfiram, dopamine, doxycycline, estrogens†, felbamate, fluconazole, fluoxetine, folic acid, furosemide, haloperidol, ibuprofen, imipramine, isoniazid, itraconazole, ketoconazole, levodopa, lidocaine, loxapine, mebendazole, meperidine, methadone, metronidazole, metyrapone, miconazole, nitrofurantoin, omeprazole, oral contraceptives, phenacemide, phenothiazines†, phenylbutazone, pyridoxine, quinidine, rifampin, salicylates†, streptozocin, succinimides†, sucralfate, sulfonylureas†, theophylline, trimethoprim, thyroid hormones†, valproic acid

ALLERGIC REACTIONS AND SIDE EFFECTS

If you are allergic to any hydantoin derivative†, you may also be allergic to this drug. You should tell your doctor about all your allergies and any unexplained symptoms you may have while taking this drug.

MORE COMMON SIDE EFFECTS: Bleeding gums*, clumsiness*, confusion*, constipation, dizziness*, drowsiness*, excitement*, eye movement*, fever*, hair growth, irritability*, itching*, muscle pain*, nausea*, nervousness*, poor coordination, skin rash*, sore throat*, speech difficulties*, stuttering*, swollen glands*, tender gums*, trembling*, unsteadiness*, vomiting*

LESS COMMON SIDE EFFECTS: Breast enlargement, facial changes, sleep disorders, twitching

RARE SIDE EFFECTS: Agitation*, arm movements*, bleeding*, blurry vision*, bone deformities*, breathing changes*, broken bones*, bruising*, chest pain*, chills*, dark urine*, erection pain*, gray stools*, headache*, joint pain*, learning difficulty*, leg movements*, loss of appetite*, numbness*, restlessness*, seizures*, slow growth*, staggering*, stomach pain*, tingling*, tiredness*, weakness*, weight loss*, yellow eyes or skin*

PRECAUTIONS

§The effectiveness of this drug may vary from product to product. Do not switch from one manufacturer to another when your prescription is refilled. Talk to your pharmacist to make sure you get the same product each time.

If you have diabetes, porphyria, or systemic lupus erythematosus, this drug may make those conditions worse.

Do not open, crush, break, or chew the extended-release products.

Stopping this drug suddenly may increase the risk of developing a seizure. If you wish to stop taking this drug, ask your doctor for specific instructions.

If you are a diabetic, you may need a change in the dose of your antidiabetic drug† or insulin, since this drug may cause changes in blood sugar.

Be careful driving or handling equipment while taking this drug because it may cause dizziness and drowsiness.

This drug may cause changes to your gums and mouth. You should see your dentist every 3 months while taking this drug. Your dentist may recommend you clean your teeth and mouth differently to avoid infection.

PREGNANCY AND BREAST-FEEDING

There is evidence that this drug may harm the fetus, but the drug may be necessary to the health of the mother.

Breast-feeding while taking this drug is not recommended.

HELPFUL COMMENTS

Oral contraceptives may not work properly when taken with this drug. You need to use a barrier contraceptive, such as a condom, or other nonhormonal contraceptive to prevent pregnancy.

The dosage of this drug may change frequently over the first few months of treatment.

If you need to take an antacid, take it either 2 hours before or after taking this drug.

PIMOZIDE

Available since July 1984

COMMONLY USED TO TREAT

Tourette's syndrome

DRUG CATEGORY

antipsychotic
Class: diphenylbutylpiperidine

---

† See page 52.   * See page 53.

PRODUCTS

Brand-Name Products with No Generic Alternative
Orap 1 mg tablet (¢¢¢¢)
Orap 2 mg tablet (¢¢¢¢¢)
No generics available.
No patents, no exclusivity.

DOSING AND FOOD

Doses are taken 1 to 3 times a day.
This drug may be taken with or without food. Do not drink grapefruit juice at any time while taking this drug.

Adults and children over age 12: Up to 10 mg per day in divided doses.

Forgotten doses: Do not take a forgotten dose. Just go back to your usual schedule with the next dose.

ALCOHOL, DRUG, HERB, AND SUPPLEMENT INTERACTIONS

Alcohol should not be used while taking this drug.
Many OTC drugs used for appetite control, asthma, colds, cough, hay fever, pain, or sinus problems affect the central nervous system and may change the effects or side effects of this drug. Check with your pharmacist for products to avoid.

Taking this drug with any of the ones listed below may change the effect of either drug with the possibility of causing toxicity or decreasing effectiveness: anticonvulsants†, antifungals†, carbamazepine, phenytoin

Severe reactions are possible when this drug is taken with those listed below: amphetamines†, analgesics, anesthetics, antiarrhythmics†, antidepressants, antihistamines†, antipsychotics†, anxiolytics†, azithromycin, barbiturates†, clarithromycin, dirithromycin, disopyramide, erythromycin, indinavir, itraconazole, ketoconazole, maprotiline, methylphenidate, narcotics†, nefazodone, nelfinavir, pemoline, phenobarbital, phenothiazines†, probucol, procainamide, quinidine, ritonavir, saquinavir, troleandomycin, zileuton

Increased side effects are possible when this drug is taken with those listed below: amoxapine, anticholinergics†, metoclopramide, metyrosine, paroxetine, promethazine, rauwolfia alkaloids†

ALLERGIC REACTIONS AND SIDE EFFECTS

If you are allergic to haloperidol, you may also be allergic to this drug. You should tell your doctor about all your allergies and any unexplained symptoms you may have while taking this drug.

MORE COMMON SIDE EFFECTS: Blurry vision, breast enlargement*, breast-milk secretion*, constipation, dizziness*, drowsiness, dry mouth, expressionless face*, fainting*, irregular heartbeat*, lightheadedness, mood swings*, poor balance*, restlessness*, shaky hands*, shuffling walk*, skin discoloration, speech difficulty*, stiffness*, trembling*, vision changes

LESS COMMON SIDE EFFECTS: Bleeding*, blinking*, bruising*, chewing motion*, depression, diarrhea, eye stillness*, eyelid spasms*, facial expressions*, fever*, headache, itching*, lip smacking*, loss of appetite, menstrual changes*, muscle spasms*, nausea, puffy cheeks*, sexual dysfunction, skin rash*, sore throat*, spastic movements*, swallowing disorder*, swelling*, tiredness, tongue movements*, vomiting, weakness, weight loss, yellow eyes or skin*

RARE SIDE EFFECTS: Blood pressure changes*, breathing difficulty*, coma*, jerking*, poor bladder control*, seizures*, sweating*

PRECAUTIONS

If you have breast cancer, glaucoma, heart disease, intestinal problems, or urinary problems, this drug may make those conditions worse.

Your body may lose potassium while taking this drug, which may cause severe side effects. Potassium levels should be monitored periodically and may need to be supplemented while taking this drug. Eat food rich in potassium, such as apricots, bananas, citrus fruit, dates, and tomatoes, if you are not taking a potassium supplement or potassium-sparing diuretic†.

People with a history of seizures are at increased risk of developing seizures while taking this drug.

Stopping this drug suddenly may cause serious side effects. If you wish to stop taking this drug, ask your doctor for specific instructions.

Be careful driving or handling equipment while taking this drug because it may cause dizziness and drowsiness.

PREGNANCY AND BREAST-FEEDING

Safety during pregnancy has not been established although the drug is known to harm animal fetuses.

It is not known if this drug passes into breast milk. Talk to your doctor about the risks associated with breast-feeding while taking this drug.

HELPFUL COMMENTS

Sucking on hard sugarless candy or chewing sugarless gum may help relieve dry mouth caused by this drug.

---

† See page 52.   * See page 53.

Avoid quick movements to minimize dizziness. Dangling your legs over the side of the bed for a few minutes may help reduce dizziness when first waking up.

It may take several weeks for the effects of this drug to be noticed.

Taking your dose of this drug at bedtime may minimize sleepiness during the day.

PINDOLOL

Available since September 1982

COMMONLY USED TO TREAT

Chest pain, also known as angina
High blood pressure, also known as hypertension

DRUG CATEGORY

antianginal
antihypertensive
Class: beta blocker

PRODUCTS

Brand-Name Products with Generic Alternatives
Visken 5 mg tablet (n/a)
  Generic: pindolol 5 mg tablet (¢¢¢¢)
Visken 10 mg tablet (n/a)
  Generic: pindolol 10 mg tablet (¢¢¢¢¢)

DOSING AND FOOD

Doses are taken 1 to 3 times a day.

Taking this drug with food will help increase the absorption of the drug.

Adults: Up to 60 mg per day in divided doses.

Lower doses are used in people with renal disease, liver disease, or heart failure.

This drug is rarely used in children.

Forgotten doses: If you are scheduled to take the next dose in less than 4 hours, do not take the forgotten dose. Otherwise take the forgotten dose as soon as you remember.

ALCOHOL, DRUG, HERB, AND SUPPLEMENT INTERACTIONS

Alcohol may increase some of the side effects from this drug, depending

on the amount consumed. Ask your doctor about the risks caused by
drinking alcohol with your condition.

Several OTC drugs used for appetite control, asthma, colds, cough, hay fever,
or sinus problems may cause an increase in blood pressure when taken
with this drug. Check with your pharmacist when selecting OTC products.

**Taking this drug with any of the ones listed below may change the effect of
either drug with the possibility of causing toxicity or decreasing effectiveness:**
aminophylline, anesthetics†, antidiabetics†, caffeine, calcium channel block-
ers†, carbonic anhydrase inhibitors†, clonidine, dyphylline, epinephrine,
guanabenz, lidocaine, nonsteroidal antiinflammatories†, oxtriphylline,
pilocarpine, reserpine, theophylline

Severe reactions are possible when this drug is taken with those listed below:
allergy shots, beta blockers†, cocaine, monoamine oxidase inhibitors†,
thioridazine

**Increased effects or side effects are possible when this drug is taken with
those listed below:**
antihypertensives†

ALLERGIC REACTIONS AND SIDE EFFECTS

If you are allergic to any other beta blockers†, you may also be allergic to
this drug.

This drug may exaggerate the reaction from your current allergies. Inform
your doctor of any allergies that you have as well as the severity of the
allergic reaction before starting this drug.

MORE COMMON SIDE EFFECTS: Dizziness, drowsiness, lightheadedness, sexual dysfunction, sleeping difficulty, tiredness, weakness

LESS COMMON SIDE EFFECTS: Anxiety, breathing difficulty*, cold hands and
feet*, constipation, depression*, diarrhea, itching, nausea, nervousness,
numbness, shortness of breath*, slow heartbeat*, sore eyes, stomachache,
stuffy nose, swelling*, tingling, vivid dreams, vomiting, wheezing

RARE SIDE EFFECTS: Back pain*, bleeding*, bruising*, chest pain*, confusion*, dizziness*, fever*, hallucinations*, irregular heartbeat*, joint pain*,
lightheadedness*, rash*, scaly skin*, sore throat*

PRECAUTIONS

People with asthma, heart disease, or a heart rate that is routinely less than
60 beats per minute (bradycardia) may not be able to take this drug.

Stopping this drug suddenly may cause chest pain or heart attack. If you
wish to stop taking this drug, ask your doctor for specific instructions.

---

† *See page 52.*   * *See page 53.*

Be careful driving or handling equipment while taking this drug because the drug may cause dizziness and drowsiness.

You need to wait 2 weeks after stopping a monoamine oxidase inhibitor† before starting this drug.

If you are diabetic, this drug may increase blood sugar levels or make the symptoms of low blood sugar less noticeable.

This drug may cause nondiabetics to develop type 2 diabetes.

If you have psoriasis or myasthenia gravis, this drug may make those conditions worse.

PREGNANCY AND BREAST-FEEDING

Safety during pregnancy has not been established although the drug is known to harm animal fetuses.

Breast-feeding while taking this drug is not recommended.

HELPFUL COMMENTS

This drug may make you more sensitive to cold temperatures.

Dosage adjustments are usually made after 3 to 4 weeks of treatment if the desired effects are not seen.

If you do not treat high blood pressure, you may develop more serious problems such as heart failure, blood vessel disease, stroke, or kidney disease. Losing weight, exercising, eating more fruits and vegetables, and avoiding salty foods, such as lunchmeat and pickles, may help make drug treatment more successful.

PIOGLITAZONE HYDROCHLORIDE

Available since July 1999

COMMONLY USED TO TREAT

High blood sugar, specifically type 2 diabetes

DRUG CATEGORY

antidiabetic
Class: thiazolidinedione

PRODUCTS

Brand-Name Products with No Generic Alternative
Actos 15 mg tablet ($$$)
Actos 30 mg tablet ($$$)
Actos 45 mg tablet ($$$$)

No generics available.
Multiple patents that begin to expire in 2006.

DOSING AND FOOD

Doses are taken once a day.
This drug may be taken with or without food.

Adults: Up to 45 mg per day.

Forgotten doses: If you are scheduled to take the next dose within a few hours, do not take the forgotten dose. Otherwise take the forgotten dose as soon as you remember.

ALCOHOL, DRUG, HERB, AND SUPPLEMENT INTERACTIONS

Alcohol may cause a change in your blood sugar, altering the effects of this drug. Ask your doctor about the risks caused by drinking alcohol with your condition.

Aloe, bilberry leaf, bitter melon, burdock, dandelion, fenugreek, garlic, ginkgo biloba, and ginseng may lower blood sugar and cause the need for a dose adjustment when taken with this drug. Tell your doctor if you are taking any of these supplements.

Several OTC drugs used for asthma, colds, cough, hay fever, sleep aid, or sinus problems may seriously change the effects of this drug. Check with your pharmacist when selecting OTC products.

Taking this drug with any of the ones listed below may change the effect of either drug with the possibility of causing toxicity or decreasing effectiveness: ketoconazole, oral contraceptives

ALLERGIC REACTIONS AND SIDE EFFECTS

You should tell your doctor about all your allergies and any unexplained symptoms you may have while taking this drug.

MORE COMMON SIDE EFFECTS: Cough, fever, headache, muscle aches, runny nose, sore throat, tooth problems*

LESS COMMON SIDE EFFECTS: Swelling*

RARE SIDE EFFECTS: Abdominal pain*, dark urine*, loss of appetite*, nausea*, vomiting*, tiredness*, weakness*, yellow eyes or skin*

PRECAUTIONS

This drug is not effective when used in people with type 1 diabetes.
If you have heart disease or liver disease, this drug may make those conditions worse.

---

†See page 52.   * See page 53.

Burns, diarrhea, fever, hormonal changes, infection, malnourishment, severe stress, uncontrolled thyroid disease, and vomiting may cause changes in blood sugar that may make this drug less effective.

If you were taking troglitazone and are changing to this drug, there should be 1 week between drugs when nothing is taken.

Liver function should be tested every 2 months when taking this drug.

This drug is usually taken in combination with another antidiabetic drug† or insulin and may lower blood sugars too much.

PREGNANCY AND BREAST-FEEDING

Safety during pregnancy has not been established although the drug is known to harm animal fetuses.

Breast-feeding while taking this drug is not recommended.

HELPFUL COMMENTS

Oral contraceptives may not work properly when taken with this drug. You need to use a barrier contraceptive, such as a condom, or other nonhormonal contraceptive to prevent pregnancy.

If you do not treat high blood sugar, you may develop more serious problems such as heart failure, blood vessel disease, eye disease, or kidney disease.

PIROXICAM

Available for over 20 years

COMMONLY USED TO TREAT

Arthritis
Pain

DRUG CATEGORY

antiarthritic
antidysmenorrheal
antigout
antipyretic
Class: nonsteroidal antiinflammatory

PRODUCTS

Brand-Name Products with Generic Alternatives
Feldene 10 mg capsule ($$)

Generic: piroxicam 10 mg capsule ($)
Feldene 20 mg capsule ($$$)
Generic: piroxicam 20 mg capsule (¢¢)

DOSING AND FOOD

Doses are taken 1 to 2 times a day.
It is best to take this drug with food or antacids.

Adults: Up to 40 mg per day.

Children 46 to 55 kg: Up to 15 mg per day.

Children 31 to 45 kg: Up to 10 mg per day.

Children 15 to 30 kg: Up to 5 mg per day.

Forgotten doses: If you are scheduled to take the next dose within a few hours, do not take the forgotten dose. Otherwise take the forgotten dose as soon as you remember.

ALCOHOL, DRUG, HERB, AND SUPPLEMENT INTERACTIONS

Alcohol may increase the risk of serious side effects from this drug. Ask your doctor about the risks caused by drinking alcohol with your condition.

Do not use dong quai, feverfew, garlic, ginger, horse chestnut, red clover, or St. John's wort while taking this drug since they may increase the risk of serious side effects.

Taking this drug with any of the ones listed below may change the effect of either drug with the possibility of causing toxicity or decreasing effectiveness: acetaminophen, antihypertensives[†], digoxin, diuretics[†], furosemide, hydrochlorothiazide, nifedipine, lithium, methotrexate, phenytoin, probenecid, sulfonylureas[†], sulindac, verapamil

Severe reactions are possible when this drug is taken with those listed below: antibiotics[†], anticoagulants[†], aspirin, cefamandole, cefoperazone, cefotetan, corticosteroids[†], cyclosporine, dipyridamole, gold salts[†], heparin, mezlocillin, nonsteroidal antiinflammatories[†], penicillamine, piperacillin, plicamycin, salicylates[†], sulfinpyrazone, ticarcillin, valproic acid, warfarin

ALLERGIC REACTIONS AND SIDE EFFECTS

If you are allergic to aspirin, zomepirac, salicylates[†], or other nonsteroidal antiinflammatories[†], you may also be allergic to this drug. You should tell your doctor about all your allergies and any unexplained symptoms you may have while taking this drug.

This drug promotes the effect of sunlight on the body and may cause severe sunburn and increased sensitivity of the eyes.

[†] *See page 52.*   [*] *See page 53.*

MORE COMMON SIDE EFFECTS: Black stools*, heartburn*, indigestion*, nausea*, swelling*, weight gain*

LESS COMMON SIDE EFFECTS: Abdominal pain, bruising*, constipation, diarrhea, dizziness, drowsiness, gas, headache, high blood pressure*, itching*, mouth sores*, skin rash*, sweating, vomiting

RARE SIDE EFFECTS: Back pain*, bloody urine*, bloody vomit, blue fingernails*, blue lips*, breathing difficulty*, chest pain*, chest tightness*, chills*, confusion*, cough*, dark urine*, fainting*, fever*, hallucinations*, hearing loss*, hives*, hoarseness*, lip sores*, loss of appetite*, low blood pressure*, mood swings*, muscle cramps*, nosebleeds*, pain*, pale skin*, pale stools*, puffy eyes*, rectal bleeding*, restlessness*, ringing in ears*, runny nose*, seizures*, shortness of breath*, sore throat*, stiff neck*, thirst*, tiredness*, urinary changes*, vision changes*, weakness*, wheezing*, yellow eyes or skin*

PRECAUTIONS

This drug may cause serious stomach problems and possibly ulcers. Be careful to take this drug as directed with food, and let your doctor know if you develop any stomach-related symptoms.

Be careful driving or handling equipment while taking this drug because the drug may cause dizziness and drowsiness.

Do not lie down for about 30 minutes after taking this drug to help reduce the risk of heartburn and throat irritation.

If you use tobacco or have a history of alcohol abuse, stomach problems, intestinal problems, hemorrhoids, diabetes mellitus, severe fluid retention, or systemic lupus erythematosus, there is an increased risk that you will develop side effects while taking this drug.

PREGNANCY AND BREAST-FEEDING

Safety during pregnancy has not been established although the drug is known to harm animal fetuses.

Breast-feeding while taking this drug is not recommended.

HELPFUL COMMENTS

People with arthritis usually notice the effects of this drug within 2 weeks.

Several nonsteroidal antiinflammatories† are available without a prescription in lower, nonprescription strengths, including ibuprofen, ketoprofen, and naproxen.

POLYTHIAZIDE

Available for over 20 years

COMMONLY USED TO TREAT

Fluid retention, also known as edema
Frequent urination in people with diabetes
High blood pressure, also known as hypertension

DRUG CATEGORY

antihypertensive
Class: thiazide diuretic

PRODUCTS

Brand-Name Products with No Generic Alternative
Renese 1 mg tablet (¢¢¢¢)
Renese 2 mg tablet (¢¢¢¢)
Renese 4 mg tablet (n/a)
Combination Products That Contain This Drug
Minizide capsule (¢¢¢¢) to ($)
Renese-R tablet (n/a)

DOSING AND FOOD

Doses are taken once a day but may be taken as little as 3 times a week.
It is best to take this drug on an empty stomach, but taking this drug with
a little food may avoid the stomach upset that some people suffer. Avoid
food with excess salt.
Adults: Up to 4 mg per day.
Lower doses may be used in children.
Forgotten doses: If you are scheduled to take the next dose within a few
hours, do not take the forgotten dose. Otherwise take the forgotten dose
as soon as you remember.

ALCOHOL, DRUG, HERB, AND SUPPLEMENT INTERACTIONS

Alcohol may cause your blood pressure to rise, making this drug less effective. Ask your doctor about the risks caused by drinking alcohol with
your condition.
Licorice root may increase potassium loss and should not be used while
taking this drug.

---

† See page 52.   * See page 53.

Several OTC drugs used for appetite control, asthma, colds, cough, hay fever, or sinus problems may cause an increase in blood pressure when taken with this drug. Check with your pharmacist when selecting OTC products.

Taking this drug with any of the ones listed below may change the effect of either drug with the possibility of causing toxicity or decreasing effectiveness: antidiabetics†, cholestyramine, colestipol, digoxin, insulin, lithium

ALLERGIC REACTIONS AND SIDE EFFECTS

If you are allergic to acetazolamide, bumetanide, dichlorphenamide, furosemide, methazolamide, sulfonamides†, or thiazide diuretics†, you may also be allergic to this drug. You should tell your doctor about all your allergies and any unexplained symptoms you may have while taking this drug.

This drug promotes the effect of sunlight on the body and may cause severe sunburn and increased sensitivity of the eyes.

LESS COMMON SIDE EFFECTS: Diarrhea*, dizziness, lightheadedness, loss of appetite, sexual dysfunction, stomach upset

RARE SIDE EFFECTS: Back pain*, black stools*, bleeding*, bloody urine*, breathing difficulty*, bruising*, burning sensation*, chest pain*, chills*, confusion*, cough*, fatigue*, fever*, hives*, headache*, hoarseness*, irregular heartbeat*, joint pain*, leg pain*, muscle cramps*, nausea*, numbness*, painful urination*, shortness of breath*, skin rash*, stomach pain*, swelling*, vomiting*, weakness*, yellow eyes or skin*

PRECAUTIONS

This drug may cause your blood sugar level to rise and may lead to type 2 diabetes.

Your body may lose potassium while taking this drug, which may cause severe side effects. Potassium levels should be monitored periodically and may need to be supplemented while taking this drug. Eat food rich in potassium, such as apricots, bananas, citrus fruit, dates, and tomatoes, if you are not taking a potassium supplement or potassium-sparing diuretic†.

People with kidney disease may not be able to take this drug.

This drug may increase the level of uric acid in the body, which may lead to gout or kidney stones.

If you have lupus erythematosus or pancreatitis, this drug may make those conditions worse.

Nicotine in cigarettes may increase blood pressure, making this drug less effective.

This drug may cause an increase in the levels of cholesterol or triglyceride in the blood.

PREGNANCY AND BREAST-FEEDING

Safety during pregnancy has not been established although the drug is known to harm animal fetuses.

Breast-feeding while taking this drug is not recommended.

HELPFUL COMMENTS

Take your last dose of the day no later than 6 P.M. to avoid urination during the night.

Avoid quick movements to minimize dizziness. Dangling your legs over the side of the bed for a few minutes may help reduce dizziness when first waking up.

Record your weight twice a day, when first getting up in the morning and after the drug causes urination. A weight gain or loss of more than 2 pounds per day should be reported to your doctor.

The antihypertensive effects of this drug will last about 1 week after it is stopped.

POTASSIUM

Available for over 20 years

COMMONLY USED TO TREAT

Low potassium levels, also known as hypokalemia

Potassium loss caused by diuretics (water pills)

DRUG CATEGORY

electrolyte replacement

Class: potassium supplement

PRODUCTS

Brand-Name Products with No Generic Alternative

K-Lyte/CL 25 mEq effervescent tablet ($)

K-Lyte/CL 50 mEq effervescent tablet ($$)

K-Lyte DS 50 mEq effervescent tablet ($$)

Kaon 20 mEq/15 ml oral elixir (¢¢¢)

Kaon-CL 20% 40 mEq/15 ml oral solution (¢¢¢)

Klor-Con 25 mEq powder for suspension ($)

Micro-K 8 mEq extended-release capsule (¢¢¢)

Micro-K 10 mEq extended-release capsule (¢¢¢)

---

† See page 52.　　* See page 53.

Rum-K 30 mEq/15 ml oral solution (¢¢¢)
Urocit-K 5 mEq extended-release tablet (¢¢¢)
Urocit-K 10 mEq extended-release tablet (¢¢¢)

Brand-Name Products with Generic Alternatives

K-Lyte 25 mEq effervescent tablet ($)
  Generic: potassium bicarbonate 25 mEq effervescent tablet (¢¢¢)
K-Vescent 25 mEq effervescent tablet (¢¢¢)
  Generic: potassium bicarbonate 25 mEq effervescent tablet (¢¢¢)
Slow-K 8 mEq extended-release tablet (n/a)
  Generic: potassium chloride 8 mEq extended-release tablet (¢¢)
K-Dur 10 mEq extended-release tablet (¢¢¢)
  Generic: potassium chloride 10 mEq extended-release tablet (¢¢)
K-Dur 20 mEq extended-release tablet (¢¢¢¢)
  Generic: potassium chloride 20 mEq extended-release tablet (¢¢¢)
Kaochlor 20 mEq/15 ml oral solution (¢¢¢)
  Generic: potassium chloride 20 mEq/15 ml oral solution (¢¢¢)
K-Lor 20 mEq powder for suspension ($)
  Generic: potassium chloride 20 mEq powder for suspension (¢¢)

Other Generic Product Names

Ed K + 10, K + 8, K + 10, K + Care ET, K-Effervescent, K + Potassium, K-Tab, Kaon-CL, Kay Ciel, Klor-Con, Klor-Con/EF, Klor-Con M, Klotrix

DOSING AND FOOD

Doses are taken 1 to 6 times a day.
This drug may be taken with or without food but is best taken with food to reduce the stomach upset that some people suffer. Follow with a full glass of water.
Adults and children: Doses are based on blood levels of potassium.
Forgotten doses: If more than 2 hours have passed since the forgotten dose, do not take the dose. Otherwise take the forgotten dose as soon as you remember.

ALCOHOL, DRUG, HERB, AND SUPPLEMENT INTERACTIONS

Salt substitutes, which contain potassium, may cause increased levels of potassium in the body and should not be used when taking this drug.
Many prescription and OTC drugs contain potassium. Tell your doctor about any potassium-containing products that you routinely use and make sure not to change the amount used without an adjustment to the dose of this drug.

Taking this drug with any of the ones listed below may change the effect of either drug with the possibility of causing toxicity or decreasing effectiveness: ACE inhibitors†, amiloride, beta blockers†, heparin, nonsteroidal anti-inflammatories†, potassium-sparing diuretics†

Severe reactions are possible when this drug is taken with those listed below: digoxin, digitoxin

Increased side effects are possible when this drug is taken with those listed below: amantadine, anticholinergics†, antidepressants†, antidyskinetics†, antihistamines†, antipsychotics†, buclizine, carbamazepine, cyclobenzaprine, cyclizine, disopyramide, flavoxate, ipratropium, meclizine, methylphenidate, orphenadrine, oxybutynin, procainamide, promethazine, quinidine, trimeprazine

ALLERGIC REACTIONS AND SIDE EFFECTS

You should tell your doctor about all your allergies and any unexplained symptoms you may have while taking this drug.

MORE COMMON SIDE EFFECTS: Diarrhea, gas, nausea, stomachache, vomiting

LESS COMMON SIDE EFFECTS: Anxiety*, breathing difficulty*, confusion*, irregular heartbeat*, numbness*, shortness of breath*, tingling*, tiredness*, weakness*

RARE SIDE EFFECTS: Abdominal pain*, bloody stools*, chest pain*, stomach cramps*, throat pain*

PRECAUTIONS

Most extended-release products should not be opened, crushed, broken, or chewed although there are some exceptions with potassium products. If using an extended-release product, check with your pharmacist to determine if the product in your prescription may be broken or crushed.

If you are taking a thiazide diuretic†, do not stop taking it without an adjustment to the dose of potassium.

If you have ulcers or intestinal problems, this drug may make those conditions worse.

Drink plenty of fluids to avoid dehydration when sweating, such as in hot weather and during exercise.

If you have diarrhea that continues for more than a day, you may need a temporary adjustment to your dose of this drug.

Liquid, powder for suspension, and effervescent tablets must be diluted with at least 1/2 glass of water to minimize side effects.

Do not make a change in your exercise routine without telling your doctor since exercise may increase the amount of potassium in your blood.

---

†See page 52.   *See page 53.

PREGNANCY AND BREAST-FEEDING

Safety during pregnancy has not been established although the drug is known to harm animal fetuses.

This drug passes into breast milk, but does not appear to harm the baby. Talk to your doctor about the risks associated with breast-feeding while taking this drug.

HELPFUL COMMENTS

An empty shell from the tablet and capsule products may pass in your stool without dissolving, which is not a concern.

PRAMIPEXOLE DIPHYDROCHLORIDE

Available since July 1997

COMMONLY USED TO TREAT

Parkinson's disease

DRUG CATEGORY

antidyskinetic
Class: nonergot dopamine agonist

PRODUCTS

Brand-Name Products with No Generic Alternative
Mirapex 0.125 mg tablet (¢¢¢¢¢)
Mirapex 0.25 mg tablet ($)
Mirapex 0.5 mg tablet ($$)
Mirapex 1 mg tablet ($$)
Mirapex 1.5 mg tablet ($$)
No generics available.
Multiple patents that begin to expire in 2007.

DOSING AND FOOD

Doses are taken 3 times a day.
This drug may be taken with or without food but works faster if taken with food. Take with food if you get nauseated after taking your dose.
Adults: Up to 4.5 mg per day in divided doses.
Lower doses are used in people with kidney disease.
Forgotten doses: If you are scheduled to take the next dose within a few

hours, do not take the forgotten dose. Otherwise take the forgotten dose as soon as you remember.

ALCOHOL, DRUG, HERB, AND SUPPLEMENT INTERACTIONS

Alcohol should not be used while taking this drug.

Many OTC drugs used for appetite control, asthma, colds, cough, hay fever, pain, or sinus problems affect the central nervous system and may change the effects or side effects of taking this drug. Check with your pharmacist for products to avoid.

Taking this drug with any of the ones listed below may change the effect of either drug with the possibility of causing toxicity or decreasing effectiveness: butyrophenones†, cimetidine, diltiazem, metoclopramide, phenothiazines†, quinidine, quinine, ranitidine, thiothixenes†, triamterene, verapamil

ALLERGIC REACTIONS AND SIDE EFFECTS

You should tell your doctor about all your allergies and any unexplained symptoms you may have while taking this drug.

MORE COMMON SIDE EFFECTS: Constipation, dizziness*, drowsiness*, dry mouth, fainting*, hallucinations*, headache, heartburn, indigestion, light-headedness*, nausea*, sleep disorders*, spastic movements*, tiredness*, twitching*, weakness*

LESS COMMON SIDE EFFECTS: Abnormal dreams, breathing difficulty*, chest tightness*, confusion*, cough*, falling asleep*, fearfulness*, fever*, itching, joint pain*, loss of appetite, memory loss*, mood swings*, muscle pain*, restlessness*, runny nose, sexual dysfunction, shortness of breath*, skin rash, swallowing disorders*, sweating, swelling*, urinary changes*, vision changes*, weight loss, wheezing*

RARE SIDE EFFECTS: Abnormal thinking*, anxiety*, bloody urine*, chest pain*

PRECAUTIONS

If you are taking other drugs for Parkinson's disease, your doses may need to be adjusted while taking this drug.

If you have a history of mental illness or low blood pressure, this drug may make those conditions worse.

Be careful driving or handling equipment while taking this drug because it may cause drowsiness and dizziness.

Stopping this drug suddenly may cause severe side effects. If you wish to stop taking this drug, ask your doctor for specific instructions.

This drug may cause dry mouth, which is associated with a greater risk of

---

†See page 52.   *See page 53.

cavities. Your dentist may recommend that you clean your teeth and mouth differently to avoid infection.

People over age 65 are at increased risk of hallucinating while taking this drug.

PREGNANCY AND BREAST-FEEDING

Safety during pregnancy has not been established although the drug is known to harm animal fetuses.

It is not known if this drug passes into breast milk. Talk to your doctor about the risks associated with breast-feeding while taking this drug.

HELPFUL COMMENTS

Avoid quick movements to minimize dizziness. Dangling your legs over the side of the bed for a few minutes may help reduce dizziness when first waking up.

It takes about a week for the effects of this drug to be noticed.

PRAVASTATIN SODIUM

Available since October 1991

COMMONLY USED TO TREAT

High blood cholesterol and lipids, also known as hyperlipidemia

DRUG CATEGORY

antilipemic
Class: HMG-CoA reductase inhibitor (statin)

PRODUCTS

Brand-Name Products with No Generic Alternative
Pravachol 10 mg tablet ($$$)
Pravachol 20 mg tablet ($$$)
Pravachol 40 mg tablet ($$$)
Pravachol 80 mg tablet (n/a)
No generics available.
Multiple patents that begin to expire in 2005.

DOSING AND FOOD

Doses are taken once a day at bedtime.
This drug may be taken with or without food.

Adults: Up to 80 mg per day.

Children age 14 to 18: Up to 40 mg per day.

Children age 8 to 13: Up to 20 mg per day.

Forgotten doses: If you are scheduled to take the next dose within a few hours, do not take the forgotten dose. Otherwise take the forgotten dose as soon as you remember.

ALCOHOL, DRUG, HERB, AND SUPPLEMENT INTERACTIONS

Alcohol should not be used while taking this drug.

Red yeast rice, banned from sale in the U.S. since 2001, contains a nutrient similar to this class of drugs and may cause toxicity if used while taking this drug.

Taking this drug with any of the ones listed below may change the effect of either drug with the possibility of causing toxicity or decreasing effectiveness: cholestyramine, colestipol, isradipine, itraconazole

Severe reactions are possible when this drug is taken with those listed below: clofibrate, cyclosporine, fenofibrate, gemfibrozil, immunosuppressants†, niacin

Increased side effects are possible when this drug is taken with those listed below: acetaminophen, amiodarone, anabolic steroids†, androgens†, antibiotics†, antithyroid drugs†, carbamazepine, carmustine, chloroquine, dantrolene, daunorubicin, disulfiram, divalproex, etetinate, gold salts†, hydroxychloroquine, isoniazid, mercaptopurine, methotrexate, naltrexone, oral contraceptives, phenothiazines†, phenytoin, plicamycin, valproic acid

ALLERGIC REACTIONS AND SIDE EFFECTS

If you are allergic to any HMG-CoA reductase inhibitors†, you may also be allergic to this drug. You should tell your doctor about all your allergies and any unexplained symptoms you may have while taking this drug.

MORE COMMON SIDE EFFECTS: Muscle cramps*, fever*

LESS COMMON SIDE EFFECTS: Blurry vision, chest pain*, constipation, diarrhea, dizziness, gas, hair loss, headache, heartburn, itching, nausea, numbness, skin rash, sleeping difficulty, stomach pain*, tingling, tiredness*, vomiting, weakness*

RARE SIDE EFFECTS: Sexual dysfunction

PRECAUTIONS

People with liver disease may not be able to take this drug.

Liver function should be tested every 1 to 6 months while taking this drug.

---

† See page 52.   * See page 53.

PREGNANCY AND BREAST-FEEDING

This drug may cause birth defects and should not be used during pregnancy. Breast-feeding while taking this drug is not recommended.

HELPFUL COMMENTS

You need to continue with a low-cholesterol diet even after this drug is started.

PRAZOSIN HYDROCHLORIDE

Available for over 20 years

COMMONLY USED TO TREAT

Enlarged prostate, also known as benign (noncancerous) prostatic hyperplasia or BPH
High blood pressure, also known as hypertension

DRUG CATEGORY

antihypertensive
Class: alpha adrenergic blocker

PRODUCTS

Brand-Name Products with No Generic Alternative
Minipress XL 2.5 mg extended-release tablet (n/a)
Minipress XL 5 mg extended-release tablet (n/a)
Brand-Name Products with Generic Alternatives
Minipress 1 mg capsule (¢¢¢)
  Generic: prazosin hydrochloride 1 mg capsule (¢¢)
Minipress 2 mg capsule (¢¢¢¢)
  Generic: prazosin hydrochloride 2 mg capsule (¢¢)
Minipress 5 mg capsule ($)
  Generic: prazosin hydrochloride 5 mg capsule (¢¢)
Combination Products That Contain This Drug
Minizide capsule (¢¢¢¢¢) to ($)

DOSING AND FOOD

Doses are taken 1 to 3 times a day. Extended-release products are taken once a day.
This drug may be taken with or without food.
Adults: Up to 20 mg per day in divided doses.

Forgotten doses: If you are scheduled to take the next dose within a few hours, do not take the forgotten dose. Otherwise take the forgotten dose as soon as you remember.

ALCOHOL, DRUG, HERB, AND SUPPLEMENT INTERACTIONS

Alcohol may cause your blood pressure to rise, making this drug less effective. Ask your doctor about the risks caused by drinking alcohol with your condition.

The herb butcher's broom may decrease the effects of this drug and should not be used.

Several OTC drugs used for appetite control, asthma, colds, cough, hay fever, or sinus problems may cause an increase in blood pressure when taken with this drug. Check with your pharmacist when selecting OTC products.

Taking this drug with any of the ones listed below may change the effect of either drug with the possibility of causing toxicity or decreasing effectiveness: aspirin, warfarin

Severe reactions are possible when this drug is taken with those listed below: antihypertensives†, diuretics†

ALLERGIC REACTIONS AND SIDE EFFECTS

If you are allergic to doxazosin or terazosin, you may also be allergic to this drug. You should tell your doctor about all your allergies and any unexplained symptoms you may have while taking this drug.

MORE COMMON SIDE EFFECTS: Dizziness*, drowsiness, fainting*, headache, lack of energy, lightheadedness*

LESS COMMON SIDE EFFECTS: Dry mouth, irregular heartbeat*, nervousness, poor bladder control*, swelling*, tiredness, weakness

RARE SIDE EFFECTS: Chest pain*, erection pain*, nausea, shortness of breath*, urinary changes

PRECAUTIONS

Do not crush, break, or chew the extended-release products.

Be careful driving or handling equipment while taking this drug because it may cause dizziness and drowsiness.

If you have chest pain or heart disease, this drug may make those conditions worse.

Drink plenty of fluids to avoid dehydration when sweating, such as in hot weather and during exercise.

Stopping this drug suddenly may cause withdrawal symptoms, including

---

†*See page 52.*   **See page 53.*

life-threatening increases in blood pressure. If you wish to stop taking this drug, ask your doctor for specific instructions.

This drug may cause lightheadedness, dizziness, and fainting, especially with the first few doses. Taking the first dose at bedtime, starting with low doses, and increasing the dose gradually, minimizes these side effects.

PREGNANCY AND BREAST-FEEDING

Safety during pregnancy has not been established although the drug is known to harm animal fetuses.

Breast-feeding while taking this drug is not recommended.

HELPFUL COMMENTS

It may take 4 to 6 weeks for the full effects of this drug to be noticed.

Avoid quick movements to minimize dizziness. Dangling your legs over the side of the bed for a few minutes may help reduce dizziness when first waking up.

If you do not treat high blood pressure, you may develop more serious problems such as heart failure, blood vessel disease, stroke, or kidney disease. Losing weight, exercising, eating more fruits and vegetables, and avoiding salty foods, such as lunchmeat and pickles, may help make drug treatment more successful.

PREDNISOLONE

Available for over 20 years

COMMONLY USED TO TREAT

Allergic reactions
Multiple sclerosis
Severe inflammation

DRUG CATEGORY

antiinflammatory
immunosuppressant
Class: corticosteroid

PRODUCTS

Brand-Name Products with No Generic Alternative
Econopred 0.125% ophthalmic suspension ($$$$$)
Pred Mild 0.12% ophthalmic suspension ($$$$$)

Brand-Name Products with Generic Alternatives
Inflamase Mild 0.125% ophthalmic solution ($$$$$)
  Generic: prednisolone sodium phosphate 0.125% ophthalmic
  solution ($$$$$)
Inflamase Forte 1% ophthalmic solution ($$$$$)
  Generic: prednisolone sodium phosphate 1% ophthalmic
  solution ($$$$$)
Orapred 15 mg/5 ml oral solution ($$)
  Generic: prednisolone sodium phosphate 15 mg/5 ml oral
  solution (n/a)
Pediapred 5 mg/5 ml oral solution ($)
  Generic: prednisolone sodium phosphate 5 mg/5 ml oral
  solution (n/a)
Pred Forte 1% ophthalmic suspension ($$$$$)
  Generic: prednisolone acetate 1% ophthalmic suspension ($$$$$)
Prelone 5 mg/5 ml oral syrup (¢¢¢¢¢)
  Generic: prednisolone 5 mg/5 ml oral syrup (n/a)
Prelone 15 mg/5 ml oral syrup ($$)
  Generic: prednisolone 15 mg/5 ml oral syrup (n/a)

Products Only Available as Generics
prednisolone 1 mg tablet (n/a)
prednisolone 2.5 mg tablet (n/a)
prednisolone 5 mg tablet (n/a)

Combination Products That Contain This Drug
Pred-G ophthalmic ointment ($$$$$)
Pred-G ophthalmic suspension ($$$$$)
Poly-Pred ophthalmic suspension ($$$$$)
Cetapred ophthalmic ointment (n/a)
Blephamide ophthalmic ointment ($$$$$)
Blephamide ophthalmic suspension ($$$$$)
Vasocidin ophthalmic ointment ($$$)
Vasocidin ophthalmic solution ($$$$$)

DOSING AND FOOD

Doses are taken 2 to 4 times a day.
The oral form of this drug should be taken with food.
Adults: Up to 60 mg per day in divided doses.
Children: Up to 2 mg/kg per day in divided doses.
Forgotten doses: Determining when to take a forgotten dose will depend

---

on your prescription schedule. If you remember the forgotten dose within a few hours of when it was due, you may take the dose immediately and continue with your regular schedule. If you are tapering the drug to avoid withdrawal symptoms you may need to evaluate the time since the last dose and the interval between the next doses. A complete change in schedule may be needed. Talk to your doctor or pharmacist for more help.

ALCOHOL, DRUG, HERB, AND SUPPLEMENT INTERACTIONS

Alcohol may increase the risk of side effects from this drug, especially stomach problems. Ask your doctor about the risks caused by drinking alcohol with your condition.

Taking this drug with any of the ones listed below may change the effect of either drug with the possibility of causing toxicity or decreasing effectiveness: aminoglutethimide, antacids, anticoagulants†, antidiabetics†, barbiturates†, carbamazepine, cholestyramine, colestipol, diuretics†, estrogens†, griseofulvin, insulin, isoniazid, mitotane, phenylbutazone, phenytoin, primidone, rifampin, salicylates†, somatrem, somatropin

Severe reactions are possible when this drug is taken with those listed below: aspirin, amphotericin B, cardiac glycosides†, immunizations, nonsteroidal antiinflammatories†, ritodrine

ALLERGIC REACTIONS AND SIDE EFFECTS

If you are allergic to any corticosteroids†, you may also be allergic to this drug. You should tell your doctor about all your allergies and any unexplained symptoms you may have while taking this drug.

This drug may cause your eyes to be more sensitive to sunlight, but there are no special risks associated with sunburn while taking this drug.

MORE COMMON SIDE EFFECTS: Excitement*, indigestion, leg pain*, nervousness, restlessness, seizures*, sleeping difficulty*, stomach pain*, swelling*

LESS COMMON SIDE EFFECTS: Acne*, bloody stools*, bruising*, skin discoloration, dizziness, eye pain*, flushing, frequent urination*, hair growth*, headache*, hiccups, increased appetite, irregular heartbeat*, lightheadedness, menstrual problems*, muscle cramps*, nausea*, pain*, red eyes*, rounding of the face*, skin irritation*, spinning sensation, stunted growth*, sweating, tearing of eyes*, thirst*, tiredness*, vision changes*, vomiting*, weakness*, weight gain*, wounds that will not heal*

RARE SIDE EFFECTS: Confusion*, depression*, hallucinations*, hives*, mood swings*, skin rash*

PRECAUTIONS

The eye products work only on the eye and are not absorbed very well into the body. Most of the interactions and warnings in this summary do not apply.

This drug may cause severe and possibly fatal withdrawal symptoms if stopped abruptly. The drug must be stopped over 7 to 10 days by gradually decreasing the dose or time between doses. If you wish to stop taking this drug, ask your doctor for specific instructions.

This drug may cause an increase in blood sugar, increase in cholesterol level, calcium loss, or retention of fluid.

Avoid contact with anyone who has the chickenpox, measles, or other communicable disease since it may be easier to catch the infection while taking this drug.

Exposure to skin tests, immunizations, and people who have received immunizations may put you at a greater risk of developing the disease when you are taking this drug.

PREGNANCY AND BREAST-FEEDING

Safety during pregnancy has not been established although the drug is known to harm animal fetuses.

This drug passes into breast milk and may cause growth problems in the baby. The risk is related to the dose and route of the drug. Small amounts the drug are absorbed into the body from topical product.

HELPFUL COMMENTS

If you need to take an antacid, take it either 2 hours before or after taking this drug.

PREDNISONE

Available for over 20 years

COMMONLY USED TO TREAT

Allergic reactions
Severe inflammation

DRUG CATEGORY

antiinflammatory
immunosuppressant
Class: corticosteroid

---

† See page 52.   * See page 53.

Brand-Name Products with Generic Alternatives
Deltasone 2.5 mg tablet (¢)
  Generic: prednisone 2.5 mg tablet (¢)
Deltasone 5 mg tablet (¢)
  Generic: prednisone 5 mg tablet (¢)
Deltasone 10 mg tablet (¢)
  Generic: prednisone 10 mg tablet (¢)
Deltasone 20 mg tablet (¢¢)
  Generic: prednisone 20 mg tablet (¢)
Deltasone 50 mg tablet (¢¢¢)
  Generic: prednisone 50 mg tablet (¢¢¢)

Products Only Available as Generics
prednisone 1 mg tablet (¢¢)
prednisone 5 mg/5 ml oral solution ($$$$)

DOSING AND FOOD

Doses are taken 1 to 4 times a day.
It is best to take this drug with food or milk.
Adults: Up to 250 mg per day in divided doses.
Children: Up to 0.14 mg/kg per day in divided doses.
Forgotten doses: Determining when to take a forgotten dose will depend
  on your prescription schedule. If you remember the forgotten dose within a few hours of when it was due, you may take the dose immediately
  and continue with your regular schedule. If you are tapering the drug
  to avoid withdrawal symptoms you may need to evaluate the time since
  the last dose and the interval between the next doses. A complete
  change in schedule may be needed. Talk to your doctor or pharmacist
  for more help.

ALCOHOL, DRUG, HERB, AND SUPPLEMENT INTERACTIONS

Alcohol may increase the risk of side effects from this drug, especially
  stomach problems. Ask your doctor about the risks caused by drinking
  alcohol with your condition.
alfalfa sprouts, astragulus, echinacea, and licorice may interfere with the
  effects of this drug and should not be used during treatment.
**Taking this drug with any of the ones listed below may change the effect of
either drug with the possibility of causing toxicity or decreasing effectiveness:**
aminoglutethimide, antacids, anticoagulants†, antidiabetics†, barbiturates†,

carbamazepine, cholestyramine, colestipol, diuretics†, estrogens†, griseofulvin, insulin, isoniazid, mitotane, phenylbutazone, phenytoin, primidone, rifampin, salicylates†, somatrem, somatropin

Severe reactions are possible when this drug is taken with those listed below:
aspirin, amphotericin B, cardiac glycosides†, immunizations, nonsteroidal
antiinflammatories†, ritodrine

ALLERGIC REACTIONS AND SIDE EFFECTS

If you are allergic to any corticosteroids†, you may also be allergic to this
drug. You should tell your doctor about all your allergies and any unexplained symptoms you may have while taking this drug.

This drug may cause your eyes to be more sensitive to sunlight, but there
are no special risks associated with sunburn while taking this drug.

MORE COMMON SIDE EFFECTS: Excitement*, indigestion, leg pain*, nervousness, restlessness*, seizures*, sleeping difficulty*, stomach pain*, swelling*,

LESS COMMON SIDE EFFECTS: Acne*, bloody stools*, bruising*, dizziness,
eye pain*, flushing, frequent urination*, hair growth*, headache*, hiccups, increased appetite, irregular heartbeat*, lightheadedness, menstrual problems*, muscle cramps*, muscle weakness*, nausea*, open
wounds*, pain*, red eyes*, rounding of the face*, skin discoloration, skin
irritation*, spinning sensation, stunted growth*, sweating, tearing of
eyes*, thirst*, tiredness*, vision changes*, vomiting*, weakness*, weight
gain*

RARE SIDE EFFECTS: Confusion*, depression*, hallucinations*, hives*, mood
swings*, skin rash*

PRECAUTIONS

This drug may cause severe and possibly fatal withdrawal symptoms if
stopped abruptly. The drug must be stopped over 7 to10 days by gradually decreasing the dose or time between doses. If you wish to stop
taking this drug, ask your doctor for specific instructions.

This drug may cause an increase in blood sugar, increase in cholesterol
level, calcium loss, or retention of fluid.

Avoid contact with anyone who has the chickenpox, measles, or other
communicable disease since it may be easier to catch the infection while
taking this drug.

Exposure to skin tests, immunizations, and people who have received
immunizations may put you at a greater risk of developing the disease
when you are taking this drug.

---

† See page 52.   * See page 53.

PREGNANCY AND BREAST-FEEDING

Safety during pregnancy has not been established although the drug is known to harm animal fetuses.

This drug passes into breast milk and may cause growth problems in the baby. The risk is related to the dose and route of the drug. Talk to your doctor before breast-feeding.

HELPFUL COMMENTS

If you need to take an antacid, take it either 2 hours before or after taking this drug.

PRIMAQUINE PHOSPHATE

Available for over 20 years

COMMONLY USED TO TREAT

Malaria

DRUG CATEGORY

antimalarial
Class: 8-amino-quinoline

PRODUCTS

Brand-Name Products with No Generic Alternative
Primaquine 26.3 mg tablet (¢¢¢¢¢)
No generics available.
No patents, no exclusivity.

DOSING AND FOOD

Doses are taken once a day or once a week.

This drug should be taken with food to reduce the stomach upset that many people suffer.

Adults: Up to 79 mg per week.

Children age 6 to 10: Up to 1.6 mg/kg per week given as a single dose.

Forgotten doses: If you are scheduled to take the next dose within a few hours, do not take the forgotten dose. Otherwise take the forgotten dose as soon as you remember.

ALCOHOL, DRUG, HERB, AND SUPPLEMENT INTERACTIONS

Alcohol may increase some of the side effects from this drug, depending on the amount consumed. Ask your doctor about the risks caused by drinking alcohol with your condition.

Taking this drug with any of the ones listed below may change the effect of either drug with the possibility of causing toxicity or decreasing effectiveness: antacids, quinacrine

Increased side effects are possible when this drug is taken with those listed below: acetohydroxamic acid, antidiabetics†, dapsone, furazolidine, methyldopa, nitrofurantoin, procainamide, quinidine, quinine, sulfonamides†, sulfoxone, vitamin K

ALLERGIC REACTIONS AND SIDE EFFECTS

If you are allergic to iodoquinol, you may also be allergic to this drug. You should tell your doctor about all your allergies and any unexplained symptoms you may have while taking this drug.

MORE COMMON SIDE EFFECTS: Back pain*, cramps, dark urine*, fever*, leg pain*, loss of appetite*, nausea, pale skin*, stomach pain*, tiredness*, vomiting, weakness*

LESS COMMON SIDE EFFECTS: Blue skin*, breathing difficulty*, dizziness*, lightheadedness*

RARE SIDE EFFECTS: Sore throat*

PRECAUTIONS

People with glucose-6-phosphate dehydrogenase deficiency (G6PD), favism, hemolytic anemia, or NADH methemoglobin reductase deficiency are at greater risk of developing side effects while taking this drug.

Don't be alarmed if your prescription label has a different dose than the doctor prescribed. The dose of this drug is often stated in 2 different ways: 26.3 mg of primaquine phosphate is the same as 15 mg of primaquine base.

PREGNANCY AND BREAST-FEEDING

Safety during pregnancy has not been established although the drug is known to harm animal fetuses.

It is not known if this drug passes into breast milk. Talk to your doctor about the risks associated with breast-feeding while taking this drug.

---

†See page 52.   *See page 53.

HELPFUL COMMENTS

If you need to take an antacid, take it either 2 hours before or after taking this drug.

Do not stop treatment early if you start to feel better. It takes the full prescription for this drug to work completely.

PRIMIDONE HYDROCHLORIDE

Available for over 20 years

COMMONLY USED TO TREAT

Seizures

DRUG CATEGORY

anticonvulsant
Class: pyrimidinedione

PRODUCTS

Brand-Name Products with Generic Alternatives
Mysoline 50 mg tablet (¢¢¢)
  Generic: primidone 50 mg tablet (¢¢¢)
Mysoline 250 mg tablet ($)
  Generic: primidone 250 mg tablet (¢)

DOSING AND FOOD

Doses are taken 1 to 3 times a day.
This drug may be taken with or without food.
Adults and children over age 8: Up to 2,000 mg per day in divided doses.
Children under age 8: Up to 750 mg per day in divided doses.
Forgotten doses: If more than 2 hours have passed since the forgotten dose, do not take the dose. Otherwise take the forgotten dose as soon as you remember.

ALCOHOL, DRUG, HERB, AND SUPPLEMENT INTERACTIONS

Alcohol should not be used while taking this drug.
Many OTC drugs used for appetite control, asthma, colds, cough, hay fever, pain, or sinus problems affect the central nervous system and may change the effects or side effects of taking this drug. Check with your pharmacist for products to avoid.

Taking this drug with any of the ones listed below may change the effect of either drug with the possibility of causing toxicity or decreasing effectiveness: acetazolamide, anesthetics, anticoagulants, antihistamines†, anxiolytics†, barbiturates†, carbamazepine, corticosteroids†, narcotics†, oral contraceptives, phenytoin, succinimides†

Severe reactions are possible when this drug is taken with those listed below: Monoamine oxidase inhibitors†, valproic acid

ALLERGIC REACTIONS AND SIDE EFFECTS

If you are allergic to any barbiturate†, you may also be allergic to this drug. You should tell your doctor about all your allergies and any unexplained symptoms you may have while taking this drug.

MORE COMMON SIDE EFFECTS: Clumsiness*, dizziness*, unsteadiness*

LESS COMMON SIDE EFFECTS: Drowsiness, excitement*, loss of appetite, mood swings, nausea, restlessness*, sexual dysfunction, vomiting

RARE SIDE EFFECTS: Breathing difficulty*, confusion*, double vision*, eye movements*, skin rash*, tiredness*, weakness*

PRECAUTIONS

If you have hyperactivity, porphyria, kidney disease, liver disease, or lung disease, this drug may make those conditions worse.

Stopping this drug suddenly may cause severe seizure activity. If you wish to stop taking this drug, ask your doctor for specific instructions.

Be careful driving or handling equipment while taking this drug because it may cause dizziness.

You need to wait 2 weeks after stopping a monoamine oxidase inhibitor† before starting this drug.

PREGNANCY AND BREAST-FEEDING

There is evidence that this drug may harm the fetus, but the drug may be necessary to the health of the mother.

Breast-feeding while taking this drug is not recommended.

HELPFUL COMMENTS

Oral contraceptives may not work properly when taken with this drug. You need to use a barrier contraceptive, such as a condom, or other nonhormonal contraceptive to prevent pregnancy.

---

† See page 52. * See page 53.

PROBENECID

Available for over 20 years

COMMONLY USED TO TREAT

Gout

High uric acid levels with gout, also known as hyperuricemia

Infections (as co-therapy with antibiotics)

DRUG CATEGORY

uricosuric

Class: sulfonamide

PRODUCTS

Products Only Available as Generics
probenecid 500 mg tablet (¢¢)

Other Generic Product Names
Probalan

Combination Products That Contain This Drug
Col-Probenecid tablet (¢¢¢¢¢)

DOSING AND FOOD

Doses are taken 2 to 4 times a day.

This drug should be taken with food to reduce the stomach upset that many people suffer.

Adults and children over age 14: Up to 1,000 mg per day in divided doses.

Children age 2 to 14: Up to 40 mg/kg per day in divided doses.

Forgotten doses: If you are scheduled to take the next dose within a few hours, do not take the forgotten dose. Otherwise take the forgotten dose as soon as you remember.

ALCOHOL, DRUG, HERB, AND SUPPLEMENT INTERACTIONS

Alcohol should not be used while taking this drug.

Taking this drug with any of the ones listed below may change the effect of either drug with the possibility of causing toxicity or decreasing effectiveness: aminosalicylic acid, antibiotics†, aspirin, chlorpropamide, dapsone, diuretics†, heparin, indomethacin, ketoprofen, methotrexate, naproxen, nitrofurantoin, pyrazinamide, sulfonylureas†, zidovudine

Increased side effects are possible when this drug is taken with those listed below: antineoplastics†

ALLERGIC REACTIONS AND SIDE EFFECTS

You should tell your doctor about all your allergies and any unexplained symptoms you may have while taking this drug.

MORE COMMON SIDE EFFECTS: Headache, joint pain, loss of appetite, nausea, swelling*, vomiting

LESS COMMON SIDE EFFECTS: Back pain*, bloody urine*, dizziness, flushing, hives*, itching*, skin rash*, sore gums, urinary changes*

RARE SIDE EFFECTS: Bleeding*, breathing difficulty*, bruising*, chest tightness*, chills*, cloudy urine*, cough*, fever*, hoarseness*, irregular breathing*, mouth sores*, shortness of breath*, skin discoloration*, sore throat*, swelling*, tiredness*, weakness*, weight gain*, wheezing*, yellow eyes or skin*

PRECAUTIONS

This drug may cause changes to your gums and mouth. Your dentist may recommend that you clean your teeth and mouth differently to avoid infection.

If you have a history of ulcers, blood disease, cancer, or kidney stones, you may have a greater risk of developing side effects while taking this drug.

This drug is not used to stop a gout attack that has already started and is not used to relieve pain or inflammation.

Gout attacks may continue to occur for the first 6 to 12 of taking this drug.

This drug may interfere with several diagnostic tests including some urine glucose tests. Diabetics should use glucose oxidase tests or glucose enzyme test strips.

PREGNANCY AND BREAST-FEEDING

Safety during pregnancy has not been established although there was no evidence of harm during studies in animals.

Breast-feeding while taking this drug is not recommended.

HELPFUL COMMENTS

If you get a headache from this drug, take acetaminophen or a nonsteroidal antiinflammatory† for relief. Do not take aspirin.

Take an antacid if needed to relieve stomach upset after taking a dose of this drug.

It may take several months for the full effect of this drug to be noticed.

Do not stop treatment early if you start to feel better. It takes the full prescription for this drug to work completely.

You should drink 8 to 10 glasses of water each day while taking this drug.

---

† See page 52.   * See page 53.

PROCAINAMIDE HYDROCHLORIDE

Available for over 20 years

COMMONLY USED TO TREAT

Irregular heartbeat, also known as arrhythmias

DRUG CATEGORY

antiarrhythmic
Class: procaine derivative

PRODUCTS

Brand-Name Products with Generic Alternatives
Pronestyl 250 mg tablet (¢¢¢¢¢)
  Generic: procainamide hydrochloride 250 mg tablet (n/a)
Pronestyl 375 mg tablet ($)
  Generic: procainamide hydrochloride 375 mg tablet (n/a)
Pronestyl 500 mg tablet ($)
  Generic: procainamide hydrochloride 500 mg tablet (n/a)
Pronestyl 250 mg capsule (¢¢¢¢¢)
  Generic: procainamide hydrochloride 250 mg capsule (¢¢)
Pronestyl 375 mg capsule (n/a)
  Generic: procainamide hydrochloride 375 mg capsule (¢¢)
Pronestyl 500 mg capsule (n/a)
  Generic: procainamide hydrochloride 500 mg capsule (¢¢¢)
Procanbid 500 mg extended-release tablet (¢¢¢¢¢)
Pronestyl 500 mg extended-release tablet (¢¢¢¢¢)
  Generic: procainamide hydrochloride 500 mg extended-release
  tablet (¢¢¢)
Procanbid 1,000 mg extended-release tablet ($$)
  Generic: procainamide hydrochloride 1,000 mg extended-release
  tablet ($)

Products Only Available as Generics
procainamide hydrochloride 250 mg extended-release tablet (n/a)
procainamide hydrochloride 750 mg extended-release tablet (¢¢¢¢¢)

DOSING AND FOOD

Doses are taken 2 to 4 times a day.
It is best to take this drug on an empty stomach with a full glass of water either 1 hour before or 2 hours after meals.

Adults: Up to 4,000 mg per day in divided doses.

Forgotten doses: If more than 2 hours (4 hours if taking an extended-release product) have passed since the forgotten dose, do not take the dose. Otherwise take the forgotten dose as soon as you remember.

ALCOHOL, DRUG, HERB, AND SUPPLEMENT INTERACTIONS

Alcohol should not be used while taking this drug.

Jimsonweed and licorice may interfere with the effects of this drug and should not be used.

Many OTC drugs used for appetite control, asthma, colds, cough, hay fever, pain, or sinus problems may cause an increase in side effects when taken with this drug. Check with your pharmacist for products to avoid.

Taking this drug with any of the ones listed below may change the effect of either drug with the possibility of causing toxicity or decreasing effectiveness: antiarrhythmics†, antihypertensives†, cholinergics†, cimetidine, decamethonium, gallium, metocurine, neostigmine, pancuronium, pyridostigmine, succinylcholine, turbocurarine

Increased side effects are possible when this drug is taken with those listed below: anticholinergics†, atropine, diphenhydramine, pimozide, tricyclic antidepressants†

ALLERGIC REACTIONS AND SIDE EFFECTS

If you are allergic to procaine, lidocaine, or any other "caine" drug, you may also be allergic to this drug. You should tell your doctor about all your allergies and any unexplained symptoms you may have while taking this drug.

MORE COMMON SIDE EFFECTS: Diarrhea, loss of appetite

LESS COMMON SIDE EFFECTS: Breathing pains*, chills*, dizziness*, fever*, itching*, joint pain*, lightheadedness, skin rash*, swelling*

RARE SIDE EFFECTS: Bleeding*, bruising*, confusion*, depression*, drowsiness*, fainting*, hallucinations*, irregular heartbeat*, nausea*, sore mouth*, sore throat*, tiredness*, urinary changes*, vomiting*, weakness*

PRECAUTIONS

Do not crush, break, or chew the extended-release products.

If you have a history lupus erythematosus or myasthenia gravis, this drug may make those conditions worse.

People with a history of asthma are at greater risk of developing an allergic reaction to this drug.

---

† See page 52.   * See page 53.

Serious withdrawal symptoms may occur if this drug is stopped suddenly. If you wish to stop taking this drug, ask your doctor for specific instructions.

Be careful driving or handling equipment while taking this drug because it may cause dizziness.

PREGNANCY AND BREAST-FEEDING

Safety during pregnancy has not been established although the drug is known to harm animal fetuses.

Breast-feeding while taking this drug is not recommended.

HELPFUL COMMENTS

Avoid quick movements to minimize dizziness. Dangling your legs over the side of the bed for a few minutes may help reduce dizziness when first waking up.

Extended-release products are not usually prescribed until after treatment has been established over a couple of weeks.

PROCHLORPERAZINE

Available for over 20 years

COMMONLY USED TO TREAT

Anxiety
Mental illness, also known as psychosis
Nausea and vomiting

DRUG CATEGORY

antiemetic
antipsychotic
Class: phenothiazine: piperazine derivative

PRODUCTS

Brand-Name Products with No Generic Alternative
Compazine 10 mg extended-release capsule ($)
Compazine 15 mg extended-release capsule ($$)
Compazine 5 mg/5 ml oral syrup (¢¢¢¢)
Brand-Name Products with Generic Alternatives
Compazine 5 mg tablet (¢¢¢¢)
  Generic: prochlorperazine maleate 5 mg tablet (¢¢¢¢)

Compazine 10 mg tablet (¢¢¢¢¢)
  Generic: prochlorperazine maleate 10 mg tablet (¢¢¢)
Compazine 25 mg tablet (n/a)
  Generic: prochlorperazine maleate 25 mg tablet (n/a)
Compazine 2.5 mg rectal suppository ($)
  Generic: prochlorperazine 2.5 mg rectal suppository (¢¢¢¢¢)
Compazine 5 mg rectal suppositories ($)
  Generic: prochlorperazine 5 mg rectal suppository (¢¢¢¢¢)
Compazine 25 mg rectal suppositories ($)
  Generic: prochlorperazine 25 mg rectal suppository ($$)

Other Generic Product Names
Compro

DOSING AND FOOD

Doses are taken 3 to 4 times a day. Extended release products are taken 1
  to 2 times a day.
Taking this drug with food or a full glass of milk or water may avoid the
  stomach upset that some people suffer.
Adults: Up to 150 mg by mouth per day in divided doses.
Children age 6 to 12: Up to 25 mg by mouth per day in divided doses.
Children age 2 to 6: Up to 20 mg by mouth per day in divided doses.
Lower doses are used in people over age 65.
Forgotten doses: If you are scheduled to take the next dose within a few
  hours, do not take the forgotten dose. Otherwise take the forgotten dose
  as soon as you remember.

ALCOHOL, DRUG, HERB, AND SUPPLEMENT INTERACTIONS

Alcohol should not be used while taking this drug.
Do not use caffeine, kava, or yohimbe while taking this drug since the drug
  effects may be decreased and severe reactions may occur.
Several OTC drugs used for appetite control, asthma, colds, cough, hay
  fever, pain, or sinus problems may seriously increase the effects and
  side effects of this drug. Check with your pharmacist when selecting OTC
  products.
**Taking this drug with any of the ones listed below may change the effect of
either drug with the possibility of causing toxicity or decreasing effectiveness:**
antacids, antihypertensives†, beta blockers†, bromocriptine, caffeine, dopa-
  mine, levodopa, lithium, phenobarbital, phenytoin, warfarin

---

† *See page 52.*   * *See page 53.*

Severe reactions are possible when this drug is taken with those listed below: alcohol, amantadine, anesthetics, antiarrhythmics†, anticholinergics†, antidepressants†, antidyskinetics†, antihistamines†, antithyroid drugs†, anxiolytics†, astemizole, barbiturates†, bromocriptine, cisapride, deferoxamine, disopyramide, diuretics†, epinephrine, erythromycin, levobunolol, lithium, metipranolol, meperidine, metrizamide, monoamine oxidase inhibitors†, nabilone, narcotics†, nitrates†, pentamidine, phenothiazines†, probucol, procainamide, promethazine, propylthiouracil, quinidine, sympathomimetics†, tricyclic antidepresants†

Increased side effects are possible when this drug is taken with those listed below: antipsychotics†, metoclopramide, metyrosine, pemoline, pimozide, rauwolfia alkaloids†, trimeprazine

ALLERGIC REACTIONS AND SIDE EFFECTS

If you are allergic to any phenothiazines†, you may also be allergic to this drug. You should tell your doctor about all your allergies and any unexplained symptoms you may have while taking this drug.

This drug promotes the effect of sunlight on the body and may cause severe sunburn and increased sensitivity of the eyes.

MORE COMMON SIDE EFFECTS: Breathing difficulty*, chewing action*, congestion, constipation, decreased sweat, dizziness, drowsiness, dry mouth, eye stare*, eyelid movement*, fainting*, fever*, lip smacking*, loss of balance*, muscle stiffness*, puffy cheeks*, restlessness*, shuffling walk*, skin rash*, tongue movements*, trembling*, twitching*, urinary difficulty*, vision changes*, yellow eyes or skin*

LESS COMMON SIDE EFFECTS: Breast-milk secretion, breast swelling, dark urine*, menstrual changes, rough tongue, sexual dysfunction, watery mouth, weight gain

RARE SIDE EFFECTS: Abdominal pain*, aching muscles, agitation*, bleeding*, blood pressure change*, bruising*, chest pain*, chills*, clumsiness*, coma*, confusion*, diarrhea*, dreams*, drooling*, excitement*, hair loss*, headaches*, irregular heartbeat*, itching*, joint pain*, lack of sweat*, loss of bladder control*, mouth sores*, muscle stiffness*, nausea*, penile erection*, red hands*, seizures*, shivering*, skin discoloration*, sleep disorders*, sore throat*, speaking difficulty*, sweating*, tiredness*, vomiting*, weakness*

PRECAUTIONS

Do not crush, break, or chew the extended-release products.

If you have a history of enlarged prostate, glaucoma, ulcers, seizures, heart disease, urinary difficulty, or Parkinson's disease, this drug may make those conditions worse.

This drug may decrease the cough reflex, putting people with lung disease at greater risk of developing pneumonia.

Heavy smoking may cause this drug to be less effective.

Be careful driving or handling equipment while taking this drug because the drug may cause dizziness and drowsiness.

This drug may cause false results from several diagnostic tests, including pregnancy tests, and should be stopped for at least 4 days before the test.

This drug should not be stopped suddenly, due to an increased risk of side effects. If you wish to stop taking this drug, ask your doctor for specific instructions.

You are more likely to overheat when taking this drug and should avoid exercising in hot weather and using a sauna or hot tub.

This drug may make you more sensitive to cold temperatures.

Touching the liquid form of this drug may cause skin irritation. Make sure you do not spill the liquid, and wash your hands immediately after taking the dose.

This drug may cause dry mouth, which is associated with a greater risk of cavities. Your dentist may recommend that you clean your teeth and mouth differently to avoid infection.

PREGNANCY AND BREAST-FEEDING

Safety during pregnancy has not been established although the drug is known to harm animal fetuses.

Breast-feeding while taking this drug is not recommended.

HELPFUL COMMENTS

If using a suppository, remove the foil and run under cold water before inserting.

If you need to take an antacid, take it either 2 hours before or after taking this drug.

Sucking on hard sugarless candy or chewing sugarless gum may help relieve dry mouth caused by this drug.

This drug may cause the color of your urine to turn pink or brown.

---

† See page 52.   * See page 53.

PROCYCLIDINE HYDROCHLORIDE

Available for over 20 years

COMMONLY USED TO TREAT

Parkinson's disease

DRUG CATEGORY

antidyskinetic
Class: anticholinergic

PRODUCTS

Brand-Name Products with No Generic Alternative
Kemadrin 5 mg tablet (¢¢¢¢)
No generics available.
No patents, no exclusivity.

DOSING AND FOOD

Doses are taken 3 times a day.
This drug should be taken after meals to avoid stomach upset.

Adults: Up to 20 mg per day in divided doses.

Lower doses may be used in children.

Forgotten doses: If you are scheduled to take the next dose within a few
hours, do not take the forgotten dose. Otherwise take the forgotten dose
as soon as you remember.

ALCOHOL, DRUG, HERB, AND SUPPLEMENT INTERACTIONS

Alcohol should not be used while taking this drug.
Many OTC drugs used for appetite control, asthma, colds, cough, hay
fever, pain, or sinus problems affect the central nervous system and may
change the effects or side effects of taking this drug. Check with your
pharmacist for products to avoid.

Taking this drug with any of the ones listed below may change the effect of
either drug with the possibility of causing toxicity or decreasing effectiveness:
antacids, antidiarrheals†, haloperidol, phenothiazines†

Increased side effects are possible when this drug is taken with those listed below:
amantadine, anesthetics, anticholinergics†, antihistamines†, anxiolytics†,
barbiturates†, narcotics†, tricyclic antidepressants†

ALLERGIC REACTIONS AND SIDE EFFECTS

If you are allergic to other anticholinergic† drugs, you may also be allergic
  to this drug. You should tell your doctor about all your allergies and any
  unexplained symptoms you may have while taking this drug.

This drug may cause your eyes to be more sensitive to sunlight, but there
  are no special risks relating to sunburn while taking this drug.

MORE COMMON SIDE EFFECTS: Blurry vision, constipation, decreased sweating, difficulty urinating, drowsiness, dry mouth*, giddiness, nausea, sensitivity to light, vomiting

LESS COMMON SIDE EFFECTS: Dizziness, headache, lightheadedness, memory loss, muscle cramps, nervousness, numbness, sore mouth, stomachache, weakness*

RARE SIDE EFFECTS: Confusion*, eye pain*, skin rash*

PRECAUTIONS

This drug may cause withdrawal symptoms if stopped suddenly. If you
  wish to stop taking this drug, ask your doctor for specific instructions.

People with angle closure glaucoma may not be able to take this drug.

This drug may cause dry mouth, which is associated with a greater risk of
  cavities. Your dentist may recommend that you clean your teeth and
  mouth differently to avoid infection.

Be careful driving or handling equipment while taking this drug because
  the drug may cause drowsiness.

This drug makes you sweat less, putting you at greater risk of developing
  heat stroke. Avoid exercising in hot weather and using a hot tub or sauna.

PREGNANCY AND BREAST-FEEDING

Safety during pregnancy has not been established although the drug is
  known to harm animal fetuses.

Breast-feeding while taking this drug is not recommended.

HELPFUL COMMENTS

You may only need to take this drug for a couple of weeks if you are using
  it to treat side effects caused by another drug.

If you need to take an antacid, take it either 2 hours before or after taking
  this drug.

Sucking on hard sugarless candy or chewing sugarless gum may help relieve dry mouth caused by this drug.

---

†See page 52.   *See page 53.

PROGESTERONE

Available for over 20 years

COMMONLY USED TO TREAT

Abnormal uterine bleeding
Menstrual dysfunction

DRUG CATEGORY

progestational drug
Class: progestin

PRODUCTS

Brand-Name Products with No Generic Alternative
Prometrium 100 mg capsule (¢¢¢¢¢)
Prometrium 200 mg capsule ($$)
Crinone 4% vaginal gel (¢¢¢¢)
Crinone 8% vaginal gel ($$$)
No generics available.
No patents, no exclusivity.

DOSING AND FOOD

Oral doses are taken once a day in the evening.
Vaginal doses are used twice a day to once every other day.
This drug may be taken with or without food.
Adults: Up to 400 mg by mouth per day.
Forgotten doses: If you are scheduled to take the next dose within a few
hours, do not take the forgotten dose. Otherwise take the forgotten dose
as soon as you remember.

ALCOHOL, DRUG, HERB, AND SUPPLEMENT INTERACTIONS

Alcohol may increase some of the side effects from this drug, depending
on the amount consumed. Ask your doctor about the risks caused by
drinking alcohol with your condition.

**Taking this drug with any of the ones listed below may change the effect of
either drug with the possibility of causing toxicity or decreasing effectiveness:**
aminoglutethimide, bromocriptine, carbamazepine, phenobarbital, phenytoin, rifabutin, rifampin

ALLERGIC REACTIONS AND SIDE EFFECTS

If you are allergic to any progestins†, you may also be allergic to this drug.

You should tell your doctor about all your allergies and any unexplained symptoms you may have while taking this drug.

MORE COMMON SIDE EFFECTS: Abdominal pain, bloating, blood pressure increase, depression*, dizziness, dry mouth*, frequent urination*, loss of appetite*, headache*, mood swings, nervousness, swelling, thirst*, vaginal bleeding*, weight gain

LESS COMMON SIDE EFFECTS: Acne, breast-milk secretion*, breast pain, constipation, diarrhea, hair growth, hair loss, hot flashes, nausea, sexual dysfunction, skin rash*, skin spots, sleeping difficulty, vomiting

RARE SIDE EFFECTS: Arm pain*, chest pain*, leg pain*, migraine*, numbness*, poor coordination*, shortness of breath*, speaking difficulty*, vision loss*

PRECAUTIONS

If you are diabetic, you may need a change in the dose of your antidiabetic drug† or insulin, since this drug may cause a change in blood sugar.

People with a history of blood clots, stroke, or varicose veins are at greater risk of developing blood clots when taking this drug.

If you have a history of breast cysts, depression, high cholesterol, and liver disease, this drug may make those conditions worse.

This drug may cause fluid retention, which may increase the risk of side effects in people with asthma, seizures, heart disease, kidney disease, or migraine headaches.

This drug may cause changes to your gums and mouth. Your dentist may recommend that you clean your teeth and mouth differently to avoid infection.

Be careful driving or handling equipment while taking this drug because it may cause dizziness.

If using more than one vaginal drug, you must wait at least 6 hours between treatments.

PREGNANCY AND BREAST-FEEDING

This drug may cause birth defects and should not be used during pregnancy. Breast-feeding while taking this drug is not recommended.

HELPFUL COMMENTS

This drug is not always given as a contraceptive. Birth control should be used unless this drug is specifically dosed as a contraceptive.

Sucking on hard sugarless candy or chewing sugarless gum may help relieve dry mouth caused by this drug.

† See page 52.   * See page 53.

PROMETHAZINE HYDROCHLORIDE

Available for over 20 years

COMMONLY USED TO TREAT

Allergies, specifically rhinitis
Motion sickness
Nausea

DRUG CATEGORY

antiemetic
antihistamine
antivertigo
Class: phenothiazine: aliphatic derivative

PRODUCTS

Brand-Name Products with No Generic Alternative
Phenergan 12.5 mg rectal suppositories
Brand-Name Products with Generic Alternatives
Phenergan 12.5 mg tablet (¢¢¢)
  Generic: promethazine hydrochloride 12.5 mg tablet (n/a)
Phenergan 25 mg tablet (¢¢¢¢)
  Generic: promethazine hydrochloride 25 mg tablet (¢)
Phenergan 50 mg tablet (¢¢¢¢¢)
  Generic: promethazine hydrochloride 50 mg tablet (¢¢)
Phenergan 6.25 mg/5 ml oral syrup (n/a)
  Generic: promethazine hydrochloride 6.25 mg/5 ml oral syrup (¢)
Phenergan 25 mg rectal suppository ($$$$)
  Generic: promethazine hydrochloride 25 mg rectal suppository ($$$)
Phenergan 50 mg rectal suppository ($$$$$)
  Generic: promethazine hydrochloride 50 mg rectal suppository ($$$$)
Other Generic Product Names
Promethacon, Promethegan, Prometh Plain, Promethazine Plain
Combination Products That Contain This Drug
Phenergan with Dextromethorphan oral syrup (n/a)
Phenergan with Codeine oral syrup ($$$$$)
Phenergan VC with Codeine oral syrup (n/a)

DOSING AND FOOD

Doses are taken 1 to 6 times a day.

Taking this drug with food or a full glass of milk or water may avoid the stomach upset that some people suffer.

Adults: Up to 150 mg per day in divided doses.

Children age 2 and older: Up to 50 mg per day in divided doses.

Lower doses are used in people over age 65.

Forgotten doses: If you are scheduled to take the next dose within a few hours, do not take the forgotten dose. Otherwise take the forgotten dose as soon as you remember.

ALCOHOL, DRUG, HERB, AND SUPPLEMENT INTERACTIONS

Alcohol should not be used while taking this drug.

Do not use kava or yohimbe while taking this drug because of the risk of developing severe side effects and potential drug toxicity.

Several OTC drugs used for appetite control, asthma, colds, cough, hay fever, pain, or sinus problems may seriously increase the effects and side effects of this drug. Check with your pharmacist when selecting OTC products.

Taking this drug with any of the ones listed below may change the effect of either drug with the possibility of causing toxicity or decreasing effectiveness:
Levodopa

Severe reactions are possible when this drug is taken with those listed below:
alcohol, anesthetics, antihistamines†, anxiolytics†, barbiturates†, contrast media, epinephrine, maprotiline, monoamine oxidase inhibitors†, narcotics†, tricyclic antidepressants†

Increased side effects are possible when this drug is taken with those listed below:
amoxapine, antipsychotics†, methyldopa, metoclopramide, metyrosine, pemoline, pimozide, promethazine, rauwolfia alkaloids†, trimeprazine

ALLERGIC REACTIONS AND SIDE EFFECTS

If you are allergic to any phenothiazines†, you may also be allergic to this drug. You should tell your doctor about all your allergies and any unexplained symptoms you may have while taking this drug.

This drug promotes the effect of sunlight on the body and may cause severe sunburn and increased sensitivity of the eyes.

MORE COMMON SIDE EFFECTS: Drowsiness, thick mucus

LESS COMMON SIDE EFFECTS: Bleeding*, bruising*, confusion, difficulty urinating, dizziness, dry mouth, excitement, fast heartbeat, fever*, increased sweating, irritability, lightheadedness, loss of appetite, nervousness, nightmares, restlessness, ringing in ears, skin rash, sore throat*, tiredness*, vision changes, weakness*

---

†See page 52.   *See page 53.

RARE SIDE EFFECTS: Clumsiness*, flushing*, hallucinations*, muscle spasms*, seizures*, shortness of breath*, shuffling walk*, sleeping disturbances*, trembling*

PRECAUTIONS

You need to wait 2 weeks after stopping a monoamine oxidase inhibitor† before starting this drug.

If you are planning an x-ray that includes an injection into the spine, beware that there may be a reaction between the injection and this drug.

If you have a history of enlarged prostate, glaucoma, ulcers, seizures, heart disease, or urinary difficulty, this drug may make those conditions worse.

Be careful driving or handling equipment while taking this drug because the drug may cause drowsiness.

Tell your doctor if you take large doses of aspirin on a regular basis since this drug may mask the symptoms of aspirin toxicity.

This drug may cause false results from several diagnostic tests, including pregnancy tests, and should be stopped for at least 4 days before the test.

PREGNANCY AND BREAST-FEEDING

Safety during pregnancy has not been established although the drug is known to harm animal fetuses.

Breast-feeding while taking this drug is not recommended.

HELPFUL COMMENTS

If using a suppository, remove the foil and run under cold water before inserting.

Take this drug 30 to 60 minutes before travel if using for motion sickness.

Sucking on hard sugarless candy or chewing sugarless gum may help relieve dry mouth caused by this drug.

PROPAFENONE HYDROCHLORIDE

Available since November 1989

COMMONLY USED TO TREAT

Irregular heartbeat, also known as arrhythmia

DRUG CATEGORY

antiarrhythmic
Class: unclassified

PRODUCTS

Brand-Name Products with Generic Alternatives
Rythmol 150 mg tablet ($$)
  Generic: propafenone hydrochloride 150 mg tablet ($$)
Rythmol 225 mg tablet ($$$)
  Generic: propafenone hydrochloride 255 mg tablet ($$)
Rythmol 300 mg tablet ($$$)
  Generic: propafenone hydrochloride 300 mg tablet ($$$)

DOSING AND FOOD

Doses are taken 3 to 4 times a day.
This drug may be taken with or without food.
Adults: Up to 900 mg per day in divided doses.
Lower doses may be used in people with kidney or liver disease.
Forgotten doses: If more than 4 hours have passed since the forgotten
  dose, do not take the dose. Just go back to your usual schedule with the
  next dose.

ALCOHOL, DRUG, HERB, AND SUPPLEMENT INTERACTIONS

Alcohol may increase some of the side effects from this drug, depending
  on the amount consumed. Ask your doctor about the risks caused by
  drinking alcohol with your condition.
Several OTC drugs used for asthma, colds, cough, hay fever, sleep aid, or
  sinus problems may seriously affect your condition. Check with your
  pharmacist when selecting OTC products.
Taking this drug with any of the ones listed below may change the effect of
either drug with the possibility of causing toxicity or decreasing effectiveness:
  beta blockers†, cimetidine, cyclosporine, desipramine, digoxin, quinidine,
  rifampin, theophylline, warfarin
Increased side effects are possible when this drug is taken with those listed below:
  anesthetics

ALLERGIC REACTIONS AND SIDE EFFECTS

You should tell your doctor about all your allergies and any unexplained
  symptoms you may have while taking this drug.
MORE COMMON SIDE EFFECTS: Taste changes
LESS COMMON SIDE EFFECTS: Blurry vision, chest pain*, constipation, diarrhea, dizziness*, dry mouth, fainting*, headache, irregular heartbeat*,

---

†See page 52.   * See page 53.

nausea, shortness of breath*, skin rash, swelling*, tiredness, vomiting, weakness*, weight gain*

RARE SIDE EFFECTS: Chills*, fever*, joint pain*, shaking*, trembling*

PRECAUTIONS

If you have myasthenia gravis, low blood pressure, congestive heart failure, or electrolyte imbalances, this drug may make those conditions worse.

People with asthma, bronchitis, or emphysema may have more trouble breathing while taking this drug.

If you have a pacemaker, the setting may need to be adjusted while taking this drug.

This drug causes changes in your blood that put you at greater risk of getting an infection. Be careful not to cut yourself or get bruised. Tell your doctor if you develop signs of infection, such as fever or sore throat. Your dentist may recommend that you clean your teeth and mouth differently to avoid infection.

It is possible to develop new arrhythmias while taking this drug.

This drug may cause dry mouth, which is associated with a greater risk of cavities.

PREGNANCY AND BREAST-FEEDING

Safety during pregnancy has not been established although the drug is known to harm animal fetuses.

Breast-feeding while taking this drug is not recommended.

HELPFUL COMMENTS

It takes about 4 to 5 days for the full effects of this drug to be noticed.

PROPANTHELINE BROMIDE

Available for over 20 years

COMMONLY USED TO TREAT

Intestinal cramps
Irritable bowel syndrome (IBS)
Ulcers

DRUG CATEGORY

antispasmodic
Class: anticholinergic

PRODUCTS

Brand-Name Products with Generic Alternatives
Pro-Banthine 7.5 mg tablet (n/a)
  Generic: propantheline bromide 7.5 mg tablet (¢¢¢¢)
Pro-Banthine 15 mg tablet (n/a)
  Generic: propantheline bromide 15 mg tablet (¢¢¢¢)

DOSING AND FOOD

Doses are taken 3 to 6 times a day.
It is best to take this drug on an empty stomach at least 30 minutes before meals.
Adults: Up to 240 mg per day in divided doses.
Children: Up to 3 mg/kg per day in divided doses.
Lower doses are used in people over age 65.
Forgotten doses: If you are scheduled to take the next dose within a few hours, do not take the forgotten dose. Otherwise take the forgotten dose as soon as you remember.

ALCOHOL, DRUG, HERB, AND SUPPLEMENT INTERACTIONS

Alcohol may increase some of the side effects from this drug, depending on the amount consumed. Ask your doctor about the risks caused by drinking alcohol with your condition.
OTC drugs used to treat diarrhea may contain an ingredient that can interfere with the effects of this drug. Ask your pharmacist for help when selecting an OTC product.
Taking this drug with any of the ones listed below may change the effect of either drug with the possibility of causing toxicity or decreasing effectiveness: antacids, anticholinergics[†], atenolol, attapulgite, digoxin, kaolin, ketoconazole, levodopa, tricyclic antidepressants[†]
Increased side effects are possible when this drug is taken with those listed below: amantadine, antihistamines[†], antidyskinetics[†], disopyramide, glutethimide, meperidine, phenothiazines, potassium supplements, procainamide, quinidine

ALLERGIC REACTIONS AND SIDE EFFECTS

If you are allergic to any belladonna alkaloids[†], you may also be allergic to this drug. You should tell your doctor about all your allergies and any unexplained symptoms you may have while taking this drug.
This drug may cause your eyes to be more sensitive to sunlight, but there are no special risks associated with sunburn while taking this drug.

[†] See page 52.   * See page 53.

MORE COMMON SIDE EFFECTS: Blurry vision, confusion*, constipation, decreased sweating, dry mouth*, dry skin*, excitement*, irregular heartbeat*, urinary difficulty

LESS COMMON SIDE EFFECTS: Bloated feeling, decreased breast milk, drowsiness*, headache, memory loss, nausea, swallowing difficulty, tiredness*, vomiting, weakness*

RARE SIDE EFFECTS: Breathing difficulty*, clumsiness*, dizziness*, eye pain*, fainting*, fast heartbeat*, fever*, flushing*, hallucinations, hives*, irritability*, lightheadedness*, nervousness*, restlessness*, seizures*, skin rash*, slurry speech*, unsteadiness*, vision changes*

PRECAUTIONS

Be careful driving or handling equipment while taking this drug because it may cause blurry vision and sensitivity of the eyes to light.

If you have colitis, enlarged prostate, fever, glaucoma, heart disease, hernia, high blood pressure, intestinal blockage, lung disease, myasthenia gravis, or urinary difficulty, this drug may make those conditions worse.

People with hyperthyroidism or Down's syndrome may experience an increase in heart rate from this drug.

You are more likely to overheat when taking this drug and should avoid exercising in hot weather and using a sauna or hot tub.

This drug may cause dry mouth, which is associated with a greater risk of cavities. Your dentist may recommend that you clean your teeth and mouth differently to avoid infection.

PREGNANCY AND BREAST-FEEDING

Safety during pregnancy has not been established although there was no evidence of harm during studies in animals.

Breast-feeding while taking this drug is not recommended.

HELPFUL COMMENTS

If you need to take an antacid, take it either 2 hours before or after taking this drug.

Eye irritation caused by the sun may be reduced by wearing sunglasses when outside.

Sucking on hard sugarless candy or chewing sugarless gum may help relieve dry mouth caused by this drug.

You may need to drink more water to reduce the constipation that many people suffer when taking this drug.

PROPOXYPHENE

Available for over 20 years

COMMONLY USED TO TREAT

Pain

DRUG CATEGORY

analgesic
Class: narcotic analgesic/opioid

PRODUCTS

Brand-Name Products with No Generic Alternative
Darvon-N 100 mg tablet (¢¢¢¢)
Darvon-N 50 mg/5 ml oral suspension (n/a)

Brand-Name Products with Generic Alternatives
Darvon 32 mg capsule (n/a)
  Generic: propoxyphene hydrochloride 32 mg capsule (n/a)
Darvon 65 mg capsule (¢¢¢)
  Generic: propoxyphene hydrochloride 65 mg capsule (¢¢¢)

Other Generic Product Names
Dolene, Kesso-gesic

Combination Products That Contain This Drug
Darvocet-N tablet (¢¢¢) to (¢¢¢¢¢)
Darvon Compound capsule (¢¢)
Darvon Compound-65 capsule (¢¢¢)
Wygesic tablet (n/a)

DOSING*AND FOOD

Doses are taken 1 to 6 times a day.
It is best to take this drug on an empty stomach, but taking this drug with
  a little food may avoid the stomach upset that some people suffer.
Adult doses vary by product: Up to 390 mg per day in divided doses for
  Darvon and generics; up to 600 mg per day in divided doses for Darvon-
  N products.
Forgotten doses: If you are scheduled to take the next dose within a few
  hours, do not take the forgotten dose. Otherwise take the forgotten dose
  as soon as you remember.

---

† See page 52.   * See page 53.

ALCOHOL, DRUG, HERB, AND SUPPLEMENT INTERACTIONS

Alcohol should not be used while taking this drug.

Several OTC drugs used for asthma, colds, cough, hay fever, sleep aid, or sinus problems may seriously change the effects and side effects of this drug. Check with your pharmacist when selecting OTC products.

Many combination products that contain this drug also contain aspirin, which may interfere with anticoagulants†.

Taking this drug with any of the ones listed below may change the effect of either drug with the possibility of causing toxicity or decreasing effectiveness:
carbamazepine, naltrexone, rifampin

Severe reactions are possible when this drug is taken with those listed below:
anesthetics, anticholinergics†, antihistamines†, barbiturates†, benzodiazepines†, cimetidine, monoamine oxidase inhibitors†, naloxone, narcotics†, phenothiazines†, sedative-hypnotics†, skeletal muscle relaxants†, tricyclic antidepressants†

ALLERGIC REACTIONS AND SIDE EFFECTS

If you are allergic to any narcotics†, you may also be allergic to this drug. You should tell your doctor about all your allergies and any unexplained symptoms you may have while taking this drug.

MORE COMMON SIDE EFFECTS: Dizziness*, drowsiness*, irregular breathing*, nausea, vomiting

LESS COMMON SIDE EFFECTS: Blurry vision, breathing difficulty*, constipation, depression*, dry mouth, excitement*, fainting, flushing*, hallucinations*, headache, hives*, irregular heartbeat*, itching*, lightheadedness, loss of appetite, mood swings*, nervousness*, restlessness*, ringing in ears*, shortness of breath*, skin rash*, sleep disorders, spastic movements*, stomach cramps, sweating*, swelling*, tiredness, trembling*, urinary changes, vision changes, weakness*, wheezing*

RARE SIDE EFFECTS: Body aches, clammy skin*, confusion*, diarrhea, fever, goosebumps, irritability, low blood pressure*, runny nose, seizures*, shivering, small pupils*, sneezing, yawning

PRECAUTIONS

Smoking may cause this drug to be less effective.

Be careful driving or handling equipment while taking this drug because it may cause dizziness and drowsiness.

If you have a history of head injury, brain disease, emphysema, asthma, lung disease, enlarged prostate, urinary disorders, gallbladder disease, or gallstones, you may not be able to take this drug.

People with colitis, heart disease, kidney disease, liver disease, and thyroid disease are at increased risk of developing side effects.

This drug may cause withdrawal symptoms if stopped suddenly. If you wish to stop taking this drug, ask your doctor for specific instructions.

Side effects may continue to develop even after this drug is stopped.

Because this drug has a high abuse potential, your prescription quantity may be limited.

PREGNANCY AND BREAST-FEEDING

Safety during pregnancy has not been established although the drug is known to harm animal fetuses.

Breast-feeding while taking this drug is not recommended.

HELPFUL COMMENTS

If the drug does not seem to be working properly, an increase in dose may not help. Talk to your doctor about other drugs and treatment options.

Sucking on hard sugarless candy or chewing sugarless gum may help relieve dry mouth caused by this drug.

Lie down for a while after taking a dose of this drug to help reduce the nausea.

Avoid quick movements to minimize dizziness. Dangling your legs over the side of the bed for a few minutes may help reduce dizziness when first waking up.

This drug works best for treating pain when taken before the pain gets too severe.

PROPRANOLOL HYDROCHLORIDE

Available for over 20 years

COMMONLY USED TO TREAT

Chest pain, also known as angina

High blood pressure, also known as hypertension

Irregular heart rhythm, also known as arrhythmia

People at risk of developing complications after a heart attack

People at risk of developing vascular headaches, also known as migraines

---

†See page 52.　　*See page 53.

DRUG CATEGORY

antianginal
antiarrhythmic
antihypertensive
Class: beta blocker

PRODUCTS

Brand-Name Products with No Generic Alternative
Inderal LA 60 mg extended-release capsule ($)
Inderal LA 80 mg extended-release capsule ($)
Inderal LA 120 mg extended-release capsule ($$)
Inderal LA 160 mg extended-release capsule ($$)

Brand-Name Products with Generic Alternatives
Inderal 10 mg tablet (¢¢¢)
  Generic: propranolol hydrochloride 10 mg tablet (¢)
Inderal 20 mg tablet (¢¢¢)
  Generic: propranolol hydrochloride20 mg tablet (¢)
Inderal 40 mg tablet (¢¢¢¢¢)
  Generic: propranolol hydrochloride 40 mg tablet (¢)
Inderal 60 mg tablet ($)
  Generic: propranolol hydrochloride 60 mg tablet (¢)
Inderal 80 mg tablet ($)
  Generic: propranolol hydrochloride 80 mg tablet (¢)

Products Only Available as Generics
propranolol hydrochloride 90 mg tablet (n/a)
propranolol hydrochloride 20 mg/5 ml oral solution (¢¢¢)
propranolol hydrochloride 40 mg/5 ml oral solution (¢¢¢)
propranolol hydrochloride Intensol 80 mg/5 ml oral concentrate ($$$$)

Combination Products That Contain This Drug
Inderide tablet ($) to ($$)

DOSING AND FOOD

Doses are taken 1 to 4 times a day.
Taking this drug with food will help increase absorption of the drug.
Adults: Up to 640 mg per day in divided doses.
Children: Up to 16 mg/kg per day in divided doses.
Lower doses are used in people with renal disease, liver disease, and heart failure.

Forgotten doses: If you are taking an extended-release product and are scheduled to take the next dose within 8 hours, do not take the forgotten dose. Otherwise take the forgotten dose as soon as you remember. If you are taking the regular-release products and are scheduled to take the next dose within 4 hours, do not take the forgotten dose. Otherwise take the forgotten dose as soon as you remember.

ALCOHOL, DRUG, HERB, AND SUPPLEMENT INTERACTIONS

Alcohol may increase some of the side effects from this drug, depending on the amount consumed. Ask your doctor about the risks caused by drinking alcohol with your condition.

Several OTC drugs used for appetite control, asthma, colds, cough, hay fever, or sinus problems may cause an increase in blood pressure when taken with this drug. Check with your pharmacist when selecting OTC products.

The herb betel palm should not be used while taking this drug.

Taking this drug with any of the ones listed below may change the effect of either drug with the possibility of causing toxicity or decreasing effectiveness: aminophylline, antacids, anesthetics†, anticholinergics†, antidiabetics†, atropine, caffeine, calcium channel blockers†, carbonic anhydrase inhibitors†, cimetidine, clonidine, dyphylline, epinephrine, guanabenz, insulin, lidocaine, nonsteroidal antiinflammatories†, oxtriphylline, phenytoin, pilocarpine, reserpine, rifampin, theophylline, tricyclic antidepressants†, turbocurarine

Severe reactions are possible when this drug is taken with those listed below: allergy shots, beta blockers†, cocaine, monoamine oxidase inhibitors†

Increased effects or side effects are possible when this drug is taken with those listed below: antihypertensives†

ALLERGIC REACTIONS AND SIDE EFFECTS

If you are allergic to any other beta blockers†, you may also be allergic to this drug.

This drug may exaggerate the reaction from your current allergies. Inform your doctor of any allergies that you have as well as the severity of the allergic reaction before starting this drug.

MORE COMMON SIDE EFFECTS: Dizziness, drowsiness, lightheadedness*, sexual dysfunction, sleeping difficulty, tiredness, weakness

LESS COMMON SIDE EFFECTS: Anxiety, breathing difficulty*, cold hands

---

†*See page 52.*   **See page 53.*

and feet*, constipation, depression*, diarrhea, irregular heartbeat*, itching, nausea, nervousness, numbness, shortness of breath*, sore eyes, stomachache, stuffy nose, swelling*, tingling, vivid dreams, vomiting, wheezing

RARE SIDE EFFECTS: Back pain*, bleeding*, bruising*, chest pain*, confusion*, dizziness*, fever*, hallucinations*, joint pain*, rash*, scaly skin*, sore throat*

PRECAUTIONS

People with asthma, heart disease, or a heart rate that is routinely less than 60 beats per minute (bradycardia), may not be able to take this drug.

Stopping this drug suddenly may cause chest pain or heart attack. If you wish to stop taking this drug, ask your doctor for specific instructions.

Be careful driving or handling equipment while taking this drug because the drug may cause dizziness and drowsiness.

You need to wait 2 weeks after stopping a monoamine oxidase inhibitor† before starting this drug.

If you are diabetic, this drug may increase blood sugar levels or make the symptoms of low blood sugar less noticeable.

This drug may cause nondiabetics to develop type 2 diabetes.

If you have psoriasis or myasthenia gravis, this drug may make those conditions worse.

Do not crush, open, break, or chew the extended-release products.

PREGNANCY AND BREAST-FEEDING

Safety during pregnancy has not been established although the drug is known to harm animal fetuses.

Breast-feeding while taking this drug is not recommended.

HELPFUL COMMENTS

This drug may make you more sensitive to cold temperatures.

If you do not treat high blood pressure, you may develop more serious problems such as heart failure, blood vessel disease, stroke, or kidney disease. Losing weight, exercising, eating more fruits and vegetables, and avoiding salty foods, such as lunchmeat and pickles, may help make drug treatment more successful.

PROPYLTHIOURACIL

Available for over 20 years

COMMONLY USED TO TREAT

High thyroid levels, also known as hyperthyroidism

DRUG CATEGORY

antithyroid drug
Class: thyroid hormone antagonist

PRODUCTS

Products Only Available as Generics
propylthiouracil 50 mg tablet (¢)

DOSING AND FOOD

Doses are taken 1 to 4 times a day.
This drug should be taken with food to reduce the stomach upset that many people suffer. Do not eat raw oysters or other raw shellfish at any time while taking this drug.

Adults: Up to 1,200 mg per day in divided doses.

Children over age 10: Up to 300 mg per day in divided doses.

Children age 6 to 10: Up to 150 mg per day in divided doses.

Infants: Up to 10 mg/kg per day in divided doses.

Forgotten doses: Take the forgotten dose as soon as you remember even if it is time for the next dose.

ALCOHOL, DRUG, HERB, AND SUPPLEMENT INTERACTIONS

Alcohol may increase the risk of liver damage from this drug. Ask your doctor about the risks caused by drinking alcohol with your condition.
OTC drugs that contain iodine should not be used while taking this drug. Ask your pharmacist for assistance when selecting OTC products.

Taking this drug with any of the ones listed below may change the effect of either drug with the possibility of causing toxicity or decreasing effectiveness:
amiodarone, beta blocker†, corticosteroids†, corticotropin, digitoxin, digoxin, iodinated glycerol, lithium, potassium iodide

Severe reactions are possible when this drug is taken with those listed below:
anticoagulants†

---

† See page 52.   * See page 53.

Increased side effects are possible when this drug is taken with those listed below: acetaminophen, anabolic steroids†, androgens†, antibiotics†, antithyroid drugs†, carbamazepine, carmustine, chloroquine, dantrolene, daunorubicin, disulfiram, divalproex, etetinate, gold salts†, hydroxychloroquine, isoniazid, mercaptopurine, methotrexate, naltrexone, phenothiazines†, phenytoin, plicamycin, valproic acid

ALLERGIC REACTIONS AND SIDE EFFECTS

If you are allergic to methimazole, you may also be allergic to this drug. You should tell your doctor about all your allergies and any unexplained symptoms you may have while taking this drug.

MORE COMMON SIDE EFFECTS: Fever*, itching*, skin rash*

LESS COMMON SIDE EFFECTS: Chills*, cough*, dizziness, hoarseness*, joint pain*, loss of taste, mouth sores*, nausea, sore throat*, stomach pain, swelling*, vomiting, weakness*

RARE SIDE EFFECTS: Backache*, black stools*, bleeding*, bloody urine*, bruising*, coldness*, constipation*, headache*, menstrual changes*, muscle aches*, numbness*, puffy skin*, shortness of breath*, skin irritation*, sleepiness*, swollen glands*, tingling*, tiredness*, urinary changes*, weight gain*, yellow eyes or skin*

PRECAUTIONS

People with liver disease may not be able to take this drug.

This drug causes changes in your blood that put you at greater risk of getting an infection. Be careful not to cut yourself or get bruised. Tell your doctor if you develop signs of infection, such as fever or sore throat. Your dentist may recommend that you clean your teeth and mouth differently to avoid infection.

PREGNANCY AND BREAST-FEEDING

There is evidence that this drug may harm the fetus, but the drug may be necessary to the health of the mother.

Breast-feeding while taking this drug is not recommended.

HELPFUL COMMENTS

This drug is also called by the generic name PTU.

It may take several months for the full effects of this drug to be noticed.

This drug is most effective when taken in equally spaced intervals. For example, if taken 3 times a day, the dose should be scheduled for every 8 hours.

PROTRIPTYLINE HYDROCHLORIDE

Available since August 1995

COMMONLY USED TO TREAT

Depression

DRUG CATEGORY

anticataplectic
antidepressant
Class: tricyclic antidepressant

PRODUCTS

Brand-Name Products with No Generic Alternative
Vivactil 5 mg tablet (¢¢¢¢¢)
Vivactil 10 mg tablet ($)
No generics available.
No patents, no exclusivity.

DOSING AND FOOD

Doses are taken 3 to 4 times a day.
Taking this drug with food or milk may avoid the stomach upset that some people suffer.
Adults: Up to 60 mg per day in divided doses.
Lower doses are used in teens and adults over age 65.
Forgotten doses: If you are scheduled to take the next dose within a few hours, do not take the forgotten dose. Otherwise take the forgotten dose as soon as you remember.

ALCOHOL, DRUG, HERB, AND SUPPLEMENT INTERACTIONS

Alcohol should not be used while taking this drug.
Evening primrose oil, SAMe, St. John's wort, and yohimbe may cause serious reactions when taken with this drug. Tell your doctor if you are taking any of these supplements.
Several OTC drugs used for asthma, colds, cough, hay fever, sleep aid, or sinus problems may seriously change the effects and side effects of this drug. Check with your pharmacist when selecting OTC products.

Taking this drug with any of the ones listed below may change the effect of either drug with the possibility of causing toxicity or decreasing effectiveness:
anesthetics, antipsychotics†, anxiolytics†, barbiturates†, beta blockers†,

---

† See page 52.   * See page 53.

cimetidine, clonidine, fluoxetine, guanabenz, guanadrel, guanethidine, haloperidol, methyldopa, methylphenidate, narcotics†, oral contraceptives, phenothiazines†, propoxyphene, reserpine

Severe reactions are possible when this drug is taken with those listed below: amphetamines†, anticholinergics†, antidyskinetics†, antihistamines†, antithyroid drugs†, appetite suppressants†, disopyramide, disulfiram, ephedrine, epinephrine, ethchlorvynol, isoproterenol, meperidine, metrizamide, monoamine oxidase inhibitors†, phenylephrine, pimozide, procainamide, quinidine, tramadol, warfarin

Increased side effects are possible when this drug is taken with those listed below: alseroxylon, deserpidine, metoclopramide, metyrosine, pemoline, pimozide, promethazine, rauwolfia serpentine, reserpine, trimeprazine

ALLERGIC REACTIONS AND SIDE EFFECTS

If you are allergic to carbamazepine, maprotiline, trazodone, or any tricyclic antidepressants†, you may also be allergic to this drug. You should tell your doctor about all your allergies and any unexplained symptoms you may have while taking this drug.

This drug promotes the effect of sunlight on the body and may cause severe sunburn and increased sensitivity of the eyes.

MORE COMMON SIDE EFFECTS: Blurry vision*, constipation*, dizziness, drowsiness, dry mouth, headache, increased appetite, irregular heartbeat*, nausea, seizures*, sweating, taste changes, tiredness, urinary changes, weakness*, weight gain

LESS COMMON SIDE EFFECTS: Confusion*, diarrhea, expressionless face*, eye pain*, fainting*, hallucinations*, heartburn, loss of balance*, nervousness*, restlessness*, shakiness*, shuffling walk*, sleeping difficulty, slowed movements*, stiffness*, swallowing difficulty*, trembling*, urinary changes*, vomiting

RARE SIDE EFFECTS: Anxiety*, breast enlargement*, hair loss, irritability*, muscle twitching*, ringing in ears*, skin rash*, sore throat*, fever*, swelling*, teeth or gum problems*, yellow eyes or skin*

PRECAUTIONS

You need to wait 2 weeks after stopping a monoamine oxidase inhibitor† before starting this drug.

Diabetics should check their blood sugar frequently while taking this drug since changes in blood sugar may occur.

Be careful driving or handling equipment while taking this drug because it may cause drowsiness and dizziness.

Stopping this drug abruptly may result in withdrawal symptoms that include nausea, headache, and general discomfort.

If you have a history of asthma, blood disorders, seizures, enlarged prostate, glaucoma, heart disease, high blood pressure, urinary difficulty, schizophrenia, or manic depression, this drug may make those conditions worse.

This drug may cause dry mouth, which is associated with a greater risk of cavities. Your dentist may recommend that you clean your teeth and mouth differently to avoid infection.

PREGNANCY AND BREAST-FEEDING

Safety during pregnancy has not been established although the drug is known to harm animal fetuses.

Breast-feeding while taking this drug is not recommended.

HELPFUL COMMENTS

Heavy smoking may decrease the effectiveness of this drug.

It takes about one week before the effects of this drug are noticed.

Sucking on hard sugarless candy or chewing sugarless gum may help relieve dry mouth caused by this drug.

PYRAZINAMIDE

Available for over 20 years

COMMONLY USED TO TREAT

Tuberculosis

DRUG CATEGORY

antibiotic
Class: antimycobacterial

PRODUCTS

Products Only Available as Generics
pyrazinamide 500 mg tablet (¢¢¢¢¢)
Combination Products That Contain This Drug
Rifater tablet ($$)

DOSING AND FOOD

Doses are taken anywhere from twice a day to twice a week.

---

† See page 52.   * See page 53.

This drug may be taken with or without food but is best taken with food to reduce the stomach upset that some people suffer.

Adults: Up to 2,000 mg per day in divided doses.

Lower doses are used in people with kidney disease.

Forgotten doses: If you are scheduled to take the next dose within a few hours, do not take the forgotten dose. Otherwise take the forgotten dose as soon as you remember.

ALCOHOL, DRUG, HERB, AND SUPPLEMENT INTERACTIONS

Alcohol may increase some of the side effects from this drug, depending on the amount consumed. Ask your doctor about the risks caused by drinking alcohol with your condition.

Severe reactions are possible when this drug is taken with those listed below: rifampin

ALLERGIC REACTIONS AND SIDE EFFECTS

If you are allergic to ethionamide, isoniazid, or niacin, you may also be allergic to this drug. You should tell your doctor about all your allergies and any unexplained symptoms you may have while taking this drug.

This drug promotes the effect of sunlight on the body and may cause severe sunburn and increased sensitivity of the eyes.

MORE COMMON SIDE EFFECTS: Joint pain*

RARE SIDE EFFECTS: Itching, loss of appetite*, skin rash, tiredness*, weakness*, yellow eyes or skin*

PRECAUTIONS

If you have gout, this drug may make that condition worse.

This drug may cause false results from several diagnostic urine tests.

If you are diabetic, you may need to have the dose of your antidiabetic drug† or insulin adjusted while taking this drug.

PREGNANCY AND BREAST-FEEDING

Safety during pregnancy has not been established although the drug is known to harm animal fetuses.

Breast-feeding while taking this drug is not recommended.

HELPFUL COMMENTS

Contact your doctor if your symptoms do not improve after a couple of weeks.

Do not stop treatment early if you start to feel better. It takes the full prescription for this drug to work completely.

PYRIMETHAMINE

Available for over 20 years

COMMONLY USED TO TREAT

Malaria
Toxoplasmosis

DRUG CATEGORY

antimalarial
Class: folic acid antagonist

PRODUCTS

Brand-Name Products with No Generic Alternative
Daraprim 25 mg tablet (¢¢¢¢)
No generics available.
No patents, no exclusivity.
Combination Products That Contain This Drug
Fansidar tablet ($$$)

DOSING AND FOOD

Doses are taken once a week.
This drug may be taken with or without food but is best taken with food to reduce the stomach upset that some people suffer. Do not eat raw oysters or other raw shellfish at any time while taking this drug.

Adults and children over age 10: Up to 25 mg per week.

Children age 4 to 10: Up to 12.5 mg per week.

Children under age 4: Up to 6.25 mg per week.

Forgotten doses: If you are scheduled to take the next dose within a few hours, do not take the forgotten dose. Otherwise take the forgotten dose as soon as you remember.

ALCOHOL, DRUG, HERB, AND SUPPLEMENT INTERACTIONS

Alcohol may increase some of the side effects from this drug, depending on the amount consumed. Ask your doctor about the risks caused by drinking alcohol with your condition.

Taking this drug with any of the ones listed below may change the effect of either drug with the possibility of causing toxicity or decreasing effectiveness: co-trimoxazole, folic acid, para-aminobenzoic acid, sulfonamides†

---

† See page 52.   * See page 53.

Severe reactions are possible when this drug is taken with those listed below:
lorazepam

Increased side effects are possible when this drug is taken with those listed below:
amphotericin B, antineoplastics†, antithyroid drugs†, azathioprine, chloramphenicol, colchicine, cyclophosphamide, flucytosine, ganciclovir, interferon, mercaptopurine, methotrexate, plicamycin, zidovudine

ALLERGIC REACTIONS AND SIDE EFFECTS

You should tell your doctor about all your allergies and any unexplained symptoms you may have while taking this drug.

LESS COMMON SIDE EFFECTS: Back pain*, black stools*, bleeding*, bloody urine*, bruising*, chills*, cough*, diarrhea, fever*, hoarseness*, loss of appetite, nausea, skin irritation*, tongue irritation*, urinary changes*, vomiting*

RARE SIDE EFFECTS: Abdominal pain*, chest pain*, excitability*, lip sores*, mouth sores*, muscle pain*, redness, seizures*, skin rash*, sore throat*, tiredness*, weakness*

PRECAUTIONS

If you have anemia or other blood disorder, this drug may make the condition worse.

People with a history of seizures are at greater risk of developing a seizure while taking this drug.

This drug causes changes in your blood that put you at greater risk of getting an infection. Be careful not to cut yourself or get bruised. Tell your doctor if you develop signs of infection, such as fever or sore throat. Your dentist may recommend that you clean your teeth and mouth differently to avoid infection.

This drug may cause your body to lose folate, a vitamin that your doctor must prescribe if you develop symptoms.

Newer drugs are available that have made this drug a second choice for the treatment of malaria.

PREGNANCY AND BREAST-FEEDING

Safety during pregnancy has not been established although the drug is known to harm animal fetuses.

Breast-feeding while taking this drug is not recommended.

HELPFUL COMMENTS

Contact your doctor if your symptoms do not improve after a couple of days.

Do not stop treatment early if you start to feel better. It takes the full prescription for this drug to work completely.

Oral contraceptives may not work properly when taken with this drug. You need to use a barrier contraceptive, such as a condom, or other nonhormonal contraceptive to prevent pregnancy.

QUAZEPAM

Available since December 1985

COMMONLY USED TO TREAT

Sleeping difficulty, also known as insomnia

DRUG CATEGORY

sedative-hypnotic
Class: benzodiazepine

PRODUCTS

Brand-Name Products with No Generic Alternative
Doral 7.5 mg tablet ($$)
Doral 15 mg tablet ($$$)
No generics available.
No patents, no exclusivity.

DOSING AND FOOD

Doses are taken once a day.
This drug may be taken with or without food.
Adults: Up to 15 mg per day.

ALCOHOL, DRUG, HERB, AND SUPPLEMENT INTERACTIONS

Alcohol should not be used while taking this drug.

Catnip, kava, lady's slipper, lemon balm, passion flower, sassafras, skullcap, and valerian should not be used while taking this drug due to an increased sedative effect.

Taking this drug with any of the ones listed below may change the effect of either drug with the possibility of causing toxicity or decreasing effectiveness: cimetidine, disulfiram, fluvoxamine, itraconazole, ketoconazole, nefazodone

Severe reactions are possible when this drug is taken with those listed below: anesthetics†, antidepressants†, antihistamines†, barbiturates†, monoamine oxidase inhibitors†, narcotics†, phenothiazines†

---

†See page 52.   *See page 53.

Increased side effects are possible when this drug is taken with those listed below: aminophylline, theophylline

ALLERGIC REACTIONS AND SIDE EFFECTS

If you are allergic to any benzodiazepines†, you may also be allergic to this drug. You should tell your doctor about all your allergies and any unexplained symptoms you may have while taking this drug.

MORE COMMON SIDE EFFECTS: Clumsiness, dizziness, drowsiness, lightheadedness, slurry speech

LESS COMMON SIDE EFFECTS: Anxiety*, confusion*, constipation, depression*, diarrhea, difficulty urinating, dry mouth, headache, irregular heartbeat*, memory loss*, muscle spasm, nausea, sexual dysfunction, stomach cramps, thirst, trembling, vision changes, vomiting, watery mouth

RARE SIDE EFFECTS: Agitation*, behavior changes*, bleeding*, bruising*, chills*, delusions*, disorientation*, excitement*, eye movement*, fever*, hallucinations*, irritability*, low blood pressure*, mouth sores*, muscle weakness*, nervousness*, seizures*, skin irritation*, sleeping difficulty*, sore throat*, spastic movements*, tiredness*, weakness*, yellow eyes or skin*

PRECAUTIONS

This drug may be habit forming and will cause severe withdrawal symptoms if stopped abruptly. If you wish to stop this drug, ask your doctor for specific instructions.

You need to wait 2 weeks after stopping a monoamine oxidase inhibitor† before starting this drug.

If you have difficulty swallowing, emphysema, asthma, bronchitis, glaucoma, hyperactivity, mental depression, mental illness, myasthenia gravis, porphyria, or sleep apnea, this drug may make those conditions worse.

Heavy smoking may cause this drug to be less effective.

Be careful driving or handling equipment while taking this drug because the drug may cause dizziness and drowsiness.

PREGNANCY AND BREAST-FEEDING

There is evidence that this drug may harm the fetus, but the drug may be necessary to the health of the mother.

Breast-feeding while taking this drug is not recommended.

HELPFUL COMMENTS

Dangling your legs over the side of the bed for a few minutes may help reduce dizziness when first waking up.

QUETIAPINE FUMARATE

Available since September 1997

COMMONLY USED TO TREAT

Mental disturbances, also known as psychosis

DRUG CATEGORY

sedative-hypnotic
Class: benzothiazepine

PRODUCTS

Brand-Name Products with No Generic Alternative
Seroquel 25 mg tablet ($)
Seroquel 100 mg tablet ($$$)
Seroquel 150 mg tablet (n/a)
Seroquel 200 mg tablet ($$$$)
Seroquel 300 mg tablet ($$$$)
No generics available.
Patent expires in 2011.

DOSING AND FOOD

Doses are taken 2 to 3 times a day.
It is best to take this drug on an empty stomach.
Adults: Up to 800 mg per day in divided doses.
Lower doses are used in people with liver disease and people over age 65.
Forgotten doses: If you are scheduled to take the next dose within a few
   hours, do not take the forgotten dose. Otherwise take the forgotten dose
   as soon as you remember.

ALCOHOL, DRUG, HERB, AND SUPPLEMENT INTERACTIONS

Alcohol should not be used while taking this drug.
Many OTC drugs used for appetite control, asthma, colds, cough, hay
   fever, pain, or sinus problems affect the central nervous system and may
   result in an increase in effects or side effects when taken with this drug.
   Check with your pharmacist for products to avoid.

Taking this drug with any of the ones listed below may change the effect of
either drug with the possibility of causing toxicity or decreasing effectiveness:
   antihypertensives†, carbamazepine, cimetidine, clarithromycin, diltiazem,
   erythromycin, fluconazole, griseofulvin, itraconazole, levodopa, lorazepam,

†See page 52.   *See page 53.

nefazodone, phenylbutazone, phenytoin, primidone, rifampin, saquinavir, thioridazine, toconazole, troglitazone, verapamil

Severe reactions are possible when this drug is taken with those listed below: alcohol, anesthetics, antihistamines†, anxiolytics†, barbiturates†, narcotics†

ALLERGIC REACTIONS AND SIDE EFFECTS

You should tell your doctor about all your allergies and any unexplained symptoms you may have while taking this drug.

MORE COMMON SIDE EFFECTS: Constipation, drowsiness*, dry mouth, indigestion, weight gain*

LESS COMMON SIDE EFFECTS: Abdominal pain, aching muscles*, chills*, decrease in appetite, dizziness*, expressionless face*, ear pain, fainting*, headache, irregular heartbeat*, lack of energy, lightheadedness*, poor balance*, runny nose, shaky hands*, shuffling walk*, skin rash*, sore throat*, sweating*, swelling*, trembling*, vision changes

RARE SIDE EFFECTS: Blood pressure changes*, breast-milk secretion*, dry skin*, fever*, loss of appetite*, menstrual changes*, pale skin*, poor bladder control*, seizures*, stiffness*, tiredness*, weakness*

PRECAUTIONS

If you have breast cancer, heart disease, stroke, or hypothyroidism, this drug may make those conditions worse.

People with a history of seizures or with Alzheimer's disease are at greater risk of developing a seizure while taking this drug.

Drink plenty of fluids to avoid dehydration when sweating, such as in hot weather and during exercise.

Be careful driving or handling equipment while taking this drug because the drug may cause drowsiness.

This drug may cause your body to lose thyroid hormones. Your doctor will need to check thyroid levels regularly, and some people taking this drug may need to start taking thyroid replacement hormones.

This drug may cause dry mouth, which is associated with a greater risk of cavities. Your dentist may recommend that you clean your teeth and mouth differently to avoid infection.

Your eyes should be checked for cataracts every 6 months while taking this drug.

PREGNANCY AND BREAST-FEEDING

Safety during pregnancy has not been established although the drug is known to harm animal fetuses.

Breast-feeding while taking this drug is not recommended.

HELPFUL COMMENTS

Avoid quick movements to minimize dizziness. Dangling your legs over the side of the bed for a few minutes may help reduce dizziness when first waking up.

Lower doses cause fewer side effects.

QUINAPRIL HYDROCHLORIDE

Available since December 1999

COMMONLY USED TO TREAT

Heart failure
High blood pressure, also known as hypertension

DRUG CATEGORY

antihypertensive
Class: ACE inhibitor

PRODUCTS

Brand-Name Products with No Generic Alternative
Accupril 5 mg tablet ($)
Accupril 10 mg tablet ($)
Accupril 20 mg tablet ($)
Accupril 40 mg tablet ($)
No generics available.
Multiple patents that began to expire in 2002.
Combination Products That Contain This Drug
Accuretic tablet ($)

DOSING AND FOOD

Doses are taken 1 to 2 times a day.
It is best to take this drug on an empty stomach.
Adults: Up to 80 mg per day in divided doses.
Lower doses are used in people with kidney disease.
This drug is rarely used in children.
Forgotten doses: If you are scheduled to take the next dose within a few hours, do not take the forgotten dose. Otherwise take the forgotten dose as soon as you remember.

---

† See page 52.   * See page 53.

ALCOHOL, DRUG, HERB, AND SUPPLEMENT INTERACTIONS

Alcohol may cause your blood pressure to rise, making this drug less effective. Ask your doctor about the risks caused by drinking alcohol with your condition. .

Licorice may interfere with the effects of this drug.

Capsaicin and other foods or supplements, including hot peppers, sweet peppers, paprika, and chili powder, derived from the capsicum family of plants may increase the risk of developing a cough and should not be taken with this drug.

Several OTC drugs used for appetite control, asthma, colds, cough, hay fever, or sinus problems may cause an increase in blood pressure when taken with this drug. Check with your pharmacist when selecting OTC products.

Taking this drug with any of the ones listed below may change the effect of either drug with the possibility of causing toxicity or decreasing effectiveness: antidiabetics†, antihypertensives†, diuretics†, insulin, lithium, potassium supplements, tetracycline

ALLERGIC REACTIONS AND SIDE EFFECTS

If you are allergic to any ACE inhibitors†, you may also be allergic to this drug. You should tell your doctor about all your allergies and any unexplained symptoms you may have while taking this drug.

MORE COMMON SIDE EFFECTS: Breathing difficulty*, dry cough, headache, skin rash*, swallowing difficulty*, swelling*

LESS COMMON SIDE EFFECTS: Diarrhea, dizziness*, fainting*, fever*, joint pain*, lightheadedness*, loss of taste, nausea, tiredness

RARE SIDE EFFECTS: Abdominal pain*, chest pain*, chills*, confusion*, hoarseness*, irregular heartbeat*, itching*, nausea*, nervousness*, numbness*, stomach pain*, vomiting*, weakness*, yellow eyes or skin*

PRECAUTIONS

Be careful driving or handling equipment while taking this drug because the drug may cause dizziness.

People with systemic lupus erythematosus may be at greater risk of developing blood problems while taking this drug.

Do not use potassium-containing products, including salt substitutes, while taking this drug.

Diuretics† should be stopped 2 to 3 days prior to starting this drug. If it is not possible to stop the diuretic, the dose of this drug should be lowered.

Drink plenty of fluids to avoid dehydration when sweating, such as in hot weather and during exercise.

PREGNANCY AND BREAST-FEEDING

Safety during pregnancy has not been established although the drug is known to harm animal fetuses.

Breast-feeding while taking this drug is not recommended.

HELPFUL COMMENTS

A persistent dry cough may appear while taking this drug, but it will go away when the drug is stopped.

Avoid quick movements to minimize dizziness. Dangling your legs over the side of the bed for a few minutes may help reduce dizziness when first waking up.

QUINIDINE SULFATE

Available for over 20 years

COMMONLY USED TO TREAT

Irregular heartbeat, also known as arrhythmias
Malaria

DRUG CATEGORY

antiarrhythmic
Class: cinchona alkaloid

PRODUCTS

Brand-Name Products with Generic Alternatives
Quinidex 300 mg extended-release tablet§ ($)
  Generic: quinidine sulfate 300 mg extended-release tablet§ (¢¢¢¢¢)
Products Only Available as Generics
quinidine sulfate 100 mg tablet (n/a)
quinidine sulfate 200 mg tablet (¢¢)
quinidine sulfate 300 mg tablet (¢¢¢)
quinidine gluconate 324 mg extended-release tablet§ (¢¢¢¢)

DOSING AND FOOD

Doses are taken 3 to 5 times a day. Extended-release tablets are taken 2 to 3 times a day.

---

†See page 52.   *See page 53.   § See "Precautions" in this entry.

This drug should be taken with food to reduce the stomach upset that many people suffer. Do not drink grapefruit juice while taking this drug.

Adults: Up to 1,800 mg per day in divided doses.

Children: Up to 30 mg/kg per day in divided doses.

Lower doses are used in people with heart failure or liver disease.

Forgotten doses: If more than 2 hours have passed since the forgotten dose, do not take the dose. Otherwise take the forgotten dose as soon as you remember.

ALCOHOL, DRUG, HERB, AND SUPPLEMENT INTERACTIONS

Alcohol may increase some of the side effects from this drug, depending on the amount consumed. Ask your doctor about the risks caused by drinking alcohol with your condition.

Jimsonweed and licorice may both interfere with the effects of this drug and should not be used.

Several OTC drugs used for appetite control, asthma, colds, cough, hay fever, pain, or sinus problems may seriously interfere with the effects of this drug. Check with your pharmacist when selecting OTC products.

Taking this drug with any of the ones listed below may change the effect of either drug with the possibility of causing toxicity or decreasing effectiveness: acetazolamide, amiodarone, antacids, antiarrhythmics†, anticonvulsants†, antidepressants†, astemizole, beta blockers†, chloroquine, cholinergics†, cisapride, clarithromycin, co-trimoxazole, dichlorphenamide, digitoxin, digoxin, diphenhydramine, erythromycin, fludrocortisone, halofantrine, haloperidol, indapamide, maprotiline, mefloquine, methazolamide, nifedipine, pentamidine, phenobarbital, phenytoin, pimozide, rifampin, risperidone, sodium bicarbonate, sparfloxacin, tamoxifen, thiazide diuretics†, thiothixene, verapamil

Severe reactions are possible when this drug is taken with those listed below: phenothiazines†, reserpine

Increased side effects are possible when this drug is taken with those listed below: anticholinergics†, neuromuscular blockers†

ALLERGIC REACTIONS AND SIDE EFFECTS

If you are allergic to quinine, tonic water, or bitter lemon, you may also be allergic to this drug. You should tell your doctor about all your allergies and any unexplained symptoms you may have while taking this drug.

This drug may cause your eyes to be more sensitive to sunlight, but there are no special risks associated with sunburn while taking this drug.

MORE COMMON SIDE EFFECTS: Diarrhea, dizziness*, fever*, headache*, lightheadedness*, loss of appetite, nausea*, ringing in ears*, vomiting*, weakness*

LESS COMMON SIDE EFFECTS: Abdominal pain*, blurry vision*, color blindness*, confusion*, delirium*, eye sensitivity*, fainting*, yellow eyes or skin*

RARE SIDE EFFECTS: Bleeding gums*, chest pain*, joint pain*, muscle pain*, nosebleeds*, pale skin*, skin rash*, tiredness*

PRECAUTIONS

§The doses of quinidine sulfate and quinidine gluconate are not the same and cannot be substituted without a new prescription.

Do not open, break, crush, or chew the extended-release products.

Tell your doctor if you take large doses of aspirin on a regular basis since this drug may mask the symptoms of aspirin toxicity.

If you have heart disease or myasthenia gravis, this drug may make those conditions worse.

Be careful driving or handling equipment while taking this drug because it may cause dizziness and fainting spells.

This drug may cause changes to your gums and mouth. Your dentist may recommend that you clean your teeth and mouth differently to avoid infection.

When this drug is used to stabilize heart rhythm after electric shock, a blood-thinning drug may be started several weeks before taking this drug to reduce the risk of blood clots.

People with glucose-6-phosphate dehydrogenase deficiency (G6PD) are at greater risk of developing damage to red blood cells.

Liver function should be measured regularly while taking this drug, especially during the first 2 months.

PREGNANCY AND BREAST-FEEDING

Safety during pregnancy has not been established although the drug is known to harm animal fetuses.

Breast-feeding while taking this drug is not recommended.

HELPFUL COMMENTS

Avoid quick movements to minimize dizziness. Dangling your legs over the side of the bed for a few minutes may help reduce dizziness when first waking up.

Stomach and intestinal side effects, especially diarrhea, may be a sign of toxicity from this drug and should be reported to your doctor right away.

---

†See page 52.   *See page 53.

QUININE SULFATE

Available for over 20 years

COMMONLY USED TO TREAT

Leg cramps during the night
Malaria

DRUG CATEGORY

antimalarial
Class: cinchone alkaloid

PRODUCTS

Products Only Available as Generics
quinine sulfate 260 mg tablet (¢)
quinine sulfate 200 mg capsule (¢¢)
quinine sulfate 324 mg capsule (¢¢)
quinine sulfate 325 mg capsule (¢¢)

DOSING AND FOOD

Doses are taken 1 to 3 times a day.
It is best to take this drug right after a meal to avoid the stomach upset that
  some people suffer.
Adults: Up to 1,950 mg per day in divided doses.
Children: Up to 30 mg/kg per day in divided doses.
Forgotten doses: If you are scheduled to take the next dose within a few
  hours, do not take the forgotten dose. Otherwise take the forgotten dose
  as soon as you remember.

ALCOHOL, DRUG, HERB, AND SUPPLEMENT INTERACTIONS

Alcohol may increase some of the side effects from this drug, depending
  on the amount consumed. Ask your doctor about the risks caused by
  drinking alcohol with your condition.

Taking this drug with any of the ones listed below may change the effect of
either drug with the possibility of causing toxicity or decreasing effectiveness:
acetazolamide, anesthetics, antacids, digitoxin, digoxin, sodium bicarbonate, warfarin

Severe reactions are possible when this drug is taken with those listed below:
mefloquine

ALLERGIC REACTIONS AND SIDE EFFECTS

If you are allergic to quinidine, tonic water, or bitter lemon, you may also be allergic to this drug. You should tell your doctor about all your allergies and any unexplained symptoms you may have while taking this drug.

MORE COMMON SIDE EFFECTS: Abdominal pain*, diarrhea*, nausea*, vomiting*

LESS COMMON SIDE EFFECTS: Anxiety*, back pain*, behavior change*, black stools*, bleeding*, bloody urine*, blurry vision*, bruising*, chills*, cold sweats*, coma*, confusion*, cough*, drowsiness*, fever*, headache*, hoarseness*, hunger*, irregular heartbeat*, nervousness*, nightmares*, pale skin*, poor concentration*, seizures*, shakiness*, skin irritation*, sleep disorders*, slurry speech*, sore throat*, tiredness*, urinary changes*, weakness*

RARE SIDE EFFECTS: Blindness*, breathing difficulty*, chest pain*, color blindness*, dizziness*, fainting*, hives*, lightheadedness*, muscle aches*, red ears*, ringing in ears*, sleepiness*, swallowing disorders*, sweating*, swelling*, vision changes*

PRECAUTIONS

People with blackwater fever, glucose-6-phosphate dehydrogenase deficiency (G6PD), or purpura have a greater risk of developing side effects while taking this drug.

If you are a diabetic, you may need a change in the dose of your antidiabetic drug† or insulin, since this drug may cause a decrease in blood sugar.

If you have myasthenia gravis, this drug may make that condition worse.

Be careful driving or handling equipment while taking this drug because it may cause blurry vision and drowsiness.

This drug may cause false results from some diagnostic urine tests.

Tell your doctor if you take large doses of aspirin on a regular basis since this drug may mask the symptoms of aspirin toxicity.

PREGNANCY AND BREAST-FEEDING

There is evidence that this drug may harm the fetus, but the drug may be necessary to the health of the mother.

This drug passes into breast milk, but does not appear to harm the baby. Talk to your doctor about the risks associated with breast-feeding while taking this drug.

---

† See page 52.   * See page 53.

HELPFUL COMMENTS

If you are taking this drug to treat malaria, do not stop treatment early if you start to feel better. It takes the full prescription for this drug to work completely.

If you need to take an antacid, ask your pharmacist to help select a product that will not interfere with the effects of this drug.

RABEPRAZOLE SODIUM

Available since August 1999

COMMONLY USED TO TREAT

Heartburn, specifically gastroesophageal reflux disease (GERD)
Ulcers

DRUG CATEGORY

antiulcer
Class: proton pump inhibitor

PRODUCTS

Brand-Name Products with No Generic Alternative
Aciphex 20 mg extended-release tablet ($$$)
No generics available.
Multiple patents that begin to expire in 2008.

DOSING AND FOOD

Doses are taken 1 to 2 times a day.

This drug may be taken with or without food.

Adults: Up to 120 mg per day in divided doses.

Forgotten doses: If you are scheduled to take the next dose within a few hours, do not take the forgotten dose. Otherwise take the forgotten dose as soon as you remember.

ALCOHOL, DRUG, HERB, AND SUPPLEMENT INTERACTIONS

You should ask your doctor about the risks caused by drinking alcohol with your condition.

Taking St. John's wort at the same time as this drug increases the risk of developing severe sunburn.

Taking this drug with any of the ones listed below may change the effect of either drug with the possibility of causing toxicity or decreasing effectiveness: cyclosporine, digoxin, ketoconazole

ALLERGIC REACTIONS AND SIDE EFFECTS

If you are allergic to lansoprazole or omeprazole, you may also be allergic to this drug. You should tell your doctor about all your allergies and any unexplained symptoms you may have while taking this drug.

MORE COMMON SIDE EFFECTS: Headache

LESS COMMON SIDE EFFECTS: Constipation, diarrhea, dizziness, drowsiness, gas, heartburn, itching, nausea, numbness, pain, tingling, vomiting, weakness*

RARE SIDE EFFECTS: Bleeding*, bloody urine*, bruising*, chills*, fever*, irregular breathing*, mouth sores*, seizures*, sore throat*, tiredness*, yellow eyes or skin*

PRECAUTIONS

Do not crush, break, or chew the extended-release products.

PREGNANCY AND BREAST-FEEDING

Safety during pregnancy has not been established although there was no evidence of harm during studies in animals.
Breast-feeding while taking this drug is not recommended.

HELPFUL COMMENTS

This drug is usually used for less than 8 weeks although people who do not respond to the treatment during that time continue for a total of 16 weeks.

RALOXIFENE HYDROCHLORIDE

Available since December 1997

COMMONLY USED TO TREAT

Osteoporosis

DRUG CATEGORY

antiosteoporotic
Class: selective estrogen receptor modulator

---

† See page 52.   * See page 53.

PRODUCTS

Brand-Name Products with No Generic Alternative
Evista 60 mg tablet ($$$)
No generics available.
Multiple patents that begin to expire in 2003.

DOSING AND FOOD

Doses are taken once a day.
This drug may be taken with or without food.

Adults: Up to 60 mg per day.

Forgotten doses: Do not take a forgotten dose. Just go back to your usual schedule with the next dose.

ALCOHOL, DRUG, HERB, AND SUPPLEMENT INTERACTIONS

Alcohol may increase some of the side effects from this drug, depending on the amount consumed. Ask your doctor about the risks caused by drinking alcohol with your condition.

Taking this drug with any of the ones listed below may change the effect of either drug with the possibility of causing toxicity or decreasing effectiveness: aspirin, cholestyramine, clofibrate, diazepam, diazoxide, estrogens†, ibuprofen, indomethacin, naproxen, warfarin

ALLERGIC REACTIONS AND SIDE EFFECTS

You should tell your doctor about all your allergies and any unexplained symptoms you may have while taking this drug.

MORE COMMON SIDE EFFECTS: Bloody urine*, chest pain*, congestion*, cough*, depression, dry throat*, fever*, gas, hot flashes, infection*, joint pain, leg cramps*, loss of voice*, muscle pain, runny nose*, skin rash*, stomachache, sweating, swelling*, swollen joints, sleeping difficulty, urinary changes*, vaginal discharge, vaginal itch*, vomiting, weight gain

LESS COMMON SIDE EFFECTS: Abdominal pain*, body aches*, breathing difficulty*, diarrhea*, hoarseness*, loss of appetite*, nausea*, swallowing difficulty*, vision changes*, weakness

RARE SIDE EFFECTS: Coughing up blood*, headache*, numbness*, poor coordination*, shortness of breath*, speech changes*

PRECAUTIONS

If you are inactive, confined to bed, having surgery, taking a long trip, or spend a lot of time sitting, you may have a greater risk of developing blood clots while taking this drug. Talk to your doctor at least 3 days in advance of any scheduled periods of inactivity.

PREGNANCY AND BREAST-FEEDING

This drug may cause birth defects and should not be used during pregnancy. Breast-feeding while taking this drug is not recommended.

HELPFUL COMMENTS

Taking calcium supplements and vitamin D should continue while on this drug.

RAMIPRIL

Available since January 1991

COMMONLY USED TO TREAT

Heart failure
High blood pressure, also known as hypertension

DRUG CATEGORY

antihypertensive
Class: ACE inhibitor

PRODUCTS

Brand-Name Products with No Generic Alternative
Altace 1.25 mg capsule (¢¢¢¢¢)
Altace 2.5 mg capsule ($)
Altace 5 mg capsule ($)
Altace 10 mg capsule ($)
No generics available.
Multiple patents that begin to expire in 2005.

DOSING AND FOOD

Doses are taken 1 to 2 times a day.
This drug may be taken with or without food.
Adults: Up to 20 mg per day in divided doses.
Lower doses are used in people with kidney disease.
This drug is rarely used in children.
Forgotten doses: If you are scheduled to take the next dose within a few

---

† See page 52. * See page 53.

hours, do not take the forgotten dose. Otherwise take the forgotten dose as soon as you remember.

ALCOHOL, DRUG, HERB, AND SUPPLEMENT INTERACTIONS

Alcohol may cause your blood pressure to rise, making this drug less effective. Ask your doctor about the risks caused by drinking alcohol with your condition.

Licorice may interfere with the effects of this drug.

Capsaicin and other foods or supplements, including hot peppers, sweet peppers, paprika, and chili powder, derived from the capsicum family of plants may increase the risk of developing a cough and should not be taken with this drug.

Several OTC drugs used for appetite control, asthma, colds, cough, hay fever, or sinus problems may cause an increase in blood pressure when taken with this drug. Check with your pharmacist when selecting OTC products.

Taking this drug with any of the ones listed below may change the effect of either drug with the possibility of causing toxicity or decreasing effectiveness: antidiabetics†, antihypertensives†, diuretics†, insulin, lithium, potassium supplements

ALLERGIC REACTIONS AND SIDE EFFECTS

If you are allergic to any ACE inhibitors†, you may also be allergic to this drug. You should tell your doctor about all your allergies and any unexplained symptoms you may have while taking this drug.

This drug promotes the effect of sunlight on the body and may cause severe sunburn and increased sensitivity of the eyes.

MORE COMMON SIDE EFFECTS: Dry cough, headache, seizures*

LESS COMMON SIDE EFFECTS: Diarrhea, dizziness*, fainting*, fever*, joint pain*, lightheadedness*, loss of taste, nausea, skin rash*, tiredness

RARE SIDE EFFECTS: Abdominal pain*, breathing difficulty*, chest pain*, chills*, confusion*, hoarseness*, irregular heartbeat*, itching*, nausea*, nervousness*, numbness*, stomach pain*, swallowing difficulty*, swelling*, vomiting*, weakness*, yellow eyes or skin*

PRECAUTIONS

Be careful driving or handling equipment while taking this drug because the drug may cause dizziness.

People with systemic lupus erythematosus may be at greater risk of developing blood problems while taking this drug.

Do not use potassium-containing products, including salt substitutes, while taking this drug.

Diuretics should be stopped 2 to 3 days prior to starting this drug. If it is not possible to stop the diuretic, the dose of this drug should be lowered.

Drink plenty of fluids to avoid dehydration when sweating, such as in hot weather and during exercise.

PREGNANCY AND BREAST-FEEDING

Safety during pregnancy has not been established although the drug is known to harm animal fetuses.

Breast-feeding while taking this drug is not recommended.

HELPFUL COMMENTS

A persistent dry cough may appear while taking this drug, but it will go away when the drug is stopped.

Avoid quick movements to minimize dizziness. Dangling your legs over the side of the bed for a few minutes may help reduce dizziness when first waking up.

RANITIDINE HYDROCHLORIDE

Available for over 20 years

COMMONLY USED TO TREAT

Ulcers, specifically duodenal ulcers and gastric ulcers

DRUG CATEGORY

antiulcer
Class: H2 receptor antagonist

PRODUCTS

Brand-Name Products with No Generic Alternative
Zantac 15 mg/ml oral syrup ($$)
Zantac 150 mg effervescent tablet ($$)
Zantac 150 mg effervescent granules ($$)
Brand-Name Products with Generic Alternatives
Zantac 150 mg tablet ($$)
  Generic: ranitidine hydrochloride 150 mg tablet (¢¢)
Zantac 300 mg tablet ($$$)
  Generic: ranitidine hydrochloride 300 mg tablet (¢)

---

† See page 52. * See page 53.

DOSING AND FOOD

Doses are taken 1 to 2 times a day.
This drug may be taken with or without food.
Adults: Up to 6 g per day in divided doses.
Children: Up to 10 mg/kg (maximum 300 mg) per day in divided doses.
Lower doses are used in people with kidney disease.
Forgotten doses: If you are scheduled to take the next dose within a few hours, do not take the forgotten dose. Otherwise take the forgotten dose as soon as you remember.

ALCOHOL, DRUG, HERB, AND SUPPLEMENT INTERACTIONS

Alcohol may increase some of the side effects from this drug, depending on the amount consumed. Ask your doctor about the risks caused by drinking alcohol with your condition.

Taking this drug with any of the ones listed below may change the effect of either drug with the possibility of causing toxicity or decreasing effectiveness: antacids, diazepam, glipizide, procainamide, warfarin

ALLERGIC REACTIONS AND SIDE EFFECTS

If you are allergic to any H2 receptor antagonists†, you may also be allergic to this drug. You should tell your doctor about all your allergies and any unexplained symptoms you may have while taking this drug.

MORE COMMON SIDE EFFECTS: Abdominal pain*, agitation*, anxiety*, bleeding*, breathing difficulty*, chest tightness*, fever*, hives*, irregular heartbeat*, shallow breathing*, shortness of breath*, swallowing difficulty*, sweating, vomiting*, weakness*, wheezing*

LESS COMMON SIDE EFFECTS: Dizziness*, vision changes*

RARE SIDE EFFECTS: Back pain*, blisters*, bruising*, chills*, confusion*, constipation, cough*, dark urine*, drowsiness, dry mouth, fainting*, itching*, joint pain*, leg pain*, loss of appetite*, mood swings*, muscle cramps*, nausea*, nervousness*, pain*, pale stools*, ringing in ears, runny nose, skin irritation*, sleep disorders, sore eyes*, sore lips*, sore throat*, swelling*, tiredness*, urinary changes, yellow eyes or skin*

PRECAUTIONS

Smoking may increase stomach acids, making your condition worse.
Nonprescription strengths of this drug should not be taken for longer than 2 weeks unless recommended by your doctor.

PREGNANCY AND BREAST-FEEDING

Safety during pregnancy has not been established although there was no evidence of harm during studies in animals.

Breast-feeding while taking this drug is not recommended.

HELPFUL COMMENTS

Once-a-day doses should be taken at bedtime.

This drug is available in 75 mg tablets without a prescription under the trade name Zantac or generic name ranitidine hydrochloride.

If you need to take an antacid, take it either 2 hours before or after taking this drug.

REPAGLINIDE

Available since December 1997

COMMONLY USED TO TREAT

High blood sugar levels, specifically type 2 diabetes

DRUG CATEGORY

antidiabetic
Class: biguanide: meglitinide

PRODUCTS

Brand-Name Products with No Generic Alternative
Prandin 0.5 mg tablet (¢¢¢¢¢)
Prandin 1 mg tablet (¢¢¢¢¢)
Prandin 2 mg tablet (¢¢¢¢¢)
No generics available.
Multiple patents that begin to expire in 2006.

DOSING AND FOOD

Doses are taken 2 to 4 times a day.

It is best to take this drug on an empty stomach 15 to 30 minutes before a meal.

Adults: Up to 16 mg per day in divided doses.

Forgotten doses: Do not take a forgotten dose. Just go back to your usual schedule with the next dose.

† See page 52.   * See page 53.

ALCOHOL, DRUG, HERB, AND SUPPLEMENT INTERACTIONS

Alcohol may cause a change in your blood sugar, altering the effects of this drug. Ask your doctor about the risks caused by drinking alcohol with your condition.

Aloe, bilberry leaf, bitter melon, burdock, dandelion, fenugreek, garlic, ginkgo biloba, and ginseng may lower blood sugar and cause the need for a dose adjustment when taken with this drug. Tell your doctor if you are taking any of these supplements.

Several OTC drugs used for asthma, colds, cough, hay fever, sleep aid, or sinus problems may change the effects of this drug. Check with your pharmacist when selecting OTC products.

Taking this drug with any of the ones listed below may change the effect of either drug with the possibility of causing toxicity or decreasing effectiveness: aspirin, barbiturates†, beta blockers†, calcium channel blockers†, carbamazepine, chloramphenicol, corticosteroids†, diuretics†, erythromycin, estrogens†, isoniazid, ketoconazole, miconazole, monoamine oxidase inhibitors†, nicotinic acid, nonsteroidal antiinflammatories†, oral contraceptives, phenothiazines†, phenytoin, probenecid, rifampin, sulfonamides†, sympathomimetics†, thyroid hormones†, warfarin

ALLERGIC REACTIONS AND SIDE EFFECTS

You should tell your doctor about all your allergies and any unexplained symptoms you may have while taking this drug.

MORE COMMON SIDE EFFECTS: Anxiety*, back pain, blurry vision*, chest pain*, confusion*, congestion*, cough*, diarrhea, drowsiness*, fever*, headache*, hunger*, irregular heartbeat*, joint pain, low blood sugar*, nausea*, nervousness*, nightmares*, pale skin*, poor concentration*, runny nose*, seizures*, shakiness*, shortness of breath*, sleep disorders*, slurry speech*, sneezing*, sore throat*, sweating*, tiredness*, unconsciousness*, weakness*

LESS COMMON SIDE EFFECTS: Bloody urine*, breathing difficulty*, chest tightness*, chills*, constipation, hives*, indigestion, itching*, numbness, skin rash*, teary eyes*, tightness, tingling, tooth problems*, urinary changes*, vomiting*, wheezing*

RARE SIDE EFFECTS: Back pain*, black stools*, bleeding*, bloody stools*, bruising*, hoarseness*, irregular heartbeat*

PRECAUTIONS

Make sure your doctor or pharmacist has explained the symptoms associated with high and low blood sugars, as well as the action you should take if you develop symptoms.

Burns, diarrhea, fever, hormonal changes, infection, malnourishment, severe stress, uncontrolled thyroid disease, and vomiting may cause changes in blood sugar that may make this drug less effective.

PREGNANCY AND BREAST-FEEDING

Safety during pregnancy has not been established although the drug is known to harm animal fetuses.

Breast-feeding while taking this drug is not recommended.

HELPFUL COMMENTS

If you do not treat high blood sugar, you may develop more serious problems such as heart failure, blood vessel disease, eye disease, or kidney disease.

RIBAVIRIN

Available since December 1985

COMMONLY USED TO TREAT

Hepatitis C virus (when given with another drug)
Viral infection in children, specifically respiratory syncytial virus (RSV)

DRUG CATEGORY

antiviral
Class: synthetic nucleoside

PRODUCTS

Brand-Name Products with No Generic Alternative
Copegus 200 mg tablet (n/a)
Rebetol 200 mg capsule ($$$$$)
Virazole 6 g solution for inhalation ($$$$$)
No generics available.
Exclusivity until 2005.

Combination Products That Contain This Drug
Rebetron kits ($$$$$)

DOSING AND FOOD

Oral doses are taken twice a day. Inhalation therapy is used 12 to 18 hours a day.

---

†See page 52.   *See page 53.

Taking this drug by mouth with fatty foods will help increase the absorption of the drug. Be careful not to eat too much fatty food. Inhalation products are not affected by food.

Adults: Oral doses up to 1,200 mg per day in divided doses.

Oral products are not used in children.

Inhalation products are only intended for use in children and require a Viratek Small Particle Aerosol Generator.

Forgotten doses: If you are scheduled to take the next dose within a few hours, do not take the forgotten dose. Otherwise take the forgotten dose as soon as you remember.

ALCOHOL, DRUG, HERB, AND SUPPLEMENT INTERACTIONS

Alcohol may increase some of the side effects from this drug, depending on the amount consumed. Ask your doctor about the risks caused by drinking alcohol with your condition.

Taking this drug with any of the ones listed below may change the effect of either drug with the possibility of causing toxicity or decreasing effectiveness: didanosine, stavudine, zidovudine

ALLERGIC REACTIONS AND SIDE EFFECTS

You should tell your doctor about all your allergies and any unexplained symptoms you may have while taking this drug.

MORE COMMON SIDE EFFECTS: Blood sugar changes*, depression*, shortness of breath*, suicidal thoughts*

LESS COMMON SIDE EFFECTS: Low blood pressure

RARE SIDE EFFECTS: Headache, itching, red eyes, skin rash

PRECAUTIONS

The oral and inhalation products are used for different reasons and cannot be substituted for one another.

When used orally to treat hepatitis C infections, this drug is not effective unless given in combination with another antiviral† drug. Ask your pharmacist about the type of drug interaction that may occur between antiretroviral drugs† to coordinate the administration times of multiple drugs.

If you have thalassemia major or sickle cell anemia, this drug may make those conditions worse.

People with liver disease may not be able to take this drug.

PREGNANCY AND BREAST-FEEDING

This drug may cause birth defects and should not be used during pregnancy. Any exposure to the drug, including touching broken tablets or having intercourse with a man taking the drug, may also be associated with birth defects.

Breast-feeding while taking this drug is not recommended.

HELPFUL COMMENTS

This drug may also be called by the generic name tribavirin.

Contact your doctor if your symptoms do not improve after a couple of days.

Do not stop treatment early if you start to feel better. It takes the full prescription for this drug to work completely.

RIFABUTIN

Available since December 1992

COMMONLY USED TO TREAT

People with HIV to prevent mycobacterium avium complex (MAC)

DRUG CATEGORY

antibiotic
Class: semisynthetic ansamycin

PRODUCTS

Brand-Name Products with No Generic Alternative
Mycobutin 150 mg capsule ($$$$)
No generics available.
No patents, no exclusivity.

DOSING AND FOOD

Doses are taken 1 to 2 times a day.

This drug may be taken with or without food but is best taken with food to reduce the stomach upset that some people suffer.

Adults: Up to 300 mg per day in divided doses.

Forgotten doses: If you are scheduled to take the next dose within a few hours, do not take the forgotten dose. Otherwise take the forgotten dose as soon as you remember.

---

† See page 52.   * See page 53.

ALCOHOL, DRUG, HERB, AND SUPPLEMENT INTERACTIONS

Alcohol may increase some of the side effects from this drug, depending on the amount consumed. Ask your doctor about the risks caused by drinking alcohol with your condition.

Taking this drug with any of the ones listed below may change the effect of either drug with the possibility of causing toxicity or decreasing effectiveness: amprenavir, delavirdine, efavirenz, indinavir, nelfinavir, nevirapine, oral contraceptives, ritonavir, saquinavir, zidovudine

ALLERGIC REACTIONS AND SIDE EFFECTS

If you are allergic to rifampin or rifapentine, you may also be allergic to this drug. You should tell your doctor about all your allergies and any unexplained symptoms you may have while taking this drug.

MORE COMMON SIDE EFFECTS: Abdominal pain, bad taste in mouth, belching, bloating, chest pain, diarrhea*, fever*, gas, headache, heartburn*, indigestion*, itching*, loss of appetite*, nausea*, skin rash*, sleep disorders, sore throat*, taste changes*, vomiting*

LESS COMMON SIDE EFFECTS: Lack of energy*, muscle pain*

RARE SIDE EFFECTS: Back pain*, black stools*, bleeding*, bruising*, chills*, cough*, eye pain*, joint pain*, mouth sores*, muscle pain*, pale skin*, shortness of breath*, tiredness*, urinary pain*, vision loss*, weakness*, yellow eyes or skin*

PRECAUTIONS

This drug may cause your body fluids to turn reddish or brown in color. This includes urine, stools, saliva, sweat, and tears. Clothes may become permanently stained, and soft contact lenses may become permanently discolored.

This drug may cause changes to your gums and mouth. Your dentist may recommend that you clean your teeth and mouth differently to avoid infection.

PREGNANCY AND BREAST-FEEDING

Safety during pregnancy has not been established although there was no evidence of harm during studies in animals.

Breast-feeding while taking this drug is not recommended.

HELPFUL COMMENTS

Oral contraceptives may not work properly when taken with this drug. You need to use a barrier contraceptive, such as a condom, or other nonhormonal contraceptive to prevent pregnancy.

Contact your doctor if your symptoms do not improve after a couple of days.

Do not stop treatment early if you start to feel better. It takes the full prescription for this drug to work completely.

The capsules may be opened and mixed with applesauce for easier swallowing.

Hard contact lenses will not discolor due to the effects of this drug.

RIFAMPIN

Available for over 20 years

COMMONLY USED TO TREAT

Leprosy
People exposed to *H. influenzae* type B
Tuberculosis

DRUG CATEGORY

antibiotic
Class: antimycobacterial

PRODUCTS

Brand-Name Products with Generic Alternatives
Rifadin 150 mg capsule ($$)
  Generic: rifampin 150 mg capsule ($)
Rifadin 300 mg capsule ($$)
  Generic: rifampin 300 mg capsule ($$)

Other Generic Product Names
Rimactane

Combination Products That Contain This Drug
Rifamate capsule ($$$)
Rifater tablet ($$)

DOSING AND FOOD

Doses are taken 1 to 2 times a day.

It is best to take this drug on an empty stomach, with a full glass of water at least 1 hour before or 2 hours after meals. Do not eat raw oysters or other raw shellfish at any time while taking this drug.

---

† See page 52.   * See page 53.

Adults and children: Up to 600 mg per day in divided doses.

Lower doses are used in people with liver disease.

Forgotten doses: If you are scheduled to take the next dose within a few hours, do not take the forgotten dose. Otherwise take the forgotten dose as soon as you remember.

ALCOHOL, DRUG, HERB, AND SUPPLEMENT INTERACTIONS

Alcohol may increase the risk of liver damage from this drug. Ask your doctor about the risks caused by drinking alcohol with your condition.

Taking this drug with any of the ones listed below may change the effect of either drug with the possibility of causing toxicity or decreasing effectiveness: aminophylline, amprenavir, anticoagulants†, antidiabetics†, barbiturates†, beta blockers†, chloramphenicol, clofibrate, corticosteroids†, cyclosporine, dapsone, delavirdine, digitoxin, digoxin, disopyramide, efavirenz, estramustine, estrogens†, fluconazole, indinavir, itraconazole, ketoconazole, methadone, mexiletine, nelfinavir, nevirapine, oral contraceptives, oxtriphylline, para-aminosalicylate, phenytoin, quinidine, ritonavir, saquinavir, sulfonylureas†, theophylline, tocainide, verapamil

Increased side effects are possible when this drug is taken with those listed below: acetaminophen, amiodarone, anabolic steroids†, androgens†, antithyroid drugs†, carbamazepine, carmustine, chloroquine, dantrolene, daunorubicin, disulfiram, divalproex, etretinate, gold salts, hydroxychloroquine, isoniazid, mercaptopurine, methotrexate, methyldopa, naltrexone, phenothiazines†, plicamycin, valproic acid

ALLERGIC REACTIONS AND SIDE EFFECTS

If you are allergic to rifabutin or rifapentine, you may also be allergic to this drug. You should tell your doctor about all your allergies and any unexplained symptoms you may have while taking this drug.

MORE COMMON SIDE EFFECTS: Diarrhea, stomach cramps

LESS COMMON SIDE EFFECTS: Breathing difficulty*, chills*, dizziness*, fever*, headache*, itching*, mouth sores, muscle pain*, shivering*, skin rash*

RARE SIDE EFFECTS: Behavior changes*, bleeding*, bloody urine*, bruising*, loss of appetite*, nausea*, sore throat*, swelling*, tiredness*, urinary changes*, vomiting*, weakness*, yellow eyes or skin*

PRECAUTIONS

People with a history of liver disease or alcohol abuse may not be able to take this drug.

Capsules may be opened and mixed with applesauce or jelly for easier swallowing.

This drug may cause your body fluids to turn reddish or brown in color. This includes urine, stools, saliva, sweat, and tears. Clothes may become permanently stained, and soft contact lenses may become permanently discolored.

This drug causes changes in your blood that put you at greater risk of getting an infection. Be careful not to cut yourself or get bruised. Tell your doctor if you develop signs of infection, such as fever or sore throat. Your dentist may recommend that you clean your teeth and mouth differently to avoid infection.

PREGNANCY AND BREAST-FEEDING

Safety during pregnancy has not been established although the drug is known to harm animal fetuses.

This drug passes into breast milk, but does not appear to harm the baby. Talk to your doctor about the risks associated with breast-feeding while taking this drug.

HELPFUL COMMENTS

Oral contraceptives may not work properly when taken with this drug. You need to use a barrier contraceptive, such as a condom, or other nonhormonal contraceptive to prevent pregnancy.

Contact your doctor if your symptoms do not improve after a couple of weeks.

Do not stop treatment early if you start to feel better. It takes the full prescription for this drug to work completely. It may be necessary to take this drug for 1 to 2 years or more.

Hard contact lenses will not discolor due to the effects of this drug.

RIFAPENTINE

Available since June 1998

COMMONLY USED TO TREAT

Tuberculosis

DRUG CATEGORY

antibiotic
Class: antimycobacterial

---

† See page 52.   * See page 53.

PRODUCTS

Brand-Name Products with No Generic Alternative
Priftin 150 mg tablet ($$$)
No generics available.
No patents. Exclusivity until 2005.

DOSING AND FOOD

Doses are taken 1 to 2 times a week.

This drug may be taken with or without food but is best taken with food to reduce the stomach upset that some people suffer. Do not eat raw oysters or other raw shellfish at any time while taking this drug.

Adults: Up to 1,200 mg per week with at least 3 days between each 600 mg dose.

Forgotten doses: If you are scheduled to take the next dose within a few hours, do not take the forgotten dose. Otherwise take the forgotten dose as soon as you remember.

ALCOHOL, DRUG, HERB, AND SUPPLEMENT INTERACTIONS

Alcohol may increase the risk of liver damage from this drug. Ask your doctor about the risks caused by drinking alcohol with your condition.

Taking this drug with any of the ones listed below may change the effect of either drug with the possibility of causing toxicity or decreasing effectiveness:
antiarrhythmics†, antibiotics†, anticonvulsants†, antidiabetics†, antifungals†, barbiturates†, benzodiazepines†, beta blockers†, calcium channel blockers†, chloramphenicol, ciprofloxacin, clarithromycin, clofibrate, corticosteroids†, delavirdine, digitoxin, digoxin, diltiazem, disopyramide, doxycycline, fluconazole, haloperidol, immunosuppressants†, itraconazole, ketoconazole, levothyroxine, methadone, mexiletine, narcotics†, nifedipine, oral contraceptives, phenytoin, progestins†, protease inhibitors†, quinidine, quinine, reverse transcriptase inhibitors (NNRTIs, NsRTIs, and NtRTIs)†, sildenafil, theophylline, tocainide, tricyclic antidepressants†, verapamil, warfarin, zidovudine

ALLERGIC REACTIONS AND SIDE EFFECTS

If you are allergic to rifabutin or rifampin, you may also be allergic to this drug. You should tell your doctor about all your allergies and any unexplained symptoms you may have while taking this drug.

MORE COMMON SIDE EFFECTS: Back pain*, bloody urine*, joint pain*, swelling*

LESS COMMON SIDE EFFECTS: Abdominal pain*, acne, aggressiveness*, black stools*, bleeding*, bloody stools*, bruising*, constipation, fever*, loss of appetite, nausea*, skin irritation*, sore throat*, tiredness*, vomiting*, weakness*, yellow eyes or skin*

RARE SIDE EFFECTS: Diarrhea*, dizziness*, headache*, increased blood pressure*

PRECAUTIONS

People with a history of liver disease or alcohol abuse may not be able to take this drug.

This drug may cause your body fluids to turn reddish or brown in color. This includes urine, stools, saliva, sweat, and tears. Clothes may become permanently stained, and soft contact lenses may become permanently discolored.

This drug causes changes in your blood that put you at greater risk of getting an infection. Be careful not to cut yourself or get bruised. Tell your doctor if you develop signs of infection, such as fever or sore throat. Your dentist may recommend that you clean your teeth and mouth differently to avoid infection.

PREGNANCY AND BREAST-FEEDING

Safety during pregnancy has not been established although the drug is known to harm animal fetuses.

Breast-feeding while taking this drug is not recommended.

HELPFUL COMMENTS

Oral contraceptives may not work properly when taken with this drug. You need to use a barrier contraceptive, such as a condom, or other non-hormonal contraceptive to prevent pregnancy.

Contact your doctor if your symptoms do not improve after a couple of weeks.

Do not stop treatment early if you start to feel better. It takes the full prescription for this drug to work completely. It may be necessary to take this drug for 1 to 2 years or more.

Hard contact lenses will not discolor due to the effects of this drug.

---

†See page 52.   * See page 53.

RILUZOLE

Available since December 1995

COMMONLY USED TO TREAT

Lou Gehrig's disease, also known as amyotrophic lateral sclerosis (ALS)

DRUG CATEGORY

neuroprotector
Class: benzothiazole

PRODUCTS

Brand-Name Products with Generic Alternatives
Rilutek 50 mg tablet ($$$$$)
  Generic: riluzole 50 mg tablet (n/a)

DOSING AND FOOD

Doses are taken twice a day.
It is best to take this drug on an empty stomach at least 1 hour before or 2
  hours after a meal. Do not eat charbroiled food since it speeds up the
  elimination of this drug from the body.
Adults: Up to 100 mg per day in divided doses.
Forgotten doses: Do not take a forgotten dose. Just go back to your usual
  schedule with the next dose.

ALCOHOL, DRUG, HERB, AND SUPPLEMENT INTERACTIONS

Alcohol may increase the risk of liver damage from this drug. Ask your
  doctor about the risks caused by drinking alcohol with your condition.

**Taking this drug with any of the ones listed below may change the effect of
either drug with the possibility of causing toxicity or decreasing effectiveness:**
allopurinol, methyldopa, sulfasalazine

ALLERGIC REACTIONS AND SIDE EFFECTS

You should tell your doctor about all your allergies and any unexplained
  symptoms you may have while taking this drug.
MORE COMMON SIDE EFFECTS: Abdominal pain, diarrhea*, dizziness,
  drowsiness, gas, loss of appetite, nausea*, spastic movements*, tingling,
  tiredness*, vomiting*, weakness*
LESS COMMON SIDE EFFECTS: Back pain, breathing difficulty*, constipation,

cough*, dry mouth, hair loss, headache, itching, pneumonia*, runny nose, skin rash, sleep disorders, sore mouth, tooth problems*

RARE SIDE EFFECTS: Bloody urine*, chills*, depression*, fever*, high blood pressure*, irregular heartbeat*, lack of energy*, mood swings*, mouth sores*, muscle pain*, poor coordination*, seizures*, skin irritation*, swallowing difficulty*, swelling*, thirst*, urinary changes*, yellow eyes or skin*

PRECAUTIONS

Heavy smoking may cause this drug to be less effective.

Be careful driving or handling equipment while taking this drug because it may cause dizziness and drowsiness.

Liver function tests must be performed regularly to ensure safe use of this drug.

PREGNANCY AND BREAST-FEEDING

Safety during pregnancy has not been established although the drug is known to harm animal fetuses.

Breast-feeding while taking this drug is not recommended.

HELPFUL COMMENTS

Avoid quick movements to minimize dizziness. Dangling your legs over the side of the bed for a few minutes may help reduce dizziness when first waking up.

Sucking on hard sugarless candy or chewing sugarless gum may help relieve dry mouth caused by this drug.

Make sure to call your doctor if you develop a fever.

RIMANTADINE HYDROCHLORIDE

Available since September 1993

COMMONLY USED TO TREAT

The flu, also known as influenza A virus

DRUG CATEGORY

antiviral
Class: nucleoside analogue

PRODUCTS

Brand-Name Products with No Generic Alternative
Flumadine 50 mg/5 ml oral syrup (¢¢¢¢¢)

†See page 52.   *See page 53.

Brand-Name Products with Generic Alternatives
Flumadine 100 mg tablet ($$)
 Generic: rimantadine hydrochloride 100 mg tablet ($$)

DOSING AND FOOD

Doses are taken 1 to 2 times a day.
This drug may be taken with or without food.

Adults and children over age 10: Up to 200 mg per day in divided doses.

Children under age 10: Up to 5 mg/kg (maximum 150 mg) per day in divided doses.

Lower doses may be used in people with kidney disease or liver disease.

Forgotten doses: If you are scheduled to take the next dose within a few hours, do not take the forgotten dose. Otherwise take the forgotten dose as soon as you remember.

ALCOHOL, DRUG, HERB, AND SUPPLEMENT INTERACTIONS

Alcohol may increase some of the side effects from this drug, depending on the amount consumed. Ask your doctor about the risks caused by drinking alcohol with your condition.

Taking this drug with any of the ones listed below may change the effect of either drug with the possibility of causing toxicity or decreasing effectiveness: acetaminophen, aspirin, cimetidine

ALLERGIC REACTIONS AND SIDE EFFECTS

You should tell your doctor about all your allergies and any unexplained symptoms you may have while taking this drug.

LESS COMMON SIDE EFFECTS: Abdominal pain, dizziness, dry mouth, headache, loss of appetite, nausea, nervousness, poor concentration, sleep disorders, tiredness, vomiting

PRECAUTIONS

People with a history of seizures are at greater risk of developing a seizure while taking this drug.

This drug works best to prevent the flu if started right after exposure to a person sick with the flu or within 48 hours of the first flu symptoms.

Be careful driving or handling equipment while taking this drug because it may cause dizziness.

You are still contagious and may spread the flu to other people while taking this drug.

PREGNANCY AND BREAST-FEEDING

Safety during pregnancy has not been established although the drug is known to harm animal fetuses.

Breast-feeding while taking this drug is not recommended.

HELPFUL COMMENTS

Contact your doctor if your symptoms do not improve after a couple of days.

Do not stop treatment early if you start to feel better. It takes the full prescription for this drug to work completely.

Do not measure doses of the oral syrup with anything but a measuring cup intended for use with prescription drugs. Slight inaccuracy from other measuring spoons may result in over- or under-dosing.

Take the last dose of the day by 6 P.M. so the drug does not keep you awake at night.

RISEDRONATE SODIUM

Available since March 1998

COMMONLY USED TO TREAT

Low bone density, also known as osteoporosis

DRUG CATEGORY

antiosteoporotic
Class: bisphosphonate

PRODUCTS

Brand-Name Products with No Generic Alternative
Actonel 5 mg tablet ($)
Actonel 30 mg tablet ($$$$$)
Actonel 35 mg tablet (n/a)
No generics available.
Multiple patents that begin to expire in 2013.

DOSING AND FOOD

Doses are taken once a day to once a week, in the morning.

Take this drug on an empty stomach with a full glass of water at least 30 minutes before eating or drinking anything but water. More drug is absorbed if you take the dose 60 minutes before eating or drinking.

---

† See page 52.   * See page 53.

Adults: Up to 30 mg per day.

Forgotten doses: Do not take a forgotten dose. Just go back to your usual schedule with the next daily dose. If taking the drug weekly, take the forgotten dose the next day then wait a full week before taking the next scheduled dose.

ALCOHOL, DRUG, HERB, AND SUPPLEMENT INTERACTIONS

Alcohol may increase some of the side effects from this drug, depending on the amount consumed. Ask your doctor about the risks caused by drinking alcohol with your condition.

Taking this drug with any of the ones listed below may change the effect of either drug with the possibility of causing toxicity or decreasing effectiveness: antacids, calcium supplements, mineral supplements

ALLERGIC REACTIONS AND SIDE EFFECTS

You should tell your doctor about all your allergies and any unexplained symptoms you may have while taking this drug.

MORE COMMON SIDE EFFECTS: Abdominal pain*, diarrhea, heartburn*, joint pain, skin rash*, swallowing difficulty*

LESS COMMON SIDE EFFECTS: Belching*, blurry vision, bone pain*, chest pain, constipation, cough, dizziness, dry eyes, fever, headache, leg cramps, nausea, ringing in ears, stomach cramps*, swelling, vision changes, weakness

RARE SIDE EFFECTS: Red eyes*

PRECAUTIONS

Do not lie down for 30 minutes after taking a dose of this drug.

If you have a swallowing disorder, esophageal or intestinal problems, this drug may make those conditions worse.

Chewing or sucking on tablets may cause irritation of the mouth or throat.

PREGNANCY AND BREAST-FEEDING

Safety during pregnancy has not been established although the drug is known to harm animal fetuses.

Breast-feeding while taking this drug is not recommended.

HELPFUL COMMENTS

Calcium and vitamin D supplements should continue but must be taken either 2 hours before or after taking this drug to prevent interference with drug absorption.

Antacids may interfere with the absorption of this drug and should be taken either 2 hours before or after taking this drug.

RISPERIDONE

Available since December 1993

COMMONLY USED TO TREAT

Mental disturbances, specifically known as psychosis

DRUG CATEGORY

antipsychotic
Class: benzisoxazole derivative

PRODUCTS

Brand-Name Products with No Generic Alternative
Risperdal 0.25 mg tablet ($$$)
Risperdal 0.5 mg tablet ($$$)
Risperdal 1 mg tablet ($$$)
Risperdal 2 mg tablet ($$$)
Risperdal 3 mg tablet ($$$$)
Risperdal 4 mg tablet ($$$$)
Risperdal 1 mg/ml oral solution ($$$$$)
No generics available.
Patent expires in 2007. Exclusivity until 2005.

DOSING AND FOOD

Doses are taken twice a day.
This drug may be taken with or without food.
Adults: Up to 6 mg per day in divided doses.
Lower doses are used in people with kidney disease, liver disease, low blood pressure, and people over age 65.
Forgotten doses: If you are scheduled to take the next dose within a few hours, do not take the forgotten dose. Otherwise take the forgotten dose as soon as you remember.

ALCOHOL, DRUG, HERB, AND SUPPLEMENT INTERACTIONS

Alcohol should not be used while taking this drug.

---

† See page 52.   * See page 53.

Many OTC drugs used for appetite control, asthma, colds, cough, hay fever, pain, or sinus problems affect the central nervous system and may change the effects or side effects of this drug. Check with your pharmacist for products to avoid.

Taking this drug with any of the ones listed below may change the effect of either drug with the possibility of causing toxicity or decreasing effectiveness: anesthetics, antihistamines†, antihypertensives†, anxiolytics†, barbiturates†, bromocriptine, carbamazepine, clozapine, levodopa, narcotics†, pergolide

ALLERGIC REACTIONS AND SIDE EFFECTS

You should tell your doctor about all your allergies and any unexplained symptoms you may have while taking this drug.

This drug promotes the effect of sunlight on the body and may cause severe sunburn and increased sensitivity of the eyes.

MORE COMMON SIDE EFFECTS: Aggressiveness*, agitation*, anxiety*, blurry vision*, constipation, cough, diarrhea*, drowsiness*, dry mouth, expressionless face*, eye stillness*, headache*, heartburn, itching*, memory loss*, menstrual changes*, mood swings*, muscle spasms*, nausea, nervousness*, poor balance*, poor concentration, restlessness*, runny nose, sexual dysfunction*, shuffling walk*, skin rash*, sleep disorders*, sore throat, spastic movements*, stiffness*, swallowing difficulty*, tiredness*, trembling*, urinary changes*, vision changes*, weakness*, weight gain

LESS COMMON SIDE EFFECTS: Back pain*, breast-milk secretion*, chest pain*, dandruff*, dry skin, joint pain, oily skin*, skin discoloration, stomach pain, vomiting, watery mouth, weight loss

RARE SIDE EFFECTS: Bleeding*, blinking*, blood pressure changes*, bruising*, chewing motion*, confusion*, excessive talking*, excitement*, eyelid spasms*, facial expressions*, fever*, irregular breathing*, irregular heartbeat*, lip smacking*, loss of appetite*, muscle cramps*, pale skin*, penile erection*, poor bladder control*, poor coordination*, puffy cheeks*, seizures*, shivering*, sweating*, thirst*, tongue movements*

PRECAUTIONS

People with a history of seizures are at greater risk of developing a seizure while taking this drug.

If you have Parkinson's disease, breast cancer, or blood vessel disease, this drug may make those conditions worse.

Stopping this drug suddenly may cause your original condition to return with more severe symptoms. If you wish to stop taking this drug, ask your doctor for specific instructions.

Be careful driving or handling equipment while taking this drug because the drug may cause drowsiness.

Drink plenty of fluids to avoid dehydration when sweating, such as in hot weather and during exercise.

This drug may cause dry mouth, which is associated with a greater risk of cavities. Your dentist may recommend that you clean your teeth and mouth differently to avoid infection.

PREGNANCY AND BREAST-FEEDING

Safety during pregnancy has not been established although the drug is known to harm animal fetuses.

Breast-feeding while taking this drug is not recommended.

HELPFUL COMMENTS

This drug makes you more sensitive to hot and cold temperatures.

It takes about a week for the effects of this drug to be noticed.

Avoid quick movements to minimize dizziness. Dangling your legs over the side of the bed for a few minutes may help reduce dizziness when first waking up.

RITONAVIR

Available since March 1996

COMMONLY USED TO TREAT

HIV infection

DRUG CATEGORY

antiretroviral
Class: protease inhibitor (PI)

PRODUCTS

Brand-Name Products with No Generic Alternative
Norvir 100 mg capsule ($$)
Norvir 80 mg/ml oral solution ($$$$)
No generics available.
Multiple patents that begin to expire in 2012.

---

† See page 52.   * See page 53.

Combination Products That Contain This Drug
Kaletra capsule
Kaletra oral solution

DOSING AND FOOD

Doses are taken twice a day.
It is best to take this drug with food.
Adults: Up to 1,200 mg per day in divided doses.
Children age 2 and older: Up to 800 mg/m^2 per day in divided doses.
Forgotten doses: If you are scheduled to take the next dose within a few hours, do not take the forgotten dose. Otherwise take the forgotten dose as soon as you remember.

ALCOHOL, DRUG, HERB, AND SUPPLEMENT INTERACTIONS

Alcohol may increase some of the side effects from this drug, depending on the amount consumed. Ask your doctor about the risks caused by drinking alcohol with your condition.
St. John's wort may noticeably interfere with the effects of this drug and should not be used at any time during treatment.

Taking this drug with any of the ones listed below may change the effect of either drug with the possibility of causing toxicity or decreasing effectiveness: amprenavir, anticoagulants†, carbamazepine, clarithromycin, delavirdine, desipramine, dexamethasone, didanosine, disopyramide, disulfiram, efavirenz, immunosuppressants†, indinavir, ketoconazole, meperidine, methadone, metronidazole, nelfinavir, nevirapine, oral contraceptives, phenobarbital, phenytoin, rifabutin, rifampin, sildenafil, saquinavir, theophylline

Severe reactions are possible when this drug is taken with those listed below: alprazolam, amiodarone, bepridil, cisapride, clorazepate, diazepam, dihydroergotamine, ergonovine, ergot alkaloids†, estazolam, flecainide, flurazepam, HMG-CoA inhibitors†, lovastatin, methylergonovine, midazolam, pimozide, propafenone, quinidine, simvastatin, triazolam, zolpidem

ALLERGIC REACTIONS AND SIDE EFFECTS

You should tell your doctor about all your allergies and any unexplained symptoms you may have while taking this drug.
MORE COMMON SIDE EFFECTS: Abdominal pain*, belching, diarrhea, dizziness, drowsiness, heartburn, nausea*, numbness, prickling, sleep disorders, sour stomach, taste changes, tingling, vomiting*, weakness

LESS COMMON SIDE EFFECTS: Behavior changes, bloating*, body aches, congestion, dizziness*, dry mouth, fainting*, fear, flushing*, gas, headache*, hoarseness, irritability, joint pain, lack of appetite, lightheadedness*, mood swings, nervousness, nighttime urination, poor concentration, runny nose, sore throat, stiffness, swallowing difficulty, sweating*, swollen glands, tiredness, voice changes

RARE SIDE EFFECTS: Bad breath*, breathing difficulty*, chest tightness*, chills*, confusion*, constipation*, cough*, dark urine*, dehydration*, dry skin*, fatigue*, fever*, hives*, hunger*, indigestion*, irregular heartbeat*, itching*, loss of appetite*, seizures*, shortness of breath*, skin irritation*, thirst*, urinary changes*, weight loss*, wheezing*, yellow eyes or skin*

PRECAUTIONS

This drug does not prevent the spread of the HIV virus.

If you are diabetic, you may need an adjustment to the dose of your antidiabetic drug† or insulin therapy while taking this drug.

Hemophiliacs may be at greater risk of bleeding while taking this drug.

This drug is usually prescribed in combination with another antiretroviral drug†. Ask your pharmacist about the type of drug interaction that may occur between antiretroviral drugs† to coordinate the administration times of multiple drugs.

PREGNANCY AND BREAST-FEEDING

Safety during pregnancy has not been established although there was no evidence of harm during studies in animals.

Breast-feeding while taking this drug is not recommended.

HELPFUL COMMENTS

Oral contraceptives may not work properly when taken with this drug. You need to use a barrier contraceptive, such as a condom, or other nonhormonal contraceptive to prevent pregnancy.

Contact your doctor if your symptoms do not improve after a couple of days.

Do not stop treatment early if you start to feel better. It takes the full prescription for this drug to work completely.

Do not measure doses of the oral solution with anything but a measuring cup intended for use with prescription drugs. Slight inaccuracy from other measuring spoons may result in over- or under-dosing.

Take the last dose of the day before 6 P.M. to reduce the chance of having to urinate during the night.

---

†See page 52.   *See page 53.

RIVASTIGMINE TARTRATE

Available since April 2000

COMMONLY USED TO TREAT

Alzheimer's disease

DRUG CATEGORY

antidementia
Class: cholinesterase inhibitor

PRODUCTS

Brand-Name Products with No Generic Alternative
Exelon 1.5 mg capsule ($$)
Exelon 3 mg capsule ($$)
Exelon 4.5 mg capsule ($$)
Exelon 6 mg capsule ($$)
Exelon 2 mg/ml oral solution ($$$$$)
No generics available.
Multiple patents that begin to expire in 2007.

DOSING AND FOOD

Doses are taken twice a day.
It is best to take this drug with food or milk.
Adults: Up to 12 mg per day in divided doses.
Forgotten doses: If you are scheduled to take the next dose within a few
  hours, do not take the forgotten dose. Otherwise take the forgotten dose
  as soon as you remember.

ALCOHOL, DRUG, HERB, AND SUPPLEMENT INTERACTIONS

Alcohol may increase some of the side effects from this drug, depending
  on the amount consumed. Ask your doctor about the risks caused by
  drinking alcohol with your condition.
Many OTC drugs used to relieve pain, including aspirin, may cause an increase in side effects while taking this drug. Check with your pharmacist
  for products to avoid.

**Taking this drug with any of the ones listed below may change the effect of
either drug with the possibility of causing toxicity or decreasing effectiveness:**
anticholinergics†, bethanechol, succinylcholine

Increased side effects are possible when this drug is taken with those listed below: aspirin, nonsteroidal antiinflammatories†

ALLERGIC REACTIONS AND SIDE EFFECTS

You should tell your doctor about all your allergies and any unexplained symptoms you may have while taking this drug.

MORE COMMON SIDE EFFECTS: Abdominal pain, bloating, confusion, constipation, depression, diarrhea*, dizziness, fatigue, hallucinations, headache, indigestion*, lack of strength*, loss of appetite*, nausea*, sleep disorders, vomiting*, weight loss*

LESS COMMON SIDE EFFECTS: Fainting*, high blood pressure*, runny nose, sweating*

RARE SIDE EFFECTS: Aggression*, irregular breathing*, large pupils*, seizures*, trembling*, urinary changes*, watery mouth*, weakness*

PRECAUTIONS

People with a history of seizures, thyroid disease, or diabetes may be at greater risk of developing seizures while taking this drug.

If you have asthma, intestinal problems, stomach problems, urinary disorders, or heart disease, this drug may make those conditions worse.

Be careful driving or handling equipment while taking this drug because it may cause dizziness.

Stopping this drug suddenly may cause serious behavioral and mental changes. If you wish to stop taking this drug, ask your doctor for specific instructions.

Heavy smoking may cause this drug to be less effective.

PREGNANCY AND BREAST-FEEDING

Safety during pregnancy has not been established although there was no evidence of harm during studies in animals.

It is not known if this drug passes into breast milk. Talk to your doctor about the risks associated with breast-feeding while taking this drug.

HELPFUL COMMENTS

This drug is used to slow the advancement of Alzheimer's disease, but is not likely to help recover memory.

Avoid quick movements to minimize dizziness. Dangling your legs over the side of the bed for a few minutes may help reduce dizziness when first waking up.

---

† See page 52.   * See page 53.

RIZATRIPTAN BENZOATE

Available since June 1998

COMMONLY USED TO TREAT

Migraine headache

DRUG CATEGORY

antimigraine
Class: triptan

PRODUCTS

Brand-Name Products with No Generic Alternative
Maxalt 5 mg tablet ($$$$$)
Maxalt 10 mg tablet ($$$$$)
Maxalt-MLT 5 mg disintegrating tablet ($$$$$)
Maxalt-MLT 10 mg disintegrating tablet ($$$$$)
No generics available.
Multiple patents that begin to expire in 2012.

DOSING AND FOOD

Doses are taken at the first sign that a migraine headache is starting.
Taking this drug on an empty stomach will lead to quicker results.
Adults: Up to 30 mg per day in divided doses.

ALCOHOL, DRUG, HERB, AND SUPPLEMENT INTERACTIONS

Alcohol may make your headache worse. You should ask your doctor about
the risks caused by drinking alcohol with your condition.

Taking this drug with any of the ones listed below may change the effect of
either drug with the possibility of causing toxicity or decreasing effectiveness:
propranolol

Severe reactions are possible when this drug is taken with those listed below:
ergot alkaloids†, monoamine oxidase inhibitors†,

Increased side effects are possible when this drug is taken with those listed below:
SSRIs†

ALLERGIC REACTIONS AND SIDE EFFECTS

If you are allergic to aspartame, you may also be allergic to the disintegrating tablets. You should tell your doctor about all your allergies and any unexplained symptoms you may have while taking this drug.

MORE COMMON SIDE EFFECTS: Chest pain*, chest pressure*, dizziness*, dry mouth, hot flashes, irregular heartbeat*, nausea*, numbness*, shortness of breath*, sleepiness*, tingling*, tiredness*, vomiting*, weakness*

LESS COMMON SIDE EFFECTS: Agitation, anxiety, blurry vision, chills, confusion, constipation, depression, diarrhea, dry eyes, eye irritation, fainting*, gas, headache*, heartburn, irritability, itching, muscle pain, ringing in ears, stiffness, swallowing difficulty, sweating, thirst, trembling, urinary changes

PRECAUTIONS

You need to wait 2 weeks after stopping a monoamine oxidase inhibitor† before starting this drug.

This drug should only be used to treat migraine headaches. It is not effective if taken in advance to prevent a migraine or used to treat any other type of headache.

Be careful driving or handling equipment while taking this drug because it may cause dizziness.

This drug is most effective if taken at the first warning signal that a migraine headache is starting.

The oral disintegrating tablets contain phenylalanine, which should not be taken by people with phenylketonuria (PKU).

If you have high blood pressure or heart disease, you may not be able to take this drug.

This drug may cause dry mouth, which is associated with a greater risk of cavities. Your dentist may recommend that you clean your teeth and mouth differently to avoid infection.

PREGNANCY AND BREAST-FEEDING

Safety during pregnancy has not been established although the drug is known to harm animal fetuses.

Breast-feeding while taking this drug is not recommended.

HELPFUL COMMENTS

Disintegrating tablets may fall apart if pushed through the foil when removing from the packaging. Instead, the foil should be peeled back to open.

---

† See page 52.   * See page 53.

ROFECOXIB

Available since May 1999

COMMONLY USED TO TREAT

Arthritis pain
Menstrual pain
Surgical pain
Swelling

DRUG CATEGORY

analgesic
antiinflammatory
Class: nonsteroidal antiinflammatory: COX-2 inhibitor

PRODUCTS

Brand-Name Products with No Generic Alternative
Vioxx 12.5 mg tablet ($$$)
Vioxx 25 mg tablet ($$$)
Vioxx 50 mg tablet ($$$)
Vioxx 12.5 mg/5 ml oral suspension ($$$)
Vioxx 25 mg/5 ml oral suspension ($$$)
No generics available.
Multiple patents that begin to expire in 2013.

DOSING AND FOOD

Doses are taken once a day only as needed to relieve pain.
This drug may be taken with or without food but is best taken with food to
reduce the stomach upset that some people suffer.
Adults: Up to 50 mg per day.

ALCOHOL, DRUG, HERB, AND SUPPLEMENT INTERACTIONS

Alcohol may increase some of the side effects from this drug, depending
on the amount consumed. Ask your doctor about the risks caused by
drinking alcohol with your condition.
Do not use dong quai, feverfew, garlic, ginger, horse chestnut, red clover,
or St. John's wort while taking this drug since they may increase the risk
of serious side effects.

Taking this drug with any of the ones listed below may change the effect of either drug with the possibility of causing toxicity or decreasing effectiveness: ACE inhibitors†, furosemide, lithium, methotrexate, rifampin, thiazide diuretics†, warfarin

Severe reactions are possible when this drug is taken with those listed below: aspirin

ALLERGIC REACTIONS AND SIDE EFFECTS

If you are allergic to aspirin or any nonsteroidal antiinflammatory†, you may also be allergic to this drug. You should tell your doctor about all your allergies and any unexplained symptoms you may have while taking this drug.

MORE COMMON SIDE EFFECTS: Back pain, congestion*, cough*, diarrhea, dizziness, fever*, headache, heartburn, loss of energy, nausea, sneezing*, sore throat*, stuffy nose, swelling, weakness

LESS COMMON SIDE EFFECTS: Black stools*, blurry vision, burning sensation*, chills*, constipation, hives*, loss of appetite*, muscle pain*, shortness of breath*, skin rash*, stomachache*, vomiting*, weight gain*

PRECAUTIONS

This drug may cause serious stomach problems and possibly ulcers. Be careful to take this drug with food, and let your doctor know if you develop any stomach-related symptoms.

People with a history of smoking, alcohol abuse, bleeding disorders, or stomach problems are at increased risk of developing side effects.

If you have anemia, asthma, dehydration, swelling, heart disease, high blood pressure, kidney disease, or liver disease, this drug may make those conditions worse.

PREGNANCY AND BREAST-FEEDING

Safety during pregnancy has not been established although the drug is known to harm animal fetuses.

Breast-feeding while taking this drug is not recommended.

HELPFUL COMMENTS

Several nonsteroidal antiinflammatories† are available without a prescription in lower, nonprescription strengths, including ibuprofen, ketoprofen, and naproxen.

---

†See page 52.　　*See page 53.

ROPINIROLE HYDROCHLORIDE

Available since September 1997

COMMONLY USED TO TREAT

Parkinson's disease

DRUG CATEGORY

antidyskinetic
Class: nonergot dopamine agonist

PRODUCTS

Brand-Name Products with No Generic Alternative
Requip 0.25 mg tablet ($)
Requip 0.5 mg tablet ($)
Requip 1 mg tablet ($)
Requip 2 mg tablet ($)
Requip 3 mg tablet ($$)
Requip 4 mg tablet ($$)
Requip 5 mg tablet ($$)
No generics available.
Multiple patents that begin to expire in 2007.

DOSING AND FOOD

Doses are taken 3 times a day.

This drug may be taken with or without food but is best taken with food to reduce the stomach upset that some people suffer.

Adults: Up to 24 mg per day in divided doses.

Forgotten doses: If you are scheduled to take the next dose within a few hours, do not take the forgotten dose. Otherwise take the forgotten dose as soon as you remember.

ALCOHOL, DRUG, HERB, AND SUPPLEMENT INTERACTIONS

Alcohol should not be used while taking this drug.

Many OTC drugs used for appetite control, asthma, colds, cough, hay fever, pain, or sinus problems affect the central nervous system and may change the effects or side effects of this drug. Check with your pharmacist for products to avoid.

Taking this drug with any of the ones listed below may change the effect of either drug with the possibility of causing toxicity or decreasing effectiveness: butyrophenone, ciprofloxacin, estrogens†, fluvoxamine, levodopa, meto-clopramide, mexiletine, norfloxacin, phenothiazines†, thioxanthenes†

Severe reactions are possible when this drug is taken with those listed below: anesthetics, antihistamines†, anxiolytics†, barbiturates†, benzodiazepines†, narcotics†

ALLERGIC REACTIONS AND SIDE EFFECTS

You should tell your doctor about all your allergies and any unexplained symptoms you may have while taking this drug.

More Common Side Effects: Confusion*, dizziness*, drowsiness*, faint-ing*, falling*, hallucinations*, lightheadedness*, nausea*, spastic move-ments*, swelling*, tiredness*, weakness*

Less Common Side Effects: Abdominal pain*, blood pressure changes*, bloody urine*, breathing difficulty*, chest pain*, chest tightness*, consti-pation, cough*, depression*, diarrhea, dreams, dry mouth, flushing, gas, headache*, heartburn, hot flashes, irregular heartbeat*, loss of appetite, memory loss*, numbness*, pain*, poor concentration*, sexual dysfunc-tion, shortness of breath*, sore throat, sweating, tingling*, tremor, urinary changes*, vision changes*, vomiting*, weight loss, wheezing*, yawning

Rare Side Effects: Agitation*, anxiety*, chills*, congestion*, cough*, fever*, joint pain*, nervousness*, poor bladder control*, ringing in ears*, runny nose*, sneezing*, swallowing difficulty*

PRECAUTIONS

If you have low blood pressure or a history of hallucinations, this drug may make those conditions worse.

The dose of this drug should be increased and decreased slowly over several weeks to prevent severe side effects from developing.

Be careful driving or handling equipment while taking this drug because it may cause dizziness and drowsiness.

If you have high blood pressure, you may need an adjustment to the dose of your antihypertensive† therapy while taking this drug.

Heavy smoking may cause this drug to be less effective.

PREGNANCY AND BREAST-FEEDING

Safety during pregnancy has not been established although the drug is known to harm animal fetuses.

Breast-feeding while taking this drug is not recommended.

---

†See page 52.   *See page 53.

HELPFUL COMMENTS

Sucking on hard sugarless candy or chewing sugarless gum may help relieve dry mouth caused by this drug.

Avoid quick movements to minimize dizziness. Dangling your legs over the side of the bed for a few minutes may help reduce dizziness when first waking up.

When taking this drug, the elderly seem to hallucinate more frequently than younger people.

ROSIGLITAZONE MALEATE

Available since May 1999

COMMONLY USED TO TREAT

High blood sugar, specifically type 2 diabetes

DRUG CATEGORY

antidiabetic
Class: thiazolidinedione

PRODUCTS

Brand-Name Products with No Generic Alternative
Avandia 2 mg tablet ($$)
Avandia 4 mg tablet ($$$)
Avandia 8 mg tablet ($$$)
No generics available.
Multiple patents that begin to expire in 2008.
Combination Products That Contain This Drug
Avandamet tablet

DOSING AND FOOD

Doses are taken 1 to 2 times a day.
This drug may be taken with or without food.
Adults: Up to 8 mg per day.
Forgotten doses: If you are scheduled to take the next dose within a few hours, do not take the forgotten dose. Otherwise take the forgotten dose as soon as you remember.

ALCOHOL, DRUG, HERB, AND SUPPLEMENT INTERACTIONS

Alcohol may cause a change in your blood sugar, altering the effects of this drug. Ask your doctor about the risks caused by drinking alcohol with your condition.

Aloe, bilberry leaf, bitter melon, burdock, dandelion, fenugreek, garlic, ginkgo biloba, and ginseng may lower blood sugar and cause the need for a dose adjustment when taken with this drug. Tell your doctor if you are taking any of these supplements.

Several OTC drugs used for asthma, colds, cough, hay fever, sleep aid, or sinus problems may change the effects of this drug. Check with your pharmacist when selecting OTC products.

Severe reactions are possible when this drug is taken with those listed below: insulin

ALLERGIC REACTIONS AND SIDE EFFECTS

You should tell your doctor about all your allergies and any unexplained symptoms you may have while taking this drug.

MORE COMMON SIDE EFFECTS: Back pain, fever*, headache, runny nose*, swelling*

LESS COMMON SIDE EFFECTS: Dizziness, lightheadedness, weight gain*

RARE SIDE EFFECTS: Abdominal pain*, dark urine*, loss of appetite*, nausea*, shortness of breath*, tiredness*, vomiting*, weakness*

PRECAUTIONS

If you have heart disease or liver disease, this drug may make those conditions worse.

People who regularly retain fluid are at greater risk of developing side effects while taking this drug.

Record your weight twice a day, when first getting up in the morning and at the end of the day. A weight gain or loss of more than 2 pounds per day should be reported to your doctor.

This drug is often given in combination with another antidiabetic drug†.

Burns, diarrhea, fever, hormonal changes, infection, malnourishment, severe stress, uncontrolled thyroid disease, and vomiting may cause changes in blood sugar that may make this drug less effective.

PREGNANCY AND BREAST-FEEDING

Safety during pregnancy has not been established although the drug is known to harm animal fetuses.

Breast-feeding while taking this drug is not recommended.

---

† *See page 52.*   * *See page 53.*

HELPFUL COMMENTS

Blood sugar levels should be checked if you experience any side effects. If you do not treat high blood sugar, you may develop more serious problems such as heart failure, blood vessel disease, eye disease, or kidney disease.

SAQUINAVIR

Available since December 1995

COMMONLY USED TO TREAT

HIV infection

DRUG CATEGORY

antiretroviral
Class: protease inhibitor (PI)

PRODUCTS

Brand-Name Products with No Generic Alternative
Fortovase 200 mg capsule§ ($)
Invirase 200 mg capsule§ ($$)
No generics available.
Patent expires in 2010.

DOSING AND FOOD

Doses are taken 3 times a day.
This drug should be taken within 2 hours after a meal. Do not take this drug with grapefruit juice.
Adults: Up to 3,600 mg per day of Fortovase in divided doses.
Adults: Up to 1,800 mg per day of Invirase in divided doses.
Forgotten doses: If you are scheduled to take the next dose within a few hours, do not take the forgotten dose. Otherwise take the forgotten dose as soon as you remember.

ALCOHOL, DRUG, HERB, AND SUPPLEMENT INTERACTIONS

Alcohol may increase some of the side effects from this drug, depending on the amount consumed. Ask your doctor about the risks caused by drinking alcohol with your condition.
Garlic and St. John's wort may reduce the effectiveness of this drug.

§ *See "Precautions" in this entry.*

Taking this drug with any of the ones listed below may change the effect of either drug with the possibility of causing toxicity or decreasing effectiveness: amprenavir, astemizole, calcium channel blockers†, carbamazepine, cisapride, delavirdine, dexamethasone, efavirenz, ergot alkaloids†, HMG-CoA inhibitors†, indinavir, ketoconazole, lopinavir, macrolides†, midazolam, nelfinavir, nevirapine, phenobarbital, phenytoin, rifabutin, rifampin, ritonavir, sildenafil, terfenadine, triazolam

ALLERGIC REACTIONS AND SIDE EFFECTS

You should tell your doctor about all your allergies and any unexplained symptoms you may have while taking this drug.

LESS COMMON SIDE EFFECTS: Abdominal pain, diarrhea, headache, mouth sores, weakness

RARE SIDE EFFECTS: Bad breath*, burning sensation*, confusion*, dehydration*, dry skin*, hunger*, itching*, nausea*, skin rash*, thirst*, tiredness*, urinary changes*, vomiting*, weight loss*

PRECAUTIONS

§Fortovase and Invirase are formulated differently and cannot be substituted for one another. The product Invirase is being phased out and replaced by Fortovase, which is formulated for better results.

Fortovase capsules are not good after 3 months from the time your prescription is filled and should be thrown out.

Hemophiliacs may be at greater risk of developing bleeding while taking this drug.

This drug is usually prescribed in combination with another antiretroviral drug†. Ask your pharmacist about the type of drug interaction that may occur between antiretroviral drugs† to coordinate the administration times of multiple drugs.

If you are taking sildenafil while on this drug, there may be an increased risk of low blood pressure, visual changes, and prolonged penile erection.

PREGNANCY AND BREAST-FEEDING

Safety during pregnancy has not been established although there was no evidence of harm during studies in animals.

Breast-feeding while taking this drug is not recommended.

HELPFUL COMMENTS

Do not stop treatment early if you start to feel better. It takes the full prescription for this drug to work completely.

This drug may cause you to gain or redistribute body fat.

---

†See page 52.   *See page 53.

SECOBARBITAL SODIUM

Available for over 20 years

COMMONLY USED TO TREAT

Sleeping difficulty, also known as insomnia

DRUG CATEGORY

sedative-hypnotic
Class: barbiturate

PRODUCTS

Brand-Name Products with No Generic Alternative
Seconal Sodium 50 mg capsule (n/a)
Brand-Name Products with Generic Alternatives
Seconal Sodium 100 mg capsule (¢¢¢¢)
  Generic: secobarbital sodium 100 mg capsule (n/a)

DOSING AND FOOD

Doses are taken 1 to 4 times a day.
It is best to take this drug on an empty stomach with a full glass of water at
  least 1 hour before or 2 hours after meals.
Adults: Up to 200 mg per day in divided doses.
Children: Up to 6 mg/kg (maximum 100 mg) per day in divided doses.
Forgotten doses: Do not take a forgotten dose. Just go back to your usual
  schedule with the next dose.

ALCOHOL, DRUG, HERB, AND SUPPLEMENT INTERACTIONS

Alcohol should not be used while taking this drug.
Several OTC drugs used for appetite control, asthma, colds, cough, hay
  fever, pain, or sinus problems may seriously increase the side effects of
  this drug. Check with your pharmacist when selecting OTC products.
Taking this drug with any of the ones listed below may change the effect of
either drug with the possibility of causing toxicity or decreasing effectiveness:
anticoagulants†, carbamazepine, corticosteroids†, corticotropin, divalproex
  sodium, oral contraceptives†, valproic acid
Increased side effects are possible when this drug is taken with those listed below:
anesthetics, antihistamines†, anxiolytics†, barbiturates†, tricyclic antide-
  pressants†

ALLERGIC REACTIONS AND SIDE EFFECTS

Allergic reactions are more likely to occur in people with a history of asthma or allergies to other drugs. You should tell your doctor about all your allergies and any unexplained symptoms you may have while taking this drug.

MORE COMMON SIDE EFFECTS: Clumsiness, dizziness, drowsiness, lightheadedness, unsteadiness

LESS COMMON SIDE EFFECTS: Anxiety, confusion*, constipation, depression*, excitement*, fainting, headache, irritability, nausea, nervousness, sleep disorders, vomiting

RARE SIDE EFFECTS: Bleeding*, bone pain*, bruising*, chest pain*, chest tightness*, fever*, hallucinations*, hives*, loss of appetite*, mouth sores*, muscle pain*, skin rash*, sore throat*, swelling*, tiredness*, weakness*, weight loss*, wheezing*, yellow eyes or skin*

PRECAUTIONS

Be careful driving or handling equipment while taking this drug because the drug may cause dizziness and drowsiness.

Children and people over age 65 often become hyperactive while taking this drug.

If you have anemia, asthma, high blood sugar, hyperactivity, depression, thyroid problems, liver disease, kidney disease, or porphyria, this drug may make those conditions worse.

This drug may be habit forming when taken for a long time. It should be stopped slowly to avoid withdrawal symptoms. It may take 2 weeks for the body to adjust after the drug is stopped. If you wish to stop taking this drug, ask your doctor for specific instructions.

PREGNANCY AND BREAST-FEEDING

There is evidence that this drug may harm the fetus, but the drug may be necessary to the health of the mother.

This drug passes into breast milk, and may cause drowsiness, slow heartbeat, and breathing difficulty in the baby.

HELPFUL COMMENTS

If used regularly for more than 2 weeks, this drug may lose the ability to make you sleep.

Oral contraceptives may not work properly when taken with this drug. You need to use a barrier contraceptive, such as a condom, or other nonhormonal contraceptive to prevent pregnancy.

---

†See page 52. *See page 53.

This drug has a calming effect and is also used to treat anxiety.

You may need to increase the fiber in your diet since this drug may cause constipation.

SELEGILINE HYDROCHLORIDE

Available since June 1989

COMMONLY USED TO TREAT

Symptoms of Parkinson's disease

DRUG CATEGORY

antidyskinetic

Class: monoamine oxidase inhibitor

PRODUCTS

Brand-Name Products with Generic Alternatives

Eldepryl 5 mg capsule ($$$)

   Generic: selegiline hydrochloride 5 mg capsule ($$$)

Products Only Available as Generics

selegiline hydrochloride 5 mg tablet (¢¢¢)

DOSING AND FOOD

Doses are taken twice a day.

This drug should be taken with breakfast and lunch. Do not eat or drink caffeine, cocoa, or high-tyramine foods while taking this drug. Foods that are high in tyramine may interact with the drug causing elevation in blood pressure. Foods prepared by aging, fermentation, pickling, or smoking, such as aged cheese, red wine, soy sauce, tap beer (including alcohol-free beer), sauerkraut, bologna, pepperoni, salami, summer sausage, and dried meats, are considered high in tyramine.

Adults: Up to 10 mg per day in divided doses.

Forgotten doses: If you are scheduled to take the next dose within a few hours, do not take the forgotten dose. Otherwise take the forgotten dose as soon as you remember.

ALCOHOL, DRUG, HERB, AND SUPPLEMENT INTERACTIONS

Alcohol should not be used while taking this drug.

Ginseng may increase the risk of developing side effects when taken with this drug.

Taking this drug with any of the ones listed below may change the effect of either drug with the possibility of causing toxicity or decreasing effectiveness: adrenergics†

Severe reactions are possible when this drug is taken with those listed below: meperidine

Increased side effects are possible when this drug is taken with those listed below: antidepressants†, fluoxetine, fluvoxamine, nefazodone, paroxetine, sertraline, venlafaxine

ALLERGIC REACTIONS AND SIDE EFFECTS

You should tell your doctor about all your allergies and any unexplained symptoms you may have while taking this drug.

This drug promotes the effect of sunlight on the body and may cause severe sunburn and increased sensitivity of the eyes.

MORE COMMON SIDE EFFECTS: Abdominal pain, dizziness*, dry mouth, fainting*, mood swings*, nausea*, sleep disorders, spastic movements*, vomiting*

LESS COMMON SIDE EFFECTS: Anxiety, back pain, black stools*, bloody vomit*, blurry vision, breathing difficulty*, burning mouth, chest tightness*, chewing motion*, chills, constipation, diarrhea, drowsiness, hallucinations*, headache*, heartburn, irregular heartbeat*, irritability*, lightheadedness*, lip smacking*, loss of appetite, memory loss, nervousness, numbness, poor balance*, puffy cheeks*, restlessness*, ringing in ears, skin irritation, speaking difficulty*, stomach pain*, sweating*, swelling*, taste changes, tiredness, tongue movements*, urinary changes*, weakness, weight loss, wheezing*

RARE SIDE EFFECTS: Agitation*, blood pressure changes*, bruxism, chest pain*, fever*, large pupils*, lockjaw*, seizures*, sore neck*

PRECAUTIONS

If you have a history of stomach ulcers, this drug may make that condition worse.

Be careful driving or handling equipment while taking this drug because it may cause dizziness.

Doses higher than 10 mg per day have not demonstrated any additional benefit and are associated with more side effects.

This drug may cause dry mouth, which is associated with a greater risk of cavities. Your dentist may recommend that you clean your teeth and mouth differently to avoid infection.

---

† See page 52.   * See page 53.

PREGNANCY AND BREAST-FEEDING

Safety during pregnancy has not been established although the drug is known to harm animal fetuses.

It is not known if this drug passes into breast milk. Talk to your doctor about the risks associated with breast-feeding while taking this drug.

HELPFUL COMMENTS

This drug may also be called by the generic name L-deprenyl hydrochloride.

The effects of this drug should be noticed within 2 to 3 days.

Eye irritation caused by the sun may be reduced by wearing sunglasses when outside.

It takes about 2 weeks for this drug to be removed from the body after it is stopped. All restrictions on food and drug intake should continue during that period.

Sucking on hard sugarless candy or chewing sugarless gum may help relieve dry mouth caused by this drug.

Take the last dose of the day by 1:00 P.M. to reduce the chance of insomnia during the night.

SERTRALINE HYDROCHLORIDE

Available since December 1991

COMMONLY USED TO TREAT

Depression

Panic attacks

Premature ejaculation

DRUG CATEGORY

antidepressant

Class: selective serotonin reuptake inhibitor (SSRI)

PRODUCTS

Brand-Name Products with No Generic Alternative

Zoloft 25 mg tablet ($$$)

Zoloft 50 mg tablet ($$$)

Zoloft 100 mg tablet ($$$)

Zoloft 20 mg/ml oral concentrate ($$$)

No generics available.

Multiple patents that begin to expire in 2005.

DOSING AND FOOD

Doses are taken once a day.

Taking this drug with food will help increase absorption of the drug.

Adults and children over age 6: Up to 200 mg per day.

Lower doses are used in people with liver disease.

Forgotten doses: Do not take a forgotten dose unless told to do so by your doctor.

ALCOHOL, DRUG, HERB, AND SUPPLEMENT INTERACTIONS

Alcohol should not be used while taking this drug.

St. John's wort may cause serious side effects when taken with this drug.

Many OTC drugs used for appetite control, asthma, colds, cough, hay fever, pain, or sinus problems affect the central nervous system and may change the effects or side effects of this drug. Check with your pharmacist for products to avoid.

Taking this drug with any of the ones listed below may change the effect of either drug with the possibility of causing toxicity or decreasing effectiveness: aspirin, cimetidine, diazepam, digitoxin, tolbutamide, warfarin

Severe reactions are possible when this drug is taken with those listed below: astemizole, bromocriptine, buspirone, dextromethorphan, disulfiram, levodopa, lithium, LSD, MDMA (ecstasy), meperidine, moclobemide, monoamine oxidase inhibitors†, nefazodone, pentazocine, SSRIs†, sumatriptan, terfenadine, tramadol, trazodone, tricyclic antidepressants†, tryptophan, venlafaxine

ALLERGIC REACTIONS AND SIDE EFFECTS

You should tell your doctor about all your allergies and any unexplained symptoms you may have while taking this drug.

MORE COMMON SIDE EFFECTS: Diarrhea, dizziness, drowsiness*, dry mouth*, gas, headache, loss of appetite, nausea*, sexual dysfunction*, shaking*, sleep disorders, stomach cramps, sweating*, tiredness, trembling, weakness, weight loss

LESS COMMON SIDE EFFECTS: Agitation, anxiety*, blurry vision, breast enlargement*, breast-milk secretion*, confusion*, constipation, diarrhea*, fever*, flushing, increased appetite, hives*, irregular heartbeat*, itching*, lack of energy*, large pupils*, mood swings*, nervousness, nosebleeds*, restlessness*, seizures*, shivering*, skin irritation*, spastic movements*, thirst*, vision changes, vomiting*

---

†*See page 52.*   **See page 53.*

PRECAUTIONS

You need to wait 2 weeks after stopping a monoamine oxidase inhibitor†
and 1 week after stopping moclobemide before starting this drug.

People with a history of seizures, brain damage, or mental disorders are at
greater risk of developing a seizure while taking this drug.

If you have a history of mania, this drug may make that condition worse.

Be careful driving or handling equipment while taking this drug because
the drug may cause drowsiness.

Stopping this drug suddenly may cause severe side effects. If you wish to
stop taking this drug, ask your doctor for specific instructions.

The dropper that comes with the oral concentrate product may contain
latex and should not be used in people with a latex allergy.

This drug may cause dry mouth, which is associated with a greater risk of
cavities. Your dentist may recommend that you clean your teeth and
mouth differently to avoid infection.

PREGNANCY AND BREAST-FEEDING

Safety during pregnancy has not been established although the drug is
known to harm animal fetuses.

This drug passes into breast milk, but does not appear to harm the baby.
Talk to your doctor about the risks associated with breast-feeding while
taking this drug.

HELPFUL COMMENTS

It takes a week for this drug to begin to take effect and up to 4 weeks before the full effects are noticed.

Oral concentrate products may be mixed with $1/2$ cup of water, ginger ale,
lemonade, orange juice, or lemon-lime soda. Do not measure doses of
the oral concentrate with anything but a measuring cup intended for use
with prescription drugs or the dropper provided. Slight inaccuracy from
other measuring spoons may result in over- or under-dosing.

SEVELAMER HYDROCHLORIDE

Available since October 1998

COMMONLY USED TO TREAT

High phosphate levels in the blood, also known as hyperphosphatemia

DRUG CATEGORY

antihyperphosphatemic
Class: polymeric phosphate binder

PRODUCTS

Brand-Name Products with No Generic Alternative
Renagel 403 mg capsule (¢¢¢¢)
Renagel 400 mg tablet (¢¢¢¢)
Renagel 800 mg tablet ($)
No generics available.
Multiple patents that begin to expire in 2013.

DOSING AND FOOD

Doses are taken 3 times a day.
It is best to take this drug with meals.
Adults and children: Doses are based on blood levels of phosphate.
Forgotten doses: If you are scheduled to take the next dose within a few
  hours, do not take the forgotten dose. Otherwise take the forgotten dose
  as soon as you remember.

ALCOHOL, DRUG, HERB, AND SUPPLEMENT INTERACTIONS

Alcohol may increase some of the side effects from this drug, depending
  on the amount consumed. Ask your doctor about the risks caused by
  drinking alcohol with your condition.
No significant interactions with this drug have been found.

ALLERGIC REACTIONS AND SIDE EFFECTS

You should tell your doctor about all your allergies and any unexplained
  symptoms you may have while taking this drug.
LESS COMMON SIDE EFFECTS: Bloating, constipation, diarrhea, gas, heartburn, nausea, vomiting

PRECAUTIONS

People with difficulty swallowing or intestinal disorders may not be able to
  take this drug.
Do not open, crush, break, or chew the capsule products.
This drug should be used in combination with a low-phosphate diet for
  best results.

---

†*See page 52.*   **See page 53.*

PREGNANCY AND BREAST-FEEDING

Safety during pregnancy has not been established although the drug is known to harm animal fetuses.

This drug passes into breast milk, but does not appear to harm the baby. Talk to your doctor about the risks associated with breast-feeding while taking this drug.

HELPFUL COMMENTS

Yogurt, nuts, milk, cheese, peanut butter, bran cereal, dried beans, dried peas, pizza, pudding, oatmeal, brown rice, and cola are all considered high-phosphate foods and should be avoided while taking this drug.

SIBUTRAMINE HYDROCHLORIDE

Available since November 1997

COMMONLY USED TO TREAT

Obesity

DRUG CATEGORY

appetite suppressant
Class: neurotransmitter reuptake inhibitor

PRODUCTS

Brand-Name Products with No Generic Alternative
Meridia 5 mg capsule ($$$)
Meridia 10 mg capsule ($$$)
Meridia 15 mg capsule ($$$)
No generics available.
Multiple patents that begin to expire in 2007.

DOSING AND FOOD

Doses are taken once a day.
This drug may be taken with or without food.
Adults: Up to 15 mg per day.

Forgotten doses: If more than 3 hours have passed since the forgotten dose, do not take the dose. Otherwise take the forgotten dose as soon as you remember.

ALCOHOL, DRUG, HERB, AND SUPPLEMENT INTERACTIONS

Alcohol should not be used while taking this drug.

L-tryptophan may trigger serious side effects when taken with this drug and should not be used.

Many OTC drugs used for appetite control, asthma, colds, cough, hay fever, pain, or sinus problems affect the central nervous system and may change the effects or side effects of this drug. Check with your pharmacist for products to avoid.

Severe reactions are possible when this drug is taken with those listed below: bromocriptine, buspirone, dextromethorphan, dihydroergotamine, fentanyl, fluoxetine, fluvoxamine, levodopa, lithium, LSD, marijuana, meperidine, moclobemide, monoamine oxidase inhibitors†, MDMA (ecstasy), nefazodone, paroxetine, pentazocine, sertraline, SSRIs†, sumatriptan, tramadol, trazodone, tricyclic antidepressants†, venlafaxine

Increased side effects are possible when this drug is taken with those listed below: analgesics, anesthetics, antihistamines†, anxiolytics†, barbiturates†, epinephrine, narcotics†, pseudoephedrine

ALLERGIC REACTIONS AND SIDE EFFECTS

You should tell your doctor about all your allergies and any unexplained symptoms you may have while taking this drug.

MORE COMMON SIDE EFFECTS: Anxiety, constipation, dizziness, dry mouth, headache, irritability, nervousness, sleep disorders, stuffy nose

LESS COMMON SIDE EFFECTS: Abdominal pain, back pain, body aches* burning, chills*, depression*, diarrhea, drowsiness, flushing, increased appetite, increased blood pressure*, indigestion, irregular heartbeat*, itching, menstrual pain*, nausea, sweating, swelling*, taste changes, thirst, tingling

RARE SIDE EFFECTS: Bleeding*, bruising*, headache*, mood swings*, seizures*, skin irritation*, weight gain*

PRECAUTIONS

If you have glaucoma, gallstones, high blood pressure, or an eating disorder, this drug may make those conditions worse.

People with a history of mental retardation, brain disease, or seizures are at a greater risk of developing a seizure while taking this drug.

If you are being treated for high blood pressure, you may need to have your dose adjusted while taking this drug.

---

†See page 52.   *See page 53.

You need to wait 2 weeks after stopping a monoamine oxidase inhibitor†
and 1 week after stopping moclobemide before starting this drug.

Be careful driving or handling equipment while taking this drug because it
may cause dizziness.

This drug may cause dry mouth, which is associated with a greater risk of
cavities. Your dentist may recommend that you clean your teeth and
mouth differently to avoid infection.

PREGNANCY AND BREAST-FEEDING

Safety during pregnancy has not been established although the drug is
known to harm animal fetuses.

Breast-feeding while taking this drug is not recommended.

HELPFUL COMMENTS

Sucking on hard sugarless candy or chewing sugarless gum may help relieve dry mouth caused by this drug.

Avoid quick movements to minimize dizziness. Dangling your legs over the
side of the bed for a few minutes may help reduce dizziness when first
waking up.

You should lose at least 4 pounds in the first 4 weeks of taking this drug. If
not, this drug may not be the best treatment option.

SILDENAFIL CITRATE

Available since March 1998

COMMONLY USED TO TREAT

Impotence, also known as erectile dysfunction

DRUG CATEGORY

impotence agent
Class: phosphodiesterase delayer

PRODUCTS

Brand-Name Products with No Generic Alternative
Viagra 25 mg tablet ($$$$)
Viagra 50 mg tablet ($$$$)
Viagra 100 mg tablet ($$$$)
No generics available.
Multiple patents that begin to expire in 2012.

DOSING AND FOOD

Doses are taken once a day 1 hour before sexual activity.

It is best to take this drug on an empty stomach.

Adults: Up to 100 mg per day.

Lower doses are used in people over age 65 and people with kidney disease or liver disease.

ALCOHOL, DRUG, HERB, AND SUPPLEMENT INTERACTIONS

Alcohol may increase some of the side effects from this drug, depending on the amount consumed. Ask your doctor about the risks caused by drinking alcohol with your condition.

Taking this drug with any of the ones listed below may change the effect of either drug with the possibility of causing toxicity or decreasing effectiveness: delavirdine, rifampin

Severe reactions are possible when this drug is taken with those listed below: nitrates†

Increased side effects are possible when this drug is taken with those listed below: cimetidine, erythromycin, itraconazole, ketoconazole, mibefradil, ritonavir, saquinavir

ALLERGIC REACTIONS AND SIDE EFFECTS

You should tell your doctor about all your allergies and any unexplained symptoms you may have while taking this drug.

This drug may cause your eyes to be more sensitive to sunlight, but there are no special risks associated with sunburn while taking this drug.

MORE COMMON SIDE EFFECTS: Congestion, flushing, headache, stomachache

LESS COMMON SIDE EFFECTS: Bladder pain*, bloody urine*, blurry vision*, diarrhea, dizziness*, urinary changes*, vision changes*

RARE SIDE EFFECTS: Anxiety, eye bleeding*, eye swelling*, painful penile erection*, seizures*, temporary blindness*

PRECAUTIONS

People with a history of arrhythmias, heart attack, high blood pressure, low blood pressure, stroke, bleeding disorders, retinitis pigmentosa, or coronary artery disease may not be able to take this drug.

If you have leukemia, multiple myeloma, polycythemia, sickle cell disease, thrombocythemia, or a history of priapism, you may be at greater risk

---

†See page 52.   *See page 53.

of developing painful, prolonged penile erection. Call the doctor right away if your erection lasts longer than 4 hours.

This drug does not prevent the spread of sexually transmitted diseases.

A full examination of the heart should be conducted before this drug is used.

PREGNANCY AND BREAST-FEEDING

Safety during pregnancy has not been established although there was no evidence of harm during studies in animals.

Breast-feeding while taking this drug is not recommended.

HELPFUL COMMENTS

It may take anywhere from 30 minutes to 4 hours for the effects of this drug to be noticed, although 2 hours is most common.

SIMVASTATIN

Available since December 1991

COMMONLY USED TO TREAT

High blood cholesterol and lipids, also known as hyperlipidemia

DRUG CATEGORY

antilipemic
Class: HMG-CoA reductase inhibitor (statin)

PRODUCTS

Brand-Name Products with No Generic Alternative
Zocor 5 mg capsule ($$)
Zocor 10 mg capsule ($$$)
Zocor 20 mg capsule ($$$)
Zocor 40 mg capsule ($$$)
Zocor 80 mg capsule ($$$)
No generics available.
Multiple patents that begin to expire in 2005.

DOSING AND FOOD

Doses are taken once a day in the evening.

This drug may be taken with or without food. Do not take this drug with grapefruit juice.

Adults: Up to 80 mg per day.

Forgotten doses: If you are scheduled to take the next dose within a few hours, do not take the forgotten dose. Otherwise take the forgotten dose as soon as you remember.

ALCOHOL, DRUG, HERB, AND SUPPLEMENT INTERACTIONS

Alcohol should not be used while taking this drug.

Red yeast rice, banned from sale in the U.S. since 2001, contains a nutrient similar to this class of drugs and may cause toxicity if used while taking this drug.

Taking this drug with any of the ones listed below may change the effect of either drug with the possibility of causing toxicity or decreasing effectiveness: digoxin, warfarin

Severe reactions are possible when this drug is taken with those listed below: cimetidine, clofibrate, erythromycin, fenofibrate, fibric acid derivatives†, gemfibrozil, immunosuppressants†, ketoconazole, protease inhibitors†, spironolactone, verapamil

Increased side effects are possible when this drug is taken with those listed below: acetaminophen, amiodarone, anabolic steroids†, androgens†, antibiotics†, antithyroid drugs†, carbamazepine, carmustine, chloroquine, dantrolene, daunorubicin, disulfiram, divalproex, etretinate, gold salts†, hydroxychloroquine, isoniazid, mercaptopurine, methotrexate, naltrexone, oral contraceptives, phenothiazines†, phenytoin, plicamycin, valproic acid

ALLERGIC REACTIONS AND SIDE EFFECTS

If you are allergic to any HMG-CoA reductase inhibitors†, you may also be allergic to this drug. You should tell your doctor about all your allergies and any unexplained symptoms you may have while taking this drug.

MORE COMMON SIDE EFFECTS: Fever*, muscle cramps*

LESS COMMON SIDE EFFECTS: Blurry vision, chest pain*, constipation, diarrhea, dizziness, gas, hair loss, headache, heartburn, itching, nausea, numbness, skin rash, sleeping difficulty, stomach pain*, tingling, tiredness*, vomiting, weakness*

RARE SIDE EFFECTS: Sexual dysfunction

PRECAUTIONS

People with liver disease may not be able to take this drug.

Liver function should be tested every 1 to 6 months while taking this drug.

---

† See page 52.   * See page 53.

PREGNANCY AND BREAST-FEEDING

This drug may cause birth defects and should not be used during pregnancy. Breast-feeding while taking this drug is not recommended.

HELPFUL COMMENTS

You need to continue with a low-cholesterol diet even after this drug is started.

It takes about 4 weeks for the effects of this drug to be noticed.

SIROLIMUS

Available since August 2000

COMMONLY USED TO TREAT

Kidney transplant recipients to reduce the risk of rejection

DRUG CATEGORY

immunosuppressant
Class: macrocyclic lactone

PRODUCTS

Brand-Name Products with No Generic Alternative
Rapamune 1 mg tablet ($$$$)
Rapamune 2 mg tablet (n/a)
Rapamune 1 mg/ml oral solution ($$$$$)
No generics available.
Multiple patents that begin to expire in 2009.

DOSING AND FOOD

Doses are taken once a day.

This drug may be taken with or without food, but should be taken the same way with each dose. Do not drink grapefruit juice or eat grapefruit while taking this drug. Do not eat raw oysters or other raw shellfish at any time while taking this drug.

Adults and children over age 13 and more than 88 pounds: Up to 2 mg per day.

Children over age 10 and less than 88 pounds: Up to 1 mg/m^2 per day.

Lower doses are used in people with liver disease.

Forgotten doses: If more than 12 hours have passed since the forgotten dose, do not take the dose. Otherwise take the forgotten dose as soon as you remember.

ALCOHOL, DRUG, HERB, AND SUPPLEMENT INTERACTIONS

Alcohol should not be used while taking this drug.

St. John's wort may decrease the effects of this drug and should not be used.

Taking this drug with any of the ones listed below may change the effect of either drug with the possibility of causing toxicity or decreasing effectiveness: bromocriptine, carbamazepine, cimetidine, clarithromycin, clotrimazole, cyclosporine, danazol, diltiazem, erythromycin, fluconazole, indinavir, itraconazole, ketoconazole, live virus vaccines, metoclopramide, nicardipine, phenobarbital, phenytoin, rifabutin, rifampin, rifapentine, ritonavir, verapamil

Severe reactions are possible when this drug is taken with those listed below: tacrolimus

Increased side effects are possible when this drug is taken with those listed below: aminoglycosides†, amphotericin B

ALLERGIC REACTIONS AND SIDE EFFECTS

You should tell your doctor about all your allergies and any unexplained symptoms you may have while taking this drug.

MORE COMMON SIDE EFFECTS: Abdominal pain*, acne, anxiousness*, back pain*, black stools*, bleeding*, bloody urine*, bone pain*, breathing difficulty*, bruising*, chest pain*, chills*, confusion*, constipation, cough*, diarrhea, fever*, headache, irregular heartbeat*, lack of energy, loss of appetite*, mood swings*, mouth sores*, muscle pain*, nausea*, numbness*, seizures*, shortness of breath*, skin rash*, sleep disorders, sore throat*, stiffness, swelling*, swollen glands*, thirst*, tingling*, tiredness*, trembling, urinary changes*, vomiting*, weakness*, weight loss*, yellow eyes or skin*

LESS COMMON SIDE EFFECTS: Nosebleeds, skin sores*

RARE SIDE EFFECTS: Poor wound healing*, weight gain*

PRECAUTIONS

If cyclosporine is taken in addition to this drug, the doses should be separated by at least 4 hours to avoid a drug interaction.

Avoid contact with anyone who has the chickenpox, measles, or other communicable disease since it may be easier to catch the infection while taking this drug.

---

†*See page 52.*   **See page 53.*

Exposure to skin tests, immunizations, and people who have received immunizations may put you at a greater risk of developing the disease when you are taking this drug.

If you have cancer or high cholesterol, this drug may make those conditions worse.

Use only a glass or plastic container for mixing the oral solution product.

This drug may cause changes to your gums and mouth. Your dentist may recommend that you clean your teeth and mouth differently to avoid infection.

This drug causes changes in your blood that put you at greater risk of getting an infection. Be careful not to cut yourself or get bruised. Tell your doctor if you develop signs of infection, such as fever or sore throat.

Touching these tablets may cause skin irritation. You should wash your hands immediately after taking the dose.

PREGNANCY AND BREAST-FEEDING

Safety during pregnancy has not been established although the drug is known to harm animal fetuses.

Breast-feeding while taking this drug is not recommended.

HELPFUL COMMENTS

Do not stop treatment early if you start to feel better. You may need to stay on this drug for life.

Oral solution products should be mixed with $1/4$ cup of water or orange juice before taking.

The oral solution may get hazy when stored in the refrigerator. This does not affect the drug and will go away when the solution returns to room temperature and is gently shaken.

This drug may stay in your body for as long as 4 months after it is stopped. You should continue to avoid foods, supplements, and drugs that may interact with this drug. Watch for side effects during this period and make sure to avoid pregnancy.

SOTALOL HYDROCHLORIDE

Available since October 1992

COMMONLY USED TO TREAT

Chest pain, also known as angina
High blood pressure, also known as hypertension

Irregular heart rhythm, also known as arrhythmia
Preventable complications after a heart attack

DRUG CATEGORY

antianginal
antiarrhythmic
antihypertensive
Class: beta blocker

PRODUCTS

Brand-Name Products with No Generic Alternative
Betapace AF 80 mg tablet ($$$)
Betapace AF 120 mg tablet ($$$)
Betapace AF 160 mg tablet ($$$)

Brand-Name Products with Generic Alternatives
Betapace 80 mg tablet ($$$)
   Generic: sotalol hydrochloride 80 mg tablet (¢¢¢¢¢)
Betapace 120 mg tablet ($$$)
   Generic: sotalol hydrochloride 120 mg tablet ($$$)
Betapace 160 mg tablet ($$$)
   Generic: sotalol hydrochloride 160 mg tablet ($$$)
Betapace 240 mg tablet ($$$$)
   Generic: sotalol hydrochloride 240 mg tablet ($$$$)

Other Generic Product Names
Sorine

DOSING AND FOOD

Doses are taken twice a day.
This drug should be taken on an empty stomach.
Adults: Up to 640 mg per day in divided doses.
Lower doses are used in people with renal disease.
This drug is rarely used in children.
Forgotten doses: If you are scheduled to take the next dose within 8 hours, do not take the forgotten dose. Otherwise take the forgotten dose as soon as you remember.

ALCOHOL, DRUG, HERB, AND SUPPLEMENT INTERACTIONS

Alcohol may increase some of the side effects from this drug, depending on the amount consumed. Ask your doctor about the risks caused by drinking alcohol with your condition.

---

† See page 52.   * See page 53.

Several OTC drugs used for appetite control, asthma, colds, cough, hay fever, or sinus problems may cause an increase in blood pressure when taken with this drug. Check with your pharmacist when selecting OTC products.

Taking this drug with any of the ones listed below may change the effect of either drug with the possibility of causing toxicity or decreasing effectiveness:
aminophylline, anesthetics†, antidiabetics†, caffeine, calcium channel blockers†, carbonic anhydrase inhibitors†, clonidine, dyphylline, epinephrine, guanabenz, insulin, lidocaine, nonsteroidal antiinflammatories†, oxtriphylline, pilocarpine, reserpine, theophylline

Severe reactions are possible when this drug is taken with those listed below:
allergy shots, beta blockers†, cocaine, monoamine oxidase inhibitors†

Increased effects or side effects are possible when this drug is taken with those listed below:
antihypertensives†

ALLERGIC REACTIONS AND SIDE EFFECTS

If you are allergic to any other beta blockers†, you may also be allergic to this drug.

This drug may exaggerate the reaction from your current allergies. Inform your doctor of any allergies that you have as well as the severity of the allergic reaction before starting this drug.

MORE COMMON SIDE EFFECTS: Dizziness*, drowsiness*, lightheadedness*, sexual dysfunction, sleeping difficulty, tiredness, weakness

LESS COMMON SIDE EFFECTS: Anxiety, breathing difficulty*, cold hands and feet*, constipation, depression*, diarrhea, irregular heartbeat*, itching, nausea, nervousness, numbness, shortness of breath*, sore eyes, stomachache, stuffy nose, swelling*, tingling, vivid dreams, vomiting, wheezing

RARE SIDE EFFECTS: Back pain*, bleeding*, bruising*, chest pain*, confusion*, fever*, hallucinations*, joint pain*, rash*, scaly skin*, sore throat*

PRECAUTIONS

People with heart disease or a heart rate that is routinely less than 60 beats per minute (bradycardia) may not be able to take this drug.

Stopping this drug suddenly may cause chest pain or heart attack. If you wish to stop taking this drug, ask your doctor for specific instructions.

Be careful driving or handling equipment while taking this drug because the drug may cause dizziness and drowsiness.

If you are diabetic, this drug may increase blood sugar levels or make the symptoms of low blood sugar less noticeable.

You need to wait 2 weeks after stopping a monoamine oxidase inhibitor† before starting this drug.

If you have psoriasis or myasthenia gravis, this drug may make those conditions worse.

PREGNANCY AND BREAST-FEEDING

Safety during pregnancy has not been established although the drug is known to harm animal fetuses.

Breast-feeding while taking this drug is not recommended.

HELPFUL COMMENTS

This drug is usually started in the hospital where heart rhythm can be monitored.

If you need to take an antacid, take it either 2 hours before or after taking this drug.

This drug may make you more sensitive to cold temperatures.

If you do not treat high blood pressure, you may develop more serious problems such as heart failure, blood vessel disease, stroke, or kidney disease. Losing weight, exercising, eating more fruits and vegetables, and avoiding salty foods, such as lunchmeat and pickles, may help make drug treatment more successful.

SPARFLOXACIN

Available since December 1996

COMMONLY USED TO TREAT

Infection

DRUG CATEGORY

antibiotic
Class: fluoroquinolone

PRODUCTS

Brand-Name Products with No Generic Alternative
Zagam 200 mg tablet ($$$$)
No generics available.
Patent expires in 2010.

---

† See page 52.   * See page 53.

DOSING AND FOOD

Doses are taken once a day.

It is best to take this drug on an empty stomach, 2 hours after a meal.

Adults: Up to 200 mg per day.

A single 400 mg dose is taken at the beginning of treatment.

Lower doses are used in people with kidney disease.

This drug is rarely used by mouth in children under age 18 because it may interfere with bone development.

Forgotten doses: If you are scheduled to take the next dose within a few hours, do not take the forgotten dose. Otherwise take the forgotten dose as soon as you remember.

ALCOHOL, DRUG, HERB, AND SUPPLEMENT INTERACTIONS

Alcohol may increase some of the side effects from this drug, depending on the amount consumed. Ask your doctor about the risks caused by drinking alcohol with your condition.

Taking this drug with any of the ones listed below may change the effect of either drug with the possibility of causing toxicity or decreasing effectiveness: antacids, didanosine, iron supplements, mineral supplements, sucralfate

Severe reactions are possible when this drug is taken with those listed below: amiodarone, antipsychotics†, astemizole, bepridil, cisapride, erythromycin, nonsteroidal antiinflammatories†, phenothiazines†, procainamide, quinidine, sotalol, tricyclic antidepressants†

ALLERGIC REACTIONS AND SIDE EFFECTS

If you are allergic to any fluoroquinolones†, you may also be allergic to this drug. You should tell your doctor about all your allergies and any unexplained symptoms you may have while taking this drug.

This drug promotes the effect of sunlight on the body and may cause severe sunburn and increased sensitivity of the eyes.

MORE COMMON SIDE EFFECTS: Irregular heartbeat*

LESS COMMON SIDE EFFECTS: Back pain, blisters*, diarrhea*, difficulty urinating, dizziness, dreams, drowsiness, headache, lightheadedness, muscle pain, nausea, nervousness, rash, seizures*, skin irritation*, sleep disorders, sore mouth, stomachache, taste changes, vaginal discharge, vaginal pain, vision changes, vomiting

RARE SIDE EFFECTS: Abdominal pain*, agitation*, bloody urine*, confusion*, dark urine*, fever*, flushing*, hallucinations*, joint pain*, leg pain*, loss of appetite*, pale stools*, shakiness*, shortness of breath*, sweating*, swelling*, tiredness*, tremors*, weakness*, yellow eyes or skin*

PRECAUTIONS

Be careful driving or handling equipment while taking this drug because the drug may cause dizziness and drowsiness.

If you have a history of tendinitis, this drug may make that condition worse.

PREGNANCY AND BREAST-FEEDING

Safety during pregnancy has not been established although the drug is known to harm animal fetuses.

Breast-feeding while taking this drug is not recommended.

HELPFUL COMMENTS

Contact your doctor if your symptoms do not improve after a couple of days.

Do not stop treatment early if you start to feel better. It takes the full prescription for this drug to work completely.

If you need to take an antacid, minerals, or iron supplements, take them either 2 hours before or 4 hours after taking this drug.

Drink a lot of water while taking this drug.

SPIRONOLACTONE

Available for over 20 years

COMMONLY USED TO TREAT

Abnormal hair gowth
Acne
Fluid (water) retention, also known as edema
High blood pressure, also known as hypertension

DRUG CATEGORY

antihypertensive
Class: potassium sparing diuretic

PRODUCTS

Brand-Name Products with Generic Alternatives
Aldactone 25 mg tablet (¢¢¢¢)
   Generic: spironolactone 25 mg tablet (¢)

---

† See page 52.   * See page 53.

Aldactone 50 mg tablet (¢¢¢¢¢)
  Generic: spironolactone 50 mg tablet (¢¢¢¢¢)
Aldactone 100 mg tablet ($$)
  Generic: spironolactone 100 mg tablet ($)

Combination Products That Contain This Drug
Aldactazide tablet (¢¢¢¢) to ($)

DOSING AND FOOD

Doses are taken 1 to 4 times a day.
This drug may be taken with or without food.

Adults: Up to 200 mg per day in divided doses.

Children: Up to 4 mg/kg per day in divided doses.

Forgotten doses: If you are scheduled to take the next dose within a few
  hours, do not take the forgotten dose. Otherwise take the forgotten dose
  as soon as you remember.

ALCOHOL, DRUG, HERB, AND SUPPLEMENT INTERACTIONS

Alcohol may increase some of the side effects from this drug, depending
  on the amount consumed. Talk to your doctor about the risks caused by
  drinking alcohol with your condition.

Licorice may interfere with the effects of this drug.

**Taking this drug with any of the ones listed below may change the effect of
either drug with the possibility of causing toxicity or decreasing effectiveness:**
anesthetics, antihypertensives†, aspirin, digoxin, digitoxin, lithium, norep-
inephrine

Severe reactions are possible when this drug is taken with those listed below:
ACE inhibitors†, cyclosporine, nonsteroidal antiinflammatories†, potassium-
containing drugs, potassium-sparing diuretics†

ALLERGIC REACTIONS AND SIDE EFFECTS

If you are allergic to amiloride or triamterene, you may also be allergic to
  this drug. You should tell your doctor about all your allergies and any un-
  explained symptoms you may have while taking this drug.

MORE COMMON SIDE EFFECTS: Diarrhea, nausea, stomach cramps, vomiting

LESS COMMON SIDE EFFECTS: Breast enlargement, breast tenderness, clum-
  siness, dizziness, hair growth, headache, menstrual changes, sexual dys-
  function, sweating, voice deepening

RARE SIDE EFFECTS: Back pain*, breathing difficulty*, chills*, confusion*, cough*, drowsiness*, dry mouth*, fever*, hoarseness*, irregular heartbeat*, itching*, lack of energy*, nervousness*, numbness*, shortness of breath*, skin rash*, thirst*, tingling*, tiredness*, urinary changes*, weakness*

PRECAUTIONS

This drug does not eliminate potassium from the body like other diuretics. Do not add extra potassium to your diet or use salt substitutes that contain potassium while taking this drug. Foods high in potassium include meat, fish, apricots, avocados, bananas, melons, kiwi, lima beans, milk, oranges, potatoes, prunes, spinach, tomatoes, and squash.

People with diabetes, kidney disease, or liver disease may have a greater risk of developing side effects while taking this drug.

If you have menstrual difficulties or experience breast enlargement, this drug may make those conditions worse.

Severe side effects may occur if you get dehydrated or have excess vomiting or diarrhea. Drink plenty of fluids to avoid dehydration when sweating, such as in hot weather and during exercise.

PREGNANCY AND BREAST-FEEDING

Safety during pregnancy has not been established although there was no evidence of harm during studies in animals.

This drug passes into breast milk, but does not appear to harm the baby. Talk to your doctor about the risks associated with breast-feeding while taking this drug.

HELPFUL COMMENTS

It may take 2 to 3 days for the effects of this drug to be noticed and as long as 3 weeks before the full effects are seen.

Take the last dose of the day before 6 P.M. to reduce the chance of having to urinate during the night.

If you do not treat high blood pressure, you may develop more serious problems such as heart failure, blood vessel disease, stroke, or kidney disease. Losing weight, exercising, eating more fruits and vegetables, and avoiding salty foods, such as lunchmeat and pickles, may help make drug treatment more successful.

---

† *See page 52.*   * *See page 53.*

STAVUDINE

Available since June 1994

COMMONLY USED TO TREAT

HIV infection

DRUG CATEGORY

antiretroviral
Class: nucleoside reverse transcriptase inhibitor (NsRTI)

PRODUCTS

Brand-Name Products with No Generic Alternative
Zerit 15 mg capsule ($$$)
Zerit 20 mg capsule ($$$)
Zerit 30 mg capsule ($$$$)
Zerit 40 mg capsule ($$$$)
Zerit 1 mg/ml oral solution ($)
Zerit XR 37.5 mg extended-release capsule (n/a)
Zerit XR 50 mg extended-release capsule (n/a)
Zerit XR 75 mg extended-release capsule (n/a)
Zerit XR 100 mg extended-release capsule (n/a)
No generics available.
Patents expire in 2008.

DOSING AND FOOD

Doses are taken twice a day.
This drug may be taken with or without food.

Adults and children over 132 pounds: Up to 80 mg per day in divided
doses.

Adults and children over 30 pounds: Up to 60 mg per day in divided
doses.

Children under 30 pounds: Up to 1 mg/kg per day in divided doses.
Lower doses are used in people with kidney disease.

Forgotten doses: If you are scheduled to take the next dose within a few
hours, do not take the forgotten dose. Otherwise take the forgotten dose
as soon as you remember.

ALCOHOL, DRUG, HERB, AND SUPPLEMENT INTERACTIONS

Alcohol may increase some of the side effects from this drug, depending

on the amount consumed. Ask your doctor about the risks caused by drinking alcohol with your condition.

Taking this drug with any of the ones listed below may change the effect of either drug with the possibility of causing toxicity or decreasing effectiveness: zidovudine

Severe reactions are possible when this drug is taken with those listed below: didanosine, hydroxyurea

Increased side effects are possible when this drug is taken with those listed below: chloramphenicol, cisplatin, dapsone, ethambutol, ethionamide, hydralazine isoniazid, lithium, metronidazole, nitrofurantoin, phenytoin, vincristine, zalcitabine

ALLERGIC REACTIONS AND SIDE EFFECTS

You should tell your doctor about all your allergies and any unexplained symptoms you may have while taking this drug.

MORE COMMON SIDE EFFECTS: Chills, fever, loss of appetite, numbness*, tingling*, weight loss

LESS COMMON SIDE EFFECTS: Chest tightness*, cough*, diarrhea, dizziness*, fast heartbeat*, headache, hives*, itching*, joint pain*, lack of energy, lack of strength, muscle pain*, shortness of breath*, skin rash*, sleep disorders, stomach pain*, swallowing difficulty*, swollen eyes*, swollen mouth*, tiredness*, weakness*, wheezing*

RARE SIDE EFFECTS: Nausea*, vomiting*

PRECAUTIONS

This drug is not a cure for HIV and does not prevent the transmission of the HIV virus.

People with a history of alcohol abuse or liver disease are at greater risk of developing liver damage while taking this drug.

If you have peripheral neuropathy, this drug may make that condition worse.

This drug is usually prescribed in combination with another antiretroviral drug†. Ask your pharmacist about the type of drug interaction that may occur between antiretroviral drugs† to coordinate the administration times of multiple drugs.

Do not open, crush, break, or chew the extended-release products.

PREGNANCY AND BREAST-FEEDING

Safety during pregnancy has not been established although the drug is known to harm animal fetuses.

---

† See page 52.   * See page 53.

Breast-feeding while taking this drug is not recommended.

HELPFUL COMMENTS

This drug is also called by the generic name d4T.

Do not stop treatment early if you start to feel better. It takes the full prescription for this drug to work completely.

If you develop tingling, numbness, or burning in the hands or feet while taking this drug, you may not be able to continue with this therapy.

SUCCIMER

Available since January 1991

COMMONLY USED TO TREAT

Lead poisoning in children

DRUG CATEGORY

chelating drug
Class: heavy metal antagonist

PRODUCTS

Brand-Name Products with No Generic Alternative
Chemet 100 mg capsule ($$$)
No generics available.
No patents, no exclusivity.

DOSING AND FOOD

Doses are taken 2 to 3 times a day.
This drug may be taken with or without food.

Children: Up to 30 mg/kg per day in divided doses.

Forgotten doses: If you are scheduled to take the next dose within a few hours, do not take the forgotten dose. Otherwise take the forgotten dose as soon as you remember.

ALCOHOL, DRUG, HERB, AND SUPPLEMENT INTERACTIONS

Taking this drug with any of the ones listed below may change the effect of either drug with the possibility of causing toxicity or decreasing effectiveness: penicillamine

ALLERGIC REACTIONS AND SIDE EFFECTS

You should tell your doctor about all your allergies and any unexplained symptoms you may have while taking this drug.

MORE COMMON SIDE EFFECTS: Diarrhea, loss of appetite, nausea, skin rash, vomiting

LESS COMMON SIDE EFFECTS: Chills*, fever

PRECAUTIONS

If you have liver disease, this drug may make that condition worse.

This drug has an unusual smell that makes the capsule difficult to swallow. The contents of the capsule may be mixed with a spoonful of food or fruit juice and taken right away.

Drink 8 to 10 glasses of water each day while taking this drug to reduce the risk of developing serious side effects.

This drug may cause false results from several diagnostic tests.

Liver function should be tested at least every week while taking this drug.

PREGNANCY AND BREAST-FEEDING

Safety during pregnancy has not been established although the drug is known to harm animal fetuses.

Breast-feeding while taking this drug is not recommended.

HELPFUL COMMENTS

This drug may cause an unusual body odor when you sweat and may cause your stools and urine to smell bad.

This drug will not work properly if the source of lead poising has not been identified and removed.

Do not stop treatment early if you start to feel better. It takes the full 19-day prescription for this drug to work completely.

SUCRALFATE

Available for over 20 years

COMMONLY USED TO TREAT

Stomach problems caused by aspirin
Ulcers

DRUG CATEGORY

antiulcer

---

† See page 52. * See page 53.

Class: pepsin inhibitor

PRODUCTS

Brand-Name Products with No Generic Alternative
Carafate 1 g/10 ml oral suspension (¢¢¢)
Brand-Name Products with Generic Alternatives
Carafate 1 g tablet (¢¢¢¢¢)
　Generic: sucralfate 1 g tablet (¢¢¢¢)

DOSING AND FOOD

Doses are taken 2 to 4 times a day.
This drug works best if taken 1 hour before meals.
Adults: Up to 4 g per day in divided doses.
Forgotten doses: If you are scheduled to take the next dose within a few
　hours, do not take the forgotten dose. Otherwise take the forgotten dose
　as soon as you remember.

ALCOHOL, DRUG, HERB, AND SUPPLEMENT INTERACTIONS

Alcohol may make your stomach problems worse. You should ask your
　doctor about the risks caused by drinking alcohol with your condition.
**Taking this drug with any of the ones listed below may change the effect of
either drug with the possibility of causing toxicity or decreasing effectiveness:**
antacids, cimetidine, ciprofloxacin, digoxin, norfloxacin, ofloxacin, phenytoin, quinidine, ranitidine, tetracycline, theophylline, vitamin A, vitamin
D, vitamin E, vitamin K

ALLERGIC REACTIONS AND SIDE EFFECTS

You should tell your doctor about all your allergies and any unexplained
　symptoms you may have while taking this drug.
MORE COMMON SIDE EFFECTS: Constipation
LESS COMMON SIDE EFFECTS: Back pain, diarrhea, dizziness, dry mouth,
　indigestion, itching, lightheadedness, nausea, skin rash, stomach pain
RARE SIDE EFFECTS: Drowsiness*, seizures*

PRECAUTIONS

If you have a history of intestinal obstruction, this drug may make that
　condition worse.
This drug contains aluminum, which may become toxic in people with kid-
　ney disease.

This drug is not taken longer than 8 weeks because of the risk of developing aluminum toxicity.

PREGNANCY AND BREAST-FEEDING

Safety during pregnancy has not been established although there was no evidence of harm during studies in animals.

This drug passes into breast milk, but does not appear to harm the baby.

HELPFUL COMMENTS

If you need to take an antacid, take it either 2 hours before or after taking this drug.

Do not stop treatment early if you start to feel better. It takes the full prescription for this drug to work completely.

If you have difficulty swallowing, the tablets can be made into a suspension by crushing and dissolving them in 1 to 2 tablespoons of water. Make sure you rinse the mixing container and drink to get the full dose.

SULFADIAZINE

Available for over 20 years

COMMONLY USED TO TREAT

Infection
People at risk of developing rheumatic fever
Urinary tract infections

DRUG CATEGORY

antibiotic
Class: sulfonamide

PRODUCTS

Products Only Available as Generics
sulfadiazine 500 mg tablet (n/a)
Combination Products That Contain This Drug
Triple Sulfoid tablet (n/a)

DOSING AND FOOD

Doses are taken 3 to 6 times a day.

---

†See page 52.　　*See page 53.

This drug may be taken with or without food but should always be taken with a full glass of water. Do not eat raw oysters or other raw shellfish at any time while taking this drug.

Adults: Up to 8,000 mg per day in divided doses.

Children: Up to 150 mg/kg (maximum 6,000 mg) per day in divided doses. This drug is not used in children under 2 months old.

Forgotten doses: If you are scheduled to take the next dose within a few hours, do not take the forgotten dose. Otherwise take the forgotten dose as soon as you remember.

ALCOHOL, DRUG, HERB, AND SUPPLEMENT INTERACTIONS

Alcohol may increase some of the side effects from this drug, depending on the amount consumed. Ask your doctor about the risks caused by drinking alcohol with your condition.

Taking this drug with any of the ones listed below may change the effect of either drug with the possibility of causing toxicity or decreasing effectiveness: anticoagulants†, antidiabetics†, sulfonylureas†

Severe reactions are possible when this drug is taken with those listed below: para-aminobenzoic acid, trimethoprim, pyrimethamine

Increased side effects are possible when this drug is taken with those listed below: acetaminophen, acetohydroxamic acid, amiodarone, ammonium chloride, anabolic steroids†, androgens†, antibiotics†, antithyroid drugs†, carbamazepine, carmustine, chloroquine, dantrolene, dapsone, daunorubicin, disulfiram, divalproex, estrogens†, ethotoin, etretinate, furazolidone, gold salts†, hydroxychloroquine, mephenytoin, mercaptopurine, methenamine, methotrexate, methyldopa, naltrexone, nitrofurantoin, oral contraceptives, phenothiazines†, phenytoin, plicamycin, primaquine, procainamide, quinidine, quinine, sulfoxone, valproic acid, vitamin C, vitamin K

ALLERGIC REACTIONS AND SIDE EFFECTS

If you are allergic to furosemide, dichlorphenamide, methazolamide, thiazide diuretics†, antidiabetics†, antiglaucoma drugs†, or any sulfa drugs, you may also be allergic to this drug. You should tell your doctor about all your allergies and any unexplained symptoms you may have while taking this drug.

This drug promotes the effect of sunlight on the body and may cause severe sunburn and increased sensitivity of the eyes.

MORE COMMON SIDE EFFECTS: Diarrhea*, dizziness, headache, itching*, loss of appetite, nausea, skin rash*, tiredness*, vomiting

LESS COMMON SIDE EFFECTS: Bleeding*, bruising*, fever*, joint pain*, muscle pain*, pale skin*, seizures*, skin irritation*, sore throat*, swallowing difficulty*, weakness*, yellow eyes or skin*

RARE SIDE EFFECTS: Abdominal pain*, back pain*, bloody urine*, mood swings*, swelling*, thirst*, urinary changes*

PRECAUTIONS

People with anemia, glucose-6-phosphate dehydrogenase deficiency (G6PD) are at greater risk of developing side effects.

If you have porphyria, this drug may make that condition worse.

This drug may interfere with several diagnostic tests including some urine glucose tests. Diabetics should use glucose oxidase tests or glucose enzyme test strips.

Drink 8 to 10 glasses of water each day while taking this drug to prevent crystals from forming in the kidneys.

This drug causes changes in your blood that put you at greater risk of getting an infection. Be careful not to cut yourself or get bruised. Tell your doctor if you develop signs of infection, such as fever or sore throat. Your dentist may recommend that you clean your teeth and mouth differently to avoid infection.

Be careful driving or handling equipment while taking this drug because it may cause dizziness.

PREGNANCY AND BREAST-FEEDING

Safety during pregnancy has not been established although the drug is known to harm animal fetuses.

Breast-feeding while taking this drug is not recommended.

HELPFUL COMMENTS

Contact your doctor if your symptoms do not improve after a couple of days.

Do not stop treatment early if you start to feel better. It takes the full prescription for this drug to work completely.

Avoid quick movements to minimize dizziness. Dangling your legs over the side of the bed for a few minutes may help reduce dizziness when first waking up.

Eye irritation caused by the sun may be reduced by wearing sunglasses when outside.

---

† See page 52.   * See page 53.

SULFASALAZINE

Available for over 20 years

COMMONLY USED TO TREAT

Arthritis
Intestinal disease, specifically ulcerative colitis

DRUG CATEGORY

antiinflammatory
antirheumatic
Class: sulfonamide

PRODUCTS

Brand-Name Products with No Generic Alternative
Azulfidine 250 mg/5 ml oral suspension (n/a)
Brand-Name Products with Generic Alternatives
Azulfidine 500 mg tablet (¢¢¢)
   Generic: sulfasalazine 500 mg tablet (¢¢)
Azulfidine 500 mg delayed-release tablet (¢¢¢)
   Generic: sulfasalazine 500 mg delayed-release tablet (¢¢¢)
Other Generic Product Names
Sulfazine EC

DOSING AND FOOD

Doses are taken 3 to 6 times a day.
This drug should be taken after a meal. Do not eat raw oysters or other raw
   shellfish at any time while taking this drug.
Adults: Up to 4,000 mg per day in divided doses.
Children over age 2: Up to 60 mg/kg (maximum 2,000 mg) per day in di-
   vided doses.
This drug may cause brain damage in children under age 2.
Forgotten doses: If you are scheduled to take the next dose within a few
   hours, do not take the forgotten dose. Otherwise take the forgotten dose
   as soon as you remember.

ALCOHOL, DRUG, HERB, AND SUPPLEMENT INTERACTIONS

Alcohol may increase some of the side effects from this drug, depending
   on the amount consumed. Ask your doctor about the risks caused by
   drinking alcohol with your condition.

Taking antacids with this drug may result in toxicity.

Taking this drug with any of the ones listed below may change the effect of either drug with the possibility of causing toxicity or decreasing effectiveness: ammonium chloride, antacids, antibiotics†, anticoagulants†, antidiabetics†, digoxin, folic acid, sulfonylureas†, vitamin C

Increased side effects are possible when this drug is taken with those listed below: acetaminophen, acetohydroxamic acid, amiodarone, anabolic steroids†, androgens†, carbamazepine, carmustine, dantrolene, dapsone, daunorubicin, disulfiram, divalproex, estrogens†, ethionamide, ethotoin, etretinate, fluconazole, furazolidone, gold salts†, labetalol, lovastatin, menadiol, mephenytoin, mercaptopurine, methimazole, methotrexate, methyldopa, naltrexone, niacin, nitrofurantoin, nonsteroidal antiinflammatories†, phenothiazines†, phenytoin, plicamycin, pravastatin, primaquine, procainamide, propylthiouracil, quinidine, quinine, simvastatin, sulfoxone, troleandomycin, valproic acid, vitamin A

ALLERGIC REACTIONS AND SIDE EFFECTS

If you are allergic to aspirin, furosemide, dichlorphenamide, methazolamide, thiazide diuretics†, antidiabetics†, antiglaucoma drugs†, or any sulfa or salicylate† drugs, you may also be allergic to this drug. You should tell your doctor about all your allergies and any unexplained symptoms you may have while taking this drug.

This drug promotes the effect of sunlight on the body and may cause severe sunburn and increased sensitivity of the eyes.

MORE COMMON SIDE EFFECTS: Abdominal pain, diarrhea, fever*, headache*, itching*, joint pain*, loss of appetite*, nausea, skin rash*, vomiting*

LESS COMMON SIDE EFFECTS: Bleeding*, bloody diarrhea*, blue skin*, breathing difficulty*, bruising*, chest pain*, chills*, cough*, muscle pain*, pale skin*, skin irritation*, sore throat*, swallowing difficulty*, tiredness*, weakness*, yellow eyes or skin*

PRECAUTIONS

People with severe allergies or asthma may be at greater risk of developing an allergic reaction to this drug.

If you have porphyria, this drug may make that condition worse.

Drink 8 to 10 glasses of water each day while taking this drug to prevent crystals from forming in the kidneys.

Do not crush, break, or chew the coated tablets or extended-release products.

---

†See page 52.   *See page 53.

This drug causes changes in your blood that put you at greater risk of getting an infection. Be careful not to cut yourself or get bruised. Tell your doctor if you develop signs of infection, such as fever or sore throat. Your dentist may recommend that you clean your teeth and mouth differently to avoid infection.

Your urine may turn orange-yellow in color and the color of your skin may change while taking this drug. The drug may also stain soft contact lenses.

This drug may interfere with several diagnostic tests including some urine glucose tests. Diabetics should use glucose oxidase tests or glucose enzyme test strips.

PREGNANCY AND BREAST-FEEDING

Safety during pregnancy has not been established although there was no evidence of harm during studies in animals.

Breast-feeding while taking this drug is not recommended.

HELPFUL COMMENTS

Contact your doctor if your symptoms do not improve after 1 to 2 months.

Eye irritation caused by the sun may be reduced by wearing sunglasses when outside.

Hard contact lenses will not discolor due to the effects of this drug.

SULFINPYRAZONE

Available for over 20 years

COMMONLY USED TO TREAT

Gouty arthritis
High uric acid levels, also known as hyperuricemia
People at risk of developing blood clots

DRUG CATEGORY

uricosuric
Class: sulfonamide

PRODUCTS

Brand-Name Products with Generic Alternatives
Anturane 100 mg capsule (n/a)
  Generic: sulfinpyrazone 100 mg capsule (¢¢¢¢)

Anturane 200 mg capsule (n/a)
Generic: sulfinpyrazone 200 mg capsule (n/a)

DOSING AND FOOD

Doses are taken twice a day.

This drug should be taken with food and a full glass of water to reduce the stomach upset that many people suffer. Do not eat raw oysters or other raw shellfish at any time while taking this drug.

Adults: Up to 800 mg per day in divided doses.

Forgotten doses: If you are scheduled to take the next dose within a few hours, do not take the forgotten dose. Otherwise take the forgotten dose as soon as you remember.

ALCOHOL, DRUG, HERB, AND SUPPLEMENT INTERACTIONS

Alcohol should not be used while taking this drug.

Taking this drug with any of the ones listed below may change the effect of either drug with the possibility of causing toxicity or decreasing effectiveness:
antidiabetics†, aspirin, bismuth subsalicylate, cefamandole, cefoperazone, cefotetan, cholestyramine, diazoxide, diuretics†, moxalactam, nitrofurantoin, penicillin, probenecid, pyrazinamide, salicylates†, warfarin

Increased side effects are possible when this drug is taken with those listed below:
anticoagulants†, antineoplastics†, dipyridamole, divalproex, heparin, nonsteroidal antiinflammatories†, pentoxifylline, plicamycin, ticarcillin, valproic acid

ALLERGIC REACTIONS AND SIDE EFFECTS

If you are allergic to aspirin, oxyphenbutazone, phenylbutazone, or other antiinflammatories†, you may also be allergic to this drug. You should tell your doctor about all your allergies and any unexplained symptoms you may have while taking this drug.

MORE COMMON SIDE EFFECTS: Back pain*, joint pain, nausea*, stomach pain*, urinary changes*, vomiting*

LESS COMMON SIDE EFFECTS: Skin rash*

RARE SIDE EFFECTS: Bleeding*, bloody vomit*, bloody stools*, breathing difficulty*, bruising*, chest tightness*, chills*, clumsiness*, diarrhea*, fever*, increased blood pressure*, mouth sores*, seizures*, shortness of breath*, skin irritation*, sore throat*, swelling*, swollen glands*, tiredness*, unsteadiness*, weakness*, weight gain*

---

† *See page 52.*   * *See page 53.*

PRECAUTIONS

People with blood disease, cancer, kidney stones, stomach problems, or intestinal disorders may be at increased risk of developing serious side effects while taking this drug.

Drink 8 to 10 glasses of water each day while taking this drug to reduce the risk of developing kidney stones.

This drug is used to prevent a gout attack but is not effective in treating an attack that has already started.

This drug causes changes in your blood that put you at greater risk of getting an infection. Be careful not to cut yourself or get bruised. Tell your doctor if you develop signs of infection, such as fever or sore throat. Your dentist may recommend that you clean your teeth and mouth differently to avoid infection.

PREGNANCY AND BREAST-FEEDING

Safety during pregnancy has not been established although the drug is known to harm animal fetuses.

Breast-feeding while taking this drug is not recommended.

HELPFUL COMMENTS

It may take 6 to 12 months before the effects of this drug are noticed. Do not stop treatment early if you start to feel better. This drug is usually taken for long periods of time.

SULFISOXAZOLE

Available for over 20 years

COMMONLY USED TO TREAT

Infection
Urinary tract infection

DRUG CATEGORY

antibiotic
Class: sulfonamide

PRODUCTS

Brand-Name Products with No Generic Alternative
Gantrisin Pediatric 500 mg/5 ml oral suspension (¢¢¢)

Products Only Available as Generics
sulfisoxazole 500 mg tablet (¢)

Other Generic Product Names
Sosol

Combination Products That Contain This Drug
Eryzole oral suspension (¢¢¢¢)
Pediazole oral suspension (¢¢¢¢¢)

DOSING AND FOOD

Doses are taken 4 to 6 times a day.

This drug may be taken with or without food but should always be taken with a full glass of water. Do not eat raw oysters or other raw shellfish at any time while taking this drug.

Adults: Up to 8,000 mg per day in divided doses.

Children: Up to 150 mg/kg (maximum 6,000 mg) per day in divided doses. This drug is not used in children under 2 months old.

Forgotten doses: If you are scheduled to take the next dose within a few hours, do not take the forgotten dose. Otherwise take the forgotten dose as soon as you remember.

ALCOHOL, DRUG, HERB, AND SUPPLEMENT INTERACTIONS

Alcohol may increase some of the side effects from this drug, depending on the amount consumed. Ask your doctor about the risks caused by drinking alcohol with your condition.

Taking this drug with any of the ones listed below may change the effect of either drug with the possibility of causing toxicity or decreasing effectiveness: anticoagulants†, antidiabetics†, sulfonylureas†

Severe reactions are possible when this drug is taken with those listed below: para-aminobenzoic acid, trimethoprim, pyrimethamine

Increased side effects are possible when this drug is taken with those listed below: acetaminophen, acetohydroxamic acid, amiodarone, ammonium chloride, anabolic steroids†, androgens†, antibiotics†, antithyroid drugs†, carbamazepine, carmustine, chloroquine, dantrolene, dapsone, daunorubicin, disulfiram, divalproex, estrogens†, ethotoin, etretinate, furazolidone, gold salts†, hydroxychloroquine, mephenytoin, mercaptopurine, methenamine, methotrexate, methyldopa, naltrexone, nitrofurantoin, oral contraceptives, phenothiazines†, phenytoin, plicamycin, primaquine, procainamide, quinidine, quinine, sulfoxone, valproic acid, vitamin C, vitamin K

---

† See page 52.   * See page 53.

ALLERGIC REACTIONS AND SIDE EFFECTS

If you are allergic to furosemide, dichlorphenamide, methazolamide, thiazide diuretics†, antidiabetics†, antiglaucoma drugs†, or any sulfa drugs, you may also be allergic to this drug. You should tell your doctor about all your allergies and any unexplained symptoms you may have while taking this drug.

This drug promotes the effect of sunlight on the body and may cause severe sunburn and increased sensitivity of the eyes.

LESS COMMON SIDE EFFECTS: Bleeding*, bruising*, diarrhea*, dizziness, fever*, headache, itching*, joint pain*, loss of appetite, muscle pain*, nausea, pale skin*, seizures*, skin irritation*, skin rash*, sore throat*, swallowing difficulty*, tiredness*, vomiting, weakness*, yellow eyes or skin*

RARE SIDE EFFECTS: Abdominal pain*, back pain*, bloody urine*, mood swings*, swelling*, thirst*, urinary changes*

PRECAUTIONS

People with anemia, glucose-6-phosphate dehydrogenase deficiency (G6PD) are at greater risk of developing side effects.

If you have porphyria, this drug may make that condition worse.

This drug may interfere with several diagnostic tests including some urine glucose tests. Diabetics should use glucose oxidase tests or glucose enzyme test strips.

Drink 8 to 10 glasses of water each day while taking this drug to prevent crystals from forming in the kidneys.

This drug causes changes in your blood that put you at greater risk of getting an infection. Be careful not to cut yourself or get bruised. Tell your doctor if you develop signs of infection, such as fever or sore throat. Your dentist may recommend that you clean your teeth and mouth differently to avoid infection.

Be careful driving or handling equipment while taking this drug because it may cause dizziness.

PREGNANCY AND BREAST-FEEDING

Safety during pregnancy has not been established although the drug is known to harm animal fetuses.

Breast-feeding while taking this drug is not recommended.

HELPFUL COMMENTS

Contact your doctor if your symptoms do not improve after a couple of days.

Do not stop treatment early if you start to feel better. It takes the full pre-scription for this drug to work completely.

Eye irritation caused by the sun may be reduced by wearing sunglasses when outside.

SULINDAC

Available for over 20 years

COMMONLY USED TO TREAT

Arthritis

DRUG CATEGORY

antiarthritic
antigout
antiinflammatory
antipyretic
Class: nonsteroidal antiinflammatory

PRODUCTS

Brand-Name Products with Generic Alternatives
Clinoril 150 mg tablet ($)
  Generic: sulindac 150 mg tablet (¢¢¢)
Clinoril 200 mg tablet ($$)
  Generic: sulindac 200 mg tablet (¢¢¢)

DOSING AND FOOD

Doses are taken twice a day.

It is best to take this drug on an empty stomach, but taking this drug with a little food may avoid the stomach upset that some people suffer.

Adults: Up to 400 mg per day in divided doses.

Forgotten doses: If you are scheduled to take the next dose within a few hours, do not take the forgotten dose. Otherwise take the forgotten dose as soon as you remember.

ALCOHOL, DRUG, HERB, AND SUPPLEMENT INTERACTIONS

Alcohol may increase the risk of serious side effects from this drug. Ask your doctor about the risks caused by drinking alcohol with your condition.

Do not use dong quai, feverfew, garlic, ginger, horse chestnut, red clover,

---

or St. John's wort while taking this drug since they may increase the risk of serious side effects.

Taking this drug with any of the ones listed below may change the effect of either drug with the possibility of causing toxicity or decreasing effectiveness: ACE inhibitors†, acetaminophen, antacids, antihypertensives†, digoxin, diflunisal, dimethylsulfoxide, diuretics†, furosemide, hydrochlorothiazide, nifedipine, lithium, methotrexate, phenytoin, probenecid, sulfonylureas†, sulindac, verapamil

Severe reactions are possible when this drug is taken with those listed below: antibiotics†, anticoagulants†, aspirin, cefamandole, cefoperazone, cefotetan, corticosteroids†, cyclosporine, dipyridamole, gold salts, heparin, mezlocillin, nonsteroidal antiinflammatories†, penicillamine, piperacillin, plicamycin, salicylates†, sulfinpyrazone, ticarcillin

ALLERGIC REACTIONS AND SIDE EFFECTS

If you are allergic to aspirin, zomepirac, salicylates†, or other nonsteroidal antiinflammatories†, you may also be allergic to this drug. You should tell your doctor about all your allergies and any unexplained symptoms you may have while taking this drug.

This drug promotes the effect of sunlight on the body and may cause severe sunburn and increased sensitivity of the eyes.

MORE COMMON SIDE EFFECTS: Abdominal pain, indigestion*, itching*, shortness of breath*, skin rash*, swelling*, weight gain*

LESS COMMON SIDE EFFECTS: Bruising*, constipation, diarrhea, dizziness, drowsiness, gas, headache, heartburn*, high blood pressure*, nausea*, sweating, vomiting

RARE SIDE EFFECTS: Back pain*, black stools*, bloody urine*, bloody vomit, blue fingernails*, blue lips*, breathing difficulty*, chest pain*, chest tightness*, chills*, confusion*, cough*, dark urine*, fainting*, fever*, hallucinations*, hearing loss*, hives*, hoarseness*, lip sores*, loss of appetite*, low blood pressure*, mood swings*, mouth sores*, muscle cramps*, nosebleeds*, pain*, pale skin*, pale stools*, puffy eyes*, rectal bleeding*, restlessness*, ringing in ears*, runny nose*, seizures*, sore throat*, stiff neck*, swollen glands*, swollen tongue*, thirst*, tiredness*, urinary changes*, vision changes*, weakness*, wheezing*, yellow eyes or skin*

PRECAUTIONS

This drug may cause serious stomach problems and possibly ulcers. Be careful to take this drug as directed with food, and let your doctor know if you develop any stomach-related symptoms.

Be careful driving or handling equipment while taking this drug because it may cause changes in attentiveness.

Do not lie down for about 30 minutes after taking this drug to help reduce the risk of heartburn and throat irritation.

If you use tobacco or have a history of alcohol abuse, stomach problems, intestinal problems, hemorrhoids, diabetes mellitus, severe fluid retention, or systemic lupus erythematosus, there is an increased risk that you will develop side effects while taking this drug.

Measure your weight every 2 to 3 days. Weight gain of more than 3 pounds in a week may be a sign of a serious reaction and should be reported to your doctor.

PREGNANCY AND BREAST-FEEDING

Safety during pregnancy has not been established although the drug is known to harm animal fetuses.

Breast-feeding while taking this drug is not recommended.

HELPFUL COMMENTS

If you need to take an antacid, take it either 2 hours before or after taking this drug.

Avoid quick movements to minimize dizziness. Dangling your legs over the side of the bed for a few minutes may help reduce dizziness when first waking up.

It may take 7 or more days for the effects of this drug to be noticed.

Several nonsteroidal antiinflammatories† are available without a prescription in lower, nonprescription strengths, including ibuprofen, ketoprofen, and naproxen.

SUMATRIPTAN SUCCINATE

Available since December 1992

COMMONLY USED TO TREAT

Migraine headache

DRUG CATEGORY

antimigraine
Class: triptan

---

† *See page 52.*   * *See page 53.*

PRODUCTS

Brand-Name Products with No Generic Alternative
Imitrex 25 mg tablet ($$$$$)
Imitrex 50 mg tablet ($$$$$)
Imitrex 100 mg tablet ($$$$$)
Imitrex 5 mg nasal spray ($$$$$)
Imitrex 20 mg nasal spray ($$$$$)
No generics available.
Multiple patents that begin to expire in 2006.

DOSING AND FOOD

Oral doses are taken as needed every 2 hours until maximum daily dose is reached or headache subsides.

Inhalation doses are used as needed twice a day with at least 2 hours between doses.

This drug may be taken with or without food but should be taken with a full glass of water.

Adults: Up to 300 mg orally per day in divided doses.

Adults: Up to 40 mg inhaled per day in divided doses.

ALCOHOL, DRUG, HERB, AND SUPPLEMENT INTERACTIONS

Alcohol may make your headache worse. You should ask your doctor about the risks caused by drinking alcohol with your condition.

Horehound should not be used while taking this drug.

Severe reactions are possible when this drug is taken with those listed below:
ergot alkaloids†, monoamine oxidase inhibitors†

ALLERGIC REACTIONS AND SIDE EFFECTS

You should tell your doctor about all your allergies and any unexplained symptoms you may have while taking this drug.

MORE COMMON SIDE EFFECTS: Chills*, dizziness*, drowsiness*, flushing*, lightheadedness*, muscle aches*, nausea*, numbness*, sinus irritation*, sore nose*, stiffness*, taste changes*, tingling*, vomiting*, warmth*

LESS COMMON SIDE EFFECTS: Anxiety, chest pain*, chest pressure*, hives*, irregular heartbeat*, itching*, skin rash*, swallowing difficulty*, tiredness, vision changes

RARE SIDE EFFECTS: Breathing difficulty*, irregular breathing*, seizures*, shortness of breath*, skin discoloration*, swelling*, wheezing*

PRECAUTIONS

You need to wait 2 weeks after stopping a monoamine oxidase inhibitor†
  before starting this drug.

People with a history of heart disease, high blood pressure, kidney disease,
  or liver disease are at greater risk of developing side effects while taking
  this drug.

This drug is only effective in treating an active migraine headache and will
  not work to prevent a migraine or relieve other types of headache pain.

Do not crush, break, or chew the tablet products.

Be careful driving or handling equipment while taking this drug because it
  may cause dizziness and drowsiness.

Inhalation products are absorbed into the body and carry the same warnings and precautions that apply to tablets.

PREGNANCY AND BREAST-FEEDING

Safety during pregnancy has not been established although the drug is
  known to harm animal fetuses.

Breast-feeding while taking this drug is not recommended.

HELPFUL COMMENTS

This drug may take 2 to 4 hours before the effects are fully noticed regard-
  less of whether a tablet or inhaler was used. The drug is also available as
  an injection for home use that starts to work 10 to 20 minutes after taking.

Take the dose of this drug at the first sign of a migraine headache.

TACRINE HYDROCHLORIDE

Available since September 1993

COMMONLY USED TO TREAT

Alzheimer's disease

DRUG CATEGORY

antidementia
Class: cholinesterase inhibitor

PRODUCTS

Brand-Name Products with No Generic Alternative
Cognex 10 mg capsule ($)
Cognex 20 mg capsule ($)

---

† *See page 52.*   * *See page 53.*

Cognex 30 mg capsule ($)
Cognex 40 mg capsule ($)
No generics available.
Multiple patents that begin to expire in 2004.

DOSING AND FOOD

Doses are taken 4 times a day.

It is best to take this drug on an empty stomach more than 1 hour before or at least 2 hours after a meal.

Adults: Up to 160 mg per day in divided doses.

Lower doses may be needed in people with liver disease.

Forgotten doses: If you are scheduled to take the next dose within a few hours, do not take the forgotten dose. Otherwise take the forgotten dose as soon as you remember.

ALCOHOL, DRUG, HERB, AND SUPPLEMENT INTERACTIONS

Alcohol may increase the risk of liver damage from this drug. Ask your doctor about the risks caused by drinking alcohol with your condition.

Taking this drug with any of the ones listed below may change the effect of either drug with the possibility of causing toxicity or decreasing effectiveness: anticholinergics†, cholinergics†, cholinesterase inhibitors†, cimetidine, nonsteroidal antiinflammatories†, skeletal muscle relaxants†, theophylline

ALLERGIC REACTIONS AND SIDE EFFECTS

You should tell your doctor about all your allergies and any unexplained symptoms you may have while taking this drug.

MORE COMMON SIDE EFFECTS: Abdominal pain, clumsiness*, diarrhea*, dizziness, headache, indigestion, loss of appetite*, nausea*, unsteadiness*, vomiting*

LESS COMMON SIDE EFFECTS: Belching, blood pressure changes*, fainting*, fast breathing, fever*, flushing, irregular heartbeat*, runny nose, skin rash*, sleep disorders, sweating*, swelling, urinary changes*, watery eyes, watery mouth*

RARE SIDE EFFECTS: Aggression*, breathing difficulty*, chest tightness*, cough*, irritability*, nervousness*, seizures*, shaky hands*, stiffness*, trembling*, weakness*, wheezing*, yellow eyes or skin*

PRECAUTIONS

Heavy smoking may cause this drug to be less effective.

If you have asthma, heart disease, intestinal problems, liver disease, Parkinson's disease, urinary difficulty, or ulcers, this drug may make those conditions worse.

People with a history of seizure, head injury, or brain disease are at greater risk of developing a seizure while taking this drug.

It is necessary to have liver function tested every 2 to 12 weeks while taking this drug to make sure that you may continue to safely use the drug.

Be careful driving or handling equipment while taking this drug because it may cause dizziness.

Stopping this drug suddenly may cause severe withdrawal symptoms. If you wish to stop taking this drug, ask your doctor for specific instructions.

Women are at greater risk than men of developing liver disease while taking this drug.

PREGNANCY AND BREAST-FEEDING

Safety during pregnancy has not been established although the drug is known to harm animal fetuses.

Breast-feeding while taking this drug is not recommended.

HELPFUL COMMENTS

This drug is also called by the generic names THA or tetrahydroaminoacridine.

TACROLIMUS

Available since April 1994

COMMONLY USED TO TREAT

Organ transplant recipients to reduce the risk of rejection
Severe skin irritation, specifically atopic dermatitis

DRUG CATEGORY

immunosuppressant
Class: macrolide

PRODUCTS

Brand-Name Products with No Generic Alternative
Prograf 0.5 mg capsule ($$)

---

† See page 52.   * See page 53.

Prograf 1 mg capsule ($$$)
Prograf 5 mg capsule ($$$$$)
Prograf 0.03% topical ointment (n/a)
Prograf 0.1% topical ointment (n/a)
No generics available.
No patents, no exclusivity.

DOSING AND FOOD

Doses are taken twice a day.

It is best to take this drug on an empty stomach. Do not eat grapefruit or drink grapefruit juice while taking this drug. Do not eat raw oysters or other raw shellfish at any time while taking this drug.

Adults and children: Up to 0.2 mg/kg per day in divided doses.

Forgotten doses: If you are scheduled to take the next dose within a few hours, do not take the forgotten dose. Otherwise take the forgotten dose as soon as you remember.

ALCOHOL, DRUG, HERB, AND SUPPLEMENT INTERACTIONS

Alcohol should not be used while taking this drug.

Taking this drug with any of the ones listed below may change the effect of either drug with the possibility of causing toxicity or decreasing effectiveness: antifungals†, bromocriptine, calcium channel blockers†, carbamazepine, cimetidine, clarithromycin, cyclosporine, danazol, diltiazem, erythromycin, fluconazole, itraconazole, ketoconazole, methylprednisolone, metoclopramide, phenobarbital, phenytoin, rifampin

Severe reactions are possible when this drug is taken with those listed below: amiloride, amphotericin B, cisplatin, immunosuppressants†, spironolactone, triamterene, vaccines

ALLERGIC REACTIONS AND SIDE EFFECTS

You should tell your doctor about all your allergies and any unexplained symptoms you may have while taking this drug.

MORE COMMON SIDE EFFECTS: Abdominal pain*, agitation*, anxiety*, bleeding*, bruising*, chills*, confusion*, depression*, diarrhea*, dizziness*, fever*, hallucinations*, headache*, high potassium levels*, infection*, itching*, loss of appetite*, loss of energy*, low magnesium levels*, nausea*, nervousness*, pale skin*, seizures*, shaky hands*, shortness of breath*, skin rash*, sleep disorders*, sore throat*, swelling*, tingling*, tiredness*, trembling*, twitching*, urinary changes*, vomiting*, weakness*

LESS COMMON SIDE EFFECTS: Blurry vision*, chest pain*, high blood pressure*, high cholesterol*, muscle cramps*, numbness*, ringing in ears*, sweating*

RARE SIDE EFFECTS: Flushing*, weight loss*, wheezing*

PRECAUTIONS

If you have cancer, diabetes, liver disease, kidney disease, nervousness, or high potassium levels, this drug may make those conditions worse.

Your body may retain potassium while taking this drug, which may cause severe side effects if the level gets too high. Potassium levels should be monitored periodically and may need to be treated while taking this drug. Avoid food rich in potassium, such as apricots, bananas, citrus fruit, dates, and tomatoes.

This drug causes changes in your blood that put you at greater risk of getting an infection. Be careful not to cut yourself or get bruised. Tell your doctor if you develop signs of infection, such as fever or sore throat. Your dentist may recommend that you clean your teeth and mouth differently to avoid infection.

Avoid contact with anyone who has the chickenpox, measles, or other communicable disease since it may be easier to catch the infection while taking this drug.

Exposure to skin tests, immunizations, and people who have received immunizations may put you at a greater risk of developing the disease when you are taking this drug.

Be careful driving or handling equipment while taking this drug because it may cause dizziness.

If you have high blood pressure or diabetes, you may need an adjustment in your antihypertensive or antidiabetic† therapy while taking this drug.

PREGNANCY AND BREAST-FEEDING

Safety during pregnancy has not been established although the drug is known to harm animal fetuses.

Breast-feeding while taking this drug is not recommended.

HELPFUL COMMENTS

If you are traveling outside the United States, make sure to have a full prescription supply on hand since this drug is not available in all countries.

†See page 52.   *See page 53.

TAMOXIFEN CITRATE

Available for over 20 years

COMMONLY USED TO TREAT

Breast cancer
Breast pain
Infertility due to high estrogen levels

DRUG CATEGORY

antineoplastic
Class: nonsteroidal antiestrogen

PRODUCTS

Brand-Name Products with Generic Alternatives
Nolvadex 10 mg tablet ($$)
  Generic: tamoxifen citrate 10 mg tablet ($$)
Nolvadex 20 mg tablet ($$$)
  Generic: tamoxifen citrate 20 mg tablet ($$$)

DOSING AND FOOD

Doses are taken 1 to 2 times a day.
This drug may be taken with or without food.
Adults: Up to 80 mg per day in divided doses.
Forgotten doses: Do not take a forgotten dose. Just go back to your usual
  schedule with the next dose.

ALCOHOL, DRUG, HERB, AND SUPPLEMENT INTERACTIONS

Alcohol may increase some of the side effects from this drug, depending
  on the amount consumed. Ask your doctor about the risks caused by
  drinking alcohol with your condition.

**Taking this drug with any of the ones listed below may change the effect of
either drug with the possibility of causing toxicity or decreasing effectiveness:**
antacids, bromocriptine, estrogens†, warfarin, oral contraceptives

Increased side effects are possible when this drug is taken with those listed below:
antineoplastics†

ALLERGIC REACTIONS AND SIDE EFFECTS

You should tell your doctor about all your allergies and any unexplained
  symptoms you may have while taking this drug.

MORE COMMON SIDE EFFECTS: Hot flashes, weight gain

LESS COMMON SIDE EFFECTS: Bone pain, dry skin, hair loss, headache, itching, menstrual changes, nausea, sexual dysfunction, skin rash, vaginal discharge, vomiting

RARE SIDE EFFECTS: Blurry vision*, cataracts*, confusion*, liver problems*, mouth irritation*, pelvic pain*, shortness of breath*, skin irritation*, sleepiness*, swelling*, vaginal bleeding*, vaginal discharge*, weakness*, yellow eyes or skin*

PRECAUTIONS

People with a history of cataracts, eye problems, high cholesterol, or other blood disorders may not be able to take this drug.

If you have a history of blood clots, this drug may make that condition worse.

Women of childbearing age may become more fertile while taking this drug and should use a barrier contraceptive or other nonhormonal contraceptive to prevent pregnancy.

Do not open, crush, break, or chew these products.

PREGNANCY AND BREAST-FEEDING

There is evidence that this drug may harm the fetus, but the drug may be necessary to the health of the mother.

Breast-feeding while taking this drug is not recommended.

HELPFUL COMMENTS

It is very important to continue taking this drug as ordered by your doctor even if the side effects make you feel ill.

This drug may need to be taken continuously for up to 5 years.

It takes about 3 to 4 weeks for this drug to start working.

If you need to take an antacid, take it either 2 hours before or after taking this drug.

TAMSULOSIN HYDROCHLORIDE

Available since April 1997

COMMONLY USED TO TREAT

Enlarged prostate, also known as benign (noncancerous) prostatic hypertrophy or BPH

---

†See page 52.   *See page 53.

DRUG CATEGORY

smooth muscle relaxant
Class: alpha adrenergic blocker

PRODUCTS

Brand-Name Products with No Generic Alternative
Flomax 0.4 mg capsule ($$)
No generics available.
Multiple patents that begin to expire in 2006.

DOSING AND FOOD

Doses are taken once a day.
This drug should be taken 30 minutes after the same meal each day.

Adults: Up to 0.8 mg per day.

Forgotten doses: Do not take a forgotten dose. Just go back to your usual
schedule with the next dose.

ALCOHOL, DRUG, HERB, AND SUPPLEMENT INTERACTIONS

Alcohol may increase some of the side effects from this drug, depending
on the amount consumed. Ask your doctor about the risks caused by
drinking alcohol with your condition.

**Taking this drug with any of the ones listed below may change the effect of
either drug with the possibility of causing toxicity or decreasing effectiveness:**
cimetidine, doxazosin, labetalol, phentolamine, prazosin, terazosin, tolazo-
line, warfarin

ALLERGIC REACTIONS AND SIDE EFFECTS

You should tell your doctor about all your allergies and any unexplained
symptoms you may have while taking this drug.

MORE COMMON SIDE EFFECTS: Back pain, diarrhea, dizziness, ejaculation
disorders, headache, stuffy nose, weakness

LESS COMMON SIDE EFFECTS: Chest pain, drowsiness, fainting, lighthead-
edness, nausea, sexual dysfunction, sleep disorders

PRECAUTIONS

Do not open, crush, break, or chew the capsule products.
Be careful driving or handling equipment while taking this drug because it
may cause dizziness.

If you are being treated for high blood pressure, the dose of your antihypertensive† therapy may need to change while taking this drug.

PREGNANCY AND BREAST-FEEDING

This drug is only used in men.
Safety during pregnancy has not been established although there was no evidence of harm during studies in animals.

HELPFUL COMMENTS

It takes about 2 to 4 weeks before the effects of this drug are noticed.
Avoid quick movements to minimize dizziness. Dangling your legs over the side of the bed for a few minutes may help reduce dizziness when first waking up.

TEGASEROD MALEATE

Available since July 2002

COMMONLY USED TO TREAT

Women with irritable bowel syndrome (IBS) suffering from constipation

DRUG CATEGORY

gastrointestinal stimulant
Class: 5-HT4 receptor agonist

PRODUCTS

Brand-Name Products with No Generic Alternative
Zelnorm 2 mg tablet (n/a)
Zelnorm 6 mg tablet (n/a)
No generics available.
Patent expires in 2013. Exclusivity until 2007.

DOSING AND FOOD

Doses are taken twice a day.
It is best to take this drug on an empty stomach at least 30 minutes before a meal.
Adults over age 18: Up to 12 mg per day in divided doses.
Lower doses are used in people with kidney disease or liver disease.
Forgotten doses: Do not take a forgotten dose. Just go back to your usual schedule with the next dose.

---

† See page 52.   * See page 53.

ALCOHOL, DRUG, HERB, AND SUPPLEMENT INTERACTIONS

Alcohol may increase some of the side effects from this drug, depending
on the amount consumed. Ask your doctor about the risks caused by
drinking alcohol with your condition.

There may be additional drug interactions that have not yet been identified since this drug is relatively new. Check with your pharmacist for the
current list of drug interactions.

**Taking this drug with any of the ones listed below may change the effect of
either drug with the possibility of causing toxicity or decreasing effectiveness:**
digoxin

ALLERGIC REACTIONS AND SIDE EFFECTS

You should tell your doctor about all your allergies and any unexplained
symptoms you may have while taking this drug.

MORE COMMON SIDE EFFECTS: Abdominal pain*, diarrhea, gas, headache

LESS COMMON SIDE EFFECTS: Nausea, vomiting

RARE SIDE EFFECTS: Back pain, belching, blurry vision, breathing difficul-
ty*, chest pain, depression*, dizziness, fainting*, flushing, increased appetite, irregular heartbeat*, itching, low blood pressure, menstrual
changes, muscle cramps, poor concentration*, shortness of breath*, sleep
disorders, suicidal thoughts*, sweating, swelling*, urinary changes*

PRECAUTIONS

People with diarrhea, kidney disease, liver disease, intestinal problems, or
gallbladder disorders may not be able to take this drug.

This drug is not effective in treating irritable bowel syndrome (IBS). It is
only effective in relieving constipation cause by IBS in women. This drug
has NOT been shown to be helpful in men with constipation from IBS.

PREGNANCY AND BREAST-FEEDING

Safety during pregnancy has not been established although there was no
evidence of harm during studies in animals.

Breast-feeding while taking this drug is not recommended.

HELPFUL COMMENTS

This drug is usually taken for 4 to 6 weeks, but people who do not respond during that time may need another 4 to 6 weeks of treatment.

Your symptoms may return 1 or 2 weeks after this drug is stopped.

Diarrhea usually occurs early in treatment and decreases the longer you
take the drug.

TELMISARTAN

Available since November 1998

COMMONLY USED TO TREAT

High blood pressure, also known as hypertension

DRUG CATEGORY

antihypertensive
Class: angiotensin II receptor antagonist

PRODUCTS

Brand-Name Products with No Generic Alternative
Micardis 20 mg tablet ($)
Micardis 40 mg tablet ($)
Micardis 80 mg tablet ($$)
No generics available.
Multiple patents that begin to expire in 2014.

Combination Products That Contain This Drug
Micardis HCT ($$)

DOSING AND FOOD

Doses are taken once a day.
This drug may be taken with or without food.
Adults: Up to 80 mg per day.
Lower doses are used in people with liver disease.
This drug is rarely used in children.
Forgotten doses: If you are scheduled to take the next dose within a few
hours, do not take the forgotten dose. Otherwise take the forgotten dose
as soon as you remember.

ALCOHOL, DRUG, HERB, AND SUPPLEMENT INTERACTIONS

Alcohol should not be used while taking this drug.
Several OTC drugs used for appetite control, asthma, colds, cough, hay fever,
or sinus problems may cause an increase in blood pressure when taken
with this drug. Check with your pharmacist when selecting OTC products.

**Taking this drug with any of the ones listed below may change the effect of
either drug with the possibility of causing toxicity or decreasing effectiveness:**
digoxin, diuretics†, warfarin

---

† See page 52.   * See page 53.

ALLERGIC REACTIONS AND SIDE EFFECTS

You should tell your doctor about all your allergies and any unexplained symptoms you may have while taking this drug.

LESS COMMON SIDE EFFECTS: Abdominal pain, appetite changes, back pain, cough, diarrhea, dizziness*, dry mouth, ear pain, fever, gas, headache, heartburn, muscle pain, nausea, nervousness, painful urination, runny nose, sinus congestion, skin rash, sneezing, sore throat, sweating, swelling, tiredness, weakness

RARE SIDE EFFECTS: Fainting*, fast heartbeat*, hives*, lightheadedness*, vision changes*

PRECAUTIONS

If you are dehydrated, the blood-pressure-lowering effect of this drug may be increased. Drink plenty of fluids to avoid dehydration when sweating, such as in hot weather and during exercise.

Be careful driving or handling equipment while taking this drug because the drug may cause dizziness.

If you have kidney disease, this drug may make that condition worse.

PREGNANCY AND BREAST-FEEDING

There is evidence that this drug may harm the fetus, but the drug may be necessary to the health of the mother.

Breast-feeding while taking this drug is not recommended.

HELPFUL COMMENTS

It may take 4 weeks before the full effects of this drug are noticed.

People of African American descent do not respond as well to this drug as Caucasians.

TEMAZEPAM

Available for over 20 years

COMMONLY USED TO TREAT

Sleeping difficulty, also known as insomnia

DRUG CATEGORY

sedative-hypnotic
Class: benzodiazepine

PRODUCTS

Brand-Name Products with No Generic Alternative
Restoril 7.5 mg capsule ($)

Brand-Name Products with Generic Alternatives
Restoril 15 mg capsule ($$)
  Generic: temazepam 15 mg capsule (¢¢)
Restoril 30 mg capsule ($$)
  Generic: temazepam 30 mg capsule (¢¢¢)

DOSING AND FOOD

Doses are taken once a day.
This drug may be taken with or without food.
Adults: Up to 30 mg per day.
Lower doses are used in people over age 65.

ALCOHOL, DRUG, HERB, AND SUPPLEMENT INTERACTIONS

Alcohol should not be used while taking this drug.
Catnip, kava, lady's slipper, lemon balm, passion flower, sassafras, skullcap, and valerian should not be used while taking this drug due to an increased sedative effect.

Taking this drug with any of the ones listed below may change the effect of either drug with the possibility of causing toxicity or decreasing effectiveness:
fluvoxamine, haloperidol, itraconazole, ketoconazole, levodopa, nefazodone

Severe reactions are possible when this drug is taken with those listed below:
anesthetics†, antidepressants†, antihistamines†, barbiturates†, monoamine oxidase inhibitors†, narcotics†, phenothiazines†

Increased side effects are possible when this drug is taken with those listed below:
aminophylline, theophylline

ALLERGIC REACTIONS AND SIDE EFFECTS

If you are allergic to any benzodiazepines†, you may also be allergic to this drug. You should tell your doctor about all your allergies and any unexplained symptoms you may have while taking this drug.

MORE COMMON SIDE EFFECTS: Clumsiness, dizziness, drowsiness, lightheadedness, slurry speech

LESS COMMON SIDE EFFECTS: Anxiety*, confusion*, constipation, depression*, diarrhea, difficulty urinating, dry mouth, headache, irregular heartbeat*, memory loss*, muscle spasm, nausea, sexual dysfunction,

† See page 52.   * See page 53.

stomach cramps, thirst, trembling, vision changes, vomiting, watery mouth

RARE SIDE EFFECTS: Agitation*, behavior changes*, bleeding*, bruising*, chills*, delusions*, disorientation*, excitement*, eye movement*, fever*, hallucinations*, irritability*, low blood pressure*, mouth sores*, muscle weakness*, nervousness*, seizures*, skin irritation*, sore throat*, spastic movements*, tiredness*, weakness*, yellow eyes or skin*

PRECAUTIONS

This drug may be habit forming and will cause severe withdrawal symptoms if stopped abruptly. If you wish to stop taking this drug, ask your doctor for specific instructions.

You need to wait 2 weeks after stopping a monoamine oxidase inhibitor† before starting this drug.

If you have difficulty swallowing, emphysema, asthma, bronchitis, glaucoma, hyperactivity, mental depression, mental illness, myasthenia gravis, porphyria, or sleep apnea, this drug may make those conditions worse.

Heavy smoking may cause this drug to be less effective.

Be careful driving or handling equipment while taking this drug because the drug may cause dizziness and drowsiness.

PREGNANCY AND BREAST-FEEDING

There is evidence that this drug may harm the fetus, but the drug may be necessary to the health of the mother.

Breast-feeding while taking this drug is not recommended.

HELPFUL COMMENTS

Dangling your legs over the side of the bed for a few minutes may help reduce dizziness when first waking up.

TENOFOVIR DISOPROXIL FUMARATE

Available since October 2001

COMMONLY USED TO TREAT

HIV infection

DRUG CATEGORY

antiretroviral
Class: nucleotide reverse transcriptase inhibitor (NtRTI)

PRODUCTS

Brand-Name Products with No Generic Alternative

Viread 300 mg tablet ($$$$$)

No generics available.

Multiple patents that begin to expire in 2006. Exclusivity until 2006.

DOSING AND FOOD

Doses are taken once a day.

It is best to take this drug with a high-fat meal to improve drug absorption. Be careful not to eat too much fatty food.

Adults: Up to 300 mg per day.

Forgotten doses: If you are scheduled to take the next dose within a few hours, do not take the forgotten dose. Otherwise take the forgotten dose as soon as you remember.

ALCOHOL, DRUG, HERB, AND SUPPLEMENT INTERACTIONS

Alcohol may increase the risk of liver damage from this drug. Ask your doctor about the risks caused by drinking alcohol with your condition.

Taking this drug with any of the ones listed below may change the effect of either drug with the possibility of causing toxicity or decreasing effectiveness: acyclovir, cidofovir, didanosine, ganciclovir, valacyclovir, valganciclovir

ALLERGIC REACTIONS AND SIDE EFFECTS

You should tell your doctor about any allergies and any unexplained symptoms you may have while taking this drug.

MORE COMMON SIDE EFFECTS: Loss of strength, vomiting

LESS COMMON SIDE EFFECTS: Gas, weight loss

RARE SIDE EFFECTS: Abdominal pain*, diarrhea*, irregular breathing*, loss of appetite*, muscle cramps*, nausea*, shortness of breath*, sleepiness*, tiredness*, weakness*

PRECAUTIONS

This drug may increase the absorption of didanosine to dangerously high levels. If you are taking both drugs, take this drug 2 hours before or 1 hour after the dose of didanosine.

People with kidney disease or liver disease may not be able to take this drug.

Since this drug is still relatively new, ask your pharmacist about any additional precautions each time you get your prescription refilled.

---

† See page 52.   * See page 53.

This drug is usually prescribed in combination with another antiretroviral drug. Ask your pharmacist about the type of drug interaction that may occur between antiretroviral drugs† to coordinate the administration times of multiple drugs.

Severe and sometime fatal liver disease may occur while taking this drug. Make sure to contact your doctor right away if you notice any abdominal discomfort, drowsiness, loss of appetite, breathing difficulty, tiredness, or weakness.

This drug does not prevent transmission of the HIV virus.

Many people notice the redistribution and accumulation of fat on the body while taking this drug.

PREGNANCY AND BREAST-FEEDING

Safety during pregnancy has not been established although there was no evidence of harm during studies in animals.

Breast-feeding while taking this drug is not recommended.

HELPFUL COMMENTS

Do not stop treatment early if you start to feel better. It takes the full prescription for this drug to work completely.

If you are taking this drug for over a year, watch for possible changes to your bones and tell your doctor of any you notice.

TERAZOSIN HYDROCHLORIDE

Available since December 1994

COMMONLY USED TO TREAT

Enlarged prostate, also known as benign (noncancerous) prostatic hypertrophy or BPH

High blood pressure, also known as hypertension

DRUG CATEGORY

antihypertensive
Class: alpha adrenergic blocker

PRODUCTS

Brand-Name Products with Generic Alternatives
Hytrin 1 mg capsule ($$)
  Generic: terazosin hydrochloride 1 mg capsule ($$)

Hytrin 2 mg capsule ($$)
  Generic: terazosin hydrochloride 2 mg capsule (¢¢¢¢)
Hytrin 5 mg capsule ($$)
  Generic: terazosin hydrochloride 5 mg capsule (¢¢¢¢)
Hytrin 10 mg capsule ($$)
  Generic: terazosin hydrochloride 10 mg capsule (¢¢¢¢)
Hytrin 1 mg tablet (n/a)
  Generic: terazosin hydrochloride 1 mg tablet ($$)
Hytrin 2 mg tablet (n/a)
  Generic: terazosin hydrochloride 2 mg tablet ($$)
Hytrin 5 mg tablet (n/a)
  Generic: terazosin hydrochloride 5 mg tablet ($$)
Hytrin 10 mg tablet (n/a)
  Generic: terazosin hydrochloride 10 mg tablet ($$)

DOSING AND FOOD

Doses are taken 1 to 2 times a day.
This drug may be taken with or without food.
Adults: Up to 20 mg per day in divided doses.
Forgotten doses: If you are scheduled to take the next dose within a few
  hours, do not take the forgotten dose. Otherwise take the forgotten dose
  as soon as you remember.

ALCOHOL, DRUG, HERB, AND SUPPLEMENT INTERACTIONS

Alcohol may cause your blood pressure to rise, making this drug less effec-
  tive. Ask your doctor about the risks caused by drinking alcohol with
  your condition.
Butcher's broom may interfere with the effects of this drug and should not
  be used.
Several OTC drugs used for appetite control, asthma, colds, cough, hay fever,
  or sinus problems may cause an increase in blood pressure when taken
  with this drug. Check with your pharmacist when selecting OTC products.
**Taking this drug with any of the ones listed below may change the effect of
either drug with the possibility of causing toxicity or decreasing effectiveness:**
antihypertensives†, clonidine

ALLERGIC REACTIONS AND SIDE EFFECTS

If you are allergic to prazosin or doxazosin, you may also be allergic to this
  drug. You should tell your doctor about all your allergies and any unex-
  plained symptoms you may have while taking this drug.

---

†*See page 52.*   **See page 53.*

MORE COMMON SIDE EFFECTS: Dizziness*, headache, tiredness, weakness

LESS COMMON SIDE EFFECTS: Back pain, blurry vision, chest pain*, drowsiness, fainting*, irregular heartbeat*, joint pain, lightheadedness*, nausea, shortness of breath*, stuffy nose, swelling*, vomiting

RARE SIDE EFFECTS: Weight gain*

PRECAUTIONS

If you have a history of chest pain or heart disease, this drug may make those conditions worse.

Be careful driving or handling equipment while taking this drug because it may cause dizziness.

PREGNANCY AND BREAST-FEEDING

Safety during pregnancy has not been established although the drug is known to harm animal fetuses.

Breast-feeding while taking this drug is not recommended.

HELPFUL COMMENTS

Avoid quick movements to minimize dizziness. Dangling your legs over the side of the bed for a few minutes may help reduce dizziness when first waking up.

If you do not treat high blood pressure, you may develop more serious problems such as heart failure, blood vessel disease, stroke, or kidney disease. Losing weight, exercising, eating more fruits and vegetables, and avoiding salty foods, such as lunchmeat and pickles, may help make drug treatment more successful.

If you are taking this drug for an enlarged prostate, it may take 6 weeks before you notice the effects of this drug. This drug will relieve symptoms, but will not shrink the prostate.

Take the first dose of this drug at bedtime since drowsiness is more common at the start of therapy.

TERBINAFINE HYDROCHLORIDE

Available since December 1992

COMMONLY USED TO TREAT

Athlete's foot
Fingernail and toenail infections

Fungal infections
Jock itch
Ringworm

DRUG CATEGORY

antifungal
Class: synthetic allylamine derivative

PRODUCTS

Brand-Name Products with No Generic Alternative
Lamisil 250 mg tablet ($$$$)
Lamisil 1% topical cream (¢¢¢¢¢)
Lamisil 1% topical solution ($)
No generics available.
Patent expires in 2006.

DOSING AND FOOD

Doses are taken once a day.
This drug may be taken with or without food.
Adults and teens: Up to 250 mg per day.
Forgotten doses: If you are scheduled to take the next dose within a few hours, do not take the forgotten dose. Otherwise take the forgotten dose as soon as you remember.

ALCOHOL, DRUG, HERB, AND SUPPLEMENT INTERACTIONS

Alcohol may increase the risk of liver damage from this drug. Ask your doctor about the risks caused by drinking alcohol with your condition.

Taking this drug with any of the ones listed below may change the effect of either drug with the possibility of causing toxicity or decreasing effectiveness: carbamazepine, corticosteroids†, griseofulvin, phenobarbital, phenylbutazone, phenytoin, primidone, rifampin

Increased side effects are possible when this drug is taken with those listed below: acetaminophen, amiodarone, anabolic steroids†, androgens†, antibiotics†, antifungals†, antithyroid drugs†, carmustine, chloramphenicol, chloroquine, cimetidine, clarithromycin, dantrolene, daunorubicin, diltiazem, disulfiram, divalproex, erythromycins†, estrogens†, etretinate, gold salts†, hydroxychloroquine, isoniazid, mercaptopurine, methotrexate, methyldopa, naltrexone, oral contraceptives, phenothiazines†, plicamycin, quinine, ranitidine, valproic acid, verapamil

†See page 52.   *See page 53.

ALLERGIC REACTIONS AND SIDE EFFECTS

You should tell your doctor about all your allergies and any unexplained symptoms you may have while taking this drug.

MORE COMMON SIDE EFFECTS: Diarrhea, nausea, stomachache, vomiting*

LESS COMMON SIDE EFFECTS: Itching*, skin rash*, taste changes

RARE SIDE EFFECTS: Bleeding*, bruising*, chills*, dark urine*, fever*, headache*, joint pain*, loss of appetite*, muscle pain*, pale skin*, pale stools*, skin irritation*, sore throat*, stomach pain*, swallowing difficulty*, tiredness*, weakness*, yellow eyes or skin*

PRECAUTIONS

People with a history of alcohol abuse, kidney disease, or liver disease may not be able to take this drug.

Very little of the topical form of this drug is absorbed into the body. Most warnings and precautions in the summary do not apply.

Topical products should be applied in a thin layer over the entire affected area. Do not bandage or wrap the affected area after applying this drug.

PREGNANCY AND BREAST-FEEDING

Safety during pregnancy has not been established although there was no evidence of harm during studies in animals.

Breast-feeding while taking this drug is not recommended.

HELPFUL COMMENTS

Contact your doctor if your symptoms do not improve after a couple of days if taking the oral product, or a week if using a topical product.

Do not stop treatment early if you start to feel better. It takes the full prescription for this drug to work completely.

TERBUTALINE SULFATE

Available for over 20 years

COMMONLY USED TO TREAT

Breathing difficulty
Premature labor

DRUG CATEGORY

bronchodilator
tocolytic

Class: adrenergic

PRODUCTS

Brand-Name Products with Generic Alternatives
Brethine 2.5 mg tablet (¢¢¢)
  Generic: terbutaline sulfate 2.5 mg tablet (¢¢¢)
Brethine 5 mg tablet (¢¢¢¢)
  Generic: terbutaline sulfate 5 mg tablet (¢¢¢)

DOSING AND FOOD

Doses are taken 3 to 4 times a day.
This drug may be taken with or without food.

Adults and children over age 15: Up to 15 mg per day in divided doses.

Children age 12 to 15: Up to 7.5 mg per day in divided doses.

Children under age 6: Up to 2.6 mg/kg per day in divided doses.

Higher doses are used in pregnant women.

Forgotten doses: If more than 1 hour has passed since the forgotten dose, do not take the dose. Otherwise take the forgotten dose as soon as you remember.

ALCOHOL, DRUG, HERB, AND SUPPLEMENT INTERACTIONS

Alcohol may increase some of the side effects from this drug, depending on the amount consumed. Ask your doctor about the risks caused by drinking alcohol with your condition.

Many OTC drugs used for appetite control, asthma, colds, cough, hay fever, pain, or sinus problems affect the central nervous system and may change the severity of side effects when taken with this drug. Check with your pharmacist for products to avoid.

Taking this drug with any of the ones listed below may change the effect of either drug with the possibility of causing toxicity or decreasing effectiveness: beta blockers†, monoamine oxidase inhibitors†, thyroid hormones†

Severe reactions are possible when this drug is taken with those listed below: aminophylline, cocaine, digoxin, levodopa, quinidine, sympathomimetics†, theophylline, tricyclic antidepressants†

Increased side effects are possible when this drug is taken with those listed below: amphetamines†

ALLERGIC REACTIONS AND SIDE EFFECTS

If you are allergic to albuterol, ephedrine, epinephrine, isoproterenol, or

†See page 52.   *See page 53.

metoproterenol, you may also be allergic to this drug. You should tell your doctor about all your allergies and any unexplained symptoms you may have while taking this drug.

MORE COMMON SIDE EFFECTS: Dizziness, drowsiness, headache, irregular heartbeat*, nausea*, nervousness, tremor, vomiting*

LESS COMMON SIDE EFFECTS: Cough, rash*, heartburn, sweating, shortness of breath*, weakness*

RARE SIDE EFFECTS: Chest pain*, difficulty urinating*, dry mouth, hives*, mental problems*, muscle pain*, seizures*, tiredness*

PRECAUTIONS

People with cardiovascular disease, high blood pressure, hyperthyroidism, or diabetes may not be able to take this drug.

If you have a history of seizures, you may be at greater risk of developing a seizure while taking this drug.

You need to wait 2 weeks after stopping a monoamine oxidase inhibitor† before starting this drug.

If you are diabetic, you may need a change in the dose of your antidiabetic drug† or insulin, since this drug may cause changes in blood sugar.

PREGNANCY AND BREAST-FEEDING

Safety during pregnancy has not been established although there was no evidence of harm during studies in animals.

This drug passes into breast milk in small quantities. Talk to your doctor about the risks associated with breast-feeding while taking this drug.

HELPFUL COMMENTS

It takes about 30 minutes after taking this drug by mouth for the effects to be noticed.

If you are taking this drug to stop preterm labor, make sure the on-call doctor knows about the drug so they may monitor the baby appropriately.

TESTOSTERONE

Available for over 20 years

COMMONLY USED TO TREAT

Delayed puberty
Testosterone deficiency

DRUG CATEGORY

antineoplastic
male hormone replacement
Class: androgen

PRODUCTS

Brand-Name Products with No Generic Alternative
Androderm 2.5 mg/24-hour extended-release patch ($$)
Androderm 5 mg/24-hour extended-release patch ($$)
Androgel 1% topical gel ($$$$$)
Striant 30 mg extended-release buccal tablet (n/a)
Testoderm 4 mg/24-hour extended-release patch ($$$)
Testoderm TTS 5 mg/24-hour extended-release patch ($$$)
Testoderm 6 mg/24-hour extended-release patch ($$$)
Testim 1% topical gel (n/a)
No generics available.
Multiple patents that begin to expire in 2004.

DOSING AND FOOD

Patches are applied once a day.
Men over age 18: Up to 6 mg per day.
Forgotten doses: Do not apply a forgotten dose. Just go back to your
usual schedule with the next dose. If your patch falls off in less than
12 hours, try to stick it back on. If it will not stay on, then skip the rest
of the dose and start again with your next scheduled dose.

ALCOHOL, DRUG, HERB, AND SUPPLEMENT INTERACTIONS

Alcohol may increase some of the side effects from this drug, depending
on the amount consumed. Ask your doctor about the risks caused by
drinking alcohol with your condition.

Taking this drug with any of the ones listed below may change the effect of
either drug with the possibility of causing toxicity or decreasing effectiveness:
anticoagulants†, carbamazepine, oxyphenbutazone, tacrolimus

Increased side effects are possible when this drug is taken with those listed below:
acetaminophen, amiodarone, anabolic steroids†, antibiotics†, antithyroid
drugs†, carmustine, chloroquine, dantrolene, daunorubicin, disulfiram,
divalproex, estrogens†, etretinate, gold salts†, hydroxychloroquine, mer-
captopurine, methotrexate, methyldopa, naltrexone, oral contraceptives,
phenothiazines†, phenytoin, plicamycin, valproic acid

†See page 52.   *See page 53.

ALLERGIC REACTIONS AND SIDE EFFECTS

If you are allergic to any androgenst, ethanol, or anabolic steroidst, you may also be allergic to this drug. You should tell your doctor about all your allergies and any unexplained symptoms you may have while taking this drug.

LESS COMMON SIDE EFFECTS: Acne, breast enlargement, breast tenderness, breathing difficulty*, headache, increased sex drive, itching, muscle pain, nausea*, penile erection*, skin discoloration*, skin irritation, swelling*, vomiting*, weakness

PRECAUTIONS

If you are a diabetic, you may need a change in the dose of your antidiabetic drugt or insulin, since this drug may cause changes in blood sugar.

There is a small risk of developing painful, prolonged erection of the penis, which requires treatment by a doctor. If this happens, go to your doctor or the nearest emergency room immediately.

There are 2 different types of patches, each of which must be applied to particular places on the body to be effective. Androderm and Testoderm TTS patches may be applied to the back, abdomen, upper arms, or thighs, but Testoderm patches are only effective when applied to genital skin in the scrotal area.

This drug may be transferred during sexual intercourse to your female partner and may cause masculine characteristics to develop.

PREGNANCY AND BREAST-FEEDING

This drug may cause birth defects and should not be used during pregnancy.

Breast-feeding while taking this drug is not recommended.

HELPFUL COMMENTS

It takes about 8 weeks for the full effects of this drug to be noticed.

This drug has been used to increase athletic performance without adequate safety information and is classified by the FDA as a controlled substance. The International Olympic Committee and World Anti-Doping Agency have banned this drug from use in competitive sports.

TETRACYCLINE

Available for over 20 years

COMMONLY USED TO TREAT

Infection

DRUG CATEGORY

antibiotic
Class: tetracycline

PRODUCTS

Brand-Name Products with No Generic Alternative
Sumycin 125 mg/5 ml oral suspension (¢¢¢¢)
Tetrex 100 mg capsule (n/a)
Tetrex 250 mg capsule (n/a)
Tetrex 500 mg capsule (n/a)

Brand-Name Products with Generic Alternatives
Sumycin 250 mg tablet (¢)
  Generic: tetracycline hydrochloride 250 mg tablet (¢)
Sumycin 500 mg tablet (¢¢)
  Generic: tetracycline hydrochloride 500 mg tablet (¢)

Other Generic Product Names
Achromycin V, Bristacycline

Combination Products That Contain This Drug
Helidac chewable tablet ($$)

DOSING AND FOOD

Doses are taken 2 to 4 times a day.

It is better to take this drug on an empty stomach with a full glass of water, but taking this drug with a little food may avoid the stomach upset that some people suffer. Do not drink milk or eat dairy products within 2 hours of taking this drug.

Adults: Up to 2,000 mg per day in divided doses.

Children over age 8: Up to 50 mg/kg per day in divided doses.

This drug is not used in children under age 8 because of potential damage to developing teeth and bones.

Forgotten doses: If you are scheduled to take the next dose within a few hours, do not take the forgotten dose. Otherwise take the forgotten dose as soon as you remember.

---

† See page 52.   * See page 53.

ALCOHOL, DRUG, HERB, AND SUPPLEMENT INTERACTIONS

Alcohol may increase some of the side effects from this drug, depending on the amount consumed. Ask your doctor about the risks caused by drinking alcohol with your condition.

Many OTC drugs, including antacids, laxatives, and mineral supplements such as calcium, magnesium, or iron, may decrease the effects of this drug when taken at the same time as the drug. If you need to take an OTC drug take it either 2 hours before or after taking this drug.

Taking this drug with any of the ones listed below may change the effect of either drug with the possibility of causing toxicity or decreasing effectiveness: antacids, anticoagulants†, calcium supplements, cholestyramine, cimetidine, colestipol, digoxin, iron supplements, mineral supplements, oral contraceptives, penicillins†, sodium bicarbonate, zinc

Severe reactions are possible when this drug is taken with those listed below: methoxyflurane

ALLERGIC REACTIONS AND SIDE EFFECTS

If you are allergic to any tetracyclines†, you may also be allergic to this drug. You should tell your doctor about all your allergies and any unexplained symptoms you may have while taking this drug.

This drug promotes the effect of sunlight on the body and may cause severe sunburn and increased sensitivity of the eyes. This effect may continue as long as 2 to 4 weeks after the drug is stopped.

MORE COMMON SIDE EFFECTS: Diarrhea, irregular heartbeat*, stomach cramps, sun sensitivity*

LESS COMMON SIDE EFFECTS: Genital itch, rectal itch, sore mouth

RARE SIDE EFFECTS: Abdominal pain*, headache*, loss of appetite*, nausea*, vomiting*, visual changes*, yellow eyes or skin*

PRECAUTIONS

This drug may interfere with urine glucose tests, providing false negative results.

People with kidney disease have a greater risk of developing side effects.

This drug decomposes after the expiration date and may be harmful if taken. Make sure you destroy any leftover tablets as soon as you are done with the prescription.

Some people get a discolored tongue when taking this drug, but the coloring will return to normal when the drug is stopped.

PREGNANCY AND BREAST-FEEDING

This drug may cause toxic effects to the fetus and should not be used during pregnancy.

Breast-feeding while taking this drug is not recommended.

HELPFUL COMMENTS

Oral contraceptives may not work properly when taken with this drug. You need to use a barrier contraceptive, such as a condom, or other nonhormonal contraceptive to prevent pregnancy.

Contact your doctor if your symptoms do not improve after a couple of days.

Do not stop treatment early if you start to feel better. It takes the full prescription for this drug to work completely.

THALIDOMIDE

Available since July 1998

COMMONLY USED TO TREAT

Graft-versus-host disease after transplant

Skin disease caused by leprosy, also known as erythema nodosum leprosum (ENL)

DRUG CATEGORY

antileprotic

Class: immunomodulator

PRODUCTS

Brand-Name Products with No Generic Alternative

Thalomid 50 mg capsule ($$$$$)

Thalomid 100 mg capsule (n/a)

Thalomid 200 mg capsule (n/a)

No generics available.

Multiple patents that begin to expire in 2018.

DOSING AND FOOD

Doses are taken once a day usually in the evening.

It is best to take this drug with a full glass of water at least 1 hour after a meal.

Adults: Up to 1,600 mg per day.

Forgotten doses: If you are scheduled to take the next dose within a few

---

hours, do not take the forgotten dose. Otherwise take the forgotten dose as soon as you remember.

ALCOHOL, DRUG, HERB, AND SUPPLEMENT INTERACTIONS

Alcohol should not be used while taking this drug.

Many OTC drugs used for appetite control, asthma, colds, cough, hay fever, pain, or sinus problems affect the central nervous system and may change the effects or side effects of this drug. Check with your pharmacist for products to avoid.

Severe reactions are possible when this drug is taken with those listed below: anesthetics, antihistamines†, anxiolytics†, barbiturates†, chlorpromazine, narcotics†, reserpine

Increased side effects are possible when this drug is taken with those listed below: chloramphenicol, cisplatin, dapsone, didanosine, ethambutol, ethionamide, hydralazine, isoniazid, lithium, nitrofurantoin, nitrous oxide, phenytoin, stavudine, vincristine, zalcitabine

ALLERGIC REACTIONS AND SIDE EFFECTS

You should tell your doctor about all your allergies and any unexplained symptoms you may have while taking this drug.

MORE COMMON SIDE EFFECTS: Constipation, diarrhea, dizziness, drowsiness, nausea, numbness*, stomach pain, tingling*, weakness*

LESS COMMON SIDE EFFECTS: Dry mouth, dry skin, headache, increased appetite, mood swings, swelling

RARE SIDE EFFECTS: Bloody urine*, chills*, fever*, irregular heartbeat*, itching*, jerking motions*, low blood pressure*, mouth sores*, red eyes*, seizures*, skin irritation*, skin rash*, sore throat*, unconsciousness*, urinary changes*

PRECAUTIONS

Women of childbearing age must have a pregnancy test no more than 24 hours before starting and every 2 to 4 weeks while taking this drug. Two forms of birth control are recommended, starting 1 month before the drug is begun and for 1 month after the drug is stopped. Even men that have had a vasectomy may pass this drug to women through sexual intercourse.

People with a history of seizures may be at greater risk of developing a seizure while taking this drug.

If you have peripheral neuropathy or a low white blood count, this drug may make those conditions worse.

PREGNANCY AND BREAST-FEEDING

This drug may cause birth defects and should not be used during pregnancy. Any exposure to the drug, including touching broken tablets or having intercourse with a man taking the drug, may also be associated with birth defects.

Breast-feeding while taking this drug is not recommended.

HELPFUL COMMENTS

Avoid quick movements to minimize dizziness. Dangling your legs over the side of the bed for a few minutes may help reduce dizziness when first waking up.

THEOPHYLLINE

Available for over 20 years

COMMONLY USED TO TREAT

Asthma
Bronchitis
Emphysema

DRUG CATEGORY

bronchodilator
Class: xanthine derivative

PRODUCTS

Brand-Name Products with No Generic Alternative
Aerolate III 65 mg extended-release capsule (¢¢)
Aerolate JR 130 mg extended-release capsule (¢¢)
Aerolate SR 260 mg extended-release capsule (¢¢)
Aerolate 150 mg/15 ml oral solution (n/a)
Quibron-T 300 mg tablet (n/a)
Slo-Bid 50 mg extended-release capsule (n/a)
Slo-Bid 75 mg extended-release capsule (n/a)
Slo-Phyllin 100 mg tablet (n/a)
Slo-Phyllin 200 mg tablet (¢¢¢)
Slo-Phyllin 80 mg/15 ml oral syrup (n/a)
Theolair 125 mg tablet (¢¢¢¢)
Theolair 250 mg tablet (¢¢¢¢¢)
Theolair-SR 250 mg extended-release tablet (n/a)

Theolair-SR 500 mg extended-release tablet (n/a)
Uniphyl 400 mg extended-release tablet ($)
Uniphyl 600 mg extended-release tablet ($)

Brand-Name Products with Generic Alternatives§
Elixophyllin 80 mg/15 ml oral elixir (¢¢¢¢¢)
   Generic: theophylline 80 mg/15 ml oral elixir (¢)
Theolair 80 mg/15 ml oral solution (n/a)
   Generic: theophylline 80 mg/15 ml oral solution (¢)
Slo-Bid 100 mg extended-release capsule (n/a)
   Generic: theophylline 100 mg extended-release capsule (n/a)
Slo-Bid 125 mg extended-release capsule (n/a)
   Generic: theophylline 125 mg extended-release capsule (¢¢¢)
Slo-Bid 200 mg extended-release capsule (n/a)
Theolair-SR 200 mg extended-release tablet (n/a)
   Generic: theophylline 200 mg extended-release tablet (¢)
Slo-Bid 300 mg extended-release capsule (n/a)
Theolair-SR 300 mg extended-release tablet (n/a)
   Generic: theophylline 300 mg extended-release tablet (¢¢)

Products Only Available as Generics§
theophylline 100 mg extended-release tablet (¢¢¢¢)
theophylline 300 mg extended-release capsule (¢¢)
theophylline 450 mg extended-release tablet (¢¢¢)

Other Generic Product Names
Quibron-T/SR, T-Phyl, Theo-24, Theo-Dur, Theochron, Uni-Dur, Uniphyl

DOSING AND FOOD

Doses are taken 3 to 4 times a day. Extended-release products are taken 1
to 2 times a day.

It is better to take this drug on an empty stomach, but taking this drug
with food may avoid the stomach upset that some people suffer.

Adults and children: Doses are individualized based on patient weight and
the product.

Forgotten doses: If you are scheduled to take the next dose within a few
hours, do not take the forgotten dose. Otherwise take the forgotten dose
as soon as you remember.

ALCOHOL, DRUG, HERB, AND SUPPLEMENT INTERACTIONS

Alcohol may increase some of the side effects from this drug, depending
on the amount consumed. Ask your doctor about the risks caused by
drinking alcohol with your condition.

§ *See "Precautions" in this entry.*

Cacao and St. John's wort may decrease the effects of this drug and should not be used.

Caffeine, guarana, and ephedra increase the risk of side effects of this drug and should not be used.

Taking this drug with any of the ones listed below may change the effect of either drug with the possibility of causing toxicity or decreasing effectiveness:
allopurinol, barbiturates†, beta blockers†, carbamazepine, charcoal, cimetidine, corticosteroids†, enoxacin, erythromycin, fluvoxamine, interferon, isoniazid, ketoconazole, lithium, loop diuretics, mexiletine, moricizine, oral contraceptives, pentoxifylline, phenytoin, propranolol, quinolones†, rifampin, tacrine, thiabendazole, ticlopidine, troleandomycin

ALLERGIC REACTIONS AND SIDE EFFECTS

If you are allergic to aminophylline, ethylenediamine, or oxtriphylline, you may also be allergic to this drug. You should tell your doctor about all your allergies and any unexplained symptoms you may have while taking this drug.

LESS COMMON SIDE EFFECTS: Frequent urination, headache, heartburn*, irregular heartbeat*, nausea, nervousness*, sleep disorders, trembling*, vomiting*

RARE SIDE EFFECTS: Abdominal pain*, behavior changes*, bloody vomit*, confusion*, diarrhea*, dizziness*, lightheadedness*, restlessness*, seizures*

PRECAUTIONS

§The effectiveness of this drug may vary from product to product. Do not switch from one manufacturer to another when your prescription is refilled. Talk to your pharmacist to make sure you get the same product each time.

Smoking cigarettes or marijuana may cause this drug to be less effective.

If you have a history of seizures, you may have an increased risk of developing a seizure while taking this drug.

People with heart failure, liver disease, or low thyroid levels may not be able to take this drug.

Most extended-release products should not be opened, crushed, broken, or chewed, although there are exceptions with this drug. Ask your pharmacist about the brand used to fill your prescription.

It is easy for this drug to reach toxic levels. Call your doctor if you even suspect that you are not tolerating this drug.

---

† See page 52.   * See page 53.

PREGNANCY AND BREAST-FEEDING

Safety during pregnancy has not been established although the drug is known to harm animal fetuses.

Breast-feeding while taking this drug is not recommended.

HELPFUL COMMENTS

Do not measure doses of the oral elixir or solution with anything but a measuring cup intended for use with prescription drugs. Slight inaccuracy from other measuring spoons may result in over- or under-dosing.

THIOGUANINE

Available for over 20 years

COMMONLY USED TO TREAT

Leukemia, specifically nonlymphocytic leukemia

DRUG CATEGORY

antineoplastic
Class: antimetabolite

PRODUCTS

Products Only Available as Generics
thioguanine 40 mg tablet ($$$)

DOSING AND FOOD

Doses are taken once a day.

This drug may be taken with or without food. Do not eat raw oysters or other raw shellfish at any time while taking this drug.

Adults and children: Up to 3 mg/kg per day.

Forgotten doses: Do not take a forgotten dose. Just go back to your usual schedule with the next dose. Talk to your doctor when the prescription is first written so you know what to do if you vomit after taking a dose.

ALCOHOL, DRUG, HERB, AND SUPPLEMENT INTERACTIONS

Alcohol may increase some of the side effects from this drug, depending on the amount consumed. Ask your doctor about the risks caused by drinking alcohol with your condition.

Taking this drug with any of the ones listed below may change the effect of either drug with the possibility of causing toxicity or decreasing effectiveness: antithyroid drugs†, azathioprine, chloramphenicol, colchicine, flucytosine, interferon, plicamycin, probenecid, sulfinpyrazone, zidovudine

Severe reactions are possible when this drug is taken with those listed below: busulfan

ALLERGIC REACTIONS AND SIDE EFFECTS

You should tell your doctor about all your allergies and any unexplained symptoms you may have while taking this drug.

LESS COMMON SIDE EFFECTS: Back pain*, black stools*, bleeding*, bloody urine*, bruising*, chills*, cough*, diarrhea, fever*, hoarseness*, itching, joint pain*, loss of appetite, nausea, skin irritation*, skin rash, swelling*, unsteadiness*, urinary changes*, vomiting

RARE SIDE EFFECTS: Mouth sores*, yellow eyes or skin*

PRECAUTIONS

Avoid contact with anyone who has the chickenpox, measles, or other communicable disease since it may be easier to catch the infection while taking this drug.

Exposure to skin tests, immunizations, and people who have received immunizations may put you at a greater risk of developing the disease when you are taking this drug.

People with a history of gout or kidney stones may be at greater risk of recurrence of their condition since this drug increases uric acid levels in the body.

Drink 8 to 10 glasses of water each day while taking this drug to reduce kidney-related problems.

This drug causes changes in your blood that put you at greater risk of getting an infection. Be careful not to cut yourself or get bruised. Tell your doctor if you develop signs of infection, such as fever or sore throat. Your dentist may recommend that you clean your teeth and mouth differently to avoid infection.

PREGNANCY AND BREAST-FEEDING

There is evidence that this drug may harm the fetus, but the drug may be necessary to the health of the mother.

Breast-feeding while taking this drug is not recommended.

---

† See page 52.   * See page 53.

HELPFUL COMMENTS

This drug is also called by the generic name 6-thioguanine or 6-TG.
It is very important to continue taking this drug as ordered by the doctor even if the side effects make you feel ill.

THIORIDAZINE HYDROCHLORIDE

Available for over 20 years

COMMONLY USED TO TREAT

Mental illness, also known as psychosis

DRUG CATEGORY

antipsychotic
Class: phenothiazine: piperidine derivative

PRODUCTS

Products Only Available as Generics
thioridazine hydrochloride 10 mg tablet (¢)
thioridazine hydrochloride 15 mg tablet (¢)
thioridazine hydrochloride 25 mg tablet (¢)
thioridazine hydrochloride 50 mg tablet (¢¢)
thioridazine hydrochloride 100 mg tablet (¢¢)
thioridazine hydrochloride 150 mg tablet (¢¢¢)
thioridazine hydrochloride 200 mg tablet (¢¢¢)
thioridazine hydrochloride 30 mg/ml oral concentrate (¢¢¢¢)
thioridazine hydrochloride 100 mg/ml oral concentrate ($$)

DOSING AND FOOD

Doses are taken 2 to 4 times a day.
Taking this drug with food or a full glass of milk or water may avoid the stomach upset that some people suffer.

Adults: Up to 800 mg per day in divided doses.

Children age 2 to 12: Up to 3 mg/kg per day in divided doses.

Lower doses are used in people over age 65.

Forgotten doses: If you are scheduled to take the next dose within a few hours, do not take the forgotten dose. Otherwise take the forgotten dose as soon as you remember.

ALCOHOL, DRUG, HERB, AND SUPPLEMENT INTERACTIONS

Alcohol should not be used while taking this drug.

Do not use caffeine while taking this drug since the drug effects may be decreased.

Several OTC drugs used for appetite control, asthma, colds, cough, hay fever, pain, or sinus problems may seriously increase the effects and side effects of this drug. Check with your pharmacist when selecting OTC products.

Taking this drug with any of the ones listed below may change the effect of either drug with the possibility of causing toxicity or decreasing effectiveness: antacids, antihypertensives†, barbiturates†, beta blockers†, bromocriptine, caffeine, dopamine, fluoxetine, levodopa, lithium, paroxetine, phenobarbital, phenytoin, warfarin

Severe reactions are possible when this drug is taken with those listed below: alcohol, amantadine, antiarrhythmics†, anticholinergics†, antidepressants†, antihistamines†, antiparkinson drugs†, antithyroid drugs†, anxiolytics†, astemizole, bromocriptine, cisapride, deferoxamine, disopyramide, diuretics†, epinephrine, erythromycin, levobunolol, lithium, metipranolol, meperidine, metrizamide, monoamine oxidase inhibitors†, nabilone, narcotics†, nitrates, pentamidine, phenothiazines†, probucol, procainamide, promethazine, propylthiouracil, quinidine, sympathomimetics†; tricyclic antidepressants†

Increased side effects are possible when this drug is taken with those listed below: antipsychotics†, metoclopramide, metyrosine, pemoline, pimozide, rauwolfia alkaloids†, trimeprazine

ALLERGIC REACTIONS AND SIDE EFFECTS

If you are allergic to any phenothiazines†, you may also be allergic to this drug. You should tell your doctor about all your allergies and any unexplained symptoms you may have while taking this drug.

This drug promotes the effect of sunlight on the body and may cause severe sunburn and increased sensitivity of the eyes.

MORE COMMON SIDE EFFECTS: Breathing difficulty* chewing action*, congestion, constipation, decreased sweating, dizziness, drowsiness, dry mouth, eye stare*, eyelid movement*, fainting*, irregular heartbeat*, lip smacking*, loss of balance*, puffy cheeks*, restlessness*, shuffling walk*, stiffness*, tongue movements*, trembling*, twitching*, urinary difficulty*, vision changes*

LESS COMMON SIDE EFFECTS: Breast-milk secretion, breast swelling, dark

---

†*See page 52.*   ** See page 53.*

urine*, menstrual changes, rough tongue, sexual dysfunction, skin rash*, watery mouth, weight gain

RARE SIDE EFFECTS: Abdominal pain*, aching muscles, agitation*, bleeding*, blood pressure change*, bruising*, chest pain*, chills*, clumsiness*, coma*, confusion*, diarrhea*, dreams*, drooling*, excitement*, fever*, hair loss*, headaches*, increased sweating*, itching*, joint pain*, lack of sweating*, loss of bladder control*, mouth sores*, nausea*, penile erection*, red hands*, seizures*, shivering*, skin discoloration*, sleep disorders*, sore throat*, speaking difficulty*, tiredness*, vomiting*, weakness*, yellow eyes or skin*

PRECAUTIONS

If you have a history of enlarged prostate, glaucoma, ulcers, seizures, heart disease, urinary difficulty, or Parkinson's disease, this drug may make those conditions worse.

This drug may decrease the cough reflex, putting people with lung disease at greater risk of developing pneumonia.

Heavy smoking may cause this drug to be less effective.

This drug may cause false results from several diagnostic tests, including pregnancy tests, and should be stopped for at least 4 days before the test.

This drug should not be stopped suddenly, due to an increased risk of side effects. If you wish to stop taking this drug, ask your doctor for specific instructions.

Be careful driving or handling equipment while taking this drug because the drug may cause dizziness and drowsiness.

You are more likely to overheat when taking this drug and should avoid exercising in hot weather and using a sauna or hot tub.

This drug may make you more sensitive to cold temperatures.

Touching the liquid form of this drug may cause skin irritation. Make sure you do not spill the liquid, and wash your hands immediately after taking the dose.

This drug may cause dry mouth, which is associated with a greater risk of cavities. Your dentist may recommend that you clean your teeth and mouth differently to avoid infection.

PREGNANCY AND BREAST-FEEDING

Safety during pregnancy has not been established although the drug is known to harm animal fetuses.

Breast-feeding while taking this drug is not recommended.

HELPFUL COMMENTS

This drug may cause the color of your urine to turn pink or brown.

If you need to take an antacid, take it either 2 hours before or after taking this drug.

Sucking on hard sugarless candy or chewing sugarless gum may help relieve dry mouth caused by this drug.

The liquid form of this drug should be mixed in $1/4$ to $1/2$ cup of applesauce, caffeine-free carbonated beverage, fruit juice, milk, pudding, soup, tomato juice, or water just before taking the dose.

THIOTHIXENE

Available for over 20 years

COMMONLY USED TO TREAT

Agitation

Mental illness, also known as psychosis

DRUG CATEGORY

antipsychotic

Class: phenothiazine: thioxanthene

PRODUCTS

Brand-Name Products with Generic Alternatives

Navane 1 mg capsule (¢¢¢)
  Generic: thiothixene 1 mg capsule (¢¢)
Navane 2 mg capsule (¢¢¢¢)
  Generic: thiothixene 2 mg capsule (¢¢)
Navane 5 mg capsule (¢¢¢¢¢)
  Generic: thiothixene 5 mg capsule (¢¢)
Navane 10 mg capsule ($)
  Generic: thiothixene 10 mg capsule (¢¢¢¢)
Navane 20 mg capsule ($$)
  Generic: thiothixene 20 mg capsule (n/a)
Navane 5 mg/ml oral concentrate (n/a)
  Generic: thiothixene 5 mg/ml oral concentrate ($)

DOSING AND FOOD

Doses are taken twice a day.

Taking this drug with food or a full glass of milk or water may avoid the stomach upset that some people suffer.

Adults: Up to 60 mg per day in divided doses.

Lower doses are used in people over age 65.

Forgotten doses: If you are scheduled to take the next dose within a few hours, do not take the forgotten dose. Otherwise take the forgotten dose as soon as you remember.

ALCOHOL, DRUG, HERB, AND SUPPLEMENT INTERACTIONS

Alcohol should not be used while taking this drug.

Do not use caffeine or nutmeg while taking this drug since the drug effects may be decreased.

Several OTC drugs used for asthma, colds, cough, hay fever, sleep aid, or sinus problems may seriously increase the side effects of this drug. Check with your pharmacist when selecting OTC products.

Taking this drug with any of the ones listed below may change the effect of either drug with the possibility of causing toxicity or decreasing effectiveness: antacids, caffeine, levodopa

Severe reactions are possible when this drug is taken with those listed below: alcohol, anesthetics, antihistamines†, anxiolytics†, epinephrine, narcotics†, quinidine, tricyclic antidepressants†

Increased side effects are possible when this drug is taken with those listed below: amoxapine, antipsychotics†, methyldopa, metoclopramide, metyrosine, pemoline, pimozide, promethazine, rauwolfia alkaloids†, trimeprazine

ALLERGIC REACTIONS AND SIDE EFFECTS

If you are allergic to any phenothiazines†, you may also be allergic to this drug. You should tell your doctor about all your allergies and any unexplained symptoms you may have while taking this drug.

This drug promotes the effect of sunlight on the body and may cause severe sunburn and increased sensitivity of the eyes.

MORE COMMON SIDE EFFECTS: Chewing action*, constipation, dizziness, drowsiness, dry mouth, expressionless face*, eye stare*, fainting, increased appetite, lack of sweating*, lightheadedness, lip smacking*, muscle spasms*, poor balance*, puffy cheeks*, restlessness*, shuffling walk*, stiffness*, stuffy nose, swallowing difficulty*, tongue movements*, trembling*, weight gain

LESS COMMON SIDE EFFECTS: Breast swelling, breast-milk secretion, difficulty urinating*, eye problems*, fainting*, menstrual changes, sexual dysfunction, skin discoloration*, skin rash*, vision changes*

RARE SIDE EFFECTS: Bleeding*, blood pressure change, body spasms*, breathing difficulty*, bruising*, excitement*, eyelid spasms*, facial spasms*, fast heartbeat*, fever*, sweating*, poor bladder control*, muscle weakness*, pale complexion*, seizures*, small pupils*, sore throat*, tiredness*, yellow eyes or skin*

PRECAUTIONS

If you have a history of enlarged prostate, glaucoma, ulcers, seizures, heart disease, urinary difficulty, or Parkinson's disease, this drug may make those conditions worse.

This drug may cause false results from several diagnostic tests, including pregnancy tests, and should be stopped for at least 4 days before the test.

This drug should not be stopped suddenly, due to an increased risk of side effects. If you wish to stop taking this drug, ask your doctor for specific instructions.

Be careful driving or handling equipment while taking this drug because the drug may cause dizziness and drowsiness.

You are more likely to overheat when taking this drug and should avoid exercising in hot weather and using a sauna or hot tub.

Touching the liquid form of this drug may cause skin irritation. Make sure you do not spill the liquid, and wash your hands immediately after taking the dose.

Heavy smoking may cause this drug to be less effective.

This drug may cause dry mouth, which is associated with a greater risk of cavities. Your dentist may recommend that you clean your teeth and mouth differently to avoid infection.

PREGNANCY AND BREAST-FEEDING

Safety during pregnancy has not been established although the drug is known to harm animal fetuses.

Breast-feeding while taking this drug is not recommended.

HELPFUL COMMENTS

The liquid form of this drug should be mixed in $1/4$ to $1/2$ cup of applesauce, caffeine-free carbonated beverage, fruit juice, milk, pudding, soup, tomato juice, or water just before taking the dose.

If you need to take an antacid, take it either 2 hours before or after taking this drug.

Sucking on hard sugarless candy or chewing sugarless gum may help relieve dry mouth caused by this drug.

---

†*See page 52.*   **See page 53.*

THYROID, DESICCATED

Available for over 20 years

COMMONLY USED TO TREAT

Goiter
Low thyroid levels, also known as hypothyroidism

DRUG CATEGORY

thyroid replacement
Class: thyroid hormone

PRODUCTS §

Brand-Name Products with No Generic Alternative
Armour Thyroid 300 mg tablet (¢¢¢¢)
Brand-Name Products with Generic Alternatives
Armour Thyroid 15 mg tablet (¢¢)
 Generic: thyroid, desiccated 15 mg tablet (¢)
Armour Thyroid 30 mg tablet (¢¢)
 Generic: thyroid, desiccated 30 mg tablet (¢)
Armour Thyroid 60 mg tablet (¢¢)
 Generic: thyroid, desiccated 60 mg tablet (¢)
Armour Thyroid 90 mg tablet (¢¢)
 Generic: thyroid, desiccated 90 mg tablet (¢)
Armour Thyroid 120 mg tablet (¢¢¢)
 Generic: thyroid, desiccated 120 mg tablet (¢)
Armour Thyroid 180 mg tablet (¢¢¢)
 Generic: thyroid, desiccated 180 mg tablet (¢)
Armour Thyroid 240 mg tablet (¢¢¢¢)
 Generic: thyroid, desiccated 240 mg tablet (¢¢)
Products Only Available as Generics
thyroid, desiccated 32.4 mg tablet (¢)
thyroid, desiccated 32.5 mg tablet (¢)
thyroid, desiccated 64.8 mg tablet (¢)
thyroid, desiccated 65 mg tablet (¢)
thyroid, desiccated 130 mg tablet (¢)
Other Generic Product Names
Nature-Throid, Westhroid

DOSING AND FOOD

Doses are taken once a day before breakfast.
§ *See "Precautions" in this entry.*

It is best to take this drug on an empty stomach at least 1 hour before a meal.

Adults: Up to 300 mg per day.

Lower doses are used in children.

Forgotten doses: If you are scheduled to take the next dose within a few hours, do not take the forgotten dose. Otherwise take the forgotten dose as soon as you remember.

ALCOHOL, DRUG, HERB, AND SUPPLEMENT INTERACTIONS

Alcohol may increase some of the side effects from this drug, depending on the amount consumed. Ask your doctor about the risks caused by drinking alcohol with your condition.

Several OTC drugs used for appetite control, asthma, colds, cough, hay fever, pain, or sinus problems may cause serious side effects when taken with this drug. Check with your pharmacist when selecting OTC products.

Taking this drug with any of the ones listed below may change the effect of either drug with the possibility of causing toxicity or decreasing effectiveness: adrenocorticoids[†], anticoagulants[†], antidiabetics[†], beta blockers[†], cholestyramine, colestipol, corticotropin, estrogens[†], insulin, phenytoin, theophylline

Severe reactions are possible when this drug is taken with those listed below: amphetamines[†], appetite suppressants, sympathomimetics[†], somatrem, tricyclic antidepressants[†]

ALLERGIC REACTIONS AND SIDE EFFECTS

If you are allergic to any thyroid hormones[†], you may also be allergic to this drug. You should tell your doctor about all your allergies and any unexplained symptoms you may have while taking this drug.

MORE COMMON SIDE EFFECTS: Irregular heartbeat[*]

LESS COMMON SIDE EFFECTS: Appetite changes, diarrhea, fever, headache[*], hives[*], irritability, leg cramps, menstrual changes, nervousness, shakiness, skin rash[*], sleep disorders, sweating, vomiting, weight loss

RARE SIDE EFFECTS: Behavior changes[*], chest pain[*], confusion[*], mood swings[*], restlessness[*], shortness of breath[*], weakness[*], yellow eyes or skin[*]

PRECAUTIONS

§This drug is derived from a natural source. The effects may vary from product to product. Do not switch from one manufacturer to another when your prescription is refilled. Talk to your pharmacist to make sure you get the same product each time.

[†] See page 52.   [*] See page 53.

The dose of this drug is often referred to in the pharmacy term "grains." One grain of thyroid is equivalent to 60 mg.

If you are a diabetic, you may need a change in the dose of your antidiabetic drug† or insulin, since this drug may cause changes in blood sugar.

People with diabetes, heart disease, high blood pressure, adrenal gland deficiency, pituitary gland deficiency, or atherosclerosis may not be able to take this drug.

This drug may make you more sensitive to warm temperatures.

Hair loss may occur in the first months of treatment but hair will usually grow back.

PREGNANCY AND BREAST-FEEDING

Safety studies in pregnant women have not found a risk to the fetus.
This drug passes into breast milk, but does not appear to harm the baby.

HELPFUL COMMENTS

It takes about 2 weeks before you begin to notice the effects of this drug.
Take your dose in the morning to help reduce the sleep disorders that some people suffer.
These tablets have a strong odor.

TIAGABINE HYDROCHLORIDE

Available since September 1997

COMMONLY USED TO TREAT

Seizures

DRUG CATEGORY

anticonvulsant
Class: GABA enhancer

PRODUCTS

Brand-Name Products with No Generic Alternative
Gabitril 2 mg tablet ($)
Gabitril 4 mg tablet ($)
Gabitril 12 mg tablet ($$)
Gabitril 16 mg tablet ($$)
No generics available.
Multiple patents that begin to expire in 2011.

DOSING AND FOOD

Doses are taken 2 to 4 times a day.

It is best to take this drug with food or milk.

Adults: Up to 56 mg per day in divided doses.

Children age 12 to 13: Up to 32 mg per day in divided doses.

Lower doses are used in people with liver disease.

Forgotten doses: If you are scheduled to take the next dose within a few hours, do not take the forgotten dose. Otherwise take the forgotten dose as soon as you remember.

ALCOHOL, DRUG, HERB, AND SUPPLEMENT INTERACTIONS

Alcohol should not be used while taking this drug.

Many OTC drugs used for appetite control, asthma, colds, cough, hay fever, pain, or sinus problems affect the central nervous system and may change the effects or side effects of this drug. Check with your pharmacist for products to avoid.

Taking this drug with any of the ones listed below may change the effect of either drug with the possibility of causing toxicity or decreasing effectiveness: carbamazepine, phenobarbital, phenytoin, primidone, valproate

Severe reactions are possible when this drug is taken with those listed below: analgesics, anesthetics, antihistamines†, anxiolytics†, barbiturates†, narcotics†

ALLERGIC REACTIONS AND SIDE EFFECTS

You should tell your doctor about all your allergies and any unexplained symptoms you may have while taking this drug.

MORE COMMON SIDE EFFECTS: Chills, diarrhea, dizziness, drowsiness*, fever, headache, muscle pain, nervousness, poor concentration, skin spots*, sore throat, tiredness, tremor, vomiting, weakness*

LESS COMMON SIDE EFFECTS: Abdominal pain, burning*, clumsiness*, confusion*, cough, depression*, flushing, increased appetite, itching*, mouth sores, nausea, numbness*, sleep disorders, speaking difficulty*, tingling*, unsteadiness*, vision changes

RARE SIDE EFFECTS: Agitation*, bloody urine*, coma*, confusion*, eye movements*, hostility*, memory loss*, muscle twitching*, seizures*, skin rash*, sluggishness*, urinary changes*

PRECAUTIONS

Be careful driving or handling equipment while taking this drug because it may cause drowsiness or dizziness.

---

†See page 52.   *See page 53.

Stopping this drug suddenly may cause seizure activity to increase in frequency and severity. If you wish to stop taking this drug, ask your doctor for specific instructions.

PREGNANCY AND BREAST-FEEDING

Safety during pregnancy has not been established although the drug is known to harm animal fetuses.

It is not known if this drug passes into breast milk. Talk to your doctor about the risks associated with breast-feeding while taking this drug.

HELPFUL COMMENTS

Avoid quick movements to minimize dizziness. Dangling your legs over the side of the bed for a few minutes may help reduce dizziness when first waking up.

TICLOPIDINE HYDROCHLORIDE

Available since October 1991

COMMONLY USED TO TREAT

People at risk of developing blood clots

DRUG CATEGORY

antiplatelet
Class: ADP blocker

PRODUCTS

Brand-Name Products with Generic Alternatives
Ticlid 250 mg tablet ($$)
  Generic: ticlopidine hydrochloride 250 mg tablet ($$)

DOSING AND FOOD

Doses are taken twice a day.
Always take your dose with a meal.
Adults: Up to 500 mg per day in divided doses.
Forgotten doses: If you are scheduled to take the next dose within a few hours, do not take the forgotten dose. Otherwise take the forgotten dose as soon as you remember.

ALCOHOL, DRUG, HERB, AND SUPPLEMENT INTERACTIONS

Alcohol may increase some of the side effects from this drug, depending on the amount consumed. Ask your doctor about the risks caused by drinking alcohol with your condition.

Red clover may increase the risk of side effects while taking this drug and should not be used.

Do not take aspirin, ibuprofen, naprosyn, or other nonsteroidal anti-inflammatories† used for pain relief while taking this drug.

Taking this drug with any of the ones listed below may change the effect of either drug with the possibility of causing toxicity or decreasing effectiveness: antacids, cimetidine, phenytoin, theophylline, xanthines†

Severe reactions are possible when this drug is taken with those listed below: anticoagulants†, aspirin, carbenicillin, clopidogrel, dipyridamole, divalproex, heparin, nonsteroidal antiinflammatories†, pentoxifylline, plicamycin, sulfinpyrazone, ticarcillin, valproic acid

ALLERGIC REACTIONS AND SIDE EFFECTS

You should tell your doctor about all your allergies and any unexplained symptoms you may have while taking this drug.

MORE COMMON SIDE EFFECTS: Abdominal pain*, diarrhea, indigestion, nausea, skin rash*

LESS COMMON SIDE EFFECTS: Back pain*, behavior changes*, black stools*, bleeding*, blistering*, bloating, blood-spotted eyeball*, bloody urine*, bloody vomit*, bruising*, chills*, dizziness*, fever*, gas, headache*, hives*, itching*, joint pain*, lip sores*, menstrual changes*, mouth sores*, nosebleeds*, pale skin*, poor concentration*, poor coordination*, ringing in ears*, seizures*, skin irritation*, sore throat*, speaking difficulty*, swelling*, tiredness*, vomiting, weakness*, yellow eyes or skin*

PRECAUTIONS

People with blood disease, clotting disorders, liver disease, or ulcers are at greater risk of developing serious side effects while taking this drug.

If you have thrombotic thrombocytopenic purpura (TTP), this drug may make that condition worse.

Blood tests must be done every 2 weeks for the first 3 months of taking this drug.

This drug should be stopped 2 weeks before surgery or dental work, due to a serious risk of bleeding during the procedure.

---

†See page 52.   *See page 53.

PREGNANCY AND BREAST-FEEDING

Safety during pregnancy has not been established although there was no evidence of harm during studies in animals.

Breast-feeding while taking this drug is not recommended.

HELPFUL COMMENTS

The effects of this drug may continue for 1 to 2 weeks after the drug is stopped.

If you need to take an antacid, take it either 2 hours before or after taking this drug.

Acetaminophen may be used instead of aspirin to relieve headaches or pain that develops while taking this drug.

TILUDRONATE DISODIUM

Available since March 1997

COMMONLY USED TO TREAT

Paget's disease

DRUG CATEGORY

antiosteoporotic

Class: bisphosphonate

PRODUCTS

Brand-Name Products with No Generic Alternative

Skelid 200 mg tablet ($$$$)

No generics available.

Multiple patents that begin to expire in 2009.

DOSING AND FOOD

Doses are taken once a day.

This drug should be taken with a full glass of water on an empty stomach at least 2 hours before or after a meal. Juice, milk, coffee, tea, and soda may all interfere with absorption and should not be used in place of water when taking your dose.

Adults: Up to 400 mg per day.

Forgotten doses: If you are scheduled to take the next dose within a few

hours, do not take the forgotten dose. Otherwise take the forgotten dose
as soon as you remember.

ALCOHOL, DRUG, HERB, AND SUPPLEMENT INTERACTIONS

Alcohol may increase some of the side effects from this drug, depending
on the amount consumed. Ask your doctor about the risks caused by
drinking alcohol with your condition.

**Taking this drug with any of the ones listed below may change the effect of
either drug with the possibility of causing toxicity or decreasing effectiveness:**
antacids, aspirin, calcium, indomethacin, iron supplements

ALLERGIC REACTIONS AND SIDE EFFECTS

You should tell your doctor about all your allergies and any unexplained
symptoms you may have while taking this drug.

MORE COMMON SIDE EFFECTS: Back pain, congestion*, cough*, diarrhea,
fever*, hoarseness*, nausea, runny nose*, sneezing*, sore throat*, stomach upset

LESS COMMON SIDE EFFECTS: Blurry vision*, chest pain*, dizziness, eye
pain*, gas, headache*, joint pain, muscle pain, red eyes, skin rash,
swelling*, vision changes*, vomiting, weight gain*

PRECAUTIONS

If you have low calcium levels, vitamin D deficiency, intestinal disorders,
ulcers, swallowing difficulty, or an overactive parathyroid, this drug may
make those conditions worse.

PREGNANCY AND BREAST-FEEDING

Safety during pregnancy has not been established although the drug is
known to harm animal fetuses.

It is not known if this drug passes into breast milk. Talk to your doctor
about the risks associated with breast-feeding while taking this drug.

HELPFUL COMMENTS

This drug is usually given for only 3 months. After that time the need for
therapy is reevaluated.

If you need to take an antacid or vitamin supplement with minerals, take it
either 2 hours before or after taking this drug.

---

†See page 52.   * See page 53.

TIMOLOL

Available for over 20 years

COMMONLY USED TO TREAT

Chest pain, also known as angina
High blood pressure, also known as hypertension
Increased pressure in the eye, also known as glaucoma
Irregular heart rhythm, also known as arrhythmia
People at risk of complications after a heart attack
People at risk of developing migraine headaches

DRUG CATEGORY

antianginal
antiarrhythmic
antiglaucoma
antihypertensive
Class: beta blocker

PRODUCTS

Brand-Name Products with No Generic Alternative
Betimol 0.25% ophthalmic solution ($$$$$)
Betimol 0.5% ophthalmic solution ($$$$$)
Brand-Name Products with Generic Alternatives
Blocadren 5 mg tablet (¢¢¢¢)
  Generic: timolol maleate 5 mg tablet (¢¢¢)
Blocadren 10 mg tablet (¢¢¢¢)
  Generic: timolol maleate 10 mg tablet (¢¢¢)
Blocadren 20 mg tablet ($)
  Generic: timolol maleate 20 mg tablet (¢¢¢¢)
Timoptic 0.25% ophthalmic solution ($$$$$)
  Generic: timolol maleate 0.25% ophthalmic solution ($$$$$)
Timoptic 0.5% ophthalmic solution ($$$$$)
  Generic: timolol maleate 0.5% ophthalmic solution ($$$$$)
Timoptic-XE 0.25% ophthalmic gel drops ($$$$$)
  Generic: timolol maleate 0.25% ophthalmic gel drops ($$$$$)
Timoptic-XE 0.5% ophthalmic gel drops ($$$$$)
  Generic: timolol maleate 0.5% ophthalmic gel drops ($$$$$)
Combination Products That Contain This Drug
Cosopt ophthalmic solution ($$$$$)

Timolide 10-25 tablet (¢¢¢¢¢)

DOSING AND FOOD

Doses are given 1 to 4 times a day.

This drug may be taken with or without food.

Adults: Up to 60 mg per day in divided doses.

Lower doses may be used in people with kidney disease or liver disease, and in people over age 65.

Eyedrops: Normally 1 eyedrop is used per dose.

This drug is rarely used in children.

Forgotten doses: If you are scheduled to take the next dose within 4 hours, do not take the forgotten dose. Otherwise take the forgotten dose as soon as you remember.

ALCOHOL, DRUG, HERB, AND SUPPLEMENT INTERACTIONS

Alcohol may increase some of the side effects from this drug, depending on the amount consumed. Ask your doctor about the risks caused by drinking alcohol with your condition.

Several OTC drugs used for appetite control, asthma, colds, cough, hay fever, or sinus problems may cause an increase in blood pressure when taken with this drug. Check with your pharmacist when selecting OTC products.

Taking this drug with any of the ones listed below may change the effect of either drug with the possibility of causing toxicity or decreasing effectiveness: aminophylline, anesthetics†, antidiabetics†, caffeine, calcium channel blockers†, carbonic anhydrase inhibitors†, clonidine, dyphylline, epinephrine, guanabenz, insulin, lidocaine, nonsteroidal antiinflammatories†, oxtriphylline, pilocarpine, quinidine, reserpine, theophylline

Severe reactions are possible when this drug is taken with those listed below: allergy shots, beta blockers†, cocaine, monoamine oxidase inhibitors†

Increased effects or side effects are possible when this drug is taken with those listed below: antihypertensives†

ALLERGIC REACTIONS AND SIDE EFFECTS

If you are allergic to any other beta blockers†, you may also be allergic to this drug.

This drug may exaggerate the reaction from your current allergies. Inform your doctor of any allergies that you have as well as the severity of the allergic reaction before starting this drug.

---

† *See page 52.* * *See page 53.*

MORE COMMON SIDE EFFECTS: Dizziness*, drowsiness, lightheadedness*, sexual dysfunction, sleeping difficulty, tiredness, weakness

LESS COMMON SIDE EFFECTS: Anxiety, breathing difficulty*, cold hands and feet*, constipation, depression*, diarrhea, itching, nausea, nervousness, numbness, shortness of breath*, slow heartbeat*, sore eyes, stomachache, stuffy nose, swollen legs or feet, tingling, vivid dreams, vomiting, wheezing

RARE SIDE EFFECTS: Back pain*, bleeding*, bruising*, chest pain*, confusion*, fever*, hallucinations*, irregular heartbeat*, joint pain*, rash*, scaly skin*, sore throat*

PRECAUTIONS

People with heart disease or a heart rate that is routinely less than 60 beats per minute (bradycardia) may not be able to take this drug.

Stopping this drug suddenly may cause chest pain or heart attack. If you wish to stop taking this drug, ask your doctor for specific instructions.

Be careful driving or handling equipment while taking this drug because the drug may cause dizziness and drowsiness.

If you are diabetic, this drug may increase blood sugar levels or make the symptoms of low blood sugar less noticeable.

You need to wait 2 weeks after stopping a monoamine oxidase inhibitor† before starting this drug.

If you have psoriasis or myasthenia gravis, this drug may make those conditions worse.

When used in the eye, this drug may be absorbed into the blood stream and may cause side effects similar those listed above for the oral drug. If these occur, they should be reported to your doctor.

PREGNANCY AND BREAST-FEEDING

Safety during pregnancy has not been established although the drug is known to harm animal fetuses.

Breast-feeding while taking this drug is not recommended.

HELPFUL COMMENTS

This drug may make you more sensitive to cold temperatures.

If using the gel foaming eyedrops, the bottle should be inverted once before use.

Doses are adjusted after 7 days if the desired effect is not seen.

If you do not treat high blood pressure, you may develop more serious problems such as heart failure, blood vessel disease, stroke, or kidney disease. Losing weight, exercising, eating more fruits and vegetables, and avoiding salty foods, such as lunchmeat and pickles, may help make drug treatment more successful.

TIZANIDINE HYDROCHLORIDE

Available since August 2002

COMMONLY USED TO TREAT

Muscle spasms associated with multiple sclerosis or spinal cord injuries

DRUG CATEGORY

skeletal muscle relaxant
Class: alpha adrenergic agonist

PRODUCTS

Brand-Name Products with No Generic Alternative
Zanaflex 6 mg capsule (n/a)
Brand-Name Products with Generic Alternatives
Zanaflex 2 mg capsule ($)
  Generic: tizanidine hydrochloride 2 mg capsule (n/a)
Zanaflex 4 mg capsule ($)
  Generic: tizanidine hydrochloride 4 mg capsule (n/a)

DOSING AND FOOD

Doses are taken 3 to 4 times a day.
This drug may be taken with or without food.
Adults: Up to 36 mg per day in divided doses.
Forgotten doses: If more than 2 hours have passed since the forgotten dose, do not take the dose. Otherwise take the forgotten dose as soon as you remember.

ALCOHOL, DRUG, HERB, AND SUPPLEMENT INTERACTIONS

Alcohol should not be used while taking this drug.
Many OTC drugs used for appetite control, asthma, colds, cough, hay fever, pain, or sinus problems affect the central nervous system and may change the effects or side effects of this drug. Check with your pharmacist for products to avoid.

Taking this drug with any of the ones listed below may change the effect of either drug with the possibility of causing toxicity or decreasing effectiveness: antihypertensives†, oral contraceptives, phenytoin

---

†*See page 52.*   **See page 53.*

Severe reactions are possible when this drug is taken with those listed below: anesthetics, antihistamines†, anxiolytics†, barbiturates†, narcotics†, tricyclic antidepressants†

ALLERGIC REACTIONS AND SIDE EFFECTS

You should tell your doctor about all your allergies and any unexplained symptoms you may have while taking this drug.

MORE COMMON SIDE EFFECTS: Anxiety, back pain, constipation, depression, diarrhea, dizziness, drowsiness, dry mouth, fever*, heartburn, lightheadedness, loss of appetite*, muscle spasms, nausea*, nervousness*, prickling*, runny nose, skin irritation*, skin rash, sleepiness, sore throat*, spastic movements, speaking difficulty, stomachache, sweating, tingling*, urinary pain*, vomiting*, weakness*, yellow eyes or skin*

LESS COMMON SIDE EFFECTS: Black stools*, bloody vomit*, blurry vision*, chills*, cough*, dry skin, eye pain*, fainting*, hair loss, hallucinations*, irregular heartbeat*, joint pain, kidney stones*, migraine headache, mood swings, neck pain, seizures*, shaking, stiffness, swallowing difficulty, swelling, tiredness*, trembling, weight changes*

PRECAUTIONS

Be careful driving or handling equipment while taking this drug because it may cause dizziness and drowsiness.

Stopping this drug suddenly may cause severe withdrawal symptoms. If you wish to stop taking this drug, ask your doctor for specific instructions.

This drug may cause dry mouth, which is associated with a greater risk of cavities. Your dentist may recommend that you clean your teeth and mouth differently to avoid infection.

PREGNANCY AND BREAST-FEEDING

Safety during pregnancy has not been established although the drug is known to harm animal fetuses.

This drug passes into breast milk, but does not appear to harm the baby. Talk to your doctor about the risks associated with breast-feeding while taking this drug.

HELPFUL COMMENTS

Sucking on hard sugarless candy or chewing sugarless gum may help relieve dry mouth caused by this drug.

Avoid quick movements to minimize dizziness. Dangling your legs over the side of the bed for a few minutes may help reduce dizziness when first waking up.

TOCAINIDE HYDROCHLORIDE

Available since November 1984

COMMONLY USED TO TREAT

Irregular heartbeats, also known as arrhythmias
Myotonic dystrophy, also known as Steinert's disease
Nerve pain, specifically trigeminal neuralgia

DRUG CATEGORY

antiarrhythmic
Class: amide anesthetic analogue

PRODUCTS

Brand-Name Products with No Generic Alternative
Tonocard 400 mg tablet ($)
Tonocard 600 mg tablet ($)
No generics available.
No patents, no exclusivity.

DOSING AND FOOD

Doses are taken 1 to 3 times a day.
This drug should be taken with food to reduce the stomach upset that
  many people suffer.
Adults: Up to 2,400 mg per day in divided doses.
Lower doses are used in people with kidney disease or liver disease.
Forgotten doses: If more than 4 hours have passed since the forgotten
  dose, do not take the dose. Otherwise take the forgotten dose as soon as
  you remember.

ALCOHOL, DRUG, HERB, AND SUPPLEMENT INTERACTIONS

Alcohol may increase some of the side effects from this drug, depending
  on the amount consumed. Ask your doctor about the risks caused by
  drinking alcohol with your condition.

**Taking this drug with any of the ones listed below may change the effect of
either drug with the possibility of causing toxicity or decreasing effectiveness:**
allopurinol, antiarrhythmics[†], cimetidine, rifampin

Severe reactions are possible when this drug is taken with those listed below:
lidocaine, metoprolol

---

†*See page 52.*   **See page 53.*

ALLERGIC REACTIONS AND SIDE EFFECTS

If you are allergic to local anesthetics, you may also be allergic to this drug. You should tell your doctor about all your unexplained symptoms you may have while taking this drug.

MORE COMMON SIDE EFFECTS: Dizziness, lightheadedness, loss of appetite, nausea

LESS COMMON SIDE EFFECTS: Blurry vision, confusion, headache, nervousness, numbness, shaking*, skin rash, sweating, tingling, trembling*, vomiting

RARE SIDE EFFECTS: Bleeding*, blisters*, bruising*, chills*, cough*, fever*, irregular heartbeat*, mouth sores*, shortness of breath*, skin irritation*

PRECAUTIONS

If you have congestive heart failure, this drug may make that condition worse.
Be careful driving or handling equipment while taking this drug because it may cause dizziness.

PREGNANCY AND BREAST-FEEDING

Safety during pregnancy has not been established although the drug is known to harm animal fetuses.
Breast-feeding while taking this drug is not recommended.

HELPFUL COMMENTS

Frequent blood tests are needed while taking this drug, especially during the first 3 months.
This drug will no longer be available after December 2003.

TOLAZAMIDE

Available for over 20 years

COMMONLY USED TO TREAT

High blood sugar, specifically type 2 diabetes

DRUG CATEGORY

antidiabetic
Class: sulfonylurea: first generation

PRODUCTS

Brand-Name Products with Generic Alternatives

Tolinase 100 mg tablet (¢¢¢)
  Generic: tolazamide 100 mg tablet (¢¢)
Tolinase 250 mg tablet (¢¢¢¢¢)
  Generic: tolazamide 250 mg tablet (¢¢)
Tolinase 500 mg tablet (n/a)
  Generic: tolazamide 500 mg tablet (¢¢¢)

DOSING AND FOOD

Doses are taken 1 to 2 times a day.

It is best to take this drug just before a meal, starting with the first meal of the day.

Adults: Up to 500 mg per day in divided doses.

Lower doses are used in people over age 65.

People with kidney or liver disease may need lower doses.

Forgotten doses: If you are scheduled to take the next dose within a few hours, do not take the forgotten dose. Otherwise take the forgotten dose as soon as you remember.

ALCOHOL, DRUG, HERB, AND SUPPLEMENT INTERACTIONS

Alcohol should not be used while taking this drug since the combination may cause a severe reaction.

Aloe, bilberry leaf, bitter melon, burdock, dandelion, fenugreek, garlic, ginkgo biloba, and ginseng may lower blood sugar and cause the need for a dose adjustment when taken with this drug. Tell your doctor if you are taking any of these supplements.

Several OTC drugs used for asthma, colds, cough, hay fever, sleep aid, or sinus problems may seriously change the effects of this drug. Check with your pharmacist when selecting OTC products.

Taking this drug with any of the ones listed below may change the effect of either drug with the possibility of causing toxicity or decreasing effectiveness: anticoagulants[†], antihistamines[†], aspirin, beta blockers[†], calcium channel blockers[†], chloramphenicol, cimetidine, corticosteroids[†], cyclosporine, estrogens[†], fluconazole, fluoroquinolones[†], insulin, isoniazid, lithium, miconazole, nonsteroidal antiinflammatories[†], oral contraceptives, phenothiazines[†], probenecid, quinine, quinidine, ranitidine, salicylates[†], sulfonamides[†], sympathomimetics[†], thiazide diuretics[†], triamterene

---

[†] *See page 52.*   [*] *See page 53.*

Severe reactions are possible when this drug is taken with those listed below: guanethidine, monoamine oxidase inhibitors†, octreotide, pentamidine

ALLERGIC REACTIONS AND SIDE EFFECTS

If you are allergic to any sulfonylureas† or sulfonamides†, you may also be allergic to this drug. You should tell your doctor about all your allergies and any unexplained symptoms you may have while taking this drug.

This drug promotes the effect of sunlight on the body and may cause severe sunburn and increased sensitivity of the eyes.

MORE COMMON SIDE EFFECTS: Anxiety*, appetite changes, behavior change*, blurry vision*, chills*, confusion*, constipation, diarrhea, difficulty concentrating*, fast heartbeat*, frequent urination, gas, low blood sugar*, nervousness*, nightmares*, shakiness*, sleep disorders*, slurry speech*, stomach pain, sweating*, tiredness*, weight gain*

LESS COMMON SIDE EFFECTS: Dizziness, drowsiness*, headache*, heartburn, hunger*, nausea*, seizures*, skin irritation*, taste changes, unconsciousness*, vomiting, weakness*

RARE SIDE EFFECTS: Bleeding*, bruising*, chest pain*, coughing up blood*, dark urine*, excess sputum*, fever*, hives*, pale skin*, pale stools*, shortness of breath*, sore throat*, yellow eyes or skin*

PRECAUTIONS

Burns, diarrhea, fever, hormonal changes, infection, malnourishment, severe stress, uncontrolled thyroid disease, and vomiting may cause changes in blood sugar that may make this drug less effective.

You need to wait 2 weeks after stopping a monoamine oxidase inhibitor† before starting this drug.

This drug is not effective in treating type 1 diabetes.

PREGNANCY AND BREAST-FEEDING

Safety during pregnancy has not been established although the drug is known to harm animal fetuses.

Breast-feeding while taking this drug is not recommended.

HELPFUL COMMENTS

Blood sugar levels should be checked if you experience any side effects.

If you do not treat high blood sugar, you may develop more serious problems such as heart failure, blood vessel disease, eye disease, or kidney disease.

TOLBUTAMIDE

Available for over 20 years

COMMONLY USED TO TREAT

High blood sugar, specifically type 2 diabetes

DRUG CATEGORY

antidiabetic
Class: sulfonylurea: first generation

PRODUCTS

Products Only Available as Generics
tolbutamide 500 mg tablet (¢)

DOSING AND FOOD

Doses are taken 1 to 3 times a day.
It is best to take this drug just before a meal, starting with the first meal of
the day.
Adults: Up to 3,000 mg per day in divided doses.
Lower doses are used in people over age 65.
People with kidney or liver disease may need lower doses.
Forgotten doses: If you are scheduled to take the next dose within a few
hours, do not take the forgotten dose. Otherwise take the forgotten dose
as soon as you remember.

ALCOHOL, DRUG, HERB, AND SUPPLEMENT INTERACTIONS

Alcohol should not be used while taking this drug since the combination
may cause a severe reaction.
Aloe, bilberry leaf, bitter melon, burdock, dandelion, fenugreek, garlic,
ginkgo biloba, and ginseng may lower blood sugar and cause the need
for a dose adjustment when taken with this drug. Tell your doctor if you
are taking any of these supplements.
Several OTC drugs used for asthma, colds, cough, hay fever, sleep aid, or
sinus problems may seriously change the effects of this drug. Check with
your pharmacist when selecting OTC products.
**Taking this drug with any of the ones listed below may change the effect of
either drug with the possibility of causing toxicity or decreasing effectiveness:**
anticoagulants†, antihistamines†, aspirin, beta blockers†, calcium channel
blockers†, chloramphenicol, cimetidine, corticosteroids†, cyclosporine,

---

† *See page 52.*   * *See page 53.*

estrogens†, fluconazole, fluoroquinolones†, insulin, isoniazid, lithium, miconazole, nonsteroidal antiinflammatories†, oral contraceptives, phenothiazines†, probenecid, quinine, quinidine, ranitidine, salicylates†, sulfonamides†, sympathomimetics†, thiazide diuretics†, triamterene

Severe reactions are possible when this drug is taken with those listed below: guanethidine, monoamine oxidase inhibitors†, octreotide, pentamidine

ALLERGIC REACTIONS AND SIDE EFFECTS

If you are allergic to any sulfonylureas† or sulfonamides†, you may also be allergic to this drug. You should tell your doctor about all your allergies and any unexplained symptoms you may have while taking this drug.

This drug promotes the effect of sunlight on the body and may cause severe sunburn and increased sensitivity of the eyes.

MORE COMMON SIDE EFFECTS: Anxiety*, appetite changes, behavior change*, blurry vision*, chills*, confusion*, constipation, diarrhea, difficulty concentrating*, dizziness, drowsiness*, fast heartbeat*, frequent urination, gas, hunger*, low blood sugar*, nervousness*, nightmares*, shakiness*, sleep disorders*, slurry speech*, sweating*, tiredness*, vomiting, weakness*, weight gain*

LESS COMMON SIDE EFFECTS: Headache*, heartburn, nausea*, seizures*, skin irritation*, stomach pain, taste changes, unconsciousness*

RARE SIDE EFFECTS: Bleeding*, bruising*, chest pain*, coughing up blood*, dark urine*, depression*, excess sputum*, fever*, hives*, pale skin*, pale stools*, shortness of breath*, sore throat*, swelling*, yellow eyes or skin*

PRECAUTIONS

Burns, diarrhea, fever, hormonal changes, infection, malnourishment, severe stress, uncontrolled thyroid disease, and vomiting may cause changes in blood sugar that may make this drug less effective.

You need to wait 2 weeks after stopping a monoamine oxidase inhibitor† before starting this drug.

This drug is not effective in treating type 1 diabetes.

PREGNANCY AND BREAST-FEEDING

Safety during pregnancy has not been established although the drug is known to harm animal fetuses.

Breast-feeding while taking this drug is not recommended.

HELPFUL COMMENTS

Blood sugar levels should be checked if you experience any side effects.

If you do not treat high blood sugar, you may develop more serious problems such as heart failure, blood vessel disease, eye disease, or kidney disease.

TOLCAPONE

Available since January 1998

COMMONLY USED TO TREAT

Parkinson's disease

DRUG CATEGORY

antidyskinetic
Class: COMT inhibitor

PRODUCTS

Brand-Name Products with No Generic Alternative
Tasmar 100 mg tablet ($$)
Tasmar 200 mg tablet ($$$)
No generics available.
Patent expires in 2012.

DOSING AND FOOD

Doses are taken 3 times a day.
This drug may be taken with or without food but works faster when taken on an empty stomach.
Adults: Up to 600 mg per day in divided doses.
Lower doses are used in people with kidney disease or liver disease.
Forgotten doses: If you are scheduled to take the next dose within a few hours, do not take the forgotten dose. Otherwise take the forgotten dose as soon as you remember.

ALCOHOL, DRUG, HERB, AND SUPPLEMENT INTERACTIONS

Alcohol may increase the risk of liver damage from this drug. Ask your doctor about the risks caused by drinking alcohol with your condition.

Taking this drug with any of the ones listed below may change the effect of either drug with the possibility of causing toxicity or decreasing effectiveness:
anticoagulants†

---

† *See page 52.*   * *See page 53.*

Severe reactions are possible when this drug is taken with those listed below: monoamine oxidase inhibitors†

Increased side effects are possible when this drug is taken with those listed below: desipramine

ALLERGIC REACTIONS AND SIDE EFFECTS

You should tell your doctor about all your allergies and any unexplained symptoms you may have while taking this drug.

MORE COMMON SIDE EFFECTS: Abdominal pain*, constipation, cough*, diarrhea*, dizziness*, dreams, drowsiness*, dry mouth, fainting*, fever*, hallucinations*, headache*, lightheadedness*, nausea*, sleep disorders*, sneezing*, sore throat*, spastic movements*, stuffy nose*, sweating, twitching*, vomiting*

LESS COMMON SIDE EFFECTS: Bloody urine*, breathing difficulty*, chest pain*, chills*, confusion*, falling*, gas, heartburn, hyperactivity*, muscle pain*, poor balance*

RARE SIDE EFFECTS: Agitation*, chest tightness*, dark urine*, irritability*, itching*, joint pain*, loss of appetite*, low blood pressure*, neck ache*, pale stools*, poor concentration*, prickling*, stiffness*, tingling*, tiredness*, urinary changes*, weakness*, yellow eyes or skin*

PRECAUTIONS

This drug is used in combination with carbidopa/levodopa.

If you have a history of hallucinations, this drug may make that condition worse.

Stopping the drug suddenly may cause serious side effects. If you wish to stop taking this drug, ask your doctor for specific instructions.

Be careful driving or handling equipment while taking this drug because it may cause dizziness and drowsiness.

This drug may cause your urine to turn bright yellow, which is not harmful, and the color will return to normal when the drug is stopped.

This drug may cause dry mouth, which is associated with a greater risk of cavities. Your dentist may recommend that you clean your teeth and mouth differently to avoid infection.

You need to wait 2 weeks after stopping a monoamine oxidase inhibitor† before starting this drug.

PREGNANCY AND BREAST-FEEDING

Safety during pregnancy has not been established although the drug is known to harm animal fetuses.

Breast-feeding while taking this drug is not recommended.

HELPFUL COMMENTS

Avoid quick movements to minimize dizziness. Dangling your legs over the side of the bed for a few minutes may help reduce dizziness when first waking up.

Sucking on hard sugarless candy or chewing sugarless gum may help relieve dry mouth caused by this drug.

The full effects of this drug should be noticed within 3 weeks.

TOLMETIN SODIUM

Available for over 20 years

COMMONLY USED TO TREAT

Arthritis

DRUG CATEGORY

antiarthritic
Class: nonsteroidal antiinflammatory

PRODUCTS

Brand-Name Products with Generic Alternatives
Tolectin 200 mg capsule (n/a)
Generic: tolmetin sodium 200 mg capsule (¢¢¢¢)
Tolectin DS 400 mg capsule ($)
Generic: tolmetin sodium 400 mg capsule (¢¢¢¢¢)
Tolectin 600 mg capsule ($$)
Generic: tolmetin sodium 600 mg capsule ($)

DOSING AND FOOD

Doses are taken 3 to 4 times a day.

It is better to take this drug on an empty stomach, but taking it with a little food may avoid the stomach upset that some people suffer.

Adults: Up to 1,800 mg per day in divided doses.

Children age 2 and older: Up to 30 mg/kg per day in divided doses.

Forgotten doses: If you are scheduled to take the next dose within a few hours, do not take the forgotten dose. Otherwise take the forgotten dose as soon as you remember.

ALCOHOL, DRUG, HERB, AND SUPPLEMENT INTERACTIONS

Alcohol may increase the risk of serious side effects from this drug. Ask your doctor about the risks caused by drinking alcohol with your condition.

Do not use dong quai, feverfew, garlic, ginger, horse chestnut, red clover, or St. John's wort while taking this drug since they may increase the risk of serious side effects.

Taking this drug with any of the ones listed below may change the effect of either drug with the possibility of causing toxicity or decreasing effectiveness: acetaminophen, antihypertensives†, digoxin, diuretics†, furosemide, hydrochlorothiazide, nifedipine, lithium, methotrexate, phenytoin, probenecid, sulfonamides†, sulfonylureas†, sulindac, verapamil

Severe reactions are possible when this drug is taken with those listed below: antibiotics†, anticoagulants†, aspirin, cefamandole, cefoperazone, cefotetan, corticosteroids†, cyclosporine, gold salts†, heparin, nonsteroidal antiinflammatories†, penicillamine, plicamycin, salicylates†, valproic acid, warfarin

ALLERGIC REACTIONS AND SIDE EFFECTS

If you are allergic to aspirin, zomepirac, salicylates†, or other nonsteroidal antiinflammatories†, you may also be allergic to this drug. You should tell your doctor about all your allergies and any unexplained symptoms you may have while taking this drug.

This drug promotes the effect of sunlight on the body and may cause severe sunburn and increased sensitivity of the eyes.

MORE COMMON SIDE EFFECTS: Breathing difficulty*, nausea*, skin rash*, swelling*, weight gain*

LESS COMMON SIDE EFFECTS: Abdominal pain, bruising*, constipation, diarrhea, dizziness, drowsiness, gas, headache, heartburn*, high blood pressure*, indigestion*, itching*, mouth sores*, sweating, vomiting

RARE SIDE EFFECTS: Back pain*, black stools*, bloody urine*, bloody vomit*, blue fingernails*, blue lips*, chest pain*, chest tightness*, chills*, confusion*, cough*, dark urine*, fainting*, fever*; hallucinations*, hearing loss*, hives*, hoarseness*, lip sores*, loss of appetite*, low blood pressure*, mood swings*, muscle cramps*, nosebleeds*, pain*, pale skin*, pale stools*, puffy eyes*, rectal bleeding*, restlessness*, ringing in ears*, runny nose*, seizures*, shortness of breath*, sore throat*, stiff neck*, swollen glands*, swollen tongue*, thirst*, tiredness*, urinary changes*, vision changes*, weakness*, wheezing*, yellow eyes or skin*

PRECAUTIONS

This drug may cause serious stomach problems and possibly ulcers. Be careful to take this drug as directed with food, and let your doctor know if you develop any stomach-related symptoms.

Be careful driving or handling equipment while taking this drug because the drug may cause dizziness and drowsiness.

If you use tobacco or have a history of alcohol abuse, stomach problems, intestinal problems, hemorrhoids, diabetes mellitus, severe fluid retention, or systemic lupus erythematosus, there is an increased risk that you will develop side effects while taking this drug.

PREGNANCY AND BREAST-FEEDING

Safety during pregnancy has not been established although the drug is known to harm animal fetuses.

Breast-feeding while taking this drug is not recommended.

HELPFUL COMMENTS

People with arthritis usually notice the effects of this drug within 1 week.

Several nonsteroidal antiinflammatories† are available without a prescription in lower, nonprescription strengths, including ibuprofen, ketoprofen, and naproxen.

TOLTERODINE TARTRATE

Available since March 1998

COMMONLY USED TO TREAT

Frequent urination
Overactive bladder (OAB)
Poor bladder control

DRUG CATEGORY

antispasmodic
Class: anticholinergic

PRODUCTS

Brand-Name Products with No Generic Alternative
Detrol 1 mg tablet ($)
Detrol 2 mg tablet ($$)
Detrol LA 2 mg extended-release capsule ($$$)

---

† See page 52.   * See page 53.

Detrol LA 4 mg extended-release capsule ($$$)
No generics available.
Multiple patents that begin to expire in 2012.

DOSING AND FOOD

Doses are taken twice a day. Extended-release products are taken once a day.
This drug should be taken with food to help increase drug absorption.
Adults: Up to 4 mg per day.
Lower doses are used in people with liver disease.
Forgotten doses: If you are scheduled to take the next dose within a few hours, do not take the forgotten dose. Otherwise take the forgotten dose as soon as you remember.

ALCOHOL, DRUG, HERB, AND SUPPLEMENT INTERACTIONS

Alcohol may increase some of the side effects from this drug, depending on the amount consumed. Ask your doctor about the risks caused by drinking alcohol with your condition.

Taking this drug with any of the ones listed below may change the effect of either drug with the possibility of causing toxicity or decreasing effectiveness: antifungals†, clarithromycin, cyclosporine, erythromycin, fluoxetine, macrolides†, vinblastine

ALLERGIC REACTIONS AND SIDE EFFECTS

You should tell your doctor about all your allergies and any unexplained symptoms you may have while taking this drug.
MORE COMMON SIDE EFFECTS: Abdominal pain, bloody urine*, chest pain, constipation, diarrhea, dizziness, drowsiness, dry eyes, dry mouth, fatigue, headache, joint pain, nausea, stomach upset, urinary changes*, vision changes*

PRECAUTIONS

If you have glaucoma or stomach problems, this drug may make those conditions worse.
Be careful driving or handling equipment while taking this drug because it may cause vision changes, drowsiness, and dizziness.
This drug may cause dry mouth, which is associated with a greater risk of cavities. Your dentist may recommend that you clean your teeth and mouth differently to avoid infection.
Do not open, break, crush, or chew the extended-release products.

PREGNANCY AND BREAST-FEEDING

Safety during pregnancy has not been established although the drug is
known to harm animal fetuses.

Breast-feeding while taking this drug is not recommended.

HELPFUL COMMENTS

Sucking on hard sugarless candy or chewing sugarless gum may help relieve dry mouth caused by this drug.

Avoid quick movements to minimize dizziness. Dangling your legs over the
side of the bed for a few minutes may help reduce dizziness when first
waking up.

TOPIRAMATE

Available since December 1996

COMMONLY USED TO TREAT

Seizures

DRUG CATEGORY

anticonvulsant
Class: sulfamate-substituted monosaccharide

PRODUCTS

Brand-Name Products with No Generic Alternative
Topamax 25 mg tablet ($)
Topamax 100 mg tablet ($$$)
Topamax 200 mg tablet ($$$)
Topamax 15 mg sprinkle capsule ($)
Topamax 25 mg sprinkle capsule ($$)
No generics available.
Exclusivity begins to expire in 2004.

DOSING AND FOOD

Doses are taken twice a day.
This drug may be taken with or without food.
Adults: Up to 400 mg per day in divided doses.
Children age 2 to 16: Up to 9 mg/kg per day in divided doses.
Lower doses are used in people with kidney disease.

---

† *See page 52.*   * *See page 53.*

Forgotten doses: If you are scheduled to take the next dose within a few hours, do not take the forgotten dose. Otherwise take the forgotten dose as soon as you remember.

ALCOHOL, DRUG, HERB, AND SUPPLEMENT INTERACTIONS

Alcohol should not be used while taking this drug.

Many OTC drugs used for appetite control, asthma, colds, cough, hay fever, pain, or sinus problems affect the central nervous system and may change the effects or side effects of this drug. Check with your pharmacist for products to avoid.

Taking this drug with any of the ones listed below may change the effect of either drug with the possibility of causing toxicity or decreasing effectiveness: carbamazepine, oral contraceptives, phenytoin, primidone, valproic acid

Increased side effects are possible when this drug is taken with those listed below: acetazolamide, anesthetics, antihistamines†, anxiolytics†, barbiturates†, dichlorphenamide, narcotics†

ALLERGIC REACTIONS AND SIDE EFFECTS

You should tell your doctor about all your allergies and any unexplained symptoms you may have while taking this drug.

MORE COMMON SIDE EFFECTS: Blurry vision*, breast pain, burning*, clumsiness*, confusion*, dizziness*, drowsiness*, eye irritation*, eye movements*, eye pain*, memory loss*, menstrual changes*, nausea, nervousness*, poor concentration*, prickling*, speaking difficulty*, tingling*, tiredness*, tremors, unsteadiness*, vision changes*, weakness*

LESS COMMON SIDE EFFECTS: Abdominal pain*, aggression*, agitation*, back pain, bleeding gums*, chest pain, chills*, constipation, depression*, fever*, heartburn, hot flashes, irritability*, leg pain, loss of appetite*, mood swings*, sore throat*, sweating, weight loss*

RARE SIDE EFFECTS: Back pain*, bloody urine*, breathing difficulty*, hearing loss*, itching*, nosebleeds*, pale skin*, poor bladder control*, ringing in ears*, sexual dysfunction*, skin rash*, suicidal thoughts*, swelling*, urinary changes*

PRECAUTIONS

This drug may cause changes to your gums and mouth. Your dentist may recommend that you clean your teeth and mouth differently to avoid infection.

People with a history of kidney stones are at greater risk of developing new kidney stones while taking this drug.

Be careful driving or handling equipment while taking this drug because it may cause dizziness, drowsiness, and vision changes.

Drink 8 to 10 glasses of water each day to reduce the risk of developing kidney stones while taking this drug.

If stopped suddenly, this drug may cause severe and frequent seizures. If you wish to stop taking this drug, ask your doctor for specific instructions.

PREGNANCY AND BREAST-FEEDING

Safety during pregnancy has not been established although the drug is known to harm animal fetuses.

It is not known if this drug passes into breast milk. Talk to your doctor about the risks associated with breast-feeding while taking this drug.

HELPFUL COMMENTS

Oral contraceptives may not work properly when taken with this drug. You need to use a barrier contraceptive, such as a condom, or other nonhormonal contraceptive to prevent pregnancy.

Sprinkle capsules should be opened and sprinkled over soft food such as applesauce, custard, ice cream, oatmeal, pudding, or yogurt. Be careful not to chew the drug pellets.

The tablets have a bitter taste if kept in the mouth too long before swallowing.

TOREMIFENE CITRATE

Available since May 1997

COMMONLY USED TO TREAT

Breast cancer

DRUG CATEGORY

antineoplastic
Class: nonsteroidal antiestrogen

PRODUCTS

Brand-Name Products with No Generic Alternative
Fareston 60 mg tablet ($$$)
No generics available.
Patent expires in 2009.

---

†*See page 52.* ** See page 53.*

DOSING AND FOOD

Doses are taken once a day.

This drug may be taken with or without food. Do not eat grapefruit or drink grapefruit juice while taking this drug.

Adults: Up to 60 mg per day.

Forgotten doses: If you are scheduled to take the next dose within a few hours, do not take the forgotten dose. Otherwise take the forgotten dose as soon as you remember.

ALCOHOL, DRUG, HERB, AND SUPPLEMENT INTERACTIONS

Alcohol may increase some of the side effects from this drug, depending on the amount consumed. Ask your doctor about the risks caused by drinking alcohol with your condition.

Taking this drug with any of the ones listed below may change the effect of either drug with the possibility of causing toxicity or decreasing effectiveness: anticoagulants†, barbiturates†, carbamazepine, clarithromycin, corticosteroids†, cyclosporine, danazol, delaviridine, diltiazem, erythromycin, fluconazole, fluoxetine, fluvoxamine, griseofulvin, indinavir, isoniazid, itraconazole, ketoconazole, metronidazole, miconazole, nafcillin, nefazodone, nelfinavir, nicardipine, nifedipine, norfloxacin, omeprazole, phenobarbital, phenytoin, prednisone, quinidine, quinine, ritonavir, rifabutin, saquinavir, sertraline, troglitazone, troleandomycin, verapamil, zafirlukast

Increased side effects are possible when this drug is taken with those listed below: thiazide diuretics†

ALLERGIC REACTIONS AND SIDE EFFECTS

You should tell your doctor about all your allergies and any unexplained symptoms you may have while taking this drug.

MORE COMMON SIDE EFFECTS: Nausea, sweating

LESS COMMON SIDE EFFECTS: Blurry vision*, bone pain, confusion*, dizziness, dry eyes, liver problems*, loss of appetite*, pelvic pain*, tiredness*, urination*, vaginal bleeding*, vaginal discharge*, vision changes*, vomiting

RARE SIDE EFFECTS: Chest pain*, shortness of breath*, swelling*

PRECAUTIONS

People with a history of blood clots may not be able to take this drug.

Drink plenty of fluids to avoid dehydration when sweating, such as in hot weather and during exercise.

Symptoms of your condition may flare up during the first few weeks of treatment with this drug.

PREGNANCY AND BREAST-FEEDING

There is evidence that this drug may harm the fetus, but the drug may be necessary to the health of the mother.

It is not known if this drug passes into breast milk. Talk to your doctor about the risks associated with breast-feeding while taking this drug.

HELPFUL COMMENTS

It takes 4 to 6 weeks for the effects of this drug to be noticed.

It is very important to continue taking this drug as ordered by the doctor even if the side effects make you feel ill.

Oral contraceptives may not work properly when taken with this drug. You need to use a barrier contraceptive, such as a condom, or other nonhormonal contraceptive to prevent pregnancy.

TORSEMIDE

Available since August 1993

COMMONLY USED TO TREAT

Fluid (water) retention caused by disease
High blood pressure, also known as hypertension

DRUG CATEGORY

antihypertensive
Class: loop diuretic

PRODUCTS

Brand-Name Products with Generic Alternatives
Demadex 5 mg tablet (¢¢¢¢)
  Generic: torsemide 5 mg tablet (n/a)
Demadex 10 mg tablet (¢¢¢¢)
  Generic: torsemide 10 mg tablet (n/a)
Demadex 20 mg tablet (¢¢¢¢¢)
  Generic: torsemide 20 mg tablet (n/a)
Demadex 100 mg tablet ($$$)
  Generic: torsemide 100 mg tablet (n/a)

---

†*See page 52.*   **See page 53.*

DOSING AND FOOD

Doses are taken once a day usually in the morning.

This drug may be taken with or without food.

Adults: Up to 200 mg per day.

Forgotten doses: If you are scheduled to take the next dose within a few hours, do not take the forgotten dose. Otherwise take the forgotten dose as soon as you remember.

ALCOHOL, DRUG, HERB, AND SUPPLEMENT INTERACTIONS

Alcohol may increase some of the side effects from this drug, depending on the amount consumed. Ask your doctor about the risks caused by drinking alcohol with your condition.

Dandelion may interfere with the effects of this drug and should not be used.

Taking this drug with any of the ones listed below may change the effect of either drug with the possibility of causing toxicity or decreasing effectiveness: anticoagulants†, cholestyramine, indomethacin, lithium, probenecid

Increased side effects are possible when this drug is taken with those listed below: acetazolamide, alcohol, aldesleukin, amphotericin B, antibiotics†, aspirin, capreomycin, carbenicillin, carmustine, cisplatin, corticosteroids†, corticotropin, cyclosporine, deferoxamine, dichlorphenamide, diuretics†, gold salts†, insulin, laxatives, methazolamide, methotrexate, mezlocillin, nonsteroidal antiinflammatories†, penicillamine, pentamidine, piperacillin, plicamycin, salicylates†, sodium bicarbonate, streptozocin, ticarcillin, tiopronin, vitamin B_{12}, vitamin D

ALLERGIC REACTIONS AND SIDE EFFECTS

If you are allergic to bumetanide, ethacrynic acid, furosemide, sulfonamides†, or thiazide diuretics†, you may also be allergic to this drug. You should tell your doctor about all your allergies and any unexplained symptoms you may have while taking this drug.

MORE COMMON SIDE EFFECTS: Constipation, dizziness*, headache, upset stomach

LESS COMMON SIDE EFFECTS: Dry mouth*, irregular heartbeat*, mood swings*, muscle pain*, nausea*, thirst*, tiredness*, vomiting*, weakness*

RARE SIDE EFFECTS: Black stools*, hearing loss*, ringing in ears*, skin rash*

PRECAUTIONS

If you are a diabetic, you may need a change in the dose of your antidiabetic drug† or insulin, since this drug may cause an increase in blood sugar.

If you have gout or hearing disorders, this drug may make those conditions worse.

This drug causes you to urinate, which should start 1 to 2 hours after taking the dose.

Your body may lose potassium while taking this drug, which may cause severe side effects. Potassium levels should be monitored periodically and may need to be supplemented while taking this drug. Eat food rich in potassium, such as apricots, bananas, citrus fruit, dates, and tomatoes, if you are not taking a potassium supplement or potassium-sparing diuretic†.

Be careful driving or handling equipment while taking this drug because it may cause dizziness.

This drug may cause dry mouth, which is associated with a greater risk of cavities. Your dentist may recommend that you clean your teeth and mouth differently to avoid infection.

Tell your doctor if you take large doses of aspirin on a regular basis since this drug may mask the symptoms of aspirin toxicity.

Record your weight twice a day, when first getting up in the morning and after the drug causes urination. A weight gain or loss of more than 2 pounds per day should be reported to your doctor.

PREGNANCY AND BREAST-FEEDING

Safety during pregnancy has not been established although there was no evidence of harm during studies in animals.

It is not known if this drug passes into breast milk. Talk to your doctor about the risks associated with breast-feeding while taking this drug.

HELPFUL COMMENTS

Sucking on hard sugarless candy or chewing sugarless gum may help relieve dry mouth caused by this drug.

Avoid quick movements to minimize dizziness. Dangling your legs over the side of the bed for a few minutes may help reduce dizziness when first waking up.

If you do not treat high blood pressure, you may develop more serious problems such as heart failure, blood vessel disease, stroke, or kidney disease. Losing weight, exercising, eating more fruits and vegetables, and avoiding salty foods, such as lunchmeat and pickles, may help make drug treatment more successful.

---

† See page 52.   * See page 53.

TRAMADOL HYDROCHLORIDE

Available since March 1995

COMMONLY USED TO TREAT

Pain

DRUG CATEGORY

analgesic
Class: cyclohexanol derivative

PRODUCTS

Brand-Name Products with Generic Alternatives
Ultram 50 mg tablet (¢¢¢¢¢)
   Generic: tramadol hydrochloride 50 mg tablet (n/a)
Combination Products That Contain This Drug
Ultracet tablet (¢¢¢¢¢)

DOSING AND FOOD

Doses are taken 4 to 6 times a day as needed.
This drug may be taken with or without food but is best taken with food to reduce the stomach upset that some people suffer.

Adults and children over age 16: Up to 400 mg per day in divided doses.

Lower doses are used in people with kidney disease or liver disease.

ALCOHOL, DRUG, HERB, AND SUPPLEMENT INTERACTIONS

Alcohol should not be used while taking this drug.

Many OTC drugs used for appetite control, asthma, colds, cough, hay fever, pain, or sinus problems affect the central nervous system and may cause a change in the effects or side effects while taking this drug. Check with your pharmacist for products to avoid.

Taking this drug with any of the ones listed below may change the effect of either drug with the possibility of causing toxicity or decreasing effectiveness: carbamazepine

Severe reactions are possible when this drug is taken with those listed below: monoamine oxidase inhibitors†

Increased side effects are possible when this drug is taken with those listed below: anesthetics, antihistamines†, anxiolytics†, barbiturates†, narcotics†

ALLERGIC REACTIONS AND SIDE EFFECTS

You should tell your doctor about all your allergies and any unexplained symptoms you may have while taking this drug.

MORE COMMON SIDE EFFECTS: Abdominal pain, agitation, anxiety, constipation, diarrhea, dizziness*, drowsiness, dry mouth, headache, heartburn, itching*, loss of appetite, nausea, nervousness, skin rash, sweating, vomiting, weakness*

LESS COMMON SIDE EFFECTS: Blisters*, blurry vision*, confusion, depression, fainting*, flushing, gas, hallucinations*, hot flashes, irregular heartbeat*, lightheadedness*, memory loss*, numbness*, poor balance*, seizures*, shaky hands*, shortness of breath*, skin irritation*, sleeping difficulty, tingling*, trembling*, urinary changes*

RARE SIDE EFFECTS: Breathing difficulty*, small pupils*

PRECAUTIONS

If you have a history of seizures or are taking a monoamine oxidase inhibitor†, you may be at greater risk of developing a seizure while taking this drug.

Be careful driving or handling equipment while taking this drug because it may cause drowsiness and dizziness.

If you lie down for a while after taking a dose of this drug, you may be able to minimize the nausea or vomiting that occurs.

This drug may cause dry mouth, which is associated with a greater risk of cavities. Your dentist may recommend that you clean your teeth and mouth differently to avoid infection.

Although this drug is not considered a narcotic, it has the same potential for addiction and dependence.

Drink plenty of fluids to avoid dehydration when sweating, such as in hot weather and during exercise.

PREGNANCY AND BREAST-FEEDING

Safety during pregnancy has not been established although the drug is known to harm animal fetuses.

Breast-feeding while taking this drug is not recommended.

HELPFUL COMMENTS

Sucking on hard sugarless candy or chewing sugarless gum may help relieve dry mouth caused by this drug.

---

† See page 52.   * See page 53.

Avoid quick movements to minimize dizziness. Dangling your legs over the side of the bed for a few minutes may help reduce dizziness when first waking up.

TRANDOLAPRIL

Available since April 1996

COMMONLY USED TO TREAT

High blood pressure, also known as hypertension
Heart failure

DRUG CATEGORY

antihypertensive
Class: ACE inhibitor

PRODUCTS

Brand-Name Products with No Generic Alternative
Mavik 1 mg tablet (¢¢¢¢¢)
Mavik 2 mg tablet (¢¢¢¢¢)
Mavik 4 mg tablet (¢¢¢¢¢)
No generics available.
Multiple patents that begin to expire in 2007.
Combination Products That Contain This Drug
Tarka extended-release tablet ($$)

DOSING AND FOOD

Doses are taken 1 to 2 times a day.
It is best to take this drug on an empty stomach at least 1 hour before meals.
Adults: Up to 8 mg per day in divided doses.
Lower doses are used in people with kidney disease.
Forgotten doses: If you are scheduled to take the next dose within a few hours, do not take the forgotten dose. Otherwise take the forgotten dose as soon as you remember.

ALCOHOL, DRUG, HERB, AND SUPPLEMENT INTERACTIONS

Alcohol may cause your blood pressure to rise, making this drug less effective. Ask your doctor about the risks caused by drinking alcohol with your condition.
Licorice may interfere with the effects of this drug.

Capsaicin increases the risk of developing a cough and should not be taken at the same time as this drug.

Several OTC drugs used for appetite control, asthma, colds, cough, hay fever, or sinus problems may cause an increase in blood pressure when taken with this drug. Check with your pharmacist when selecting OTC products.

Taking this drug with any of the ones listed below may change the effect of either drug with the possibility of causing toxicity or decreasing effectiveness: antacids, antidiabetics†, antihypertensives†, diuretics†, insulin, lithium, potassium supplements

ALLERGIC REACTIONS AND SIDE EFFECTS

If you are allergic to any ACE inhibitors†, you may also be allergic to this drug. You should tell your doctor about all your allergies and any unexplained symptoms you may have while taking this drug.

MORE COMMON SIDE EFFECTS: Breathing difficulty*, swallowing difficulty*, swelling*

LESS COMMON SIDE EFFECTS: Diarrhea, dizziness*, dry cough, fainting*, fever*, headache, joint pain*, lightheadedness*, loss of taste, nausea, skin rash*, tiredness

RARE SIDE EFFECTS: Abdominal pain*, chest pain*, chills*, confusion*, hoarseness*, irregular heartbeat*, itching*, nausea*, nervousness*, numbness*, stomach pain*, vomiting*, weakness*, yellow eyes or skin*

PRECAUTIONS

Be careful driving or handling equipment while taking this drug because the drug may cause dizziness.

People with systemic lupus erythematosus may be at greater risk of developing blood problems while taking this drug.

Do not use potassium-containing products, including salt substitutes, while taking this drug.

Diuretics† should be stopped 2 to 3 days prior to starting this drug. If it is not possible to stop the diuretic, the dose of this drug should be lowered.

Drink plenty of fluids to avoid dehydration when sweating, such as in hot weather and during exercise.

PREGNANCY AND BREAST-FEEDING

Safety during pregnancy has not been established although the drug is known to harm animal fetuses.

Breast-feeding while taking this drug is not recommended.

---

† See page 52.   * See page 53.

HELPFUL COMMENTS

A persistent dry cough may appear while taking this drug, but it will go away when the drug is stopped.

If you need to take an antacid, take it either 2 hours before or after taking this drug.

African Americans usually require higher doses of this drug than Caucasians.

TRAZODONE HYDROCHLORIDE

Available for over 20 years

COMMONLY USED TO TREAT

Aggressive behavior
Depression
Panic attacks

DRUG CATEGORY

antidepressant
Class: triazolopyridine derivative

PRODUCTS

Brand-Name Products with Generic Alternatives
Desyrel 50 mg tablet ($$)
  Generic: trazodone hydrochloride 50 mg tablet (¢¢¢)
Desyrel 100 mg tablet ($$$)
  Generic: trazodone hydrochloride 100 mg tablet (¢¢¢)
Desyrel Dividose 150 mg tablet ($$$)
  Generic: trazodone hydrochloride 150 mg tablet (¢¢¢¢)
Desyrel Dividose 300 mg tablet ($$$$)
  Generic: trazodone hydrochloride 300 mg tablet ($$$)

DOSING AND FOOD

Doses are taken 1 to 2 times a day.
Taking this drug with food will help increase drug absorption.
Adults: Up to 400 mg per day in divided doses.
Forgotten doses: If more than 4 hours have passed since the forgotten dose, do not take the dose. Otherwise take the forgotten dose as soon as you remember.

ALCOHOL, DRUG, HERB, AND SUPPLEMENT INTERACTIONS

Alcohol should not be used while taking this drug.

Ginkgo biloba and St. John's wort should not be used while taking this drug, due to an increased risk of developing severe side effects.

Many OTC drugs used for appetite control, asthma, colds, cough, hay fever, pain, or sinus problems affect the central nervous system and may change the effects or side effects of this drug. Check with your pharmacist for products to avoid.

Taking this drug with any of the ones listed below may change the effect of either drug with the possibility of causing toxicity or decreasing effectiveness: antihypertensives†, digoxin, phenytoin

Severe reactions are possible when this drug is taken with those listed below: anesthetics, antihistamines†, anxiolytics†, barbiturates†, narcotics†, tricyclic antidepressants†

ALLERGIC REACTIONS AND SIDE EFFECTS

You should tell your doctor about all your allergies and any unexplained symptoms you may have while taking this drug.

MORE COMMON SIDE EFFECTS: Bad taste, dizziness, drowsiness*, dry mouth, headache, lightheadedness, nausea*, vomiting*

LESS COMMON SIDE EFFECTS: Blurry vision, confusion*, constipation, diarrhea, fainting*, muscle pains, tiredness, tremors*, weakness

RARE SIDE EFFECTS: Excitement*, irregular heartbeat*, penile erection*, poor coordination*, skin rash*

PRECAUTIONS

People with a history of alcoholism, kidney disease, or liver disease are at greater risk of developing side effects while taking this drug.

Be careful driving or handling equipment while taking this drug because it may cause drowsiness and dizziness.

This drug may cause dry mouth, which is associated with a greater risk of cavities. Your dentist may recommend that you clean your teeth and mouth differently to avoid infection.

Stopping this drug suddenly may cause severe side effects. If you wish to stop taking this drug, ask your doctor for specific instructions.

Men have a small risk of developing painful, prolonged erection of the penis, which requires treatment by a doctor. If this happens, go to your doctor or the nearest emergency room immediately.

---

† See page 52.   * See page 53.

PREGNANCY AND BREAST-FEEDING

Safety during pregnancy has not been established although the drug is known to harm animal fetuses.

Breast-feeding while taking this drug is not recommended.

HELPFUL COMMENTS

It may take 2 weeks before the effects of this drug are noticed.

Sucking on hard sugarless candy or chewing sugarless gum may help relieve dry mouth caused by this drug.

The drowsiness that occurs after taking a dose should begin to go away after this drug has been taken for more than a few weeks.

Avoid quick movements to minimize dizziness. Dangling your legs over the side of the bed for a few minutes may help reduce dizziness when first waking up.

TRIAMCINOLONE

Available for over 20 years

COMMONLY USED TO TREAT

Allergic reactions
Collagen disease
Severe inflammation

DRUG CATEGORY

antiinflammatory
immunosuppressant
Class: corticosteroid

PRODUCTS

Brand-Name Products with No Generic Alternative
Azmacort oral inhaler ($$)
Kenacort 8 mg tablet (n/a)
Kenalog topical spray (¢¢)
Nasacort AQ nasal spray ($$)
Nasacort nasal aerosol ($$$$$)
Brand-Name Products with Generic Alternatives
Kenacort 4 mg tablet (n/a)
  Generic: triamcinolone 4 mg tablet (n/a)

Kenalog 0.025% topical cream (n/a)
  Generic: triamcinolone acetonide 0.025% topical cream (¢)
Kenalog 0.1% topical cream (¢¢)
  Generic: triamcinolone acetonide 0.1% topical cream (¢)
Kenalog 0.5% topical cream ($)
  Generic: triamcinolone acetonide 0.5% topical cream (¢)
Kenalog 0.025% topical lotion (¢¢)
  Generic: triamcinolone acetonide 0.025% topical lotion (¢¢)
Kenalog 0.1% topical lotion (¢¢)
  Generic: triamcinolone acetonide 0.1% topical lotion (¢)
Kenalog 0.025% topical ointment (n/a)
  Generic: triamcinolone acetonide 0.025% topical ointment (¢)
Kenalog 0.1% topical ointment (¢¢¢)
  Generic: triamcinolone acetonide 0.1% topical ointment (¢)
Kenalog 0.1% dental paste ($$)
  Generic: triamcinolone acetonide 0.1% dental paste (¢¢¢¢)

Products Only Available as Generics
triamcinolone acetonide 0.5% topical ointment (¢)

Other Generic Product Names
Acetocot, Aristocort, Aristocort A, Clinicort, Triacet, Triamcot, Triderm, Trymex

Combination Products That Contain This Drug
Mycolog-II 0.1% topical cream (¢¢)
Mycolog-II 0.1% topical ointment (¢¢)

DOSING AND FOOD

Doses of oral tablets are taken 1 to 4 times a day.
The oral form of this drug should be taken with food.
Adults: Up to 60 mg per day in divided doses.
Children: Up to 1.7 mg/kg per day in divided doses.
Nasal doses are used once daily, up to 4 sprays per nostril in adults, 2 sprays per nostril in children.
Oral inhalers are used 3 to 4 times a day, up to 16 inhalations per day in adults, 12 inhalations per day in children.
Topical preparations should be applied in a thin layer up to 4 times a day.
Forgotten doses: Determining when to take a forgotten dose will depend on your prescription schedule. If you remember the forgotten dose within a few hours of when it was due, you may take the dose immediately and continue with your regular schedule. If you are tapering the drug to

---

avoid withdrawal symptoms, you may need to evaluate the time since the last dose and the interval between the next doses. A complete change in schedule may be needed. Talk to your doctor or pharmacist for more help.

ALCOHOL, DRUG, HERB, AND SUPPLEMENT INTERACTIONS

Alcohol may increase the risk of side effects from this drug, especially stomach problems. Ask your doctor about the risks caused by drinking alcohol with your condition.

Taking this drug with any of the ones listed below may change the effect of either drug with the possibility of causing toxicity or decreasing effectiveness: aminoglutethimide, antacids, anticoagulants†, antidiabetics†, barbiturates†, carbamazepine, cholestyramine, colestipol, diuretics†, estrogens†, griseofulvin, insulin, isoniazid, mitotane, phenylbutazone, phenytoin, primidone, rifampin, salicylates†, somatrem, somatropin

Severe reactions are possible when this drug is taken with those listed below: aspirin, amphotericin B, cardiac glycosides†, immunizations, nonsteroidal antiinflammatories†, ritodrine

ALLERGIC REACTIONS AND SIDE EFFECTS

If you are allergic to any corticosteroids†, you may also be allergic to this drug. You should tell your doctor about all your allergies and any unexplained symptoms you may have while taking this drug.

This drug may cause your eyes to be more sensitive to sunlight, but there are no special risks associated with sunburn while taking this drug.

MORE COMMON SIDE EFFECTS: Excitement*, indigestion, leg pain*, nervousness, restlessness, seizures*, sleeping difficulty*, stomach pain*, swelling*

LESS COMMON SIDE EFFECTS: Acne*, bloody stools*, bruising*, dizziness, eye pain*, flushing, frequent urination*, headache*, hiccups, increased appetite, thirst*, irregular heartbeat*, lightheadedness, menstrual problems*, muscle cramps*, muscle weakness*, nausea*, open wounds*, pain*, red eyes*, rounding of the face*, skin discoloration, skin irritation*, spinning sensation, stunted growth*, sweating, tearing eyes*, tiredness*, vision changes*, vomiting*, weakness*, weight gain*

RARE SIDE EFFECTS: Confusion*, depression*, hallucinations*, hives*, mood swings*, restlessness*, skin rash*

PRECAUTIONS

The topical and inhalation products are absorbed into the body and may carry the same warnings as the oral product. Tell your doctor if you begin to notice side effects.

This drug may cause severe and possibly fatal withdrawal symptoms if stopped abruptly. The drug must be stopped over 7 to 10 days by gradually decreasing the dose or time between doses. If you wish to stop taking this drug, ask your doctor for specific instructions.

You may experience an increase in blood sugar or cholesterol level, calcium loss, or retention of fluid while taking this drug.

Avoid contact with anyone who has the chickenpox, measles, or other communicable disease since it may be easier to catch the infection while taking this drug.

Exposure to skin tests, immunizations, and people who have received immunizations may put you at a greater risk of developing the disease when you are taking this drug.

PREGNANCY AND BREAST-FEEDING

Safety during pregnancy has not been established although the drug is known to harm animal fetuses.

This drug passes into breast milk and may cause growth problems in the baby. The risk is related to the dose and route of the drug. Talk to your doctor about the risks associated with breast-feeding while taking this drug.

HELPFUL COMMENTS

If you need to take an antacid, take it either 2 hours before or after taking this drug.

Rinse your mouth with water or mouthwash after using the oral inhaler to reduce the dry and irritated mouth that many people suffer.

TRIAMTERENE

Available for over 20 years

COMMONLY USED TO TREAT

Fluid (water) retention

DRUG CATEGORY

antihypertensive
antihypokalemic
Class: potassium-sparing diuretic

---

† See page 52.   * See page 53.

PRODUCTS

Brand-Name Products with No Generic Alternative
Dyrenium 50 mg capsule (¢¢¢¢¢)
Dyrenium 50 mg capsule ($$)
No generics available.
No patents, no exclusivity.

Combination Products That Contain This Drug
Dyazide capsule (¢¢¢¢)
Maxzide tablet (¢¢¢¢) to ($)

DOSING AND FOOD

Doses are taken twice a day.
This drug may be taken with or without food.

Adults: Up to 300 mg per day in divided doses.

Children: Up to 4 mg/kg per day in divided doses.

Forgotten doses: If you are scheduled to take the next dose within a few hours, do not take the forgotten dose. Otherwise take the forgotten dose as soon as you remember.

ALCOHOL, DRUG, HERB, AND SUPPLEMENT INTERACTIONS

Alcohol may increase some of the side effects from this drug, depending on the amount consumed. Talk to your doctor about the risks caused by drinking alcohol with your condition.

Licorice may interfere with the effects of this drug.

Taking this drug with any of the ones listed below may change the effect of either drug with the possibility of causing toxicity or decreasing effectiveness:
antihypertensives[†], cimetidine, lithium

Severe reactions are possible when this drug is taken with those listed below:
ACE inhibitors[†], cyclosporine, nonsteroidal antiinflammatories[†], potassium-containing drugs, potassium-sparing diuretics[†]

ALLERGIC REACTIONS AND SIDE EFFECTS

If you are allergic to amiloride or spironolactone, you may also be allergic to this drug. You should tell your doctor about all your allergies and any unexplained symptoms you may have while taking this drug.

This drug promotes the effect of sunlight on the body and may cause severe sunburn and increased sensitivity of the eyes.

LESS COMMON SIDE EFFECTS: Constipation, diarrhea, dizziness, dry mouth, headache, muscle cramps, nausea, sexual dysfunction, stomach cramps, tiredness, vomiting, weakness

RARE SIDE EFFECTS: Itching*, shortness of breath*, skin rash*

PRECAUTIONS

This drug does not eliminate potassium from the body like other diuretics. Do not add extra potassium to your diet or use salt substitutes that contain potassium while taking this drug. Foods high in potassium include meat, fish, apricots, avocados, bananas, melons, kiwi, lima beans, milk, oranges, potatoes, prunes, spinach, tomatoes, and squash.

People with diabetes, kidney disease, or liver disease may have a greater risk of developing side effects while taking this drug.

If you have a history of gout or kidney stones, this drug may make those conditions worse.

Stopping this drug suddenly may cause severe side effects due to potassium imbalance in the body. If you wish to stop taking this drug, ask your doctor for specific instructions.

Severe side effects may occur if you get dehydrated or experience excess vomiting or diarrhea. Call your doctor before your symptoms get too bad.

PREGNANCY AND BREAST-FEEDING

Safety during pregnancy has not been established although there was no evidence of harm during studies in animals.

This drug passes into breast milk, but does not appear to harm the baby. Talk to your doctor about the risks associated with breast-feeding while taking this drug.

HELPFUL COMMENTS

It may take 2 to 3 weeks for the full effects of this drug to be noticed.

Eye irritation caused by the sun may be reduced by wearing sunglasses when outside.

If this drug is taken alone rather than in combination with another diuretic, urination may be delayed for 2 to 3 days. Combination products should be taken before 6 P.M. to reduce the chance of having to urinate during the night.

This drug may cause your urine to turn blue.

---

†*See page 52.*   *See page 53.*

TRIAZOLAM

Available for over 20 years

COMMONLY USED TO TREAT

Sleeping difficulty, also known as insomnia

DRUG CATEGORY

sedative-hypnotic
Class: benzodiazepine

PRODUCTS

Brand-Name Products with Generic Alternatives
Halcion 0.125 mg tablet ($)
  Generic: triazolam 0.125 mg tablet (¢¢¢)
Halcion 0.25 mg tablet ($)
  Generic: triazolam 0.25 mg tablet (¢¢¢)

DOSING AND FOOD

Doses are taken once a day.
This drug may be taken with or without food. Do not drink grapefruit juice
  while taking this drug.
Adults: Up to 0.5 mg per day.
Lower doses are used in people over age 65.

ALCOHOL, DRUG, HERB, AND SUPPLEMENT INTERACTIONS

Alcohol should not be used while taking this drug.
Catnip, kava, lady's slipper, lemon balm, passion flower, sassafras, skullcap,
  and valerian should not be used while taking this drug due to an increased sedative effect.

**Taking this drug with any of the ones listed below may change the effect of
either drug with the possibility of causing toxicity or decreasing effectiveness:**
cimetidine, digoxin, disulfiram, erythromycin, fluvoxamine, haloperidol,
isoniazid, itraconazole, ketoconazole, levodopa, nefazodone, oral contraceptives, rifampin

Severe reactions are possible when this drug is taken with those listed below:
anesthetics†, antidepressants†, antihistamines†, barbiturates†, monoamine
oxidase inhibitors†, narcotics†, phenothiazines†

Increased side effects are possible when this drug is taken with those listed below:
aminophylline, theophylline

ALLERGIC REACTIONS AND SIDE EFFECTS

If you are allergic to any benzodiazepines†, you may also be allergic to this drug. You should tell your doctor about all your allergies and any unexplained symptoms you may have while taking this drug.

MORE COMMON SIDE EFFECTS: Clumsiness, dizziness, drowsiness, headache

LESS COMMON SIDE EFFECTS: Anxiety*, confusion*, constipation, depression*, diarrhea, difficulty urinating, dry mouth, irregular heartbeat*, lightheadedness, memory loss*, muscle spasm, nausea, sexual dysfunction, slurry speech, stomach cramps, thirst, trembling, vision changes, vomiting, watery mouth

RARE SIDE EFFECTS: Agitation*, behavior changes*, bleeding*, bruising*, chills*, delusions*, disorientation*, excitement*, eye movement*, fever*, hallucinations*, irritability*, low blood pressure*, mouth sores*, nervousness*, seizures*, skin irritation*, sore throat*, spastic movements*, tiredness*, weakness*, yellow eyes or skin*

PRECAUTIONS

This drug may be habit forming and will cause severe withdrawal symptoms if stopped abruptly. If you wish to stop taking this drug, ask your doctor for specific instructions.

You need to wait 2 weeks after stopping a monoamine oxidase inhibitor† before starting this drug.

If you have difficulty swallowing, emphysema, asthma, bronchitis, glaucoma, hyperactivity, mental depression, mental illness, myasthenia gravis, porphyria, or sleep apnea, this drug may make those conditions worse.

Heavy smoking may cause this drug to be less effective.

Be careful driving or handling equipment while taking this drug because the drug may cause dizziness and drowsiness.

PREGNANCY AND BREAST-FEEDING

This drug may cause birth defects and should not be used during pregnancy. Breast-feeding while taking this drug is not recommended.

HELPFUL COMMENTS

You should be in bed when you take this drug since the sedative effect works very quickly.

Dangling your legs over the side of the bed for a few minutes may help reduce dizziness when first waking up.

---

† See page 52.   * See page 53.

TRICHLORMETHIAZIDE

Available for over 20 years

COMMONLY USED TO TREAT

Fluid retention, also known as edema
Frequent urination in people with diabetes
High blood pressure, also known as hypertension

DRUG CATEGORY

antihypertensive
Class: thiazide diuretic

PRODUCTS

Brand-Name Products with Generic Alternatives
Naqua 4 mg tablet (¢¢¢¢¢)
  Generic: trichlormethiazide 4 mg tablet (¢)
Products Only Available as Generics
trichlormethiazide 2 mg tablet (n/a)
Other Generic Product Names
Metahydrin

DOSING AND FOOD

Doses are taken once a day but may be taken as little as 3 times a week.
Adults: Up to 4 mg per day.
Lower doses may be used in children.
It is best to take this drug on an empty stomach, but taking this drug with
a little food may avoid the stomach upset that some people suffer. Avoid
food with excess salt.
Forgotten doses: If you are scheduled to take the next dose within a few
hours, do not take the forgotten dose. Otherwise take the forgotten dose
as soon as you remember.

ALCOHOL, DRUG, HERB, AND SUPPLEMENT INTERACTIONS

Alcohol may cause your blood pressure to rise, making this drug less effective. Ask your doctor about the risks caused by drinking alcohol with
your condition.
Licorice root may increase potassium loss and should not be used while
taking this drug.

Several OTC drugs used for appetite control, asthma, colds, cough, hay fever, or sinus problems may cause an increase in blood pressure when taken with this drug. Check with your pharmacist when selecting OTC products.

Taking this drug with any of the ones listed below may change the effect of either drug with the possibility of causing toxicity or decreasing effectiveness: antidiabetics†, cholestyramine, colestipol, digoxin, insulin, lithium

ALLERGIC REACTIONS AND SIDE EFFECTS

If you are allergic to acetazolamide, bumetanide, dichlorphenamide, furosemide, methazolamide, sulfonamides†, or thiazide diuretics†, you may also be allergic to this drug. You should tell your doctor about all your allergies and any unexplained symptoms you may have while taking this drug.

This drug promotes the effect of sunlight on the body and may cause severe sunburn and increased sensitivity of the eyes.

LESS COMMON SIDE EFFECTS: Diarrhea*, dizziness, lightheadedness, loss of appetite, sexual dysfunction, stomach upset

RARE SIDE EFFECTS: Back pain*, black stools*, bleeding*, bloody urine*, breathing difficulty*, bruising*, burning sensation*, chest pain*, chills*, confusion*, cough*, fatigue*, fever*, hives*, headache*, hoarseness*, irregular heartbeat*, joint pain*, leg pain*, muscle cramps*, nausea*, numbness*, painful urination*, shortness of breath*, skin rash*, stomach pain*, swelling*, weakness*, vomiting*, yellow eyes or skin*

PRECAUTIONS

This drug may cause your blood sugar level to rise, leading to type 2 diabetes.

Your body may lose potassium while taking this drug, which may cause severe side effects. Potassium levels should be monitored periodically and may need to be supplemented while taking this drug. Eat food rich in potassium, such as apricots, bananas, citrus fruit, dates, and tomatoes, if you are not taking a potassium supplement or potassium-sparing diuretic.†

People with kidney disease may not be able to take this drug.

This drug may increase the level of uric acid in the body, which may lead to gout or kidney stones.

If you have lupus erythematosus or pancreatitis, this drug may make those conditions worse.

Nicotine in cigarettes may increase blood pressure, making this drug less effective.

---

† See page 52.   * See page 53.

This drug may cause an increase in the levels of cholesterol or triglyceride in the blood.

PREGNANCY AND BREAST-FEEDING

Safety during pregnancy has not been established although the drug is known to harm animal fetuses.

Breast-feeding while taking this drug is not recommended.

HELPFUL COMMENTS

Take your last dose of the day no later than 6 P.M. to avoid urination during the night.

Avoid quick movements to minimize dizziness. Dangling your legs over the side of the bed for a few minutes may help reduce dizziness when first waking up.

Record your weight twice a day, when first getting up in the morning and after the drug causes urination. A weight gain or loss of more than 2 pounds per day should be reported to your doctor.

The antihypertensive effects of this drug will last about 1 week after it is stopped.

TRIFLUOPERAZINE HYDROCHLORIDE

Available for over 20 years

COMMONLY USED TO TREAT

Anxiety
Mental illness, also known as psychosis

DRUG CATEGORY

antiemetic
antipsychotic
Class: phenothiazine: piperazine derivative

PRODUCTS

Brand-Name Products with No Generic Alternative
Stelazine 10 mg/ml oral concentrate ($$$$$)

Brand-Name Products with Generic Alternatives
Stelazine 1 mg tablet (¢¢¢¢¢)
  Generic: trifluoperazine hydrochloride 1 mg tablet (¢¢¢¢)

Stelazine 2 mg tablet ($)
   Generic: trifluoperazine hydrochloride 2 mg tablet (¢¢¢¢¢)
Stelazine 5 mg tablet ($)
   Generic: trifluoperazine hydrochloride 5 mg tablet (¢¢¢)
Stelazine 10 mg tablet ($$)
   Generic: trifluoperazine hydrochloride 10 mg tablet (¢¢¢¢)

DOSING AND FOOD

Doses are taken 2 times a day.

Taking this drug with food or a full glass of milk or water may avoid the stomach upset that some people suffer.

Adults: Up to 40 mg per day in divided doses.

Children age 6 to 12: Up to 15 mg per day in divided doses.

Lower doses are used in people over age 65.

Forgotten doses: If you are scheduled to take the next dose within a few hours, do not take the forgotten dose. Otherwise take the forgotten dose as soon as you remember.

ALCOHOL, DRUG, HERB, AND SUPPLEMENT INTERACTIONS

Alcohol should not be used while taking this drug.

Do not use caffeine, kava, or yohimbe while taking this drug since the drug effects may be decreased and severe reactions may occur.

Several OTC drugs used for appetite control, asthma, colds, cough, hay fever, pain, or sinus problems may seriously increase the effects and side effects of this drug. Check with your pharmacist when selecting OTC products.

Taking this drug with any of the ones listed below may change the effect of either drug with the possibility of causing toxicity or decreasing effectiveness: antihypertensives†, caffeine, barbiturates†, beta blockers†, levodopa, lithium, warfarin

Severe reactions are possible when this drug is taken with those listed below: alcohol, amantadine, antiarrhythmics†, anticholinergics†, antidepressants†, antithyroid drugs†, anxiolytics†, astemizole, bromocriptine, cisapride, deferoxamine, disopyramide, diuretics†, epinephrine, nabilone, narcotics†, pentamidine, procainamide, promethazine, propylthiouracil, quinidine, sympathomimetics†

Increased side effects are possible when this drug is taken with those listed below: antipsychotics†, metoclopramide, metyrosine, pemoline, pimozide, rauwolfia alkaloids†, trimeprazine

---

† See page 52.   * See page 53.

ALLERGIC REACTIONS AND SIDE EFFECTS

If you are allergic to any phenothiazines†, you may also be allergic to this drug. You should tell your doctor about all your allergies and any unexplained symptoms you may have while taking this drug.

This drug promotes the effect of sunlight on the body and may cause severe sunburn and increased sensitivity of the eyes.

MORE COMMON SIDE EFFECTS: Breathing difficulty*, chewing action*, congestion, constipation, decreased sweating*, dizziness, drowsiness, dry mouth, eye stare*, eyelid movement*, fainting*, lip smacking*, loss of balance*, puffy cheeks*, restlessness*, shuffling walk*, stiffness*, tongue movements*, trembling*, twitching*, vision changes*

LESS COMMON SIDE EFFECTS: Breast-milk secretion, breast swelling, dark urine*, menstrual changes, rough tongue, sexual dysfunction, skin rash*, urinary difficulty*, watery mouth, weight gain

RARE SIDE EFFECTS: Abdominal pain*, agitation*, bleeding*, blood pressure change*, bruising*, chest pain*, chills*, clumsiness*, coma*, confusion*, diarrhea*, dreams*, drooling*, excitement*, fever*, hair loss*, headache*, increased sweating*, irregular heartbeat*, itching*, joint pain*, loss of bladder control*, mouth sores*, nausea*, penile erection*, red hands*, seizures*, shivering*, skin discoloration*, sleep disorders*, sore throat*, speaking difficulty*, tiredness*, vomiting*, weakness*, yellow eyes or skin*

PRECAUTIONS

If you have a history of enlarged prostate, glaucoma, ulcers, seizures, heart disease, urinary difficulty, or Parkinson's disease, this drug may make those conditions worse.

This drug may decrease the cough reflex, putting people with lung disease at greater risk of developing pneumonia.

Heavy smoking may cause this drug to be less effective.

This drug may cause false results from several diagnostic tests, including pregnancy tests, and should be stopped for at least 4 days before the test.

This drug should not be stopped suddenly, due to an increased risk of side effects. If you wish to stop taking this drug, ask your doctor for specific instructions.

Be careful driving or handling equipment while taking this drug because the drug may cause dizziness and drowsiness.

You are more likely to overheat when taking this drug and should avoid exercising in hot weather and using a sauna or hot tub.

This drug may make you more sensitive to cold temperatures.

Touching the liquid form of this drug may cause skin irritation. Make sure you do not spill the liquid, and wash your hands immediately after taking the dose.

If this drug is being used to treat anxiety, do not use for longer than 12 weeks.

This drug may cause dry mouth, which is associated with a greater risk of cavities. Your dentist may recommend that you clean your teeth and mouth differently to avoid infection.

PREGNANCY AND BREAST-FEEDING

Safety during pregnancy has not been established although the drug is known to harm animal fetuses.

Breast-feeding while taking this drug is not recommended.

HELPFUL COMMENTS

If you need to take an antacid, take it either 2 hours before or after taking this drug.

Sucking on hard sugarless candy or chewing sugarless gum may help relieve dry mouth caused by this drug.

This drug may cause the color of your urine to turn pink or brown.

TRIHEXYPHENIDYL HYDROCHLORIDE

Available for over 20 years

COMMONLY USED TO TREAT

Symptoms of Parkinson's disease caused by drugs and other conditions

DRUG CATEGORY

antidyskinetic
Class: anticholinergic

PRODUCTS

Brand-Name Products with Generic Alternatives
Artane 2 mg tablet (n/a)
  Generic: trihexyphenidyl hydrochloride 2 mg tablet (¢¢)
Artane 5 mg tablet (n/a)
  Generic: trihexyphenidyl hydrochloride 5 mg tablet (¢¢)

---

† See page 52.   * See page 53.

Artane 2 mg/5 ml oral elixir (n/a)
  Generic: trihexyphenidyl hydrochloride 2 mg/5 ml oral elixir (¢¢¢)

DOSING AND FOOD

Doses are taken 3 to 4 times a day.

This drug may be taken with or without food but is best taken with food to reduce the stomach upset that some people suffer.

Adults: Up to 15 mg per day in divided doses.

Forgotten doses: If you are scheduled to take the next dose within a few hours, do not take the forgotten dose. Otherwise take the forgotten dose as soon as you remember.

ALCOHOL, DRUG, HERB, AND SUPPLEMENT INTERACTIONS

Alcohol should not be used while taking this drug.

Many OTC drugs used for appetite control, asthma, colds, cough, hay fever, pain, or sinus problems affect the central nervous system and may change the effects or side effects of this drug. Check with your pharmacist for products to avoid.

Taking this drug with any of the ones listed below may change the effect of either drug with the possibility of causing toxicity or decreasing effectiveness: antacids, antidiarrheals†, haloperidol, levodopa, phenothiazines†

Increased side effects are possible when this drug is taken with those listed below: amantadine, anesthetics, anticholinergics†, antihistamines†, anxiolytics†, barbiturates†, narcotics†, tricyclic antidepressants†

ALLERGIC REACTIONS AND SIDE EFFECTS

If you are allergic to other anticholinergic† drugs, you may also be allergic to this drug. You should tell your doctor about all your allergies and any unexplained symptoms you may have while taking this drug.

MORE COMMON SIDE EFFECTS: Dry mouth*, giddiness, nausea

LESS COMMON SIDE EFFECTS: Blurry vision, constipation, decreased sweating, dizziness, drowsiness, hallucinations, headache, lightheadedness, memory loss, muscle cramps, nervousness, numbness, sore mouth, stomachache, urinary changes*, vomiting, weakness

RARE SIDE EFFECTS: Confusion*, skin rash*

PRECAUTIONS

This drug may cause withdrawal symptoms if stopped suddenly. If you wish to stop taking this drug, ask your doctor for specific instructions.

People with glaucoma may not be able to take this drug.

Be careful driving or handling equipment while taking this drug because the drug may cause dizziness and drowsiness.

This drug may cause dry mouth, which is associated with a greater risk of cavities. Your dentist may recommend that you clean your teeth and mouth differently to avoid infection.

This drug makes you sweat less putting you at greater risk of developing heat stroke. Avoid exercising in hot weather and using a hot tub or sauna.

PREGNANCY AND BREAST-FEEDING

Safety during pregnancy has not been established although the drug is known to harm animal fetuses.

Breast-feeding while taking this drug is not recommended.

HELPFUL COMMENTS

You may only need to take this drug for a couple of weeks if you are using it to treat the side effects caused by another drug.

If you need to take an antacid, take it either 2 hours before or after taking this drug.

Sucking on hard sugarless candy or chewing sugarless gum may help relieve dry mouth caused by this drug.

TRIMIPRAMINE MALEATE

Available for over 20 years

COMMONLY USED TO TREAT

Depression
Ulcers, specifically duodenal ulcers

DRUG CATEGORY

antidepressant
antineuralgic
Class: tricyclic antidepressant

PRODUCTS

Brand-Name Products with No Generic Alternative
Surmontil 25 mg capsule (¢¢¢¢¢)
Surmontil 50 mg capsule ($$)
Surmontil 100 mg capsule ($$)

No generics available.
No patents, no exclusivity.

DOSING AND FOOD

Doses are taken once a day, usually at bedtime. Twice-a-day dosing may be
needed initially to avoid side effects.

Taking this drug with food or milk may avoid the stomach upset that some
people suffer.

Adults: Up to 200 mg per day.

Lower doses are used in teens and adults over age 65.

Forgotten doses: If you have forgotten a bedtime dose, do not take the
forgotten dose. Just go back to your usual schedule with the next dose. If
you have forgotten a daytime dose and are scheduled to take the next
dose within a few hours, do not take the forgotten dose. Otherwise take
the forgotten dose as soon as you remember.

ALCOHOL, DRUG, HERB, AND SUPPLEMENT INTERACTIONS

Alcohol should not be used while taking this drug.

Evening primrose oil, SAMe, St. John's wort, and yohimbe may cause serious reactions when taken with this drug. Tell your doctor if you are taking
any of these supplements.

Several OTC drugs used for asthma, colds, cough, hay fever, sleep aid, or
sinus problems may seriously change the effects and side effects of this
drug. Check with your pharmacist when selecting OTC products.

**Taking this drug with any of the ones listed below may change the effect of
either drug with the possibility of causing toxicity or decreasing effectiveness:**
anesthetics, antipsychotics†, anxiolytics†, barbiturates†, beta blockers†,
cimetidine, clonidine, fluoxetine, guanabenz, guanadrel, guanethidine,
haloperidol, methyldopa, methylphenidate, narcotics†, oral contraceptives, phenothiazines†, propoxyphene, reserpine, SSRIs†

Severe reactions are possible when this drug is taken with those listed below:
amphetamines†, anticholinergics†, antidepressants†, antidyskinetics†, anti-
histamines†, antithyroid drug†, anxiolytics†, appetite suppressants,
disopyramide, disulfiram, ephedrine, epinephrine, ethchlorvynol, isoproterenol, meperidine, metrizamide, monoamine oxidase inhibitors†,
phenylephrine, pimozide, procainamide, quinidine, warfarin

Increased side effects are possible when this drug is taken with those listed below:
alseroxylon, deserpidine, metoclopramide, metyrosine, pemoline, pimozide, promethazine, rauwolfia serpentine, reserpine, trimeprazine

ALLERGIC REACTIONS AND SIDE EFFECTS

If you are allergic to carbamazepine, maprotiline, trazodone, or any tricyclic antidepressants†, you may also be allergic to this drug. You should tell your doctor about all your allergies and any unexplained symptoms you may have while taking this drug.

This drug promotes the effect of sunlight on the body and may cause severe sunburn and increased sensitivity of the eyes.

MORE COMMON SIDE EFFECTS: Blurry vision*, constipation*, dizziness, drowsiness, dry mouth, irregular heartbeat*, seizures*, sweating, tiredness, urinary changes

LESS COMMON SIDE EFFECTS: Confusion*, diarrhea, expressionless face*, eye pain*, fainting*, hallucinations*, headache, heartburn, loss of balance*, nausea, nervousness*, restlessness*, shakiness*, shuffling walk*, sleeping difficulty, slow movements*, stiffness*, swallowing difficulty*, taste changes, trembling*, urinary changes*, vomiting, weakness*

RARE SIDE EFFECTS: Anxiety*, breast enlargement*, hair loss, irritability*, muscle twitching*, ringing in ears*, skin rash*, sore throat*, fever*, swelling*, teeth or gum problems*, yellow eyes or skin*

PRECAUTIONS

You need to wait 2 weeks after stopping a monoamine oxidase inhibitor† before starting this drug.

Be careful driving or handling equipment while taking this drug because it may cause drowsiness and dizziness.

Stopping this drug abruptly may result in withdrawal symptoms that include nausea, headache, and general discomfort. If you wish to stop taking this drug, ask your doctor for specific instructions.

If you have a history of asthma, blood disorders, seizures, enlarged prostate, glaucoma, heart disease, high blood pressure, urinary difficulty, schizophrenia, or manic depression, this drug may make those conditions worse.

This drug may cause dry mouth, which is associated with a greater risk of cavities. Your dentist may recommend that you clean your teeth and mouth differently to avoid infection.

PREGNANCY AND BREAST-FEEDING

Safety during pregnancy has not been established although the drug is known to harm animal fetuses. There have been reports of babies suffering from muscle spasms, heart problems, breathing difficulty, and urinary problems when the mother was taking this drug.

---

†*See page 52.*   *See page 53.*

Breast-feeding while taking this drug is not recommended.

HELPFUL COMMENTS

Heavy smoking may decrease the effectiveness of this drug.

You may need to take this drug for 2 to 6 weeks before you notice the effects.

Sucking on hard sugarless candy or chewing sugarless gum may help relieve dry mouth caused by this drug.

The drowsiness that occurs after taking a dose should begin to go away after this drug has been taken for more than a few weeks.

TRIPELENNAMINE

Available for over 20 years

COMMONLY USED TO TREAT

Allergies

DRUG CATEGORY

antihistamine
Class: H1 receptor blocker: ethylenediamine

PRODUCTS

Brand-Name Products with No Generic Alternative
PBZ 25 mg tablet (n/a)
Brand-Name Products with Generic Alternative
PBZ 50 mg tablet (n/a)
　Generic: tripelennamine 50 mg tablet (n/a)

DOSING AND FOOD

Doses are taken 4 to 6 times a day.

It is best to take this drug on an empty stomach, but taking it with a little food may avoid the stomach upset that some people suffer.

Adults: Up to 300 mg per day in divided doses.

Children: Up to 5 mg/kg per day in divided doses.

Forgotten doses: If you are scheduled to take the next dose within a few hours, do not take the forgotten dose. Otherwise take the forgotten dose as soon as you remember.

ALCOHOL, DRUG, HERB, AND SUPPLEMENT INTERACTIONS

Alcohol may increase some of the side effects from this drug, depending

on the amount consumed. Ask your doctor about the risks caused by drinking alcohol with your condition.

Several OTC drugs used for appetite control, asthma, colds, cough, hay fever, pain, or sinus problems may seriously increase the effects of this drug. Check with your pharmacist when selecting OTC products.

Taking this drug with any of the ones listed below may change the effect of either drug with the possibility of causing toxicity or decreasing effectiveness: anesthetics, anticholinergics†, antidepressants†, anxiolytics†, barbiturates†, narcotics†

Severe reactions are possible when this drug is taken with those listed below: monoamine oxidase inhibitors†

Increased side effects are possible when this drug is taken with those listed below: alcohol, antihistamines†

ALLERGIC REACTIONS AND SIDE EFFECTS

If you are allergic to other antihistamines†, you may also be allergic to this drug. You should tell your doctor about all your allergies and any unexplained symptoms you may have while taking this drug.

This drug promotes the effect of sunlight on the body and may cause severe sunburn and increased sensitivity of the eyes.

MORE COMMON SIDE EFFECTS: Drowsiness, dry mouth, headache*, nausea, stomachache, thick mucus, weight gain

LESS COMMON SIDE EFFECTS: Appetite change, belching, bleeding*, body aches, bruising*, clumsiness, confusion, congestion, constipation, cough, diarrhea, difficulty urinating, early menstruation, excitement, fatigue, fever*, heartburn, hoarseness, indigestion, irregular heartbeat*, irritability, joint pain, muscle cramps, nervousness, nightmares, painful menstruation, restlessness, ringing in ears, runny nose, skin rash, sore throat*, stiffness, sweating, swelling*, tremor, vision changes, vomiting

RARE SIDE EFFECTS: Abdominal pain*, chest tightness*, chills*, cough*, dark urine*, diarrhea*, dizziness*, hives*, itching*, pale stools*, seizures*, shortness of breath*, skin irritation*, swallowing difficulty*, tingling*, tiredness*, weakness*, wheezing*

PRECAUTIONS

If you have glaucoma, an enlarged prostate, or difficulty urinating, this drug may make those conditions worse.

This drug may interfere with skin tests used to diagnose allergies and should be stopped for at least 4 days before the test.

---

†See page 52.   *See page 53.

You need to wait 2 weeks after stopping a monoamine oxidase inhibitor†
before starting this drug.

Be careful driving or handling equipment while taking this drug because
the drug may cause drowsiness.

This drug may cause dry mouth, which is associated with a greater risk of
cavities. Your dentist may recommend that you clean your teeth and
mouth differently to avoid infection.

PREGNANCY AND BREAST-FEEDING

Safety during pregnancy has not been established although there was no
evidence of harm during studies in animals.

Breast-feeding while taking this drug is not recommended.

HELPFUL COMMENTS

Sucking on hard sugarless candy or chewing sugarless gum may help relieve dry mouth caused by this drug.

Several antihistamines are sold without a prescription by the following
generic names: brompheniramine, chlorpheniramine, clemastine, diphenhydramine, doxylamine, loratadine. Ask your pharmacist about specific
products that contain these drugs.

TROLEANDOMYCIN

Available for over 20 years

COMMONLY USED TO TREAT

Infection
Pneumonia

DRUG CATEGORY

antibiotic
Class: macrolide

PRODUCTS

Brand-Name Products with No Generic Alternative
Tao 250 mg capsule ($)
No generics available.
No patents, no exclusivity.

DOSING AND FOOD

Doses are taken 4 times a day.

It is best to take this drug on an empty stomach either 1 hour before or 2 hours after a meal.

Adults: Up to 2,000 mg per day in divided doses.

Children: Up to 11 mg/kg (maximum 1,000 mg) per day in divided doses.

Forgotten doses: If you are scheduled to take the next dose within a few hours, do not take the forgotten dose. Otherwise take the forgotten dose as soon as you remember.

ALCOHOL, DRUG, HERB, AND SUPPLEMENT INTERACTIONS

Alcohol may increase the risk of liver damage from this drug. Ask your doctor about the risks caused by drinking alcohol with your condition.

Taking this drug with any of the ones listed below may change the effect of either drug with the possibility of causing toxicity or decreasing effectiveness: carbamazepine, methylprednisolone, theophylline

Severe reactions are possible when this drug is taken with those listed below: ergotamine, oral contraceptives

ALLERGIC REACTIONS AND SIDE EFFECTS

If you are allergic to azithromycin, clarithromycin, dirithromycin, or erythromycin, you may also be allergic to this drug. You should tell your doctor about all your allergies and any unexplained symptoms you may have while taking this drug.

MORE COMMON SIDE EFFECTS: Abdominal pain*, nausea*

LESS COMMON SIDE EFFECTS: Diarrhea*, fever*, itching, skin rash, vomiting, yellow eyes or skin*

PRECAUTIONS

Heavy smoking may cause this drug to be less effective.

PREGNANCY AND BREAST-FEEDING

Safety during pregnancy has not been established although the drug is known to harm animal fetuses.

It is not known if this drug passes into breast milk. Talk to your doctor about the risks associated with breast-feeding while taking this drug.

HELPFUL COMMENTS

Contact your doctor if your symptoms do not improve after a couple of days. Do not stop treatment early if you start to feel better. It takes the full prescription for this drug to work completely.

---

† See page 52.   * See page 53.

This drug is usually taken for only 10 days. People taking the drug for longer than 10 days have a greater risk of developing severe side effects that start with nausea and abdominal pain.

TROVAFLOXACIN MESYLATE

Available since December 1997

COMMONLY USED TO TREAT

Infection

DRUG CATEGORY

antibiotic
Class: fluoroquinolone

PRODUCTS

Brand-Name Products with No Generic Alternative
Trovan 100 mg tablet ($$$$)
Trovan 200 mg tablet ($$$$)
No generics available.
Multiple patents that begin to expire in 2011.

DOSING AND FOOD

Doses are taken once a day.
This drug may be taken with or without food.
Adults: Up to 200 mg per day.
Lower doses are used in people with kidney disease.
This drug is rarely used in children under age 18 because it may interfere with bone development.
Forgotten doses: If you are scheduled to take the next dose within a few hours, do not take the forgotten dose. Otherwise take the forgotten dose as soon as you remember.

ALCOHOL, DRUG, HERB, AND SUPPLEMENT INTERACTIONS

Alcohol may increase some of the side effects from this drug, depending on the amount consumed. Ask your doctor about the risks caused by drinking alcohol with your condition.
If you need to take an antacid, vitamins, minerals, or iron supplements, take them either 6 hours before or 2 hours after taking this drug.

Taking this drug with any of the ones listed below may change the effect of either drug with the possibility of causing toxicity or decreasing effectiveness: didanosine, sucralfate, warfarin

Severe reactions are possible when this drug is taken with those listed below: aminophylline, oxtriphylline, theophylline

ALLERGIC REACTIONS AND SIDE EFFECTS

If you are allergic to any fluoroquinolones†, you may also be allergic to this drug. You should tell your doctor about all your allergies and any unexplained symptoms you may have while taking this drug.

This drug promotes the effect of sunlight on the body and may cause severe sunburn and increased sensitivity of the eyes.

MORE COMMON SIDE EFFECTS: Abdominal pain*, dark urine*, diarrhea*, dizziness, fever*, loss of appetite*, nausea*, nervousness, pale stools*, rash*, seizures*, skin irritation*, shortness of breath*, tiredness*, vomiting*, weakness*, yellow eyes or skin*

LESS COMMON SIDE EFFECTS: Back pain, blisters*, difficulty urinating, dreams, drowsiness, headache, lightheadedness, muscle pain, sleep disorders, sore mouth, stomachache, vaginal discharge, vaginal pain, taste changes, vision changes

RARE SIDE EFFECTS: Agitation*, bloody urine*, confusion*, flushing*, hallucinations*, irregular heartbeat*, joint pain*, leg pain*, shakiness*, sweating*, swelling*, tremors*

PRECAUTIONS

Be careful driving or handling equipment while taking this drug because the drug may cause dizziness and drowsiness.

If you have a history of tendonitis or liver disease, this drug may make that condition worse.

PREGNANCY AND BREAST-FEEDING

Safety during pregnancy has not been established although the drug is known to harm animal fetuses.

Breast-feeding while taking this drug is not recommended.

HELPFUL COMMENTS

Contact your doctor if your symptoms do not improve after a couple of days.

Do not stop treatment early if you start to feel better. It takes the full prescription for this drug to work completely.

Drink a lot of water while taking this drug.

---

† See page 52.   * See page 53.

VALACYCLOVIR HYDROCHLORIDE

Available since December 1995

COMMONLY USED TO TREAT

Genital herpes
Herpes simplex virus associated with HIV infection
Shingles, also known as herpes zoster

DRUG CATEGORY

antiviral
Class: synthetic purine nucleoside

PRODUCTS

Brand-Name Products with No Generic Alternative
Valtrex 500 mg tablet ($$$)
Valtrex 1 g tablet ($$$$)
No generics available.
Multiple patents that begin to expire in 2009. Exclusivity begins to expire
   2004.

DOSING AND FOOD

Doses are taken 1 to 3 times a day.
This drug may be taken with or without food but is best taken with food to
   reduce the stomach upset that some people suffer.
Adults: Up to 3,000 mg per day in divided doses.
Lower doses are used in people with kidney disease.
Forgotten doses: If you are scheduled to take the next dose within a few
   hours, do not take the forgotten dose. Otherwise take the forgotten dose
   as soon as you remember.

ALCOHOL, DRUG, HERB, AND SUPPLEMENT INTERACTIONS

Alcohol may increase some of the side effects from this drug, depending
   on the amount consumed. Ask your doctor about the risks caused by
   drinking alcohol with your condition.

**Taking this drug with any of the ones listed below may change the effect of
either drug with the possibility of causing toxicity or decreasing effectiveness:**
cimetidine, probenecid

ALLERGIC REACTIONS AND SIDE EFFECTS

If you are allergic to acyclovir, you may also be allergic to this drug. You should tell your doctor about all your allergies and any unexplained symptoms you may have while taking this drug.

MORE COMMON SIDE EFFECTS: Headache*, nausea

LESS COMMON SIDE EFFECTS: Constipation, diarrhea, dizziness, joint pain, loss of appetite, menstrual pain*, stomach pain, tiredness*, vomiting, weakness

RARE SIDE EFFECTS: Anxiety, back pain*, behavior changes*, black stools*, breathing difficulty*, chest pain*, chills*, cough*, dry mouth, fever*, hallucinations*, high blood pressure*, irregular heartbeat*, irritability, itching*, leg pains*, lightheadedness*, mood swings, nervousness, restlessness, shortness of breath*, skin irritation*, skin rash*, swallowing difficulty*, swelling*, urinary changes*, wheezing*, yellow eyes or skin*

PRECAUTIONS

Once absorbed into the body, this drug is quickly converted to acyclovir, which is responsible for the antiviral effects. Acyclovir is a separate drug that can be taken as an alternative, but the dosage is different and cannot be substituted for this drug without a new prescription.

This drug is only effective in treating the pain and discomfort of the disease and to help the sores heal more quickly.

People with bone marrow transplant, advanced HIV infection, or a kidney transplant are at greater risk of developing severe side effects.

The area with an outbreak of sores should be kept clean and dry.

PREGNANCY AND BREAST-FEEDING

Safety during pregnancy has not been established although there was no evidence of harm during studies in animals.

Breast-feeding while taking this drug is not recommended.

HELPFUL COMMENTS

This drug is most helpful if started within 48 hours of the first symptoms.

Contact your doctor if your symptoms do not improve after a couple of days.

Do not stop treatment early if you start to feel better. It takes the full prescription for this drug to work completely.

Wear loose-fitting clothes to minimize irritation of the sores.

---

† See page 52.   * See page 53.

VALDECOXIB

Available since November 2001

COMMONLY USED TO TREAT

Arthritis pain
Menstrual pain

DRUG CATEGORY

analgesic
antiinflammatory
antipyretic
Class: nonsteroidal antiinflammatory: COX-2 inhibitor

PRODUCTS

Brand-Name Products with No Generic Alternative
Bextra 10 mg tablet ($$$)
Bextra 20 mg tablet ($$$)
No generics available.
Patent expires in 2015. Exclusivity until 2006.

DOSING AND FOOD

Doses are taken 1 to 2 times a day as needed.
This drug may be taken with or without food but is best taken with food to reduce the stomach upset that some people suffer.
Adults: Up to 40 mg per day in divided doses.

ALCOHOL, DRUG, HERB, AND SUPPLEMENT INTERACTIONS

Alcohol may increase some of the side effects from this drug, depending on the amount consumed. Ask your doctor about the risks caused by drinking alcohol with your condition.

Taking this drug with any of the ones listed below may change the effect of either drug with the possibility of causing toxicity or decreasing effectiveness: dextromethorphan, fluconazole, furosemide, ketoconazole, lithium, warfarin

Increased side effects are possible when this drug is taken with those listed below: aspirin

ALLERGIC REACTIONS AND SIDE EFFECTS

If you are allergic to aspirin, nonsteroidal antiinflammatories†, sulfonamides†, or salicylates†, you may also be allergic to this drug. You should tell your doctor about all your allergies and any unexplained symptoms you may have while taking this drug.

MORE COMMON SIDE EFFECTS: Belching, cough, diarrhea, ear pressure, headache*, heartburn, indigestion, sore throat, sour stomach

LESS COMMON SIDE EFFECTS: Accident prone*, back pain, black stools*, bleeding*, bloating*, bloody urine*, bloody vomit*, blurry vision*, breathing difficulty*, bruising*, chills*, dizziness*, fever*, gas, muscle pains*, nausea*, nervousness*, pale skin*, pounding eardrums*, skin rash, stomach pain*, stuffy nose, swelling*, tingling*, tiredness*, urinary changes*, weakness*, weight gain*, yellow eyes or skin*

RARE SIDE EFFECTS: Chest tightness*, drowsiness*, shortness of breath*, thirst*, vomiting*, wheezing*

PRECAUTIONS

If you have asthma, anemia, dehydration, fluid retention, heart disease, high blood pressure, kidney disease, or liver disease, this drug may make those conditions worse.

People with a history of smoking, alcohol abuse, bleeding disorders, ulcers, or intestinal problems are at greater risk of developing side effects while taking this drug. This drug may cause serious stomach and intestinal ulcers and bleeding.

Call your doctor immediately if you have chest tightness, swelling, wheezing, or breathing difficulty, which may indicate an allergic reaction.

PREGNANCY AND BREAST-FEEDING

Safety during pregnancy has not been established although the drug is known to harm animal fetuses.

Breast-feeding while taking this drug is not recommended.

HELPFUL COMMENTS

The effects of this drug should be noticed about 3 hours after taking the first dose, but the full effects may take 4 days to notice.

VALGANCICLOVIR HYDROCHLORIDE

Available since March 2001

COMMONLY USED TO TREAT

Eye infections in those with AIDS, specifically cytomegalovirus (CMV) retinitis
Viral infections

---

† See page 52.   * See page 53.

DRUG CATEGORY

antiviral
Class: synthetic nucleoside

PRODUCTS

Brand-Name Products with No Generic Alternative
Valcyte 450 mg tablet ($$$$$)
No generics available.
Patent expires in 2014. Exclusivity until 2004.

DOSING AND FOOD

Doses are taken 1 to 2 times a day.
It is best to take this drug with food.
Adults: Up to 1,800 mg per day in divided doses.
Lower doses are used in people with kidney disease.
Forgotten doses: If you are scheduled to take the next dose within a few
hours, do not take the forgotten dose. Otherwise take the forgotten dose
as soon as you remember.

ALCOHOL, DRUG, HERB, AND SUPPLEMENT INTERACTIONS

Alcohol may increase some of the side effects from this drug, depending
on the amount consumed. Ask your doctor about the risks caused by
drinking alcohol with your condition.

Taking this drug with any of the ones listed below may change the effect of
either drug with the possibility of causing toxicity or decreasing effectiveness:
didanosine, mycophenolate, probenecid

Severe reactions are possible when this drug is taken with those listed below:
amphotericin B, antineoplastics†, antithyroid drugs†, azathioprine, chloramphenicol, colchicine, cyclophosphamide, flucytosine, interferon, mercaptopurine, methotrexate, plicamycin, zidovudine

ALLERGIC REACTIONS AND SIDE EFFECTS

If you are allergic to ganciclovir, you may also be allergic to this drug. You
should tell your doctor about all your allergies and any unexplained
symptoms you may have while taking this drug.

MORE COMMON SIDE EFFECTS: Abdominal pain, back pain*, black stools*,
bleeding*, bloody urine*, breathing difficulty*, bruising*, chills*, cough*,
diarrhea, fever*, headache, hoarseness*, mouth sores*, nausea, numb-

ness, pale skin*, skin irritation*, sleeping difficulty*, sore throat*, tingling, tiredness*, urinary changes*, visual changes*, vomiting, weakness*

LESS COMMON SIDE EFFECTS: Agitation, chest tightness*, confusion*, hallu-cinations*, hives*, irregular breathing*, itching*, runny nose*, seizures*, shortness of breath*, skin discoloration*, skin rash*, swelling*, wheezing*

PRECAUTIONS

This drug causes changes in your blood that put you at greater risk of get-ting an infection. Be careful not to cut yourself or get bruised. Tell your doctor if you develop signs of infection, such as fever or sore throat. Your dentist may recommend that you clean your teeth and mouth differently to avoid infection.

Avoid contact with anyone who has the chickenpox, measles, or other com-municable disease since it may be easier to catch the infection while tak-ing this drug.

Exposure to skin tests, immunizations, and people who have received immunizations may put you at a greater risk of developing the disease when you are taking this drug.

If you have a low blood count (platelets, white cell, or red cell), this drug may make that condition worse.

Eye exams are recommended every 4 to 6 weeks while taking this drug.

Touching these tablets may cause skin irritation. You should wash your hands immediately after taking the dose.

Once absorbed into the body, this drug is quickly converted to gancyclovir, which is responsible for the antiviral effects. Gancylovir is a separate drug that can be taken as an alternative, but the dosage is different and cannot be substituted for this drug without a new prescription.

Men should use a barrier contraceptive, such as a condom, for 90 days after this drug is stopped to prevent insemination that could lead to pregnancy.

PREGNANCY AND BREAST-FEEDING

Safety during pregnancy has not been established although the drug is known to harm animal fetuses.

Breast-feeding while taking this drug is not recommended.

HELPFUL COMMENTS

Contact your doctor if symptoms do not improve after a couple of days.

Do not stop treatment early if you start to feel better. It takes the full pre-scription for this drug to work completely.

---

† *See page 52.*   * *See page 53.*

VALPROIC ACID

Available for over 20 years

COMMONLY USED TO TREAT

People at risk of developing migraine headache
Seizures

DRUG CATEGORY

anticonvulsant
Class: carboxylic acid derivative

PRODUCTS

Brand-Name Products with Generic Alternatives
Depakene 250 mg capsule ($$)
 Generic: valproic acid 250 mg capsule (¢¢¢)
Depakene 250 mg/5 ml oral syrup ($$)
 Generic: valproic acid 250 mg/5 ml oral syrup (¢¢¢)

DOSING AND FOOD

Doses are taken 2 to 3 times a day.

This drug may be taken with or without food but is best taken with food to reduce the stomach upset that some people suffer.

Adults and children: Up to 60 mg/kg per day in divided doses.

Lower doses are used in people over age 65.

Forgotten doses: If you are scheduled to take the next dose within a few hours, do not take the forgotten dose. Otherwise take the forgotten dose as soon as you remember.

ALCOHOL, DRUG, HERB, AND SUPPLEMENT INTERACTIONS

Alcohol should not be used while taking this drug.

Many OTC drugs used for appetite control, asthma, colds, cough, hay fever, pain, or sinus problems affect the central nervous system and may change the effects or side effects of this drug. Check with your pharmacist for products to avoid.

Taking this drug with any of the ones listed below may change the effect of either drug with the possibility of causing toxicity or decreasing effectiveness:
aspirin, felbamate, lamotrigine, mefloquine, salicylates†

Severe reactions are possible when this drug is taken with those listed below:
anticoagulants, clonazepam, dipyridamole, heparin, nonsteroidal anti-
inflammatories†, pentoxifylline, sulfinpyrazone, ticarcillin

Increased side effects are possible when this drug is taken with those listed below:
acetaminophen, amiodarone, anabolic steroids†, androgens†, anesthetics,
antihistamines†, anxiolytics†, barbiturates†, carbamazepine, carmustine,
dantrolene, daunorubicin, disulfiram, estrogens†, etretinate, gold salts†,
mercaptopurine, methotrexate, methyldopa, monoamine oxidase in-
hibitors†, naltrexone, narcotics†, phenothiazines†, phenytoin, plicamycin,
primidone

ALLERGIC REACTIONS AND SIDE EFFECTS

If you are allergic to divalproex or valproate, you may also be allergic to
this drug. You should tell your doctor about all your allergies and any unexplained symptoms you may have while taking this drug.

MORE COMMON SIDE EFFECTS: Diarrhea, drowsiness, hair loss, indigestion,
loss of appetite*, menstrual changes*, nausea*, sleepiness, stomach
cramps*, trembling*, vomiting*, weight changes*

LESS COMMON SIDE EFFECTS: Behavior changes*, bleeding*, bruising*,
clumsiness, constipation, dizziness, excitement, eye movements*, headache, irritability, mood swings*, restlessness, seizures*, skin rash, swelling*, tiredness*, unsteadiness, vision changes*, weakness*, yellow eyes
or skin*

PRECAUTIONS

Be careful driving or handling equipment while taking this drug because
the drug may cause drowsiness.

People with brain disease, blood disorders, or kidney disease are at greater
risk of developing serious side effects.

Do not open, crush, break, or chew the capsule products since the drug is
very irritating to the mouth and throat.

Stopping this drug suddenly may cause severe side effects. If you wish to
stop taking this drug, ask your doctor for specific instructions.

This drug causes changes to your blood that make it harder to stop bleeding. If you are planning surgery, a dental appointment, or have an emergency injury, make sure you tell the doctor or dentist that you are taking
this drug.

This drug may interfere with several diagnostic tests including urinary
ketones and thyroid function tests.

---

† See page 52.   * See page 53.

PREGNANCY AND BREAST-FEEDING

There is evidence that this drug may harm the fetus, but the drug may be necessary to the health of the mother.

Breast-feeding while taking this drug is not recommended.

HELPFUL COMMENTS

Do not measure doses of the oral syrup with anything but a measuring cup intended for use with prescription drugs. Slight inaccuracy from other measuring spoons may result in over- or under-dosing.

The syrup product may be mixed with food or liquid for easier swallowing.

VALSARTAN

Available since July 2001

COMMONLY USED TO TREAT

High blood pressure, also known as hypertension

DRUG CATEGORY

antihypertensive
Class: angiotensin II receptor antagonist

PRODUCTS

Brand-Name Products with No Generic Alternative
Diovan 80 mg tablet ($)
Diovan 160 mg tablet ($$)
Diovan 320 mg tablet ($$)
No generics available.
Multiple patents that begin to expire in 2012.

Other Products That Contain This Drug
Diovan HCT tablet ($$)

DOSING AND FOOD

Doses are taken 1 to 2 times a day.
This drug may be taken with or without food.
Adults: Up to 320 mg per day.
Lower doses are used in people with liver disease.
This drug is rarely used in children.

Forgotten doses: If you are scheduled to take the next dose within a few hours, do not take the forgotten dose. Otherwise take the forgotten dose as soon as you remember.

ALCOHOL, DRUG, HERB, AND SUPPLEMENT INTERACTIONS

Alcohol may increase some of the side effects from this drug, depending on the amount consumed. Ask your doctor about the risks caused by drinking alcohol with your condition.

Several OTC drugs used for appetite control, asthma, colds, cough, hay fever, or sinus problems may cause an increase in blood pressure when taken with this drug. Check with your pharmacist when selecting OTC products.

Taking this drug with any of the ones listed below may change the effect of either drug with the possibility of causing toxicity or decreasing effectiveness: diuretics†

ALLERGIC REACTIONS AND SIDE EFFECTS

You should tell your doctor about all your allergies and any unexplained symptoms you may have while taking this drug.

LESS COMMON SIDE EFFECTS: Abdominal pain, back pain, cough, diarrhea, headache, muscle pain, stiffness, swelling, tiredness

RARE SIDE EFFECTS: Breathing difficulty*, chills*, dizziness*, fainting*, fever*, hoarseness*, lightheadedness*, sore throat*, swallowing difficulty, swelling

PRECAUTIONS

If you are dehydrated, the blood-pressure-lowering effect of this drug may be increased. Drink plenty of fluids to avoid dehydration when sweating, such as in hot weather and during exercise.

Be careful driving or handling equipment while taking this drug because the drug may cause dizziness.

If you have kidney disease, this drug may make that condition worse.

PREGNANCY AND BREAST-FEEDING

There is evidence that this drug may harm the fetus, but the drug may be necessary to the health of the mother.

Breast-feeding while taking this drug is not recommended.

HELPFUL COMMENTS

It may take 4 weeks before the full effects of this drug are noticed.

---

†See page 52.   *See page 53.

VANCOMYCIN HYDROCHLORIDE

Available for over 20 years

COMMONLY USED TO TREAT

Colitis
Diarrhea caused by antibiotics

DRUG CATEGORY

antibiotic
Class: glycopeptide

PRODUCTS

Brand-Name Products with No Generic Alternative
Vancocin 125 mg capsule ($$$$)
Vancocin 250 mg capsule ($$$$$)
Vancocin 500 mg/6 ml oral solution (n/a)
Brand-Name Products with Generic Alternatives
Vancocin 250 mg/5 ml oral solution (n/a)
   Generic: vancomycin hydrochloride 250 mg/5 ml oral solution (n/a)

DOSING AND FOOD

Doses are taken 3 to 4 times a day.
This drug may be taken with or without food.
Adults: Up to 2,000 mg per day in divided doses.
Children: Up to 40 mg/kg (maximum 2,000 mg) per day in divided doses.
Lower doses are used in people with kidney disease.
Forgotten doses: If you are scheduled to take the next dose within a few
   hours, do not take the forgotten dose. Otherwise take the forgotten dose
   as soon as you remember.

ALCOHOL, DRUG, HERB, AND SUPPLEMENT INTERACTIONS

Taking this drug with any of the ones listed below may change the effect of
either drug with the possibility of causing toxicity or decreasing effectiveness:
cholestyramine, colestipol

Severe reactions are possible when this drug is taken with those listed below:
skeletal muscle relaxants†

Increased side effects are possible when this drug is taken with those listed below:
aminoglycosides†, amphotericin B, capreomycin, cisplatin, colistin, methoxyflurane, polymyxin B

ALLERGIC REACTIONS AND SIDE EFFECTS

You should tell your doctor about all your allergies and any unexplained symptoms you may have while taking this drug.

MORE COMMON SIDE EFFECTS: Bad taste, mouth irritation, nausea, vomiting

LESS COMMON SIDE EFFECTS: Chills, fever, hearing loss, low blood pressure*, ringing in ears, shortness of breath, wheezing

RARE SIDE EFFECTS: Hives*, welts*, skin discoloration*, skin rash*

PRECAUTIONS

The oral form of this drug is not absorbed into the body but works directly in the intestinal tract. Different warnings and precautions apply to the intravenous form of this drug.

People with inflammatory bowel problems are at greater risk of developing side effects while taking this drug.

Tell your doctor if you take large doses of aspirin on a regular basis since this drug may mask the symptoms of aspirin toxicity.

PREGNANCY AND BREAST-FEEDING

Safety during pregnancy has not been established although the drug is known to harm animal fetuses.

It is not known if this drug passes into breast milk. Talk to your doctor about the risks associated with breast-feeding while taking this drug.

HELPFUL COMMENTS

Do not measure doses of the oral solution with anything but a measuring cup intended for use with prescription drugs. Slight inaccuracy from other measuring spoons may result in over- or under-dosing.

Contact your doctor if your symptoms do not improve after a couple of days.

Do not stop treatment early if you start to feel better. It takes the full prescription for this drug to work completely.

If you need to take cholestyramine or colestipol, take it either 3 to 4 hours before or after taking this drug.

VENLAFAXINE HYDROCHLORIDE

Available since December 1993

COMMONLY USED TO TREAT

Anxiety
Depression

---

† See page 52.   * See page 53.

DRUG CATEGORY

anxiolytic
antidepressant
Class: neurotransmitter reuptake inhibitor

PRODUCTS

Brand-Name Products with No Generic Alternative
Effexor 25 mg tablet ($)
Effexor 37.5 mg tablet ($)
Effexor 50 mg tablet ($)
Effexor 75 mg tablet ($$)
Effexor 100 mg tablet ($$)
Effexor XR 37.5 mg extended-release capsule ($$)
Effexor XR 75 mg extended-release capsule ($$$)
Effexor XR 150 mg extended-release capsule ($$$)
No generics available.
Multiple patents that begin to expire in 2007. Exclusivity until 2004.

DOSING AND FOOD

Doses are taken 2 to 3 times a day. Extended-release products are taken
  once a day.
It is best to take this drug with food or milk.
Adults: Up to 225 mg per day in divided doses.
Lower doses are used in people with kidney disease or liver disease.
Forgotten doses: If you are scheduled to take the next dose within a few
  hours, do not take the forgotten dose. Otherwise take the forgotten dose
  as soon as you remember.

ALCOHOL, DRUG, HERB, AND SUPPLEMENT INTERACTIONS

Alcohol may increase some of the side effects from this drug, depending
  on the amount consumed. Ask your doctor about the risks caused by
  drinking alcohol with your condition.
Yohimbe may seriously increase the effects of this drug and should not be
  used.
Many OTC drugs used for appetite control, asthma, colds, cough, hay
  fever, pain, or sinus problems affect the central nervous system and may
  change the effects or side effects of this drug. Check with your pharma-
  cist for products to avoid.

Taking this drug with any of the ones listed below may change the effect of either drug with the possibility of causing toxicity or decreasing effectiveness: cimetidine

Severe reactions are possible when this drug is taken with those listed below: moclobemide, monoamine oxidase inhibitors†

Increased side effects are possible when this drug is taken with those listed below: amitriptyline, bromocriptine, buspirone, clomipramine, dextromethorphan, imipramine, levodopa, lithium, LSD, marijuana, MDMA (ecstasy), meperidine, nefazodone, pentazocine, SSRI†, sumatriptan, tramadol, trazodone, tryptophan

ALLERGIC REACTIONS AND SIDE EFFECTS

You should tell your doctor about all your allergies and any unexplained symptoms you may have while taking this drug.

MORE COMMON SIDE EFFECTS: Anxiety, chills, constipation, diarrhea, dizziness, drowsiness*, dry mouth, gas, headache, heartburn, high blood pressure*, loss of appetite, nausea, nervousness, sexual dysfunction*, shaking*, sleep disorders, stuffy nose, sweating, tingling*, tiredness*, trembling*, vision changes*, vomiting, weakness*, weight loss

LESS COMMON SIDE EFFECTS: Chest pain*, irregular heartbeat*, mood swings*, ringing in ears*, taste changes, yawning

RARE SIDE EFFECTS: Agitation*, breathing difficulty*, excessive talking*, fainting*, itching*, lightheadedness*, lockjaw*, menstrual changes*, seizures*, skin rash*, swelling*, urinary changes*

PRECAUTIONS

You need to wait 2 weeks after stopping a monoamine oxidase inhibitor† and 3 days after stopping moclobemide before starting this drug.

People with a history of seizures or brain disease may be at greater risk of developing a seizure while taking this drug.

If you have heart disease, high blood pressure, low blood pressure, or mania, this drug may make those conditions worse.

Do not open, crush, break, or chew the extended-release products.

Be careful driving or handling equipment while taking this drug because it may cause drowsiness, dizziness, or vision changes.

Stopping this drug suddenly may cause severe side effects. If you wish to stop taking this drug, ask your doctor for specific instructions.

A skin rash or hives may be the first warning symptom that you are having an allergic reaction to this drug.

† See page 52.   * See page 53.

This drug may cause dry mouth, which is associated with a greater risk of cavities. Your dentist may recommend that you clean your teeth and mouth differently to avoid infection.

PREGNANCY AND BREAST-FEEDING

Safety during pregnancy has not been established although the drug is known to harm animal fetuses.

Breast-feeding while taking this drug is not recommended.

HELPFUL COMMENTS

It may take 4 weeks before the effects of this drug are noticed.

Sucking on hard sugarless candy or chewing sugarless gum may help relieve dry mouth caused by this drug.

Avoid quick movements to minimize dizziness. Dangling your legs over the side of the bed for a few minutes may help reduce dizziness when first waking up.

VERAPAMIL HYDROCHLORIDE

Available for over 20 years

COMMONLY USED TO TREAT

Chest pain, also known as angina
High blood pressure, also known as hypertension
Irregular heartbeat, also known as arrhythmias

DRUG CATEGORY

antianginal
antiarrhythmic
antihypertensive
Class: calcium channel blocker

PRODUCTS

Brand-Name Products with No Generic Alternative
Verelan 360 mg extended-release capsule ($$$)
Verelan PM 100 mg extended-release capsule ($)
Verelan PM 200 mg extended-release capsule ($$)
Verelan PM 300 mg extended-release capsule ($$$)

Brand-Name Products with Generic Alternatives

Isoptin 40 mg tablet (n/a)
  Generic: verapamil hydrochloride 40 mg tablet (¢¢¢)

Isoptin 80 mg tablet (n/a)
  Generic: verapamil hydrochloride 80 mg tablet (¢¢)

Isoptin 120 mg tablet (n/a)
  Generic: verapamil hydrochloride 120 mg tablet (¢¢)

Isoptin SR 120 mg extended-release tablet ($)
  Generic: verapamil hydrochloride 120 mg extended-release tablet (¢¢¢¢¢)

Isoptin SR 180 mg extended-release tablet ($$)
  Generic: verapamil hydrochloride 180 mg extended-release tablet (¢)

Isoptin SR 240 mg extended-release tablet ($$)
  Generic: verapamil hydrochloride 240 mg extended-release tablet (¢)

Verelan 120 mg extended-release capsule ($$)
  Generic: verapamil hydrochloride 120 mg extended-release capsule ($)

Verelan 180 mg extended-release capsule ($$)
  Generic: verapamil hydrochloride 180 mg extended-release capsule ($)

Verelan 240 mg extended-release capsule ($$)
  Generic: verapamil hydrochloride 240 mg extended-release capsule ($$)

Other Generic Product Names
Calan, Calan SR, Covera-HS,

Combination Products That Contain This Drug
Tarka extended-release tablet ($$)

DOSING AND FOOD

Doses of regular products are taken 3 to 4 times a day. Extended-release
  products are taken once a day.

It is best to take this drug with food or milk.

Adults: Up to 480 mg per day in divided doses.

Forgotten doses: If you are scheduled to take the next dose within a few
  hours, do not take the forgotten dose. Otherwise take the forgotten dose
  as soon as you remember.

ALCOHOL, DRUG, HERB, AND SUPPLEMENT INTERACTIONS

Alcohol should not be used while taking this drug.

Black catechu and yerba maté should not be used while taking this drug.

Several OTC drugs used for appetite control, asthma, colds, cough, hay fever,
  or sinus problems may cause an increase in blood pressure when taken
  with this drug. Check with your pharmacist when selecting OTC products.

---

† *See page 52.*   * *See page 53.*

Taking this drug with any of the ones listed below may change the effect of either drug with the possibility of causing toxicity or decreasing effectiveness: carbamazepine, cyclosporine, digoxin, procainamide, quinidine, rifampin

Severe reactions are possible when this drug is taken with those listed below: antihypertensives†, beta blockers†, disopyramide, flecainide

ALLERGIC REACTIONS AND SIDE EFFECTS

If you are allergic to any other calcium channel blocker†, you may also be allergic to this drug. You should tell your doctor about all your allergies and any unexplained symptoms you may have while taking this drug.

MORE COMMON SIDE EFFECTS: Breathing difficulty*, constipation, fainting*, fluid retention*, irregular heartbeat*, shortness of breath*, swelling*

LESS COMMON SIDE EFFECTS: Dizziness, flushing, headache, nausea, skin rash*, tiredness, weakness, wheezing*

RARE SIDE EFFECTS: Breast-milk secretion, chest pain*, tender gums*

PRECAUTIONS

Do not crush, break, or chew the Covera-HS or Verelan PM extended-release products. Isoptin SR and Calan SR may be broken in half, but should not be crushed or chewed.

This drug may cause changes to your gums and mouth. Your dentist may recommend that you clean your teeth and mouth differently to avoid infection.

Learn how to measure your heart rate and call your doctor if it falls below 60 beats per minute.

People with heart failure or liver disease may not be able to take this drug.

PREGNANCY AND BREAST-FEEDING

Safety during pregnancy has not been established although the drug is known to harm animal fetuses.

Breast-feeding while taking this drug is not recommended.

HELPFUL COMMENTS

If you are taking Verelan pellet-filled capsules (not Verelan PM) and having difficulty swallowing, you may sprinkle the contents of the capsules onto soft food such as applesauce. Do not chew or crush the pellets when swallowing.

WARFARIN SODIUM

Available for over 20 years

COMMONLY USED TO TREAT

People at risk of developing blood clots

DRUG CATEGORY

anticoagulant
Class: coumarin derivative

PRODUCTS

Brand-Name Products with Generic Alternatives
Coumadin 1 mg tablet (¢¢¢¢)
  Generic: warfarin sodium 1 mg tablet (¢¢¢¢)
Coumadin 2 mg tablet (¢¢¢¢)
  Generic: warfarin sodium 2 mg tablet (¢¢¢¢)
Coumadin 2.5 mg tablet (¢¢¢¢)
  Generic: warfarin sodium 2.5 mg tablet (¢¢¢¢)
Coumadin 3 mg tablet (¢¢¢¢)
  Generic: warfarin sodium 3 mg tablet (¢¢¢¢)
Coumadin 4 mg tablet (¢¢¢¢)
  Generic: warfarin sodium 4 mg tablet (¢¢¢¢)
Coumadin 5 mg tablet (¢¢¢¢)
  Generic: warfarin sodium 5 mg tablet (¢¢¢¢)
Coumadin 6 mg tablet ($)
  Generic: warfarin sodium 6 mg tablet (¢¢¢¢¢)
Coumadin 7.5 mg tablet ($)
  Generic: warfarin sodium 7.5 mg tablet (¢¢¢¢¢)
Coumadin 10 mg tablet ($)
  Generic: warfarin sodium 10 mg tablet (¢¢¢¢¢)

DOSING AND FOOD

Doses are taken once a day.
This drug may be taken with or without food. Food high in Vitamin K, including asparagus, broccoli, cabbage, lettuce, turnips, greens, spinach, watercress, pork liver, beef liver, green tea, and tomatoes, may decrease the effects of this drug.
Adults: Up to 10 mg per day based on the results of blood-clotting tests.
Forgotten doses: If you are scheduled to take the next dose within a few

---

† *See page 52.*   * *See page 53.*

hours, do not take the forgotten dose. Otherwise take the forgotten dose as soon as you remember.

ALCOHOL, DRUG, HERB, AND SUPPLEMENT INTERACTIONS

Alcohol should not be used while taking this drug.

Angelica root, anise, arnica flower, asafetida, bromelain, celery, chamomile, clover, danshen, devil's claw, dong quai, fenugreek, feverfew, garlic, ginger, ginkgo biloba, horse chestnut, licorice, meadowsweet, motherwort, onion, papain, parsley, passion flower, quassia, red clover, reishi mushroom, rue, sweet clover, and turmeric may increase the risk of bleeding while taking this drug and should not be used.

Ginseng, green tea, St. John's wort, and ubiquinon may decrease the effects of this drug and should not be used.

Several OTC drugs used for appetite control, asthma, colds, cough, hay fever, pain, or sinus problems may seriously increase the effects of this drug. Check with your pharmacist when selecting OTC products.

Taking this drug with any of the ones listed below may change the effect of either drug with the possibility of causing toxicity or decreasing effectiveness: acetaminophen, alcohol, allopurinol, amiodarone, anabolic steroids†, androgens†, antifungals†, antithyroid drugs†, aspirin, barbiturates†, carbamazepine, carbenicillin, cephalosporins†, chloral hydrate, chloramphenicol, cholestyramine, cimetidine, cinchophen, ciprofloxacin, clofibrate, corticosteroids†, danazol, dextrothyroxine, diazoxide, diflunisal, dipyridamole, disulfiram, divalproex, erythromycin, ethacrynic acid, ethychlorvynol, flu shot, fluvoxamine, glucagon, glutethimide, griseofulvin, heparin, ibuprofen, indomethacin, isoniazid, itraconazole, ketoprofen, lovastatin, mefanamic acid, methimazole, metronidazole, miconazole, moxalactam, neomycin, nonsteroidal antiinflammatories†, norfloxacin, ofloxacin, omeprazole, oral contraceptives, paroxetine, pentoxifylline, phenobarbital, phenylbutazone, phenytoin, plicamycin, primidone, propafenone, prophylthiouracil, propoxyphene, quinidine, rifampin, salicylates†, sertraline, simvastatin, streptokinase, sulfapyridine, sulfasalazine, sulfinpyrazone, sulfonamides†, sulindac, tamoxifen, tetracyclines, thiazide diuretics†, thyroid hormones†, ticarcillin, ticlopidine, tricyclic antidepressants†, urokinase, valproic acid, vitamin K, zafirlukast, zileuton

ALLERGIC REACTIONS AND SIDE EFFECTS

If you are allergic to any anticoagulant†, you may also be allergic to this drug. You should tell your doctor about all your allergies and any unexplained symptoms you may have while taking this drug.

LESS COMMON SIDE EFFECTS: Abdominal pain*, back pain*, bloating, chills*, cough*, diarrhea*, fever*, hives*, hoarseness*, itching*, loss of appetite*, nausea*, skin rash*, urinary changes*, vomiting*

RARE SIDE EFFECTS: Back pain*, black stools*, blisters*, bloody eyes*, bloody sputum*, bloody stools*, bloody urine*, bloody vomit*, blue toes*, blurry vision*, breathing difficulty*, chest pain*, confusion*, constipation*, dark urine*, dizziness*, fainting*, headache*, itching*, joint pain*, mouth sores*, nervousness*, numbness*, paralysis*, shortness of breath*, skin irritation*, stiffness*, swelling*, tingling*, toe pain*, weakness*, yellow eyes or skin*

PRECAUTIONS

This drug causes changes to your blood that make it harder to stop bleeding. If you are planning surgery, a dental appointment, or have an emergency injury, make sure you tell the doctor or dentist that you're taking this drug.

People with blood disorders, cancer, recent childbirth or miscarriage, diabetes, diverticulitis, head injury, high blood pressure, intestinal problems, liver disease, spinal anesthesia, major surgery, dental surgery, aneurysm, heart infection, ulcers, or vitamin K deficiency are at increased risk of severe bleeding while taking this drug and may need a dose adjustment.

This drug may make you more sensitive to cold temperatures.

Make sure you do not participate in activities that could lead to bruising or bleeding while taking this drug. Tell your doctor immediately if you notice any sign of bleeding or bruising, especially in hot weather when the effects of this drug may be increased.

This drug may cause your gums to bleed more easily. Your dentist may recommend that you clean your teeth and mouth differently to avoid infection.

Blood should be tested at least once a month to make sure this drug is used safely and effectively.

This drug may interfere with the blood test used to determine theophylline levels.

PREGNANCY AND BREAST-FEEDING

This drug may cause birth defects and should not be used during pregnancy. Breast-feeding while taking this drug is not recommended.

HELPFUL COMMENTS

If you skip meals or cannot eat on a regular basis, you may need an adjustment to the dose of this drug.

The effects of this drug may not be noticed for 7 days.

---

†See page 52.   * See page 53.

ZAFIRLUKAST

Available since September 1996

COMMONLY USED TO TREAT

Asthma

DRUG CATEGORY

antiasthmatic
Class: leukotriene receptor antagonist

PRODUCTS

Brand-Name Products with No Generic Alternative
Accolate 10 mg tablet ($)
Accolate 20 mg tablet ($)
No generics available.
Multiple patents that begin to expire in 2010.

DOSING AND FOOD

Doses are taken twice a day.
It is best to take this drug on an empty stomach at least 1 hour before
meals or 2 hours after a meal.
Adults and children over age 12: Up to 40 mg per day in divided doses.
Children age 7 to 11: Up to 20 mg per day in divided doses.
Forgotten doses: If you are scheduled to take the next dose within a few
hours, do not take the forgotten dose. Otherwise take the forgotten dose
as soon as you remember.

ALCOHOL, DRUG, HERB, AND SUPPLEMENT INTERACTIONS

Alcohol may increase some of the side effects from this drug, depending
on the amount consumed. Ask your doctor about the risks caused by
drinking alcohol with your condition.

**Taking this drug with any of the ones listed below may change the effect of
either drug with the possibility of causing toxicity or decreasing effectiveness:**
aspirin, erythromycin, theophylline, warfarin

ALLERGIC REACTIONS AND SIDE EFFECTS

You should tell your doctor about all your allergies and any unexplained
symptoms you may have while taking this drug.
LESS COMMON SIDE EFFECTS: Headache, nausea

RARE SIDE EFFECTS: Abdominal pain*, breathing difficulty*, diarrhea, irregular heartbeat*, itching*, numbness*, skin rash*, tingling*, tiredness*,
yellow eyes or skin*

PRECAUTIONS

This drug is used to prevent an asthma attack but is not effective in treating
an attack that has already started.
People with liver disease or a history of alcohol abuse may not be able to
take this drug.

PREGNANCY AND BREAST-FEEDING

Safety during pregnancy has not been established although there was no
evidence of harm during studies in animals.
Breast-feeding while taking this drug is not recommended.

HELPFUL COMMENTS

It takes about 3 to 4 days for the effects of this drug to be noticed.
If you get a headache while taking this drug do NOT take aspirin since it
may change the effects of the drug.

ZALCITABINE

Available since June 1992

COMMONLY USED TO TREAT

Advanced HIV infection

DRUG CATEGORY

antiretroviral
Class: nucleoside reverse transcriptase inhibitor (NsRTI)

PRODUCTS

Brand-Name Products with No Generic Alternative
Hivid 0.375 mg tablet ($$)
Hivid 0.75 mg tablet ($$$)
No generics available.
Multiple patents that begin to expire in 2006.

DOSING AND FOOD

Doses are taken 3 times a day.

---

†See page 52.   * See page 53.

It is best to take this drug on an empty stomach more than 1 hour before or 2 hours after a meal.

Adults and children over age 13: Up to 2.25 mg per day in divided doses. Lower doses are used in people with kidney disease.

Forgotten doses: If you are scheduled to take the next dose within a few hours, do not take the forgotten dose. Otherwise take the forgotten dose as soon as you remember.

ALCOHOL, DRUG, HERB, AND SUPPLEMENT INTERACTIONS

Alcohol should not be used while taking this drug.

Taking this drug with any of the ones listed below may change the effect of either drug with the possibility of causing toxicity or decreasing effectiveness: antacids, cimetidine, probenecid

Severe reactions are possible when this drug is taken with those listed below: alcohol, aminoglycosides†, amphotericin, asparaginase, azathioprine, didanosine, estrogens†, foscarnet, furosemide, methyldopa, pentamidine, stavudine, sulfonamides†, sulindac, tetracyclines, thiazide diuretics†, valproic acid

Increased side effects are possible when this drug is taken with those listed below: chloramphenicol, cisplatin, dapsone, disulfiram, ethambutol, ethionamide, glutethimide, gold salts†, hydralazine, iodoquinol, isoniazid, lithium, metronidazole, nitrofurantoin, nitrous oxide, phenytoin, ribavirin, vincristine

ALLERGIC REACTIONS AND SIDE EFFECTS

You should tell your doctor about all your allergies and any unexplained symptoms you may have while taking this drug.

MORE COMMON SIDE EFFECTS: Numbness*, tingling*

LESS COMMON SIDE EFFECTS: Diarrhea, fever*, headache, joint pain*, mouth sores*, muscle pain*, skin rash*, stomach pain*

RARE SIDE EFFECTS: Nausea*, sore throat*, vomiting*, yellow eyes or skin*

PRECAUTIONS

People with a history of alcohol abuse, high triglyceride levels, or pancreatitis may not be able to take this drug.

This drug is not a cure for HIV and does not prevent the transmission of the HIV virus.

If you have peripheral neuropathy, this drug may make that condition worse.

This drug may need to be stopped if you develop a burning, numbness, or tingling sensation in the hands, legs, arms, or feet.

PREGNANCY AND BREAST-FEEDING

Safety during pregnancy has not been established although the drug is known to harm animal fetuses.

Breast-feeding while taking this drug is not recommended.

HELPFUL COMMENTS

This drug is also called by the generic name ddC or dideoxycytidine.

If you need to take an antacid, take it either 2 hours before or after taking this drug.

Do not stop treatment early if you start to feel better. It takes the full prescription for this drug to work completely.

ZALEPLON

Available since August 1999

COMMONLY USED TO TREAT

Sleeping difficulty, also known as insomnia

DRUG CATEGORY

sedative-hypnotic
Class: pyrazolopyrimidine

PRODUCTS

Brand-Name Products with No Generic Alternative
Sonata 5 mg capsule ($$)
Sonata 10 mg capsule ($$)
No generics available.
Exclusivity until 2004.

DOSING AND FOOD

Doses are taken once a day at bedtime.

This drug may be taken with or without food but works faster when taken on an empty stomach.

Adults: Up to 20 mg per day.

Lower doses are used in people over age 65 and in people with kidney disease.

---

† *See page 52.*   * *See page 53.*

Forgotten doses: Do not take a forgotten dose. Just go back to your usual schedule with the next dose.

ALCOHOL, DRUG, HERB, AND SUPPLEMENT INTERACTIONS

Alcohol should not be used while taking this drug.

Many OTC drugs used for appetite control, asthma, colds, cough, hay fever, pain, or sinus problems affect the central nervous system and may change the effects or side effects of this drug. Check with your pharmacist for products to avoid.

Taking this drug with any of the ones listed below may change the effect of either drug with the possibility of causing toxicity or decreasing effectiveness: alcohol, barbiturates, carbamazepine, cimetidine, glutethimide, phenylbutazone, phenytoin, primidone, rifampin

Increased side effects are possible when this drug is taken with those listed below: anesthetics, antihistamines†, anxiolytics†, narcotics†, tricyclic antidepressants†

ALLERGIC REACTIONS AND SIDE EFFECTS

You should tell your doctor about all your allergies and any unexplained symptoms you may have while taking this drug.

MORE COMMON SIDE EFFECTS: Dizziness*, headache*, muscle pain, nausea

LESS COMMON SIDE EFFECTS: Abdominal pain, anxiety*, blurry vision*, breathing difficulty*, chest tightness, constipation, cough, depression, drowsiness*, dry mouth, eye pain, fever, hearing changes, heartburn, indigestion, itching, joint pain, memory loss, menstrual pain, nervousness, poor concentration, prickling, shaking, shortness of breath, skin rash, tingling, tiredness, trembling, weakness*, wheezing

RARE SIDE EFFECTS: Clumsiness*, confusion*, fainting*, hallucinations*, nosebleeds*, sluggishness*

PRECAUTIONS

This drug may be habit forming. People with a history of alcohol or drug abuse are at greater risk of developing dependence.

Stopping this drug suddenly may cause severe withdrawal side effects. If you wish to stop taking this drug, ask your doctor for specific instructions.

If you have depression or breathing problems, this drug may make those conditions worse.

Make sure you are ready to go to sleep when you take this drug since it works pretty quickly. Allow for at least 4 hours of sleep time before the drowsiness effect of the drug starts to wear off.

Be careful driving or handling equipment while taking this drug because it may cause drowsiness and dizziness.

PREGNANCY AND BREAST-FEEDING

Safety during pregnancy has not been established although the drug is known to harm animal fetuses.

Breast-feeding while taking this drug is not recommended.

HELPFUL COMMENTS

The full effects of this drug should be noticed within 2 hours.

This drug is usually taken for less than 5 weeks.

ZIDOVUDINE

Available since March 1987

COMMONLY USED TO TREAT

HIV infection

DRUG CATEGORY

antiretroviral

Class: nucleoside reverse transcriptase inhibitor (NsRTI)

PRODUCTS

Brand-Name Products with No Generic Alternative

Retrovir 100 mg capsule ($$)

Retrovir 300 mg tablet ($$$$)

Retrovir 50 mg/5 ml oral syrup (¢¢¢¢¢)

No generics available.

Patents expire in 2005.

Combination Products That Contain This Drug

Combivir tablet ($$$$$)

Trizivir tablet ($$$$$)

DOSING AND FOOD

Doses are taken 2 to 4 times a day.

This drug may be taken with or without food.

Adults and children over age 12: Up to 600 mg per day in divided doses.

Children age 3 months to 12 years: Up to 720 mg/m^2 (maximum 600 mg) per day in divided doses.

---

† *See page 52.*   * *See page 53.*

Lower doses are used in children under 3 months and in people with kidney disease.

Forgotten doses: If you are scheduled to take the next dose within a few hours, do not take the forgotten dose. Otherwise take the forgotten dose as soon as you remember.

ALCOHOL, DRUG, HERB, AND SUPPLEMENT INTERACTIONS

Alcohol may increase some of the side effects from this drug, depending on the amount consumed. Ask your doctor about the risks caused by drinking alcohol with your condition.

Taking this drug with any of the ones listed below may change the effect of either drug with the possibility of causing toxicity or decreasing effectiveness: clarithromycin, doxorubicin, fluconazole, methadone, probenecid, ribavirin, valproic acid

Severe reactions are possible when this drug is taken with those listed below: acyclovir

Increased side effects are possible when this drug is taken with those listed below: acetaminophen, amphotericin B, antineoplastics†, antithyroid drugs†, aspirin, azathioprine, chloramphenicol, colchicine, cyclophosphamide, dapsone, flucytosine, ganciclovir, indomethacin, interferon alpha, mercaptopurine, methotrexate, pentamidine, plicamycin

ALLERGIC REACTIONS AND SIDE EFFECTS

You should tell your doctor about all your allergies and any unexplained symptoms you may have while taking this drug.

MORE COMMON SIDE EFFECTS: Chills*, fever*, headache, nausea*, pale skin*, sleep disorders*, sore throat*, tiredness*, weakness*

LESS COMMON SIDE EFFECTS: Fingernail discoloration, skin discoloration

RARE SIDE EFFECTS: Abdominal pain*, confusion*, cramping*, diarrhea*, irregular breathing*, loss of appetite*, mood swings*, muscle pain*, seizures*, shortness of breath*, sleepiness*

PRECAUTIONS

If you have anemia, low folic acid, low vitamin B_{12}, or other blood disorders, this drug may make those conditions worse.

Avoid contact with anyone who has the chickenpox, measles, or other communicable disease since it may be easier to catch the infection while taking this drug.

Exposure to skin tests, immunizations, and people who have received immunizations may put you at a greater risk of developing the disease when you are taking this drug.

This drug causes changes in your blood that put you at greater risk of getting an infection. Be careful not to cut yourself or get bruised. Tell your doctor if you develop signs of infection, such as fever or sore throat. Your dentist may recommend that you clean your teeth and mouth differently to avoid infection.

This drug is not a cure for HIV and does not prevent the transmission of the HIV virus.

A blood test should be done about every 2 weeks while taking this drug to make sure your risk of developing an infection has not increased too much.

PREGNANCY AND BREAST-FEEDING

Safety during pregnancy has not been established although the drug is known to harm animal fetuses.

Breast-feeding while taking this drug is not recommended.

HELPFUL COMMENTS

Do not stop treatment early if you start to feel better. It takes the full prescription for this drug to work completely.

Side effects may continue to occur for up to 2 months after this drug is stopped.

This drug is also called by the generic name AZT.

Do not measure doses of the oral syrup with anything but a measuring cup intended for use with prescription drugs. Slight inaccuracy from other measuring spoons may result in over- or under-dosing.

ZILEUTON

Available since December 1996

COMMONLY USED TO TREAT

Asthma

DRUG CATEGORY

antiasthmatic
Class: leukotriene formation inhibitor

---

†See page 52.   *See page 53.

PRODUCTS

Brand-Name Products with No Generic Alternative
Zyflo 600 mg tablet (¢¢¢¢¢)
No generics available.
Patent expires in 2010.

DOSING AND FOOD

Doses are taken 4 times a day.
This drug may be taken with or without food.
Adults and children over age 12: Up to 2,400 mg per day in divided doses.
Forgotten doses: If you are scheduled to take the next dose within a few hours, do not take the forgotten dose. Otherwise take the forgotten dose as soon as you remember.

ALCOHOL, DRUG, HERB, AND SUPPLEMENT INTERACTIONS

Alcohol may increase some of the side effects from this drug, depending on the amount consumed. Ask your doctor about the risks caused by drinking alcohol with your condition.

Taking this drug with any of the ones listed below may change the effect of either drug with the possibility of causing toxicity or decreasing effectiveness: beta blockers†, terfenadine, theophylline, warfarin

ALLERGIC REACTIONS AND SIDE EFFECTS

You should tell your doctor about all your allergies and any unexplained symptoms you may have while taking this drug.
MORE COMMON SIDE EFFECTS: Nausea, stomachache
LESS COMMON SIDE EFFECTS: Abdominal pain*, weakness*
RARE SIDE EFFECTS: Itching*, runny nose*, tiredness*, yellow eyes or skin*

PRECAUTIONS

This drug should not be used to treat an active asthma attack. Rather, it should be used to prevent attacks from occurring.
People with a history of alcohol abuse may be at greater risk of developing side effects while taking this drug.
Liver function should be tested every 1 to 3 months while taking this drug.

PREGNANCY AND BREAST-FEEDING

Safety during pregnancy has not been established although the drug is known to harm animal fetuses.

It is not known if this drug passes into breast milk. Talk to your doctor about the risks associated with breast-feeding while taking this drug.

HELPFUL COMMENTS

Do not stop treatment early if you start to feel better.
This drug will no longer be available after 2003.

ZIPRASIDONE HYDROCHLORIDE

Available since February 2001

COMMONLY USED TO TREAT

Mental disturbances, specifically schizophrenia

DRUG CATEGORY

antipsychotic
Class: unclassified

PRODUCTS

Brand-Name Products with No Generic Alternative
Geodon 20 mg capsule ($$$)
Geodon 40 mg capsule ($$$)
Geodon 60 mg capsule ($$$)
Geodon 80 mg capsule ($$$)
No generics available.
Multiple patents that begin to expire in 2007. Exclusivity until 2006.

DOSING AND FOOD

Doses are taken twice a day.
It is best to take this drug with food.
Adults: Up to 100 mg per day in divided doses.
Forgotten doses: If you are scheduled to take the next dose within a few hours, do not take the forgotten dose. Otherwise take the forgotten dose as soon as you remember.

ALCOHOL, DRUG, HERB, AND SUPPLEMENT INTERACTIONS

Alcohol may increase some of the side effects from this drug, depending on the amount consumed. Ask your doctor about the risks caused by drinking alcohol with your condition.

---

† See page 52.　　* See page 53.

Many OTC drugs used for appetite control, asthma, colds, cough, hay fever, pain, or sinus problems affect the central nervous system and may change the effects or side effects of this drug. Check with your pharmacist for products to avoid.

Taking this drug with any of the ones listed below may change the effect of either drug with the possibility of causing toxicity or decreasing effectiveness: carbamazepine, levodopa, ketoconazole

Severe reactions are possible when this drug is taken with those listed below: antiarrhythmics†, chlorpromazine, diuretics†, dofetilide, dolasetron, droperidol, gatifloxacin, halofantrine, levomethadyl, mefloquine, mesoridazine, moxifloxacin, pentamidine, pimozide, probucol, quinidine, sotalol, sparfloxacin, tacrolimus, thioridazine

ALLERGIC REACTIONS AND SIDE EFFECTS

You should tell your doctor about all your allergies and any unexplained symptoms you may have while taking this drug.

MORE COMMON SIDE EFFECTS: Belching, constipation, diarrhea, drooling, heartburn, indigestion, jerking, nausea, poor balance, restlessness, shuffling walk, skin rash, sleepiness*, sour stomach, spastic movements, speaking difficulty*, stiffness, stomachache, trembling, weakness, weight gain

LESS COMMON SIDE EFFECTS: Blinking, breathing difficulty*, dry mouth, dry skin, eye stillness, eyelid twitching, facial expressions, fainting*, irregular heartbeat*, itching, loss of appetite, sneezing, stuffy nose, swallowing difficulty, swelling, tongue movements, vision changes, weight loss

RARE SIDE EFFECTS: Dizziness*, drowsiness*, penile erection*, seizures*, slurry speech*

PRECAUTIONS

People with a history of seizures or Alzheimer's disease may be at increased risk of developing a seizure while taking this drug.

If you have heart disease, neuroleptic malignant syndrome (NMS), or tardive dyskinesia, this drug may make those conditions worse.

Be careful driving or handling equipment while taking this drug because it may cause sleepiness.

Do not open, crush, break, or chew the capsule products.

This drug puts you at greater risk of developing irregular heartbeats if your body loses too much potassium or magnesium. Make sure to eat a balanced meal and tell your doctor if there is any change in your diet.

PREGNANCY AND BREAST-FEEDING

Safety during pregnancy has not been established although the drug is known to harm animal fetuses.

Breast-feeding while taking this drug is not recommended.

HELPFUL COMMENTS

It may take 4 to 6 weeks before the effects of this drug are noticed.

Avoid quick movements to minimize dizziness. Dangling your legs over the side of the bed for a few minutes may help reduce dizziness when first waking up.

This drug may make you less tolerant to heat and humidity.

ZOLMITRIPTAN

Available since November 1997

COMMONLY USED TO TREAT

Migraine headache

DRUG CATEGORY

antimigraine
Class: triptan

PRODUCTS

Brand-Name Products with No Generic Alternative
Zomig 2.5 mg tablet ($$$$$)
Zomig 5 mg tablet ($$$$$)
Zomig-ZMT 2.5 mg disintegrating tablet ($$$$$)
Zomig-ZMT 5 mg disintegrating tablet ($$$$$)
No generics available.
Patent expires in 2012.

DOSING AND FOOD

Doses are taken every 2 hours up to the daily maximum.

This drug may be taken with or without food.

Adults: Up to 10 mg per day in divided doses.

Lower doses are used in people with liver disease.

---

† See page 52.   * See page 53.

ALCOHOL, DRUG, HERB, AND SUPPLEMENT INTERACTIONS

Alcohol may make your headache worse. You should ask your doctor about the risks caused by drinking alcohol with your condition.

Taking this drug with any of the ones listed below may change the effect of either drug with the possibility of causing toxicity or decreasing effectiveness: cimetidine, monoamine oxidase inhibitors†, oral contraceptives

Severe reactions are possible when this drug is taken with those listed below: antimigraine drugs†, ergot alkaloids†

Increased side effects are possible when this drug is taken with those listed below: fluoxetine, fluvoxamine, paroxetine, sertraline

ALLERGIC REACTIONS AND SIDE EFFECTS

You should tell your doctor about all your allergies and any unexplained symptoms you may have while taking this drug.

MORE COMMON SIDE EFFECTS: Chest pain*, dizziness, nausea*, numbness*, sleepiness, tingling*, tiredness*, weakness*

LESS COMMON SIDE EFFECTS: Abdominal pain*, agitation, anxiety, back pain*, breathing difficulty*, chest tightness*, chills*, cough*, depression, diarrhea*, dry mouth, fainting, fever*, heartburn, hives*, hoarseness*, irregular heartbeat*, itching*, loss of appetite*, mouth discomfort, puffy eyelids*, shortness of breath*, skin discoloration*, skin irritation, skin rash*, swallowing difficulty*, sweating, swelling*, urinary changes*, wheezing*

PRECAUTIONS

The oral disintegrating tablets may contain aspartame, which should not be taken in people with phenylketonuria (PKU).

Be careful driving or handling equipment while taking this drug because it may cause dizziness.

Disintegrating tablets should be placed on top of the tongue for a few seconds, then swallowed with saliva.

This drug may cause dry mouth, which is associated with a greater risk of cavities. Your dentist may recommend that you clean your teeth and mouth differently to avoid infection.

People with a history of chest pain, arrhythmias, high blood pressure, kidney disease, liver disease, or stroke may not be able to take this drug.

This drug is only effective in treating an active migraine headache and is not used to prevent a headache from occurring.

For maximum effect, take this drug at the first sign that a headache is starting.

Do not crush, break, or chew the disintegrating tablets.
If your headache does not respond to this drug, you should talk to your doctor about other treatment.

PREGNANCY AND BREAST-FEEDING

Safety during pregnancy has not been established although the drug is known to harm animal fetuses.
It is not known if this drug passes into breast milk. Talk to your doctor about the risks associated with breast-feeding while taking this drug.

HELPFUL COMMENTS

Disintegrating tablets may fall apart if pushed through the foil when removing from the packaging. Instead, the foil should be peeled back to open.
Avoid quick movements to minimize dizziness. Dangling your legs over the side of the bed for a few minutes may help reduce dizziness when first waking up.

ZOLPIDEM TARTRATE

Available since December 1992

COMMONLY USED TO TREAT

Sleeping difficulty, also known as insomnia

DRUG CATEGORY

sedative-hypnotic
Class: imidazopyridine

PRODUCTS

Brand-Name Products with No Generic Alternative
Ambien 5 mg tablet ($$)
Ambien 10 mg tablet ($$$)
No generics available.
Patent expires in 2006.

DOSING AND FOOD

Doses are taken once a day at bedtime.
This drug may be taken with or without food but works quicker if taken on an empty stomach.
Adults: Up to 10 mg per day.

† See page 52.   * See page 53.

Lower doses are used in people over age 65 and people with liver disease.

Forgotten doses: Do not take a forgotten dose. Just go back to your usual schedule with the next dose.

ALCOHOL, DRUG, HERB, AND SUPPLEMENT INTERACTIONS

Alcohol should not be used while taking this drug.

Many OTC drugs used for appetite control, asthma, colds, cough, hay fever, pain, or sinus problems affect the central nervous system and may change the effects or side effects of this drug. Check with your pharmacist for products to avoid.

Severe reactions are possible when this drug is taken with those listed below: anesthetics, antihistamines†, anxiolytics†, barbiturates†, narcotics†, tricyclic antidepressants†

ALLERGIC REACTIONS AND SIDE EFFECTS

You should tell your doctor about all your allergies and any unexplained symptoms you may have while taking this drug.

LESS COMMON SIDE EFFECTS: Abdominal pain, clumsiness*, confusion*, depression*, diarrhea, drowsiness, dry mouth, headache, memory loss, nausea*, nightmares, unsteadiness*, vision changes*, vomiting*

RARE SIDE EFFECTS: Breathing difficulty*, Dizziness*, excitement*, fainting*, falling*, hallucinations*, irregular heartbeat*, irritability*, lightheadedness*, nervousness*, skin rash*, sleeping difficulty, swelling*, wheezing*

PRECAUTIONS

If you have emphysema, asthma, bronchitis, lung disease, depression, or sleep apnea, this drug may make those conditions worse.

This drug may be habit forming. People with a history of alcohol or drug abuse are at greater risk of developing dependence.

Make sure you are ready to go to sleep when you take this drug since it works pretty quickly. Allow for at least 7 to 8 hours of sleep time before the drowsiness effect of the drug starts to wear off.

Be careful driving or handling equipment while taking this drug because it may cause drowsiness and dizziness.

Stopping this drug suddenly may cause severe withdrawal side effects. If you wish to stop taking this drug, ask your doctor for specific instructions.

Because this drug has a high abuse potential, your prescription quantity may be limited.

PREGNANCY AND BREAST-FEEDING

Safety during pregnancy has not been established although there was no
  evidence of harm during studies in animals.
Breast-feeding while taking this drug is not recommended.

HELPFUL COMMENTS

The full effects of this drug should be noticed within 2 hours.
This drug is usually taken for less than 2 weeks.

ZONISAMIDE

Available since March 2000

COMMONLY USED TO TREAT

Seizures

DRUG CATEGORY

anticonvulsant
Class: sulfonamide

PRODUCTS

Brand-Name Products with No Generic Alternative
Zonegran 100 mg capsule ($$)
No generics available.
Patent expires in 2018. Exclusivity until 2005.

DOSING AND FOOD

Doses are taken 1 to 2 times a day.
This drug may be taken with or without food. Do not drink grapefruit juice
  or eat grapefruit while taking this drug.
Adults over age 16: Up to 400 mg per day in divided doses.
Lower doses are used in people with kidney disease or liver disease.
Forgotten doses: If you are scheduled to take the next dose within a few
  hours, do not take the forgotten dose. Otherwise take the forgotten dose
  as soon as you remember.

ALCOHOL, DRUG, HERB, AND SUPPLEMENT INTERACTIONS

Alcohol should not be used while taking this drug.
Many OTC drugs used for appetite control, asthma, colds, cough, hay fever,

---

†See page 52.   * See page 53.

pain, or sinus problems affect the central nervous system and may change the effects or side effects of this drug. Check with your pharmacist for products to avoid.

Taking this drug with any of the ones listed below may change the effect of either drug with the possibility of causing toxicity or decreasing effectiveness: barbiturates†, carbamazepine, clarithromycin, corticosteroids†, cyclosporine, danazol, delaviridine, diltiazem, erythromycin, fluconazole, fluoxetine, fluvoxamine, griseofulvin, indinavir, isoniazid, itraconazole, ketoconazole, metronidazole, miconazole, nafcillin, nefazodone, nelfinavir, nicardipine, nifedipine, norfloxacin, omeprazole, phenytoin, prednisone, primidone, quinidine, quinine, rifabutin, rifampin, ritonavir, saquinavir, sertraline, troglitazone, troleandomycin, verapamil, zafirlukast

ALLERGIC REACTIONS AND SIDE EFFECTS

If you are allergic to any sulfonamide†, you may also be allergic to this drug. You should tell your doctor about all your allergies and any unexplained symptoms you may have while taking this drug.

MORE COMMON SIDE EFFECTS: Anxiety, dizziness, drowsiness, loss of appetite, restlessness, shakiness*, sleepiness, unsteadiness*

LESS COMMON SIDE EFFECTS: Agitation*, belching, bruising*, chills, constipation, delusions*, diarrhea, double vision, dry mouth, eye movements, fever, hallucinations*, headache, heartburn, indigestion, joint pain, memory loss, mood swings*, nausea, nervousness, poor concentration, rash*, skin discoloration*, sleeping difficulty, sneezing, sour stomach, speaking difficulty, stuffy nose, taste changes, tingling, tiredness, weakness, weight loss

RARE SIDE EFFECTS: Breathing difficulty*, confusion*, fainting*, irregular heartbeat*, unconsciousness*

PRECAUTIONS

Do not open, crush, break, or chew the capsule products.

Be careful driving or handling equipment while taking this drug because it may cause dizziness.

Stopping the drug suddenly may cause severe side effects including frequent seizures. If you wish to stop taking this drug, ask your doctor for specific instructions.

Drink 8 to 10 glasses of water every day while taking this drug to reduce the risk of developing kidney stones.

This drug may make you sweat less, putting you at greater risk of developing heat stroke. Avoid exercising in hot weather and using a hot tub or sauna.

If you have a history of kidney stones or gout, this drug may make those conditions worse.

PREGNANCY AND BREAST-FEEDING

Safety during pregnancy has not been established although the drug is known to harm animal fetuses.

Breast-feeding while taking this drug is not recommended.

HELPFUL COMMENTS

Contact your doctor if the frequency of your seizures does not improve after a few weeks. The dose of this drug may be adjusted every 2 weeks if needed.

7

Index of Drugs by Category and Class

The category and class information found in the drug summaries can be used to find similar drugs, which may be less expensive prescription alternatives. These similiar drugs can also be mentioned to your doctor as possible alternatives if your current prescription is not effective or tolerated. But remember that not every drug in a class or category, despite its similarities, can be used as a therapeutic substitute. Always talk to your doctor about your prescription and follow the instructions closely. It does not hurt to talk to your doctor about other drugs, but it may hurt to take someone else's prescription.

The index is arranged alphabetically by either drug category or drug class. Each entry is followed by a list of drugs included in that catagory or class. For example, if you want to see a list of all the beta blockers, you would search in the Bs. But if you want to find all the antihypertensives, which include the beta blockers plus other drug classes, you would search under the As. Some drugs in the index are italicized, which indicates that a summary for that drug is not included in this book. These italicized drugs are not frequently prescribed for use at home.

This index does not contain the name of every drug available. Instead, the list is comprehensive relative to the drug interactions, categories, and classes referenced in this book. Drugs not included are those not taken by mouth, such as injectable and topical drugs.

Italicized drugs may not be available in an oral product
and do not have a summary included in this book.

1-Aminomethyl Cyclohexoneacetic Acid—gabapentin

4-Amino-quinoline—chloroquine phosphate,
hydroxychloroquine sulfate, *mefloquine hydrochloride*

5-HT4 Receptor Agonist—tegaserod maleate

8-Amino-quinoline—primaquine phosphate

8-Hydroxyquinolone—*iodoquinol*

AIIRBs—see Angiotensin II Receptor Antagonist

ACE Inhibitor—benazepril hydrochloride, captopril, enalapril
maleate, fosinopril sodium, lisinopril, moexipril hydrochloride,
perindopril erbumine, quinapril hydrochloride, ramipril,
trandolapril

Acetaldehyde—*chloral hydrate*

ADP Blocker—clopidogrel bisulfate, ticlopidine hydrochloride

Adrenergic—albuterol, *brimonidine tartrate, ephedrine sulfate,
epinephrine, isoetharine hydrochloride, isoproterenol,* levalbuterol
hydrochloride, metaproterenol sulfate, *pirbuterol acetate,*
terbutaline sulfate

Alcohol Deterrent—disulfiram

Aldehyde Dehydrogenase Inhibitor—disulfiram

Aldosterone Blocker—eplerenone

Alkali Metal—lithium

Alkylating Agent—*altretamine,* busulfan, *thiotepa*

- **Alkylating Agent: Estrogen**—estramustine phosphate
  sodium

- **Alkylating Agent: Nitrogen Mustard**—chlorambucil,
  cyclophosphamide, *ifosfamide, mechlorethamine
  hydrochloride,* melphalan (*phylalanine mustard*)

- **Alkylating Agent: Nitrosureas**—*carmustine,* lomustine
  (CCNU), *streptozocin*

Alpha Adrenergic Agonist—tizanidine hydrochloride

Alpha Adrenergic Blocker—doxazosin mesylate, prazosin hydrochloride, tamsulosin hydrochloride, terazosin hydrochloride

Alphaglucosidase Inhibitor—acarbose, miglitol

Altitude Sickness Agent—acetazolamide

Amebicide—chloroquine phosphate, *iodoquinol*, metronidazole, *paromomycin sulfate*

Amide Anesthetic Analogue—tocainide hydrochloride

Amino Acid Derivative—acetylcysteine

Aminoglycoside—*amikacin sulfate, gentamicin sulfate,* kanamycin sulfate, neomycin sulfate, *paromomycin sulfate, tobramycin sulfate*

Aminoketone—bupropion hydrochloride

Anabolic Steroid—*nandrolone decanoate, oxandrolone, oxymetholone, stanozolol*

Analeptic—methylphenidate hydrochloride, modafinil

Analgesic—*acetaminophen, aspirin,* celecoxib, *choline magnesium salicylate,* codeine sulfate, diclofenac, diflunisal, etodolac, fenoprofen calcium, *hydrocodone bitartrate,* hydromorphone hydrochloride, ibuprofen, ketoprofen, ketorolac tromethamine, *levomethadyl acetate hydrochloride,* levorphanol, meclofenamate sodium, mefenamic acid, meloxicam, meperidine hydrochloride, methadone hydrochloride, morphine sulfate, oxycodone hydrochloride, propoxyphene, rofecoxib, tramadol hydrochloride, valdecoxib

Androgen—danazol, fluoxymesterone, methyltestosterone, *testolactone,* testosterone

Androgen Synthesis Inhibitor—dutasteride, finasteride

Angiotensin II Receptor Antagonist—candesartan cilexetil, eprosartan mesylate, irbesartan, losartan potassium, olmesartan medoxomil, telmisartan, valsartan

Anilinoquinazoline—gefitinib

Antiacne—erythromycin, isotretinoin, *tretinoin*

Antianginal—acebutolol, amlodipine besylate, *amyl nitrate,* atenolol, bepridil hydrochloride, carteolol hydrochloride, diltiazem, felodipine, isosorbide, isradipine, metoprolol, nadolol, nicardipine hydrochloride, nifedipine, nitroglycerin, penbutolol sulfate, pindolol, propranolol, sotalol hydrochloride, timolol, verapamil hydrochloride

Antiarrhythmic—acebutolol, amiodarone hydrochloride, atenolol, digoxin, diltiazem, disopyramide phosphate, dofetilide, flecainide acetate, metoprolol, mexiletine, moricizine hydrochloride, nadolol, procainamide hydrochloride, propafenone hydrochloride, propranolol hydrochloride, quinidine sulfate, sotalol hydrochloride, timolol, tocainide hydrochloride, verapamil hydrochloride

Antiarthritic—diclofenac, diflunisal, etodolac, fenoprofen calcium, flurbiprofen, ibuprofen, indomethacin, ketoprofen, meclofenamate sodium, nabumetone, naproxen, oxaprozin, piroxicam, sulindac, tolmetin sodium

Antiasthmatic—*beclomethasone dipropionate, flunisolide,* montelukast sodium, zafirlukast, zileuton

Antibiotic—*amikacin sulfate, aminosalicylic acid,* amoxicillin, ampicillin/ampicillin trihydrate, azithromycin dihydrate, bacampicillin hydrochloride, carbenicillin indanyl sodium, cefaclor, cefadroxil, cefdinir, cefditoren pivoxil, *cefotetan, cefoxitin,* cefpodoxime proxetil, cefprozil, ceftibuten dihydrate, cefuroxime axetil, cephalexin hydrochloride, cephradine, *chloramphenicol,* ciprofloxacin hydrochloride, clarithromycin, clindamycin, cloxacillin sodium, co-trimoxazole, cycloserine, demeclocycline hydrochloride, dicloxacillin sodium, dirithromycin, doxycycline, erythromycin, ethambutol hydrochloride, *ethionamide,* fosfomycin tromethamine, gatifloxacin, *gentamicin sulfate,* isoniazid (INH), kanamycin sulfate, levofloxacin, *lincomycin,* linezolid, lomefloxacin hydrochloride, *loracarbef, methenamine hippurate,* metronidazole, *mezlocillin sodium,* minocycline hydrochloride, moxifloxacin hydrochloride, *nafcillin sodium, nalidixic acid,* neomycin sulfate, *nitrofurantoin, nitrofurazone,* norfloxacin, ofloxacin, oxacillin sodium, oxytetracycline hydrochloride, penicillin V potassium, *piperacillin,* pyrazinamide, rifabutin, rifampin, rifapentine, sparfloxacin, sulfadiazine, sulfisoxazole, tetracycline, *ticarcillin disodium, tobramycin sulfate, trimethoprim,* troleandomycin, trovafloxacin mesylate, vancomycin hydrochloride

Antibulemic—amitriptyline hydrochloride, clomipramine hydrochloride, desipramine hydrochloride, imipramine

Anticachectic—megestrol acetate

Anticataplectic—clomipramine hydrochloride, desipramine hydrochloride, imipramine, protriptyline hydrochloride

Anticholinergic—*atropine, belladonna,* benztropine mesylate, biperiden hydrochloride, *clidinium bromide, cyclopentolate hydrochloride,* dicyclomine hydrochloride, *diphenhydramine, flavoxate* hydrochloride, glycopyrrolate, *homatropine methylbromide, hyoscyamine, ipratropium bromide, mepenzolate bromide, methscopolamine bromide,* procyclidine hydrochloride, propantheline bromide, *scopolamine,* tolterodine tartrate, trihexyphenidyl hydrochloride

Anticoagulant—*anisindione,* enoxaparin sodium, warfarin sodium

Anticonvulsant—acetazolamide, *amobarbital,* carbamazepine, clonazepam, clorazepate dipotassium, diazepam, *divalproex sodium,* ethosuximide, *ethotoin,* felbamate, *fosphenytoin sodium,* gabapentin, lamotrigine, levetiracetam, mephobarbital, methsuximide, oxcarbazepine, phenobarbital, phenytoin, primidone, tiagabine hydrochloride, topiramate, *trimethadione,* valproate sodium, valproic acid, zonisamide

Antidementia—donepezil hydrochloride, ergoloid mesylates, galantamine hydrobromide, rivastigmine tartrate, tacrine hydrochloride

Antidepressant—amitriptyline hydrochloride, amoxapine, bupropion hydrochloride, citalopram hydrobromide, clomipramine hydrochloride, desipramine hydrochloride, doxepin hydrochloride, fluoxetine hydrochloride, imipramine, *isocarboxazid, maprotiline hydrochloride,* mirtazapine, nefazodone hydrochloride, nortriptyline hydrochloride, paroxetine hydrochloride, *phenelzine sulfate,* protriptyline hydrochloride, sertraline hydrochloride, *tranylcycpromine,* trazodone hydrochloride, trimipramine maleate, venlafaxine hydrochloride

Antidiabetic—acarbose, acetohexamide, chlorpropamide, glimepiride, glipizide, glyburide, metformin hydrochloride, miglitol, nateglinide, pioglitazone hydrochloride, repaglinide, rosiglitazone maleate, tolazamide, tolbutamide

Antidiarrheal—codeine sulfate, glycopyrrolate, morphine sulfate

Antidiuretic—chlorpropamide, desmopressin acetate

Antidyskinetic—amantadine hydrochloride, benztropine mesylate, biperiden hydrochloride, bromocriptine mesylate, *diphenhydramine,* entacapone, levodopa-carbidopa, pergolide mesylate, pramipexole diphydrochloride, procyclidine hydrochloride, ropinirole hydrochloride, selegiline hydrochloride (l-deprenyl hydrochloride), tolcapone, trihexyphenidyl hydrochloride

Antidysmenorrheal—diclofenac, flurbiprofen, ibuprofen, indomethacin, ketoprofen, meclofenamate sodium, mefenamic acid, naproxen, piroxicam

Antiemetic—chlorpromazine hydrochloride, dolasetron mesylate monohydrate, dronabinol, granisetron hydrochloride, meclizine hydrochloride, metoclopramide hydrochloride, ondansetron hydrochloride, perphenazine, prochlorperazine, promethazine hydrochloride, *thiethylperazine maleate,* trifluoperazine hydrochloride, *trimethobenzamide hydrochloride*

Antienuretic—amitriptyline hydrochloride, imipramine

Antifungal—*amphotericin B, butoconazole, caspofungin,*

clotrimazole, econazole nitrate, fluconazole, flucytosine, griseofulvin, itraconazole, ketoconazole, *miconazole nitrate*, nystatin, terbinafine hydrochloride, *terconazole*

Antiglaucoma Drug—acetazolamide, *bimatoprost, brimonidine tartrate, dorzolamide hydrochloride, epinephryl borate, latanoprost, levobunolol hydrochloride*, timolol, *travoprost*

Antigout—allopurinol, *colchicine*, diclofenac, diflunisal, etodolac, fenoprofen calcium, ibuprofen, indomethacin, ketoprofen, naproxen, piroxicam, sulindac

Antihelminic—albendazole, mebendazole

Antihistamine—azatadine maleate, *azelastine hydrochloride, brompheniramine maleate*, cetirizine hydrochloride, *chlorpheniramine maleate, clemastine fumarate*, cyproheptadine hydrochloride, desloratadine, dexchlorpheniramine maleate, *diphenhydramine*, fexofenadine hydrochloride, hydroxyzine, *ketotifen fumarate, loratadine*, promethazine hydrochloride, tripelennamine hydrochloride

Antihomocystinuric—betaine

Antihypercalcemic—bumetanide, ethacrynic acid, etidronate disodium, furosemide

Antihyperphosphatemic—sevelamer hydrochloride

Antihypertensive—acebutolol, amiloride hydrochloride, amlodipine besylate, atenolol, benazepril hydrochloride, bendroflumethiazide, betaxolol hydrochloride, bisoprolol fumarate, bosentan, bumetanide, candesartan cilexetil, captopril, carteolol hydrochloride, carvedilol, chlorothiazide, chlorthalidone, clonidine hydrochloride, *deserpidine*, diazoxide, diltiazem, doxazosin mesylate, enalapril maleate, eplerenone, eprosartan mesylate, ethacrynic acid, felodipine, fosinopril sodium, furosemide, guanabenz acetate, guanfacine hydrochloride, hydralazine hydrochloride, hydrochlorothiazide, hydroflumethiazide, indapamide, irbesartan, isradipine, labetalol hydrochloride, lisinopril, losartan potassium, methyclothiazide, methyldopa, metolazone, metoprolol, minoxidil, moexipril hydrochloride, nadolol, nicardipine hydrochloride, nifedipine, nisoldipine, olmesartan medoxomil, penbutolol sulfate, perindopril erbumine, pindolol, polythiazide, prazosin hydrochloride, propranolol hydrochloride, quinapril hydrochloride, ramipril, *reserpine,* sotalol hydrochloride, spironolactone, telmisartan, terazosin hydrochloride, timolol, torsemide, trandolapril, triamterene, trichlormethiazide, valsartan, verapamil hydrochloride

Antihyperuricemic—allopurinol

Antihypoglycemic—diazoxide

Antihypokalemic—amiloride hydrochloride, triamterene

Antihypotensive—*dihydroergotamine mesylate,* ergotamine tartrate, midodrine hydrochloride

Antiinflammatory—*alclometasone dipropionate, amcinonide, aspirin,* balsalazide disodium, *beclomethasone dipropionate,* betamethasone, budesonide, celecoxib, chloroquine phosphate, *choline magnesium salicylate, clobetasol propionate, clocortolone pivalate,* cortisone acetate, *desonide, desoximetasone,* dexamethasone, *diflorasone diacetate,* fenoprofen calcium, *flunisolide, fluocinolone acetonide, fluocinonide, flurandrenolide,* flurbiprofen, *fluticasone propionate, halobetasol propionate, halcinonide,* hydrocortisone, hydroxychloroquine sulfate, indomethacin, *magnesium salicylate,* mefenamic acid, meloxicam, *mesalamine (5-aminosalicylic acid),* methylprednisolone, naproxen, olsalazine sodium, prednisolone, prednisone, rofecoxib, *salsalate,* sulfasalazine, sulindac, triamcinolone, valdecoxib

Antileprotic—*clofazimine,* dapsone, thalidomide

Antilipemic—atorvastatin calcium, *cholestyramine,* clofibrate, colesevelam hydrochloride, colestipol hydrochloride, ezetimibe, fenofibrate, fluvastatin sodium, gemfibrozil, lovastatin, pravastatin sodium, simvastatin

Antimalarial—chloroquine phosphate, dapsone, halofantrine, hydroxychloroquine sulfate, *mefloquine hydrochloride,* primaquine phosphate, pyrimethamine, quinine sulfate

Antimetabolite—capecitabine, cladribine, cytarabine, floxuridine, fludarabine phosphate, fluorouracil, gemcitabine hydrochloride, mercaptopurine (6-MP), methotrexate sodium, pentostatin, thioguanine

Antimigraine—almotriptan, dihydroergotamine mesylate, ergotamine tartrate, frovatriptan succinate, methysergide maleate, naratriptan hydrochloride, rizatriptan benzoate, sumatriptan succinate, zolmitriptan

Antimycobacterial—aminosalicylic acid, cycloserine, ethambutol hydrochloride, ethionamide, isoniazid (INH), pyrazinamide, rifabutin, rifampin, rifapentine

Antineoplastic—altretamine, anastrozole, bexarotene, bicalutamide, busulfan, capecitabine, carmustine, chlorambucil, cladribine, cyclophosphamide, cytarabine, estradiol, estramustine phosphate sodium, estrogen, estropipate, ethinyl estradiol, etoposide, exemestane, floxuridine, fludarabine phosphate, fluorouracil, fluoxymesterone, flutamide, gemcitabine hydrochloride, gefitinib, hydroxyurea, ifosfamide, imatinib mesylate, letrozole, levamisole hydrochloride, lomustine (CCNU), mechlorethamine hydrochloride, medroxyprogesterone acetate, megestrol acetate, melphalan (phylalanine mustard), mercaptopurine (6-MP), methotrexate sodium, methyltestosterone, mitotane, nilutamide, pentostatin, procarbazine hydrochloride, streptozocin, tamoxifen citrate, teniposide, testolactone, testosterone, thioguanine, thiotepa, toremifene citrate, tretinoin

Antineuralgic—amitriptyline hydrochloride, carbamazepine, clomipramine hydrochloride, desipramine hydrochloride, doxepin hydrochloride, fluphenazine hydrochloride, imipramine, nortriptyline hydrochloride, trimipramine maleate

Antiobesity—orlistat

Antiosteoporotic—alendronate sodium, calcitonin, estrogen, etidronate disodium, raloxifene hydrochloride, risedronate sodium, tiludronate disodium

Antipanic—alprazolam, clomipramine hydrochloride, clonazepam, desipramine hydrochloride, diazepam, imipramine, lorazepam, nortriptyline hydrochloride, paroxetine hydrochloride

Antiplatelet—anagrelide hydrochloride, *cilostazol,* clopidogrel bisulfate, dipyridamole, ticlopidine hydrochloride

Antiprotozoal—atovaquone, dapsone, metronidazole, nitazoxanide, *pentamidine isethionate*

Antipruretic—doxepin hydrochloride, hydroxyzine

Antipsoriatic—acitretin, *calcipotriene,* methotrexate sodium

Antipsychotic—aripiprazole, chlorpromazine hydrochloride, clozapine, fluphenazine hydrochloride, haloperidol, loxapine succinate, mesoridazine besylate, molindone hydrochloride, olanzapine, perphenazine, pimozide, prochlorperazine, quetiapine fumarate, risperidone, thioridazine hydrochloride, thiothixene, trifluoperazine hydrochloride, ziprasidone

Antipyretic—celecoxib, fenoprofen calcium, ibuprofen, indomethacin, naproxen, piroxicam, sulindac, valdecoxib

Antiretroviral—abacavir sulfate, amprenavir, delavirdine mesylate, didanosine (ddl), efavirenz, indinavir sulfate, lamivudine (3TC), nelfinavir mesylate, nevirapine, ritonavir, saquinavir, stavudine (d4T), tenofovir disoproxil fumarate, zalcitabine (ddC), zidovudine (AZT)

Antirheumatic—auranofin, azathioprine, leflunomide, methotrexate sodium, penicillamine, sulfasalazine

Antispasmodic—alosetron, dicyclomine, *flavoxate hydrochloride,* glycopyrrolate, *mepenzolate bromide, methscopolamine bromide,* oxybutynin chloride, papaverine hydrochloride, propantheline bromide, tolterodine tartrate

Antithyroid Drug—methimazole, propylthiouracil (PTU), *sodium iodide*

Antitremor—alprazolam, chlordiazepoxide hydrochloride, diazepam, lorazepam

Antitussive—codeine sulfate, *dextromethorphan*, hydromorphone hydrochloride, methadone hydrochloride, morphine sulfate

Antiulcer—cimetidine, esomeprazole magnesium, famotidine, lansoprazole, misoprostol, nizatidine, omeprazole, pantoprazole, rabeprazole sodium, ranitidine hydrochloride, sucralfate

Antivertigo—meclizine hydrochloride, promethazine hydrochloride

Antiviral—acyclovir, adefovir dipivoxil, amantadine hydrochloride, famciclovir, ganciclovir, oseltamivir phosphate, ribavirin, rimantadine hydrochloride, valacyclovir hydrochloride, valganciclovir, *zanamivir* (see also Antiretroviral)

Anxiolytic—alprazolam, buspirone hydrochloride, chlordiazepoxide hydrochloride, clorazepate dipotassium, diazepam, halazepam, hydroxyzine, lorazepam, meprobamate, oxazepam, paroxetine, venlafaxine hydrochloride

Aormatic Diamidine—*pentamidine isethionate*

Appetite Stimulant—sibutramine hydrochloride

Appetite Suppressant—*amphetamine sulfate, benzphetamine hydrochloride, dextroamphetamine sulfate, diethylpropion hydrochloride, methamphetamine hydrochloride, phendimetrazine tartrate,* phentermine hydrochloride

Aromatase Inhibitor—anastrozole, exemestane, letrozole

Azaspirodecanedione Derivative—buspirone hydrochloride

Azole Derivative—fluconazole, itraconazole, ketoconazole

Barbiturate—*amobarbital, apobarbital,* butabarbital sodium, *butalbital,* mephobarbital, pentobarbital sodium, phenobarbital, secobarbital sodium

Behavioral Agent—atomoxetine hydrochloride, fluvoxamine maleate, lithium, pemoline

Belladonna Alkaloid—*atropine, belladonna, homatropine methylbromide, hyoscyamine, methscopolamine bromide, scopolamine*

Benzamide Derivative—flecainide acetate, nitazoxanide

Benzimidazole—albendazole, mebendazole

Benzisoxazole Derivative—risperidone

Benzodiazepine—alprazolam, chlordiazepoxide hydrochloride, clonazepam, clorazepate dipotassium, diazepam, estazolam, flurazepam hydrochloride, halazepam, lorazepam, oxazepam, quazepam, temazepam, triazolam

Benzofuran Derivative—amiodarone hydrochloride

Benzothiazole—riluzole

Benzoxazole Derivative—chlorzoxazone

Beta Blocker—acebutolol, atenolol, betaxolol hydrochloride, bisoprolol fumarate, carteolol hydrochloride, carvedilol, labetalol hydrochloride, *levobunolol hydrochloride, metipranolol hydrochloride*, metoprolol, nadolol, penbutolol sulfate, pindolol, propranolol hydrochloride, sotalol hydrochloride, timolol

Beta Lactam—*aztreonam, imipenem* (see also Cephalosporins)

Biguanide—metformin hydrochloride

Biguanide: Meglitinide—nateglinide, repaglinide

Bile Acid Sequestrant—*cholestyramine*, colesevelam hydrochloride, colestipol hydrochloride

Biological Response Modifier—levamisole hydrochloride

Bisphosphonate—alendronate sodium, etidronate disodium, risedronate sodium, tiludronate disodium

Bronchodilator—albuterol, aminophylline, *dyphylline, ephedrine sulfate, epinephrine, formoterol fumarate, ipratropium bromide, isoetharine hydrochloride, isoproterenol, levalbuterol hydrochloride,* metaproterenol sulfate, *oxtriphylline, pirbuterol acetate, salmeterol xinafoate,* terbutaline sulfate, theophylline

Butyrophenone—haloperidol

Calcium Channel Blocker—amlodipine besylate, bepridil

hydrochloride, diltiazem, felodipine, isradipine, nicardipine hydrochloride, nifedipine, nimodipine, nisoldipine, verapamil hydrochloride

Cannabinoid—dronabinol

Carbamate—carisoprodol, felbamate, meprobamate, methocarbamol

Carbohydrate Derivative—pentosan polysulfate sodium

Carbonic Anhydrase Inhibitor—acetazolamide, *methazolamide*

Carboxamide Derivative—oxcarbazepine

Carboxylic Acid Derivative—*divalproex sodium*, valproate sodium, valproic Acid

Cardiac Glycoside—digoxin

Centrally Acting Antiadrenergic—clonidine hydrochloride, guanabenz acetate, guanfacine hydrochloride, methyldopa

Cephalosporins—See First Generation Cephalosporin, Second Generation Cephalosporin, and Third Generation Cephalosporin

Chelating Drug—penicillamine, *succimer*

Chlorophenyl Derivative—baclofen

Chlorotrianisene Derivative—clomiphene citrate

Cholesterol Absorption Inhibitor—ezetimibe

Cholinergic Agonist (Cholinergics)—bethanechol chloride, cevimeline hydrochloride, *pilocarpine hydrochloride*

Cholinesterase Inhibitor—donepezil hydrochloride, galantamine hydrobromide, rivastigmine tartrate, tacrine hydrochloride

Cinchona Alkaloid—quinidine sulfate, quinine sulfate

CNS Stimulant—*amphetamine sulfate, dextroamphetamine sulfate, methamphetamine hydrochloride*, methylphenidate hydrochloride, modafinil, pemoline

Colchicum Autumnale Alkaloid—*colchicine*

COMT Inhibitor—entacapone, tolcapone

Corticosteroid—*alclometasone dipropionate, amcinonide, beclomethasone dipropionate,* betamethasone, budesonide, *clobetasol propionate, clocortolone pivalate,* cortisone acetate, *desonide, desoximetasone,* dexamethasone, *diflorasone diacetate,* fludrocortisone acetate, *flunisolide, fluocinolone acetonide, fluocinonide, flurandrenolide, fluticasone propionate, halobetasol propionate, halcinonide,* hydrocortisone, methylprednisolone, prednisolone, prednisone, triamcinolone

Coumarin Derivative—*anisindione,* warfarin sodium

Cyclohexane Dione—nitisinone

Cyclohexanol Derivative—tramadol hydrochloride

Decarboxylase Inhibitor/Dopamine Precursor—levodopa-carbidopa

Dibenzodiazepine—clozapine

Dibenzothiazepine—quetiapine fumarate

Dibenzoxazepine—loxapine succinate

Dichloroacetic Acid Derivative—*chloramphenicol*

Dihydroindolone—molindone hydrochloride

Diphenhydramine Analogue—orphenadrine citrate

Diphenylbutylpiperidine—pimozide

Diuretic—acetazolamide, *methazolamide* (see also Loop Diuretic, Potassium-Sparing Diuretic, and Thiazide Diuretic)

Dopaminergic Agonist—pergolide mesylate

Echinocandin—*butoconazole, caspofungin, miconazole nitrate, tioconazole*

Electrolyte Replacement—potassium

Endothelin Receptor Antagonist—bosentan

Ergot Alkaloid—bromocriptine mesylate, *dihydroergotamine mesylate,* ergoloid mesylates, ergonovine, ergotamine tartrate, methylergonovine maleate, methysergide maleate

Estrogen Hormone—*dienestrol,* estradiol, estrogen, estropipate, *ethinyl estradiol*

Estrogen Replacement—*dienestrol,* estradiol, estrogen, estropipate, *ethinyl estradiol*

Ethanolamine-Related Antihistamine—*trimethobenzamide hydrochloride*

Fibric Acid Derivative—clofibrate, gemfibrozil

Fibrinolytic Inhibitor—aminocaproic acid

Fibrotic Acid Derivative—fenofibrate

First Generation Cephalosporin—cefadroxil, cephalexin hydrochloride, cephradine

Fluorinated Pyrimidine—flucytosine

Fluoroquinolone—ciprofloxacin hydrochloride, gatifloxacin, levofloxacin, lomefloxacin hydrochloride, moxifloxacin hydrochloride, norfloxacin, ofloxacin, sparfloxacin, trovafloxacin mesylate (see also Quinolones)

Folic Acid Antagonist—pyrimethamine

GABA Enhancer—tiagabine hydrochloride

Gastric Mucosal Protectant—misoprostol

Gastrointestinal Stimulant—bethanechol chloride, metoclopramide hydrochloride, tegaserod maleate

Glycine Derivative—betaine

Glycopeptide—vancomycin hydrochloride

Gold Salt—auranofin

Gonadatropin Inhibitor—danazol

Growth Hormone Suppressant—bromocriptine mesylate

H1 Receptor Blocker—azatadine maleate, *azelastine hydrochloride, brompheniramine maleate,* cetirizine hydrochloride, *chlorpheniramine maleate, clemastine fumarate,* cyproheptadine hydrochloride, desloratadine, dexchlorpheniramine maleate, *diphenhydramine,* fexofenadine hydrochloride, hydroxyzine, *loratadine,* tripelennamine hydrochloride

H2 Receptor Antagonist—cimetidine, famotidine, nizatidine, ranitidine hydrochloride

Heavy Metal Antagonist—penicillamine, *succimer*

Hemorrheologic—pentoxifylline

Hemostatic—aminocaproic acid, desmopressin acetate

Heparin Anticoagulant—enoxaparin sodium, *heparin*

HMG-CoA Reductase Inhibitor (Statin)—atorvastatin calcium, fluvastatin sodium, lovastatin, pravastatin sodium, simvastatin

Hydantoin Derivative—dantrolene sodium, *ethotoin, fosphenytoin sodium,* phenytoin

Hydroxynapthalenedione—atovaquone

Imidazopyridine—zolpidem tartrate

Iminophenazine—*clofazimine*

Iminostilbene Derivative—carbamazepine

Immunomodulator—thalidomide

Immunosuppressant—azathioprine, betamethasone, chlorambucil, cortisone acetate, cyclophosphamide, cyclosporine, dexamethasone, hydrocortisone, methylprednisolone, mycophenolate mofetil, prednisolone, prednisone, sirolimus, tacrolimus, triamcinolone

Impotence Agent—*alprostadil,* sildenafil citrate

Influenza Virus Neuraminidase Inhibitor—oseltamivir phosphate

Inotrope—digoxin

Lactation Inhibitor—bromocriptine mesylate

Leukotriene Formation Inhibitor—zileuton

Leukotriene Receptor Antagonist—montelukast sodium, zafirlukast

Lincosamide—clindamycin, *lincomycin*

Lipase Inhibitor—orlistat

Loop Diuretic—bumetanide, ethacrynic acid, furosemide, torsemide

Macrocyclic Lactone—sirolimus

Macrolide—azithromycin dihydrate, clarithromycin, dirithromcyin, erythromycin, tacrolimus, troleandomycin

Male Hormone Replacement—fluoxymesterone, methyltestosterone, testosterone

Mast Cell Stabilizer—*ketotifen fumarate*

Megakaryocyte Disrupter—anagrelide hydrochloride

Methenamines—fosfomycin tromethamine, *methenamine hippurate*

Methylhydrazine Derivative—*procarbazine hydrochloride*

Mineralocorticoide Replacement Therapy—fludrocortisone acetate

Monoamine Oxidase (MAO) Inhibitor—*isocarboxazid, phenelzine sulfate,* selegiline hydrochloride, *tranylcypromine*

Mucolytic—acetylcysteine, *dornase alfa*

Mycophenolic Acid Derivative—mycophenolate mofetil

Narcotic Analgesic/Opioid—codeine sulfate, *difenoxin hydrochloride, hydrocodone bitartrate,* hydromorphone hydrochloride, *levomethadyl acetate hydrochloride,* levorphanol, meperidine hydrochloride, methadone hydrochloride, morphine sulfate, oxycodone hydrochloride, propoxyphene

Neuraminidase Inhibitor—*zanamivir*

Neuromuscular Blocker—see Skeletal Muscle Relaxant

Neuroprotector—riluzole

Neurotransmitter Reuptake Inhibitor—sibutramine hydrochloride, venlafaxine hydrochloride

Nitrate—*amyl nitrate*, isosorbide, nitroglycerin

Nitrofuran—*nitrofurantoin, nitrofurazone*

Nitroimidazole—metronidazole

Nonergot Dopamine Agonist—pramipexole diphydrochloride, ropinirole hydrochloride

Nonnarcotic Analgesic—*acetaminophen*

Nonnucleodise Reverse Transcriptase Inhibitor (NNRTI)—delavirdine mesylate, efavirenz, nevirapine

Nonsteroidal Antiandrogen—bicalutamide, flutamide, nilutamide

Nonsteroidal Antiestrogen—tamoxifen citrate, toremifene citrate

Nonsteroidal Antiinflammatory (NSAID)—diclofenac, etodolac, fenoprofen calcium, flurbiprofen, ibuprofen, indomethacin, ketoprofen, ketorolac tromethamine, meclofenamate sodium, mefenamic acid, meloxicam, nabumetone, naproxen, oxaprozin, piroxicam, sulindac, tolmetin sodium

- **NSAID COX-2 Inhibitor**—celecoxib, rofecoxib, valdecoxib
- **NSAID: Salicylate**—balsalazide disodium, olsalazine sodium

Norepinephrine Reuptake Inhibitor—atomoxetine hydrochloride

Nucleoside Analog—adefovir dipivoxil, rimantadine hydrochloride

Nucleoside Reverse Transcriptase Inhibitor (NsRTI)—abacavir sulfate, didanosine (ddI), lamivudine (3TC), stavudine (d4T), zalcitabine (ddC), zidovudine (AZT)

Nucleotide Reverse Transcriptase Inhibitor (NtRTI)—tenofovir disoproxil fumarate

Ovulation Stimulant—clomiphene citrate

Oxazolidinodione—*trimethadione*

Oxazolidinone Derivative—linezolid, metaxalone

Oxytocic—ergonovine, methylergonovine maleate

Para-aminobenzoic Acid Derivative—metoclopramide hydrochloride

PDE III Inhibitor—*cilostazol*

Penicillin

- **Aminopenicillin**—amoxicillin, ampicillin, bacampicillin hydrochloride
- **Extended Spectrum Penicillin**—carbenicillin indanyl sodium, *mezlocillin sodium, piperacillin, ticarcillin disodium*
- **Natural Penicillin**—penicillin V potassium
- **Penicillinase-Resistant Penicillin**—cloxacillin sodium, dicloxacillin sodium, *nafcillin sodium,* oxacillin sodium

Penicillium Antibiotic—griseofulvin

Pepsin Inhibitor—sucralfate

Peripheral Vasodilator—diazoxide, hydralazine hydrochloride, minoxidil, papaverine hydrochloride

Phenothiazine—chlorpromazine hydrochloride, fluphenazine hydrochloride, mesoridazine besylate, perphenazine, prochlorperazine, promethazine hydrochloride, *thiethylperazine maleate,* thioridazine hydrochloride, thiothixene, trifluoperazine hydrochloride

Phenylpiperazine—nefazodone hydrochloride

Phenyltriazine—lamotrigine

Phosphodiesterase Delayer—sildenafil citrate

Piperazine-Derivative Antihistamines—meclizine hydrochloride

Podophyllotoxin—etoposide, teniposide

Polyene Antibiotic—*amphotericin B*

Polyene Macrolide—nystatin

Polymeric Phosphate Binder—sevelamer hydrochloride

Polypeptide—*calcitonin*

Polypeptide Antibiotic—cyclosporine

Posterior Pituitary Hormone—desmopressin acetate

Potassium-Sparing Diuretic—amiloride hydrochloride, spironolactone, triamterene

Potassium Supplement—potassium

Procaine Derivative—procainamide hydrochloride

Progestational Drug—*levonorgestrel*, medroxyprogesterone acetate, norethindrone, norgestrel, progesterone

Progestins—*levonorgestrel*, medroxyprogesterone acetate, megestrol acetate, norethindrone, norgestrel, progesterone

Prosecretory—cevimeline hydrochloride

Prostaglandin—*alprostadil*

Prostaglandin Analogue—*bimatoprost, latanoprost, travoprost*

Prostaglandin E1 Analogue—misoprostol

Protease Inhibitor (PI)—amprenavir, indinavir sulfate, nelfinavir mesylate, ritonavir, saquinavir

Protein-Tyrosine Kinase Inhibitor—imatinib mesylate

Proton Pump Inhibitor—esomeprazole magnesium, lansoprazole, omeprazole, pantoprazole, rabeprazole sodium

Purine Antagonist—azathioprine

Pyrazolopyrimidine—zaleplon

Pyridine Derivative—disopyramide phosphate

Pyrimidine Analogue—dipyridamole

Pyrimidine Synthesis Inhibitor—leflunomide

Pyrimidinedione—primidone

Quinolone—*nalidixic acid*

Rauwolfia Alkaloid—*deserpidine, reserpine*

Respiratory Stimulant—aminophylline

Retinoid—acitretin, *adapalene, alitretinoin,* bexarotene, isotretinoin, *tazarotene, tretinoin*

RhDNase—*dornase alfa*

Salicylate—*aspirin, choline magnesium salicylate,* diflunisal, *magnesium salicylate,* mesalamine (5-aminosalicylic acid), *salsalate* (see also Nonsteroidal Antiinflammatory: Salicylate)

Second Generation Cephalosporin—cefaclor, *cefotetan, cefoxitin,* cefprozil, cefuroxime axetil, *loracarbef*

Sedative-Hypnotic—alprazolam, *amobarbital, apobarbital,* butabarbital sodium, *chloral hydrate,* chlordiazepoxide hydrochloride, clonazepam, clorazepate dipotassium, diazepam, estazolam, flurazepam hydrochloride, halazepam, lorazepam, oxazepam, pentobarbital sodium, phenobarbital, quazepam, secobarbital sodium, temazepam, triazolam, zaleplon, zolpidem tartrate

Selective 5-HT3 Receptor Antagonist—alosetron, dolasetron mesylate monohydrate, granisetron hydrochloride, ondansetron hydrochloride

Selective Beta 2 Receptor Agonist—*formoterol fumarate, salmeterol xinafoate*

Selective Estrogen Receptor Modulator—raloxifene hydrochloride

Selective Serotonin Reuptake Inhibitor (SSRI)—citalopram hydrobromide, fluoxetine hydrochloride, fluvoxamine maleate, paroxetine hydrochloride, sertraline hydrochloride

Skeletal Muscle Relaxant—baclofen, carisoprodol, chlorzoxazone, cyclobenzaprine hydrochloride, dantrolene sodium, diazepam, lorazepam, metaxalone, methocarbamol, orphenadrine citrate, tizanidine hydrochloride

Smoking Cessation Aid—bupropion hydrochloride

Smooth Muscle Relaxant—tamsulosin hydrochloride

Sodium Channel Blocker—mexiletine, moricizine hydrochloride

SSRI—see Selective Serotonin Reuptake Inhibitor

Steroid Derivative—dutasteride, finasteride

Subarachnoid Hemorrhage Therapy—nimodipine

Succinimide Derivative—ethosuximide, methsuximide

Sulfamate-Substituted Monosaccharide—topiramate

Sulfonamide—co-trimoxazole, *dorzolamide hydrochloride*, probenecid, sulfadiazine, *sulfamethizole*, sulfasalazine, sulfinpyrazone, sulfisoxazole, zonisamide

Sulfonamide and Folate Antagonist—co-trimoxazole

Sulfonylurea: First Generation—acetohexamide, chlorpropamide, tolazamide, tolbutamide

Sulfonylurea: Second Generation—glimepiride, glipizide, glyburide

Sympathomimetic—*benzphetamine hydrochloride, diethylpropion hydrochloride, phendimetrazine tartrate,* phentermine hydrochloride (see also Adrenergics)

Synthetic Acyclic Guanine Derivative—famciclovir

Synthetic Allylamine Derivative—terbinafine hydrochloride

Synthetic Cyclic Primary Amine—amantadine hydrochloride

Synthetic Folate Antagonist—*trimethoprim*

Synthetic Imidazole Derivative—*clotrimazole, econazole nitrate*

Synthetic Nucleoside—ganciclovir, ribavirin, valganciclovir hydrochloride

Synthetic Purine Nucleoside—acyclovir, valacyclovir hydrochloride

Synthetic Sulfone—dapsone

Synthetic Vitamin D$_3$ Analogue—*calcipotriene*

Tertiary Amine—oxybutynin chloride

Tetracyclic Antidepressant—*maprotiline hydrochloride,* mirtazapine

Tetracycline—demeclocycline hydrochloride, doxycycline, oxytetracycline hydrochloride, tetracycline

Thiazide Diuretic—bendroflumethiazide, chlorothiazide, hydrochlorothiazide, hydroflumethiazide, methyclothiazide, polythiazide, trichlormethiazide

Thiazidelike Diuretic—chlorthalidone, indapamide, metolazone

Thiazolidinedione—pioglitazone hydrochloride, rosiglitazone maleate

Thienobenzodiazepine Derivative—olanzapine

Third Generation Cephalosporin—cefdinir, cefditoren pivoxil, cefpodoxime proxetil, ceftibuten dihydrate

Thyroid Hormone—levothyroxine sodium, liothyronine sodium, liotrix, thyroid (desiccated)

Thyroid Hormone Antagonist—methimazole, propylthiouracil (PTU), *sodium iodide*

Thyroid Replacement—levothyroxine sodium, liothyronine sodium, liotrix, thyroid (desiccated)

Tocolytic—terbutaline sulfate

Triazole Derivative—*terconazole*

Triazolopyridine Derivative—trazodone hydrochloride

Tricyclic Antidepressant—amitriptyline hydrochloride, amoxapine, clomipramine hydrochloride, cyclobenzaprine hydrochloride, desipramine hydrochloride, doxepin hydrochloride, imipramine, nortriptyline hydrochloride, protriptyline hydrochloride, trimipramine maleate

Triptan—almotriptan, frovatriptan succinate, naratriptan hydrochloride, rizatriptan benzoate, sumatriptan succinate, zolmitriptan

Tyrosine Degradation Inhibitor—nitisinone

Urea—hydroxyurea

Uricosuric—probenecid, sulfinpyrazone

Urinary Analgesic—pentosan polysulfate sodium,

Urinary Tract Stimulant—bethanechol chloride

Vasopressor—midodrine hydrochloride

Xanthine Derivative—aminophylline, *dyphylline, oxtriphylline,* pentoxifylline, theophylline

Xanthine Oxidase Inhibitor—allopurinol

Index of Combination Drugs

Several drugs are prescribed together in combination with other drugs to improve the overall treatment outcomes. When the combinations are given frequently, a drug manufacturer will begin making a product that contains more than one active drug ingredient. These products are commonly referred to as "combination drugs."

Combination drugs do not have separate drug summaries in this book, but are listed in this index with cross-references to the individual drugs. Review each of the separate drug summaries in Chapter 6 to determine the warnings, precautions, and helpful comments associated with a combination drug. Note that the dosing information for combination drugs may differ from that for the individual drug ingredients. Also, not all active drug ingredients have a separate drug summary in Chapter 6. Ask your pharmacist if you would like more information about combination drugs.

Use this index by finding the name of your combination drug in the listing alphabetized by brand name. All the active drug ingredients are identified next to the brand name. If more than one strength of the product is available, the number of strengths is identified in parenthesis after the last drug. If the product is available as a generic, the combination drug is highlighted in bold.

Generic available if product name is **bold**.

COMBINATION DRUG PRODUCT NAME	ACTIVE INGREDIENTS (NUMBER OF DIFFERENT STRENGTHS)
Accuretic	hydrochlorothiazide, quinapril hydrochloride (3)
Activella	estradiol, norethindrone acetate
Advicor	lovastatin, niacin (3)
Aggrenox	aspirin, dipyridamole
Aldactazide	**hydrochlorothiazide, spironolactone (2)**
Aldoril	**hydrochlorothiazide, methyldopa (4)**
Alesse	ethinyl estradiol, levonorgestrel
Allegra-D	fexofenadine hydrochloride, pseudoephedrine hydrochloride
Ambenyl	**bromodiphenhydramine hydrochloride, codeine phosphate**
Apresazide	**hydralazine hydrochloride, hydrochlorothiazide (2)**
Arthrotec	diclofenac sodium, misoprostol (2)
Atacand HCT	candesartan cilexetil, hydrochlorothiazide (2)
Augmentin	amoxicillin, clavulanate potassium (wide variety)
Avalide	hydrochlorothiazide, irbesartan (2)
Avandamet	metformin hydrochloride, rosiglitazone maleate (3)
Aviane	ethinyl estradiol, levonorgestrel
Benzaclin	benzoyl peroxide, clindamycin phosphate
Blephamide	prednisolone acetate, sulfacetamide sodium
Brevicon	ethinyl estradiol, norethindrone
Cafergot	**caffeine, ergotamine tartrate**
Capital and Codeine	**acetaminophen, codeine phosphate**
Capozide	**captopril, hydrochlorothiazide (4)**
Carmol HC	**hydrocortisone acetate, urea**
Cetapred	prednisolone acetate, sulfacetamide sodium
Cipro HC	ciprofloxacin hydrochloride, hydrocortisone
Clopres	chlorthalidone, clonidine hydrochloride (3)

COMBINATION DRUG PRODUCT NAME	ACTIVE INGREDIENTS (NUMBER OF DIFFERENT STRENGTHS)
Col-Probenecid	colchicine, probenecid
Coly-Mycin S	colistin sulfate, hydrocortisone acetate, neomycin sulfate, thonzonium bromide
CombiPatch	estradiol, norethindrone acetate (2)
Combivent	albuterol sulfate, ipratropium bromide
Combivir	lamivudine, zidovudine
Cortisporin	hydrocortisone, neomycin sulfate, polymyxin B sulfate (some products also contain bacitracin zinc)
Corzide	bendroflumethiazide, nadolol (2)
Cosopt	dorzolamide hydrochloride, timolol maleate
Cryselle	ethinyl estradiol, norgestrel
Cyclessa	desogestrel, ethinyl estradiol
Darvocet-N	acetaminophen, propoxyphene napsylate (2)
Darvon Compound	aspirin, caffeine, propoxyphene hydrochloride
Darvon Compound-65	aspirin, caffeine, propoxyphene hydrochloride
Demulen	ethinyl estradiol, ethynodiol diacetate (2)
Desogen	desogestrel, ethinyl estradiol
Dexacidin	dexamethasone, neomycin sulfate, polymyxin B sulfate
Dexasporin	dexamethasone, neomycin sulfate, polymyxin B sulfate
Diovan HCT	hydrochlorothiazide, valsartan (2)
Diupres	chlorothiazide, reserpine (2)
Duac	benzoyl peroxide, clindamycin phosphate
Duoneb	albuterol sulfate, ipratropium bromide
Dyazide	hydrochlorothiazide, triamterene
Enduronyl	deserpidine, methyclothiazide (2)
Enpresse	ethinyl estradiol, levonorgestrel
Epifoam	hydrocortisone acetate, pramoxine hydrochloride
Ercatab	caffeine, ergotamine tartrate

COMBINATION DRUG PRODUCT NAME	ACTIVE INGREDIENTS (NUMBER OF DIFFERENT STRENGTHS)
Eryzole	erythromycin ethylsuccinate, sulfisoxazole acetyl
Estrostep FE	ethinyl estradiol, norethindrone acetate
Fansidar	pyrimethamine, sulfadoxine
Femhrt	ethinyl estradiol, norethindrone acetate
Fiorinal with Codeine No. 3	aspirin, butalbital, caffeine, codeine phosphate
Gencept	ethinyl estradiol, norethindrone
Glucovance	glyburide, metformin hydrochloride [3]
Helidac	bismuth subsalicylate, metronidazole, tetracycline hydrochloride
Hyzaar	hydrochlorothiazide, losartan potassium [2]
Inderide	hydrochlorothiazide, propranolol hyrochloride [2]
Kaletra	lopinavir, ritonavir [2]
Kariva	desogestrel, ethinyl estradiol
Lessina	ethinyl estradiol, levonorgestrel
Levlite	ethinyl estradiol, levonorgestrel
Levora	ethinyl estradiol, levonorgestrel
Lexxel	enalapril maleate, felodipine [2]
Limbitrol	amitriptyline hydrochloride, chlordiazepoxide
Limbitrol DS	amitriptyline hydrochloride, chlordiazepoxide
Lo/Ovral	ethinyl estradiol, norgestrel
Loestrin	ethinyl estradiol, norethindrone acetate [2]
Lopressor HCT	hydrochlorothiazide, metoprolol tartrate [3]
Lotensin HCT	benazepril hydrochloride, hydrochlorothiazide [4]
Lotrel	amlodipine besylate, benazepril hydrochloride [4]
Lotrisone	betamethasone dipropionate, clotrimazole
Low-Ogestrel	ethinyl estradiol, norgestrel
Maxitrol	dexamethasone, neomycin sulfate, polymyxin B sulfate
Maxzide	hydrochlorothiazide, triamterene

COMBINATION DRUG PRODUCT NAME	ACTIVE INGREDIENTS (NUMBER OF DIFFERENT STRENGTHS)
Metaglip	glipizide, metformin hydrochloride [3]
Micardis HCT	hydrochlorothiazide, telmisartan
Microgestin	ethinyl estradiol, norethindrone acetate [2]
Minizide	polythiazide, prazosin hydrochloride [3]
Mircette	desogestrel, ethinyl estradiol
Modicon	ethinyl estradiol, norethindrone
Moduretic	amiloride hydrochloride, hydrochlorothiazide
Monopril-HCT	fosinopril sodium, hydrochlorothiazide [2]
Mybanil	bromodiphenhydramine hydrochloride, codeine phosphate
Mycolog II	nystatin, triamcinolone acetonide
Myphetane DC	brompheniramine maleate, codeine phosphate, phenylpropanolamine hydrochloride
Neo-Cort-Dome	hydrocortisone, neomycin sulfate [eardrops also contain acetic acid]
Neosporin	bacitracin zinc, neomycin sulfate, polymyxin B sulfate
Norcept	ethinyl estradiol, norethindrone
Nordette	ethinyl estradiol, levonorgestrel
Norethin	ethinyl estradiol, norethindrone
Norgesic	aspirin, caffeine, orphenadrine citrate
Norgesic Forte	aspirin, caffeine, orphenadrine citrate
Norinyl	ethinyl estradiol, norethindrone
Nortrel	ethinyl estradiol, norethindrone [3]
Nuvaring	ethinyl estradiol, etonogestrel
Ogestrel	ethinyl estradiol, norgestrel
Ortho Cyclen	ethinyl estradiol, norgestimate
Ortho Evra	ethinyl estradiol, norelgestromin
Ortho-Cept	desogestrel, ethyinyl estradiol
Ortho-Novum	ethinyl estradiol, norethindrone [3]

COMBINATION DRUG PRODUCT NAME	ACTIVE INGREDIENTS (NUMBER OF DIFFERENT STRENGTHS)
Ortho Tricyclen	ethinyl estradiol, norgestimate (2)
Oticair	hydrocortisone, neomycin sulfate, polymyxin B sulfate
Otobiotic	hydrocortisone, polymyxin B sulfate
Ovcon	ethinyl estradiol, norethindrone
Ovral	ethinyl estradiol, norgestrel
Pediazole	erythromycin ethylsuccinate, sulfisoxazole acetyl
Pediotic	hydrocortisone, neomycin sulfate, polymyxin B sulfate
Percocet	acetaminophen, oxycodone hydrochloride (6)
Percodan	aspirin, oxycodone hydrochloride, oxycodone terephthalate (2)
Phenaphen with Codeine No. 3	acetaminophen, codeine phosphate
Phenaphen with Codeine No. 4	acetaminophen, codeine phosphate
Phenergan VC with Codeine	codeine phosphate, phenylephrine hydrochloride, promethazine hydrochloride
Phenergan with Codeine	codeine phosphate, promethazine hydrochloride
Phenergan with Dextromethorphan	dextromethorphan hydrobromide, promethazine hydrochloride
Phrenilin with Caffeine and Codeine	acetaminophen, butalbital, caffeine, codeine phosphate
Poly Pred	neomycin sulfate, polymyxin B sulfate, prednisolone acetate
Portia	ethinyl estradiol, levonorgestrel
Pramosone	hydrocortisone acetate, pramoxine hydrochloride (3)
Pred G	gentamicin sulfate, prednisolone acetate
Prefest	estadiol, norgestimate
Premphase	estrogens (conjugated), medroxyprogesterone acetate
Prempro	estrogens (conjugated), medroxyprogesterone acetate

COMBINATION DRUG PRODUCT NAME	ACTIVE INGREDIENTS (NUMBER OF DIFFERENT STRENGTHS)
Preven	ethinyl estradiol, levonorgestrel
Prevpac	amoxicillin, clarithromycin, lansoprazole
Prinzide	**hydrochlorothiazide, lisinopril (3)**
Proctofoam HC	**hydrocortisone acetate, pramoxine hydrochloride**
Prometh VC with Codeine	**codeine phosphate, phenylephrine hydrochloride, promethazine hydrochloride**
Prometh with Codeine	**codeine phosphate, promethazine hydrochloride**
Promethazine VC with Codeine	**codeine phosphate, phenylephrine hydrochloride, promethazine hydrochloride**
Rebetron	interferon alfa-2b, ribavirin
Renese-R	polythiazide, reserpine
Rifamate	isoniazid, rifampin
Rifater	isoniazid, pyrazinamide, rifampin
Robaxisal	**aspirin, methocarbamol**
Roxicet	acetaminophen, oxycodone hydrochloride (2)
Salutensin	hydroflumethiazide, reserpine
Sine-Aid IB	**ibuprofen, pseudoephedrine, hydrochloride**
Sinemet	**carbidopa, levodopa (3)**
Sinemet-CR	**carbidopa, levodopa (2)**
Soma Compound	**aspirin, carisoprodol**
Soma Compound with Codeine	**aspirin, carisoprodol, codeine phosphate**
Sprintec	**ethinyl estradiol, norgestimate**
Tarka	trandolapril, verapamil hydrochloride (4)
Teczem	diltiazem maleate, enalapril maleate
Tenoretic	**atenolol, chlorthalidone**
Terra-Cortril	hydrocortisone acetate, oxytetracycline hydrochloride
Terramycin with Polymyxin B Sulfate	oxytetracycline hydrochloride, polymyxin B sulfate
Teveten HCT	eprosartan mesylate, hydrochlorothiazide (2)

COMBINATION DRUG PRODUCT NAME	ACTIVE INGREDIENTS (NUMBER OF DIFFERENT STRENGTHS)
Timolide	hydrochlorothiazide, timolol maleate
Tobradex	dexamethasone, trobramycin
Triacin-C	codeine phosphate, pseudoephedrine hydrochloride, triprolidine hydrochloride
Trinalin	azatadine maleate, pseudoephedrine sulfate
Tri-Norinyl	ethinyl estradiol, norethindrone
Triphasil	ethinyl estradiol, levonorgestrel
Triple Sulfoid	sulfadiazine, sulfamerazine, sulfamethazine
Trivora	ethinyl estradiol, levonorgestrel
Trizivir	abacavir sulfate, lamivudine, zidovudine
Tylenol #1, #2, #3, or #4	acetaminophen, codeine phosphate (4)
Tylox	acetaminophen, oxycodone hydrochloride
Ultracet	acetaminophen, tramadol hydrochloride
Uniretic	hydrochlorothiazide, moexipril hydrochloride (3)
Vaseretic	enalapril maleate, hydrochlorothiazide (2)
Vasocidin	prednisolone sodium phosphate, sulfacetamide sodium
Vicoprofen	hydrocodone bitartrate, ibuprofen
Wygesic	acetaminophen, propoxyphene hydrochloride
Yasmin	drospirenone, ethinyl estradiol
Zestoretic	hydrochlorothiazide, lisinopril (3)
Ziac	bisoprolol fumarate, hydrochlorothiazide (3)
Zovia	ethinyl estradiol, ethynodiol diacetate (2)
Zyrtec-D	cetirizine hydrochloride, pseudoephedrine hydrochloride

Summary of Tips and Additional Resources

Getting the best price on prescription drugs is not always easy. There is a lot of information in this book that will help you understand the system, but you need to put the pieces together. The first step is to shop around for both the price and the service that you need. Get the pharmacy to tell you the price of your prescription before you have it filled. You can search the Internet for prices from on-line pharmacies to use as a point of reference. Internet pharmacies that are registered in the United States display on their homepage the VIPPS (Verified Internet Pharmacy Practice Sites) symbol, a blue oval shape with the red letters VIPPS in the center. These pharmacies must comply with the same regulations as all other pharmacies in the United States and will carry a supply of drugs that has been approved for use through the FDA. You will also find dozens of other on-line pharmacies that are willing to fill your prescription. Many people are having their prescriptions filled through Canada to save money. While this system may work, the process is not entirely without risk. U.S. customs agents have the right to confiscate drugs shipped across the border, which may result in your not getting your prepaid prescription. In addition to customs laws, there is no guarantee that the drug is safe and effective if manufactured outside the United States. You may be paying for a 10 mg tablet that only contains 8 mg because of the difference in quality standards between the United States and other countries. Or the drug may be contaminated with high levels of an unwanted ingredient such as lead or aluminum. The controls put in place by the FDA may mean higher drug costs, but they are intended to keep the public safe.

SUMMARY OF TIPS

The Right Drug

Getting the right drug is something that needs to be negotiated with your doctor. Chapter 3 emphasizes the need to talk to your doctor, an expert on disease management. Chapter 6 includes a summary of drug information that can be used to preview what to expect from the drug and to help identify alternatives. Chapters 7 and 8 provide additional information on therapeutic alternatives and combination drugs that can be used in your discussion with your doctor to make sure you get the right drug.

The Right Strength

Many drugs are available in more than one product strength. The number of products sold each year will often influence the price. So in some cases, a higher-strength product may be less expensive than a lower-strength product. This is especially true of generic products of which a manufacturer will only make the most popular strength. Use the cost-comparison symbols in Chapter 6 to find out the relative pricing of your drug. Your doctor may be able to prescribe a different strength that costs less. Just remember that it is more important for you to have treatment that will work than for you to pay less money for a less effective drug.

Some people request a prescription for a highter strength product and only take half a tablet to get their correct dose. While this might be acceptable for some drugs, it may also be unsafe for others. A pill splitter should only be used on tablets with an indentation in the center called a "score." Tablets that are scored will break in the center assuring that close to half the drug is in each half tablet. Splitting non-scored tablets may result in under- and over- dosing, causing fluctuations in blood levels of the drug and periods when the disease may be less controlled. Capsules, coated tablets, and delayed or extended-release products should not be split. Your pharmacist can tell you if your prescription drug can be split.

The Right Number of Daily Doses

The cost associated with manufacturing each dose of a drug suggests that you can save more money by taking fewer doses each day. Many of the new drugs are designed for once-a-day dosing. Older drugs have been manufactured into extended-release products for just a few cents more. Use the drug summaries in Chapter 6 to review the products that are available. Talk to your doctor if you discover a less expensive alternative that will allow you to take fewer daily doses and save money.

Optimal Fill Quantity

Chapter 2 offers tips on the prescription process that will help you determine if the number of doses in your prescription is the most cost-effective. Make sure to avoid additional pharmacy and insurance fees by getting the maximum number of doses you are allowed.

Generic Products

If there is a generic product available for your drug, it will be noted in the drug summary in Chapter 6. When a generic product is available, there are usually dozens of different companies that make the drug. Competition between generic drug companies has kept costs down and options up. If the prescription is written for a generic product, your pharmacy will decide which of the generic products to use. Ask about pricing before the prescription is filled.

Out-of-Pocket Payment

Coordination of insurance and length of treatment are key factors of out-of-pocket payment. There may be times when it is less expensive to pay for the prescription without applying an insurance benefit. Review Chapter 2 for more information.

ADDITIONAL RESOURCES

New Drug Information

Dozens of new drugs are approved for sale in the United States each year. The pharmaceutical company will give your doctor detailed drug information. The drugs have usually been tested in clinical trials on a few thousand patients before being made available to the general population. Clinical trial data is used as a basis for safety and efficacy. You will see new drugs in television commercials and magazine ads, but the information you see is created to make the drug look like something you need. In some cases, it may be great; in other cases, it may just be something different. The best way for you to get unbiased information on new drugs is through the Consumer Drug Information website managed by the FDA (http://www.fda.gov/cder/consumerinfo/). If the drug is not listed, ask your local pharmacist for more details.

Pharmacists

There are approximately 200,000 licensed pharmacists in the United States who can and should provide drug-information assistance. I have heard complaints that the pharmacist is always hidden behind the prescription counter and not available for questions, but that perception is not entirely true. Federal legislation called OBRA '90 (Omnibus Budget Reconciliation Act of 1990) requires that pharmacists keep proper patient records, evaluate the reason for drug usage before dispensing, and inform patients about their drugs. OBRA '90 was written for pharmacies that fill prescriptions for Medicaid patients, but has been adopted as a standard of practice in pharmacy. The drug-information requirement is typically met by including a drug fact sheet with every prescription. Although the fact sheet meets the minimum OBRA '90 requirements, all you have to do is ask to talk with the pharmacist. The pharmacist should offer whatever drug-information assistance you may need. However, if you ask about the price of your prescription, there are no requirements that a pharmacist must be involved. OBRA '90 only applies to providing drug information, so ask your questions.

Index

About the Author

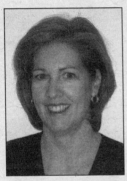

Diane Nitzki-George, RPh, MBA, BCNSP, has been a licensed pharmacist since 1980 and is currently board certified in nutrition support pharmacy and a member of the American Medical Writers Association, the American Society of Health-System Pharmacists, and the American Society for Parenteral and Enteral Nutrition. She has worked in Chicago-area hospitals, including a major teaching hospital and a government hospital with outpatient clinics. Diane Nitzki-George has developed and presented educational programs for pharmacists across the country and was a clinical support manager involved in nutrition and prescription drugs with one of the world's largest healthcare companies. Right now, she splits her time between freelance medical writing and working in pharmacy with patients receiving home infusion therapy. Diane earned her degrees in chemistry, pharmacy, and business from Northern Illinois University, Creighton University, and Keller Graduate School, respectively.